Clinical Manual of Blood and Bone Marrow Transplantation

Clinical Manual of Blood and Bone Marrow Transplantation

EDITED BY

Syed A. Abutalib, MD

Assistant Director, Hematology & Bone Marrow Transplantation Program
Director, Hematopoietic Progenitor Cell Collection Facility
Midwestern Regional Medical Center
Cancer Treatment Centers of America
Zion, IL, USA

Parameswaran Hari, MD, MRCP, MS

Armand Quick – William Stapp Professor of Hematology
Interim Division Chief, Division of Hematology and Oncology
Director, Adult Blood and Marrow Transplant Program
Medical College of Wisconsin
Milwaukee, WI, USA

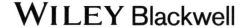

Registered Offices
John Wiley & Sons, Inc., 111 River Street, Hoboken, NJ 07030, USA
John Wiley & Sons Ltd, The Atrium, Southern Gate, Chichester, West Sussex, PO19 8SQ, UK

Editorial Office
9600 Garsington Road, Oxford, OX4 2DQ, UK

For details of our global editorial offices, customer services, and more information about Wiley products visit us at www.wiley.com.

Wiley also publishes its books in a variety of electronic formats and by print-on-demand. Some content that appears in standard print versions of this book may not be available in other formats.

Library of Congress Cataloging-in-Publication Data
Names: Abutalib, Syed A., editor. | Hari, Parameswaran, editor.
Title: Clinical manual of blood and bone marrow transplantation/edited by Dr. Syed A. Abutalib, Dr. Parameswaran Hari.
Description: Hoboken, NJ : John Wiley & Sons Inc., 2017. | Includes bibliographical references and index.
Identifiers: LCCN 2016055357| ISBN 9781119095453 (pbk.) | ISBN 9781119095460 (Adobe PDF) | ISBN 9781119095477 (epub)
Subjects: | MESH: Hematopoietic Stem Cell Transplantation | Bone marrow transplantation
Classification: LCC RD123.5 | NLM WH 380 | DDC 617.4/410592–dc23
LC record available at https://lccn.loc.gov/2016055357

Cover Design: Wiley
Cover Image: (Red Blood Cells) © Science Photo Library - SCIEPRO/Gettyimages; (White Blood Cells) © SCIEPRO/Gettyimages

Set in 8.5/10.5pt Meridien by SPi Global, Pondicherry, India

10 9 8 7 6 5 4 3 2 1

Dedication

Syed A. Abutalib

I dedicate this book to my everlasting thirst for acquiring medical knowledge, my valued mentors who I strive to emulate in their compassion and advocacy on behalf of the patient, my junior colleagues who continue to teach and remind me that there is always more to learn, and sincerest thanks to my family for their support, most especially my daughter who is the love of my life.

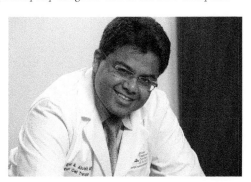

Parameswaran Hari

I dedicate this work mostly to my father who advised me that "your work is to discover your work, and then, to give yourself to it wholeheartedly." Thereafter, I remain grateful to my mentors and mentees, my family and friends, and, above all, my patients who respectively contributed wisdom, equilibrium, and sense of purpose to my work.

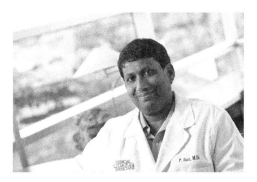

Contents

Contributors

Syed A. Abutalib, MD
Assistant Director, Hematology & Bone Marrow
Transplantation Program
Director, Hematopoietic Progenitor Cell Collection Facility
Midwestern Regional Medical Center
Cancer Treatment Centers of America
Zion, IL, USA

Syed Abbas Ali, MD
Sydney Kimmel Comprehensive Cancer Center
Division of Hematologic Malignancies
Johns Hopkins University
Baltimore, MD, USA

Emanuele Angelucci, MD
Unità Operativa Ematologia.
IRCCS Azienda Ospedaliera Universitaria San Martino -
IST - Istituto Nazionale per la Ricerca sul Cancro
Genova, Italy

Harold Atkins, MD, FRCPC
Physician, Blood and Marrow Transplant Program
The Ottawa Hospital;
Scientist, Cancer Therapeutics Program
The Ottawa Hospital Research Institute
and
Associate Professor, Division of Hematology
University of Ottawa, Ottawa, Ontario, Canada

Asad Bashey, MD, PhD
The Blood and Marrow Transplant Group of Georgia at
Northside Hospital
Atlanta, GA, USA

Ludovic Belle, PhD
Medical College of Wisconsin
Milwaukee, WI, USA

Koen van Besien, MD
Division of Hematology and Oncology
Department of Medicine
Weill Cornell Medical College
New York, NY, USA

Melinda Biernacki, MD
Fred Hutchinson Cancer Research Center and
the University of Washington
Seattle, WA, USA

Jaap Jan Boelens, MD, PhD
University Medical Center Utrecht
Pediatric Blood and Marrow Transplantation Program
and
Laboratory Translational Immunology
University Medical Center Utrecht
Utrecht, The Netherlands

Catherine M. Bollard, MBChB, MD, FRACP, FRCPA
Children's National Medical Center
and
The George Washington University
Washington, DC, USA

Adam Bryant, MD
Bone Marrow Transplant Fellow
Memorial Sloan Kettering Cancer Center
New York, NY, USA

Sonali Chaudhury, MD
Associate Professor of Pediatrics
Division of Pediatric Hematology/Oncology/Stem Cell
Transplantation
Ann & Robert H. Lurie Children's Hospital of Chicago
Northwestern University Feinberg School of Medicine
Chicago, IL, USA

Christina Cho, MD
Adult Bone Marrow Transplantation Service
Memorial Sloan Kettering Cancer Center
and
Weill Cornell Medical College
New York, NY, USA

Stefan O. Ciurea, MD
Department of Stem Cell Transplant and Cellular Therapy
The University of Texas MD Anderson Cancer Center
Houston, TX, USA

Luciano J. Costa, MD, PhD
Division of Hematology and Oncology
Department of Medicine
University of Alabama at Birmingham, Birmingham, AL, USA

Daniel R. Couriel, MD, MS
Division of Hematology and Hematologic Malignancies
Huntsman Cancer Institute
University of Utah
Salt Lake City, UT, USA

Conrad R. Cruz, MD, PhD
Children's National Medical Center
and
The George Washington University
Washington, DC, USA

Anita D'Souza, MD
Medical College of Wisconsin
Milwaukee, WI, USA

H. Joachim Deeg, MD
Fred Hutchinson Cancer Research Center and
the University of Washington
Seattle, WA, USA

Binod Dhakal, MD, MS
Medical College of Wisconsin
Milwaukee, WI, USA

Andrew C. Dietz, MD, MS
Pediatric Hematology, Oncology, & Blood and Marrow
Transplantation
Children's Hospital Los Angeles
University of Southern California
Los Angeles, CA, USA

Eva Domingo-Domenech, MD
Clinical Hematology Department
Institut Català d'Oncologia – Hospital Duran i Reynals
Barcelona, Spain

William R. Drobyski, MD
Medical College of Wisconsin
Milwaukee, WI, USA

Daniel Egan, MD
Fred Hutchinson Cancer Research Center
Seattle, WA, USA

Mahmoud Elsawy, MD, MSc
Clinical Research Division, Fred Hutchinson
Cancer Research Center
University of Washington School of Medicine, Seattle, WA, USA
and
Department of Medical Oncology
National Cancer Institute
Cairo University, Egypt

Narendranath Epperla, MD
Division of Hematology and Oncology
Medical College of Wisconsin
Milwaukee, WI, USA

Timothy S. Fenske, MD
Associate Professor of Medicine
Division of Hematology and Oncology
Medical College of Wisconsin
Milwaukee, WI, USA

Adele K. Fielding, MBBS, PhD, FRCP, FRCPath
UCL Cancer Institute
London, UK

Flore Sicre de Fontbrune, MD
Hematology Transplant Unit
Saint-Louis Hospital, APHP
and
National French Reference Center
for Bone Marrow Failure
Paris, France

Stephen J. Forman, MD
City of Hope National Medical Center
Duarte, CA, USA

Daniel Fowler, MD
Experimental Transplantation and Immunology Branch
National Cancer Institute
National Institutes of Health
Bethesda, MD, USA

Shuang Fu, MD
Blood & Marrow Transplant Program
Cleveland Clinic
Cleveland, OH, USA

Henry C. Fung, MD
Fox Chase Cancer Center
Temple Health
Philadelphia, PA, USA

Timothy Gilligan, MD, MS
Associate Professor in Medicine
Vice-Chair for Education
Cleveland Clinic Taussig Cancer Institute
Cleveland, OH, USA

Corrado Girmenia, MD
Dipartimento di Ematologia, Oncologia, Anatomia
Patologica e Medicina Rigenerativa
Azienda Policlinico Umberto I
Sapienza University of Rome
Rome, Italy

John Gribben, MD, DSc, FRCP, FRCPath, FMedSci
Centre for Haemato-Oncology
Barts Cancer Institute
Queen Mary University of London
London, UK

David C. Halverson, MD
Experimental Transplantation and Immunology Branch
National Cancer Institute
National Institutes of Health
Bethesda, MD, USA

Mehdi Hamadani, MD
Division of Hematology and Oncology
Medical College of Wisconsin
Milwaukee, WI, USA

Parameswaran Hari, MD, MRCP, MS
Armand Quick – William Stapp Professor of Hematology;
Interim Division Chief, Division of Hematology
and Oncology
and
Director, Adult Blood and Marrow Transplant Program
Medical College of Wisconsin
Milwaukee, WI, USA

Hamza Hashmi, MD
Department of Internal Medicine
Michigan State University
Grand Rapids, MI, USA

Dennis D. Hickstein, MD
Experimental Transplantation and Immunology
Branch,
National Cancer Institute
National Institutes of Health
Bethesda, MD, USA

Vincent T. Ho, MD
Dana Farber Cancer Institute
Boston, MA, USA

Amara S. Hussain, MD
Medical College of Wisconsin
Milwaukee, WI, USA

Racquel D. Innis-Shelton, MD
Division of Hematology and Oncology
Department of Medicine
University of Alabama at Birmingham
Birmingham, AL, USA

Madan Jagasia, MD, MBBS, MS
Hematology and Stem Cell Transplantation Section
Division of Hematology/Oncology
Department of Medicine,
Vanderbilt University Medical Center and Veterans Affairs
Medical Center;
Vanderbilt University School of Medicine
Nashville, TN, USA

Yogesh Jethava, MD, FACP, MRCP, FRCPath
Divison of Hematology and Oncology
University of Arkansas for Medical Sciences
Little Rock, AR, USA

Nisha S. Joseph, MD
Department of Hematology and Medical Oncology
Emory University School of Medicine
Atlanta, GA, USA

Jennifer A. Kanakry, MD
Experimental Transplantation and Immunology Branch
National Cancer Institute
National Institutes of Health
Bethesda, MD, USA

Natasha Kekre, MD, MPH, FRCPC
Blood and Marrow Transplant Program
The Ottawa Hospital and Ottawa Hospital Research Institute
Ottawa, Canada

Michael D. Keller, MD
Children's National Medical Center
and
The George Washington University
Washington, DC, USA

Vanessa E. Kennedy, MD
Vanderbilt University School of Medicine
Vanderbilt University Medical Center
Nashville, TN, USA

Piyanuch Kongtim, MD
Department of Stem Cell Transplant and Cellular Therapy
The University of Texas MD Anderson Cancer Center
Houston, TX, USA

Amrita Krishnan, MD
City of Hope National Medical Center
Duarte, CA, USA

Nicolaus Kröger, MD
Department of Stem Cell Transplantation
University Medical Center Hamburg-Eppendorf
Hamburg, Germany

Patricia Kropf, MD
Fox Chase Cancer Center
Temple Health
Philadelphia, PA, USA

Hillard M. Lazarus, MD, FACP
Department of Medicine
University Hospitals Seidman Cancer Center
Case Western Reserve University
Cleveland, OH, USA

Sagar Lonial, MD
Department of Hematology and Medical Oncology
Emory University School of Medicine
Atlanta, GA, USA

Navneet S. Majhail, MD, MS
Professor, Cleveland Clinic Lerner College of Medicine
and
Director, Blood & Marrow Transplant Program
Cleveland Clinic,
Cleveland, OH, USA

Marisa B. Marques, MD
Division of Laboratory Medicine
Department of Pathology
University of Alabama at Birmingham
Birmingham, AL, USA

Fabienne McClanahan Lucas, MD, PhD
The Ohio State University
Columbus, OH, USA

Kathryn McKay, MS, MT (ASCP)
Lineberger Comprehensive Cancer Center
University of North Carolina at Chapel Hill
Chapel Hill, NC, USA

Shin Mineishi, MD
Bone Marrow Transplant Program
Penn State Hershey Medical Center
Hershey, PA, USA

Mohamed Mohty, MD, PhD
Department of Haematology
Saint Antoine Hospital
Paris, France

Nitya Nathwani, MD
City of Hope National Medical Center
Duarte, CA, USA

Ajay K. Nooka, MD, MPH, FACP
Department of Hematology and Medical Oncology
Emory University School of Medicine
Atlanta, GA, USA

Moshe C. Ornstein, MD, MA
Fellow in Hematology-Oncology
Cleveland Clinic Taussig Cancer Institute
Cleveland, OH, USA

Anand Padmanabhan, MD, PhD
Blood Center of Wisconsin & Medical College of Wisconsin
Milwaukee, WI, USA

Philip Pancari, MD
Fox Chase Cancer Center
Temple Health
Philadelphia, PA, USA

Yara A. Park, MD
Department of Pathology and Laboratory Medicine
University of North Carolina at Chapel Hill
Chapel Hill, NC, USA

Regis Peffault de Latour, MD, PhD
Hematology Transplant Unit
Saint-Louis Hospital, APHP
and
National French Reference Center for Bone Marrow Failure
Paris, France

Miguel-Angel Perales, MD
Adult Bone Marrow Transplantation Service
Memorial Sloan Kettering Cancer Center
and
Weill Cornell Medical College
New York, NY, USA

Adrienne A. Phillips, MD, MPH
Division of Hematology and Oncology
Department of Medicine
Weill Cornell Medical College
New York, NY, USA

Federica Pilo, MD
Unità Operativa di Ematologia e Centro Trapianti.
Ospedale Oncologico di Riferimento Regionale "Armando Businco"
Cagliari, Italy

Michael A. Pulsipher, MD
Pediatric Hematology, Oncology, & Blood and Marrow Transplantation
Children's Hospital Los Angeles
University of Southern California
Los Angeles, CA, USA

Sabarinath Venniyil Radhakrishnan, MD
Division of Hematology and Hematologic Malignancies
Huntsman Cancer Institute
University of Utah
Salt Lake City, UT, USA

Jerald Radich, MD
Fred Hutchison Cancer Research Center
Seattle, WA, USA

Jay S. Raval, MD
Department of Pathology and Laboratory Medicine
University of North Carolina at Chapel Hill
Chapel Hill, NC, USA

Istvan Redei, MD
Director
Department of Hematology and Bone Marrow Transplant
Cancer Treatment Centers of America
Zion, IL, USA

Gian Maria Rossolini, MD
Dipartimento di Biotecnologie Mediche
University of Siena
Siena, Italy;
Dipartimento di Medicina Sperimentale e Clinica
University of Florence
Florence, Italy
and
SOD Microbiologia e Virologia
Azienda Ospedaliera Universitaria Careggi
Florence, Italy

Ayman Saad, MD
Blood & Marrow Transplantation and Cellular Therapy
Program
University of Alabama at Birmingham
Birmingham, AL, USA

Bipin N. Savani, MD
Hematology and Stem Cell Transplantation Section
Division of Hematology/Oncology
Department of Medicine
Vanderbilt University Medical Center and Veterans Affairs
Medical Center;
Vanderbilt University School of Medicine
Nashville, TN, USA

Bronwen E. Shaw, MD, PhD
Center for International Blood and
Marrow Transplant Research
Department of Medicine
Medical College of Wisconsin
Milwaukee, WI, USA

Shalini Shenoy, MD
Professor of Pediatrics
Teresa J Vietti Scholar in Pediatrics
Division of Pediatric Hematology/Oncology/Stem Cell
Transplantation
Washington University School of Medicine
St. Louis Children's Hospital
St. Louis, MO, USA

Melhem Solh, MD
The Blood and Marrow Transplant Group of Georgia
at Northside Hospital
Atlanta, GA, USA

Mohamed L. Sorror, MD, MSc
Clinical Research Division, Fred Hutchinson
Cancer Research Center
and
Division of Medical Oncology, Department of Medicine
University of Washington School of Medicine
Seattle, WA, USA

Jean Soulier, MD, PhD
Hematology Laboratory
Saint-Louis Hospital, APHP
University Paris Diderot; and
INSERM U944/CNRS UMR7212, University Institute
of Hematology
and
National French Reference Center for Bone Marrow Failure
Paris, France

Stephen R. Spellman, MBS
Center for International Blood and Marrow Transplant
Research
Minneapolis, MN, USA

Anna Sureda, MD, PhD
Clinical Hematology Department
Institut Català d'Oncologia – Hospital Duran i
Reynals
Barcelona, Spain

Masumi Ueda, MD, MA
Clinical Research Division
Fred Hutchinson Cancer Research Center
Seattle, WA, USA

Claudio Viscoli, MD
University of Genoa (DISSAL)
IRCCS S. Martino – IST
Genoa, Italy

Robert F. Wynn, MA, MD, MRCP, FRCPath
Royal Manchester Children's Hospital
Department of Hematology/BMT
Manchester, UK

Ghada Zakout, MBBS, MRCP, FRCPath
Royal Free London NHS Foundation Trust
London, UK

Preface

Cellular therapy in general, and hematopoietic cell transplantation in particular, has rapidly expanded in scope, practice, and basic understanding in the past 30 years. The indications now encompass a wide and diverse range of inherited and acquired disorders, malignant and non-malignant indications, conditioning therapies of varying intensities and numerous "constantly growing" strategies with novel cells, *ex vivo* processed cells and genetically re-engineered products. Concomitant advances in supportive and ancillary technologies now allow better immune matching, rapid diagnosis, and risk stratification of complications such as graft-versus-host disease and viral illnesses. Parallel development in treatments have also occurred that have reduced transplant related mortality and morbidity. Our saga of success in transplant has been built on the basis incremental small gains in technology. Assimilating and applying these new diagnostic and therapeutic modalities to daily patient care can be challenging and, often times, overwhelming.

We have attempted to describe the state of practice in hematopoietic cell transplantation in this manual. Developed with both the teacher and learner in mind, our book offers trainees and practitioners an excellent opportunity to enhance their knowledge and practice skills. Physicians in training, physicians in other disciplines who see transplant survivors, in fact all health care providers wishing to increase their knowledge in this sub-specialty area, will find the format engaging and robust with direct relevance to daily practice. Our book provides a concise "practical expert review" non-exhaustive format in 42 chapters with each chapter annotated with numerous practical headings for focused learning. Without the intention to write it as a text book, we attempted to include the diagnosis and management of as many transplant related practical questions faced by hematologists and transplant physicians. We hope that the accessible format will enable reader to become familiar with both the basics and nuances of clinical transplant care. The authors are experts in the field of hematopoietic cell transplant and cell therapy and have all followed the same basic format. Readers will find that this *Clinical Manual of Blood and Marrow Transplantation* has clear take-away points that are informative and valuable for clinical practice beyond transplant in the management of hematologic disorders. Ultimately, we hope that the professionals using this book will find the content of value and of benefit in their own interactions with patients.

Syed A. Abutalib, MD
Parameswaran Hari, MD, MRCP, MS

CHAPTER 1

Donor and graft selection strategy

Ayman Saad[1], Marisa B. Marques[2], and Shin Mineishi[3]

[1] Blood & Marrow Transplantation and Cellular Therapy Program, University of Alabama at Birmingham, Birmingham, AL, USA

[2] Division of Laboratory Medicine, Department of Pathology, University of Alabama at Birmingham, Birmingham, AL, USA

[3] Bone Marrow Transplant Program, Penn State Hershey Medical Center, Hershey, PA, USA

Introduction

A key component of the decision-making process of an allogeneic hematopoietic cell transplant is selection of the appropriate donor and graft. The best donor is an HLA-matched sibling. However, this option is available only for one third of patients. While the choice of a graft type is often determined by the transplant center preference and experience, there are advantages and disadvantages with each option.

What are the donor options?

In the absence of an HLA-matched sibling, an alternative donor is pursued. The options of donors are:

1 HLA-matched sibling (including one antigen/allelic mismatch)
2 Unrelated volunteer adult donor (MUD donor) (including one antigen/allelic mismatch).
3 Umbilical cord blood (UCB).
4 Haploidentical donor.

What are the graft sources?

Initial allogeneic transplants were done using bone marrow grafts. However, more options are currently available. The sources of hematopoietic grafts are:

1 Peripheral blood (PB).
2 Bone marrow (BM).
3 UCB.

Donor options

HLA matching is the most relevant factor when choosing a donor. Details of HLA typing are explained in Chapter 2. Some pertinent details are outlined next.

HLA matching for donor selection

HLA antigens are either "high expression" such as HLA-A, B, C (class I), DRB1 (class II), or "low expression" such as DQB1, DPB1, and DRB3/4/5 (all class II). The "high expression" antigens play a pivotal role in the transplant setting because of *high antigen density* on the cells. (We will refer to DRB1, DQB1, and DPB1 as DR, DQ, and DP, respectively, throughout this chapter.) An HLA-matched sibling is usually the preferred donor. A haploidentical donor ($\geq 4/8$ match) is defined as a first degree relative that shares at least one full haplotype with the recipient (i.e., it cannot be mismatched in both loci of any HLA alleles).

For unrelated donors, HLA matching at the allele level of HLA-A, B, C and DRB1 (8 alleles) is done according to National Marrow Donor Program (NMDP) recommendation. An ideal donor is 8/8 HLA-match. When there is more than one 8/8 HLA-matched donor, additional HLA matching at the DQ and DP may be helpful to identify a better candidate (see Chapter 2). For example, with DQ typing, 10/10 matched donors may be favored. On the other hand, DP matching is only seen in about 20% of 10/10 HLA-matched unrelated donors. Nevertheless, groups of "permissive" versus "non-permissive" mismatching have been identified based on cross-reactivity profiles. Permissive mismatching (found in ~70% of 10/10 HLA-matched donors) means two mismatched DP alleles will have a favorable outcome (less non-relapse mortality (NRM)) similar to

---

a HLA-matched DP. The use of DQ and DP matching has not been universally recommended.

Each single locus mismatching in classical HLA loci (A, B, C, and DRB1) is associated with ~10% reduction in overall survival particularly for "early stage" disease. Earlier data showed that the worst "bone marrow" mismatches were HLA-A or HLA-DRB1 alleles, and the worst PB mismatch was HLA-C antigen. However, more recent data showed that the type (allele/antigen) and locus (HLA-A, B, C, or DR) of mismatch have equal impact on survival outcome. The only exception is a favorable outcome with the permissive mismatch of C*03:03/C*03:04.

HLA matching of UCB

Due to the immaturity of UCB T-cells, HLA matching is less stringent when using this graft source. UCB should be at least a 4/6 (A/B and DRB1) match using HLA-A and B (DNA-based low resolution/antigen level) and DRB1 (DNA-based high resolution/allele level). Outcomes of 4/6 UCB transplants are comparable to that of HLA-matched unrelated donors, albeit with an increased risk of NRM. When using a "single" unit of UCB, HLA-C antigen mismatching was shown to increase transplant-related mortality (TRM), particularly, if combined with HLA-DRB1 mismatching. When using double UCB units (as in most adult patients), there are no guidelines for HLA matching *between* the two units as long as minimum requirement of 4/6 HLA matching is present of each unit with the patient's HLA. Nevertheless, some centers prefer to use at least a 4/6 matching *between* the two units.

When a HLA-matched unrelated donor or a mismatched unit is used, it is essential to test the recipient for pre-formed donor-specific anti-HLA as described next.

HLA antibodies

About one-third (33%) of recipients have antibodies directed against HLA class I or II. However, only 5–10% of those recipients have "donor-specific" HLA antibodies (DSA). High titer (>1,000–2,000 MFI; mean fluorescent intensity) of DSA is associated with risk of graft rejection. Risk of graft rejection with DSA is higher when using NMA, compared to myeloablative regimens. Testing recipients for DSA is crucial when using HLA-mismatched, unrelated, haploidentical donors or mismatched cord units. Higher CD34+ cell/kg in PB grafts compared to BM grafts may overcome negative impact of DSA, particularly when the titer is considered low, that is, <1,000 MFI.

How is DSA tested?

HLA antibody testing is done by initial screening of the recipient's serum using the "Panel Reactive Antigen" (PRA) assay. PRA determines the percentage of random people's sera against which the recipient could have antibodies. If PRA is positive, "Single Antigen Beads" (SAB) test is performed to identify whether the antibodies are against DSA or not (requires blood test from the donor). DSA may be mitigated by therapeutic plasma exchange (TPE), rituximab, bortezomib, and/or intravenous immunoglobulin.

The following is a description of the pros and cons with each of the donor options.

HLA-matched sibling

An HLA-matched sibling is favored in most cases, if available. Any full biological sibling (same biologic parents) of the patient would have a 25% chance of being fully HLA-matched, 25% of being HLA-non-matched and 50% of being HLA-haploidentical matched. DSA testing is not required in the setting of HLA-MSD. In addition, another advantage of a HLA-MSD is that he/she would be readily available for graft procurement for the potential need for future cell donations such as donor lymphocyte infusion (DLI) or a CD34+ cell boost-"graft boost".

Unrelated volunteer adult donor (MUD donor)

When a fully HLA-MSD is not available, a HLA-MUD donor is sought through registries. In the United States, the NMDP represents a major source for volunteer donors. In addition, The Bone Marrow Donors Worldwide (BMDW) organization has data for over 25 million volunteer donors. Once again, the ideal donor is 8/8 HLA-matched with the patient. HLA-MUD donors are typically available for donation after about 8 weeks but may not be available for another cell donation for DLI or graft boost. Thus, transplant centers may opt to store an extra portion of the HLA-MUD graft (if feasible) for future use.

UCB

When a fully HLA-matched donor (whether a MSD or MUD donor) is not available, an UCB donor can be considered. UCB would be promptly available, but is not available again for DLI or graft boost. More details on UCB use is outlined below under graft sources.

HLA-haploidentical donor (haplo donor)

Recent introduction of post-transplant cyclophosphamide (PTCy) made HLA-haploidentical transplant a feasible option even in a center not specialized on this type of transplant. When a fully HLA-matched donor (whether a MSD or MUD donor) is not available, a haplo donor can be considered. A haplo donor is typically a first degree relative like a parent, a child or a sibling. The majority of patients have a haplo donor (exceptions include adopted and old patients with no children). While the haplo donor would be readily available for the donation transplant centers with no adequate expertise in performing HLA-haploidentical transplants may opt to use HLA-mismatched from unrelated donors. The choice between haplo- and UCB- transplant often depends on the center preference and experience. The choice between UCB and haploidentical transplant remains controversial until the CTN 1101 clinical trial comparing haplo BM vs UCB with reduced intensity regimen, is completed.

Clinical differences among different types of donors are summarized in Table 1.1.

Graft composition

There are biological differences among the three sources of grafts (PB, BM and UCB) due to their different composition. These grafts are primarily composed of:
- CD34+ cells, which make ~1% of the entire graft composition.
- Lymphocytes (mainly T-cells, and also B-cells and natural killer (NK) cells).
- Myeloid precursors.
- Monocytes (with potential for cytokine release).
- Other cells (e.g., endothelial progenitor cells and mesenchymal cells).

The CD34+ cell dose is the primary determinant of successful engraftment. However, other components (in particular, the T-cells = CD3+ cells) play pivotal roles in transplant outcomes. Simply stated, CD3+ cells (T-cells) mediate the following four immunological processes:
1 Engraftment.
2 Immune reconstitution to prevent infection.
3 Graft-versus-tumor (GvT) effect to prevent relapse.
4 Graft-versus-host-disease (GvHD).

While engraftment, immune reconstitution, and GvT are favorable processes, GvHD is not.

PB graft

Although the initial transplants were done with BM grafts, PB grafts are now more commonly used. Main advantages of using PB grafts are faster and more secure engraftment (thus preferred for NMA and RIC regimens) and immune reconstitution, and less relapses (via GvT effect). However, chronic GvHD (cGvHD) continues to be a major long-term complication of PB grafts.

A PB graft is collected by apheresis procedure. Typically, donors receive growth factor injection for 4 days and then undergo leukapheresis for 1–2 days. The recommended CD34+ cell dose in a PB graft is at least 4×10^6 CD34+ cells/kg of recipient weight, while a dose of $< 2 \times 10^6$ CD34+ cells/kg is discouraged to avoid risk of engraftment failure (See chapters 5 and 6).

BM graft

BM was the initial graft source used for allogeneic transplantation. BM grafts, by virtue of having less T-cells, have higher risk of engraftment failure (particularly when using NMA conditioning regimens), delayed immune reconstitution, and potential risk of neoplastic disease relapse (less GvT effect). However, they are associated with less risk of cGvHD and clinical trials have shown equivalent survival outcomes when compared with PB in hematologic malignancies.

BM is harvested in the operating room under general anesthesia. It is typically a 1-day surgery with the risks of complications common to general anesthesia, as well as bleeding, pain, and, rarely, traumatic surgical injury. The recommended cell dose in a BM graft is 4×10^8 TNC

Table 1.1 Comparison of the different graft sources.

	HLA-MSD	HLA-MUD	Haplo Donor	UCB
Priority	First Priority	First alternative	Next alternative	Next alternative
Availability	Readily available	Procurement time of 4–8 weeks or longer	Readily available	Promptly available
Cost	Donor testing and collection	Registry search, donor testing and collection	Donor testing and collection	Expensive: A single UCB unit is ~ $30,000 –$50,000
DLI and graft boost	Available	May be available	Available	NOT available*
Graft manipulation trials	Donor available to consent	Requires Registry approval	Donor available to consent	NOT possible*

*Once thawed, the whole UCB unit is infused and generally not amenable for cellular manipulation in usual circumstances.

(total nucleated cells)/kg of recipient weight for hematologic malignancies. A dose of $<2\times10^8$ TNC/kg is discouraged. The TNC (rather than the CD34$^+$ cell count) is used to determinate the cell dose in the BM graft since the interim cell dose evaluation (during the harvest procedure) is routinely done using the quick hemocytometer cell counter of TNC.

Why is BM graft is preferred in children with hematologic malignancies?

In children, BM graft is used more than PB mainly to avoid the long-term complications of cGvHD. The risk of engraftment failure in children is less with BM graft as they always receive enough CD34$^+$ cells (due to their small body weight compared to the donor). Children may also tolerate infectious complications (if delayed immune reconstitution) better than adults, who often have medical comorbidities. The risk of relapse of neoplastic diseases (by virtue of less GvT) of the BM graft may be reduced by myeloablative regimens, which children can tolerate better than adults.

UCB graft

UCB units are cryopreserved (voluntarily donated) in several cord banks. UCB banking is recommended for public use. Storing UCB for personal use (i.e., reserved for the same baby if he/she develops disease in the future) is generally discouraged, because the probability of a newborn using his/her own UCB is too small, around 0.04–0.001%. While cord blood baking started in the 1980s in the United States, FDA regulations have only been imposed since 2011. Any UCB unit stored without conforming with the FDA regulations issued in late 2011 is considered "unlicensed", and its use is currently available only under FDA approval (considered investigational use). Units stored according to the FDA regulations are "licensed," and are available for routine use in the United States. One of the advantages of UCB units is that they are promptly available. They are typically of small volume with 1 log fewer TNCs and CD34$^+$ cells/recipient weight (compared to PB and BM grafts). However, for most adults, 2 units (double cord transplant) are used for a successful transplant. When double cord units are used, eventually only one UCB engrafts and the other one vanishes after providing cellular immune support during the early post-transplant time. UCB has more immature T-cells and, thus, is less immunologically reactive. Consequently, they are associated with higher risk of engraftment failure (particularly with NMA regimen), delayed immune reconstitution and potential for neoplastic disease relapse (limited GvT effect). The risk of GvHD with UCB depends on the degree of HLA disparity with the recipient. Due to the immaturity of the cord blood T-cells, HLA matching is less restrictive. An ideal

UCB unit should have at least 3×10^7 TNC/kg of recipient weight. When performing a double UCB transplant in adults, each unit has to have at least 1.5×10^7 TNC/kg of recipient weight. Since the CD34$^+$ cell dose in the UCB is about a log less than that in PB or BM graft, at an average of 3×10^5/kg (~1% of TNC) for an adult, slow engraftment is expected. It is also to be noted that UCB is typically negative for antibodies to CMV. In routine clinical practice (outside clinical trials), UCB is not available for future use (e.g., DLI).

Differences among the three sources of graft sources are summarized in Table 1.2.

Which graft type should I use?

Although several transplant centers tend to use one type of graft more than another, it is often prudent to consider several factors when selecting the type of the graft for each individual patient. As a general rule, UCB or haploidentical graft are typically reserved for recipients with no available HLA-matched donors. The decision-making to choose between PB and BM is summarized in Table 1.3.

Non-HLA factors

What if more than one HLA-matched donor is available?

HLA matching is the most relevant factor when choosing a donor. However, the following factors are to be considered when there is more than one equivalent donor. The order of preference of these factors is often based on institutional preference.

1 CMV status of the donor and patient.
2 ABO blood matching with the patient.
3 Gender of the donor.
4 Age of the donor.
5 Weight discrepancy between the donor and the patient.
6 Availability (domestic or international) and timeframe of availability.
7 Killer cell Immunoglobulin-like Receptors (KIR) status of the donor using techniques such as KIR B content score.

CMV status

Most of the population acquire CMV infection when young and remain seropositive for life. CMV remains dormant in leukocytes and can be re-activated when the host becomes immunocompromised. For a CMV negative patient, ideally, a CMV negative donor should be used, whenever possible. However, for patients who are CMV positive, either CMV negative or positive donor can be used. Some centers prefer to use CMV positive donors for CMV positive patients (i.e., CMV matching) to allow the transfer of CMV immune lymphocytes (from the donor) to the patient to combat post-transplant CMV reactivation. The latter approach, although not systematically studied, may be beneficial with T-cell depleted transplants (in particular with anti-thymocyte

Table 1.2 Comparison of the three hematopoietic graft sources.

	PB	BM	UCB
Prevalence of use	Most common	Common in pediatric transplants	Common in pediatric transplants
Feasibility	- Donor evaluation - Apheresis	- Donor evaluation - Harvesting of BM	Cryopreserved units
Donor's risks	- Central venous access (if used) - Electrolyte imbalance - Hyperviscosity (MI and CVA in high-risk donors)	- General anesthesia - Hypovolemia with big volume harvest	None
Graft composition			
Cell dose target	CD34$^+$ cells: $\geq 4 \times 10^6$/kg	TNC: $\geq 4 \times 10^8$/kg	TNC: $\geq 2.5 \times 10^7$/kg (single UCB). TNC: $\geq 3 \times 10^7$/kg (double UCB)
Average CD34$^+$ cell dose	4–6×10^6/kg	2–4×10^6/kg	3×10^5/kg
Average T-cell (CD3$^+$) dose	$\sim 3 \times 10^8$/kg	$\sim 3 \times 10^7$/kg (one log less than PB)	$< 1 \times 10^7$/kg
G-CSF primed cells	YES (at all times)	NO*	NO
CMV status	Positive or negative	Positive or negative	Negative
Clinical outcome			
Engraftment	Fast	Slow	Slowest
Immune reconstitution	Fast	Slow	Slowest
Relapse risk	Low	High	Highest
cGvHD risk	High	Low	High (if mismatched)

* Unless donor is, uncommonly, primed by G-CSF before harvest.
MI: myocardial infarction, CVA: cerebrovascular accident, cGvHD: chronic graft-versus-host-disease, TNC: total nucleated cells.

Table 1.3 Factors to consider when selecting PB or BM graft.

Factor	PB	BM
• Disease type	Appropriate for all indications, in particular: - Neoplastic diseases (better GvT).	Appropriate for severe aplastic anemia, and BM failure diseases (no GvT needed). - Thalassemia and sickle cell disease.
• Disease status	Appropriate for all disease statuses, in particular, refractory or active neoplastic disease (better GvT).	Acceptable for neoplastic diseases when in remission.
• Conditioning regimen: MA, RIC, NMA	Appropriate for all regimens, and including RIC and NMA.	Risk of engraftment failure is high with RIC or NMA regimens (less T-cells).
• Active infection (or multiple comorbidities) at the time of transplant	Preferred (faster immune reconstitution).	Better avoided because of delayed immune reconstitution.
• ABO mismatching	No need for RBC depletion.	Requires RBC depletion which may compromise CD34$^+$ cell dose.
• Children	Acceptable	Usually preferred

MA: myeloablative, NMA: non-myeloablative, RIC: Reduced intensity conditioning

Table 1.4 ABO blood matching of donor and recipient.

		Recipient			
		A	**B**	**AB**	**O**
Donor	A	compatible	MAJOR/minor	minor	MAJOR
	B	MAJOR/minor	compatible	minor	MAJOR
	AB	MAJOR	MAJOR	compatible	MAJOR
	O	minor	minor	minor	compatible

Major/minor (bi-directional) = both mismatch complications can happen.

globulin). UCB are always CMV seronegative and, thus, may be a good option for a CMV seronegative patient who does not have other HLA-matched donor options.

ABO blood type

The commonest blood group types are A and O (each is 40–45%). ABO blood type matching is not required for a successful transplant. However, ABO mismatching can result in complications. Matching between recipient and donor depends upon the interaction between the ABO antigen (on RBCs) and isohemagglutinins (anti-A and anti-B) in the plasma. Donor/recipient matching are either compatible or mismatched (major, minor or bi-directional) as outlined in Table 1.4.

Major and bi-directional (major and minor) mismatches are best avoided, if possible.

- **ABO major mismatch** (e.g., A graft and O recipient). This mismatch carries risk of two complications:
  o *Acute hemolysis* upon infusion of the graft. Clinically significant hemolytic reaction is uncommon due to routine RBC depletion of BM grafts and minimal RBC content in the PB grafts. It is recommended that volume of RBCs in the graft be < 0.3 ml/kg.
  o *Delayed erythroid engraftment and pure red cell aplasia:* This may occur when the residual recipient's plasma cells (making anti-A and anti-B) survive for several weeks and suppress the donor's erythroid engraftment. This may be treated with rituximab.
  Anti-A is typically stronger than anti-B; thus, an A graft is less desirable than a B graft when there is a major ABO mismatch.
- **ABO minor mismatch** (e.g., O graft and A recipient). This does not carry risk of significant hemolysis upon infusion of the graft due to dilution of the infused isohemagglutinins in the recipient's plasma (unless small RBCs volume in a child with very high donor isohemagglutinin titer). The primary concerns of this mismatch are two complications:
  o *Passenger lymphocyte syndrome (PLS):* This rare but serious complication can happen between days +5 and +15 of transplant. In this case, the donor's plasma cells (passenger lymphocytes) may become activated shortly (within a few days) of the transplant making high titers

of isohemagglutinins that induce hemolysis of the recipient's RBCs. This is an urgent life-threatening medical condition that causes acute anemia and requires therapeutic plasma exchange (TPE) until the high isohemagglutinin titer subsides.
  o *Delayed hemolysis* (up to 4 months) of residual recipient RBCs by donor-derived isohemagglutinins. This is often self-limiting and resolves spontaneously.

What about Rh incompatibility?

Rh incompatibility is of little clinical significance in the transplant setting. If an Rh negative recipient receives an Rh positive graft, he/she will unlikely form anti-D because of immunosuppression. However, caution is needed if an Rh negative recipient is alloimmunized (i.e., with anti-D) and receives an Rh positive graft. In that case, acute hemolysis may occur upon infusion of the graft. For example, an Rh negative recipient who is alloimmunized via prior pregnancy (has anti-D) receives a CD34+ cell graft that has RBCs which are Rh positive then the graft RBCs will undergo acute hemolysis upon infusion.

Should we check isohemagglutinin titers in all patients?

Isohemagglutinins are the IgM Anti-A or anti-B antibody that are naturally occurring and can increase with repeated transfusion. Isohemagglutinin titers of the recipient are important in case of major ABO mismatch. Some centers use TPE to decrease the titer prior to infusion of the graft. There is no well-established definition of a high titer, but titers > 1:32 may be clinically significant.

Table 1.5 summarizes the complications of ABO mismatching and measures to prevent them.

Donor gender

Female donors can impact transplant in two ways:
1 Female donor grafts may produce anti-HY antibody (HY gene of the Y chromosome) in male recipients, and this may be associated with higher risk of GvHD. Of note, anti-HY antibody is being investigated as a biomarker of cGvHD.
2 Multiparous female donors may have been alloimmunized during prior pregnancies against HLA, which also imposes a risk of cGvHD.

Table 1.5 Complications and preventive measures with ABO incompatibility.

Type of Mismatch	Risks	Prevention
Major mismatch (e.g., A graft and O recipient)	• Infusion hemolytic reaction. • Delayed erythroid engraftment. • Pure red cell aplasia (PRCA).	**RBCs depletion** of the graft can minimize infusion hemolysis. **TPE** (of recipient) can minimize infusion hemolysis and may also decrease risk of PRCA.
Minor mismatch (e.g., O graft and A recipient)	• Infusion hemolytic reaction (uncommon). • PLS (within few days of transplant), a medical emergency treated with TPE. • Delayed hemolysis (of residual recipient RBCs) of no clinical significance.	**Plasma depletion** of the graft. **Close monitoring for hemolysis** between day +5 and +15 (typical time for PLS).

TPE: therapeutic plasma exchange.

Thus, multiparous women are usually avoided as donors, and male donor is preferred for a male transplant recipient.

Donor age
The quality of the CD34+ cells may decline with age. Furthermore, older age can be associated with comorbidities that may influence the donor's safety for donation. Thus, the NMDP uses young volunteer donors whenever possible. However, there is no well-defined donor maximum age cutoff. Studies have shown that outcome of older HLA-matched sibling is not inferior to that of younger HLA-MUD donors in certain diseases.

Donor weight
The CD34+ cell yield from a donor is generally proportional to his/her body weight. Thus, a big weight discrepancy between the recipient and the donor may be clinically significant. This problem may be encountered when an adult (higher weight) recipient is receiving an haplo product from his young children (lower weight). In case of BM harvest, NMDP (and most centers) mandates that the maximum BM volume that can be harvested to be 20 ml/kg of the donor's weight. Thus, a PB product (with expected higher yield of CD34+ cells) may be preferred if the recipient's weight is significantly higher than the donor's.

Availability
The volunteer donor registries are worldwide. Extended search through international registries can be time-consuming and, thus, not appropriate for an urgent transplant (i.e., needed within 4–8 weeks). Other available donors (including haplo and UCB) may be preferred in this setting.

KIR status
KIR are expressed on NK-cells and are involved in the graft cytotoxic (GvT) effect. The KIR complex includes inhibitory (type A) and stimulatory (type B) motifs that are either centromeric (toward the chromosomal centromere) or telomeric (toward the chromosomal telomere). The higher the B content (particularly centromeric), the more stimulatory (cytotoxic), the NK-cells of the graft. Inhibitory KIR binds to KIR ligand (encoded by HLA-C) on the target cells. In case of HLA-C mismatching, this inhibitory signal does not occur, inducing NK cytotoxicity (GvT). A study has shown that patients with AML who received HLA-C mismatched graft with KIR 2DS1 had lower relapse rate. However, these findings have not been validated, and KIR status is not routinely sought when identifying an appropriate donor. This is a subject of ongoing research.

SUMMARY

The following is a summary of ideal graft and donor selection with an algorithm depicted in Figure 1.1.

• HLA typing of the patient and siblings (if available):
  ○ Matched sibling identified = best option.
  ○ If no matched sibling:
    ▪ Adult (HLA-MUD) and UCB registry search
    ▪ Identification of haplo donors.

The following are recommendations when using an alternative donor.
• MUD donor:
  ○ 8/8 HLA-matched MUD donor is next preferred if no HLA-MSD.
  ○ DP permissive mismatching and DQ matching may be considered if multiple 8/8 HLA-matched donors are available.
• Haplo donor:
  ○ Can be used if no 8/8 HLA- MUD donor is available.
  ○ DSA testing: if positive DSA → avoid use especially if titers are high.
• Cord blood:
  ○ Can be used if no 8/8 HLA-MUD donor is available.
  ○ At least ≥ 4/6 matched for HLA-A, B (low/intermediate resolution) and DRB1 (high resolution).
  ○ DSA testing: if positive DSA → → avoid use if titers are high.

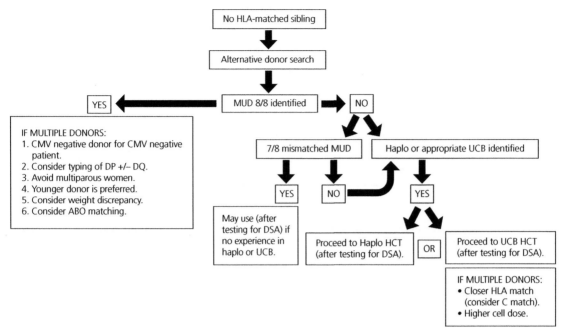

Figure 1.1 Algorithm for selection of a graft/donor for allogeneic transplant.

Abbreviations

BM:	bone marrow
FDA:	Food and Drug Administration
PBSC:	Peripheral Blood Stem Cell
UCB:	Umbilical Cord Blood
RIC:	Reduced Intensity Conditioning
TNC:	Total nucleated cells
MA:	Myeloablative
NMA:	Non-myeloablative
NMDP:	National Marrow Donor Program

Selected reading

1. Confer DL, Abress LK, Navarro W, Madrigal A. Selection of adult unrelated hematopoietic stem cell donors: beyond HLA. *Biol Blood Marrow Transplant*. 2010;**16**(1 Suppl): S8–S11.

2. Ciurea SO, Thall PF, Wang X, Wang SA, Hu Y, Cano P, et al. Donor-specific anti-HLA Abs and graft failure in matched unrelated donor hematopoietic stem cell transplantation. *Blood*. 2011;**118**(22):5957–5964.

3. Sheppard D, Tay J, Bryant A, McDiarmid S, Huebsch L, Tokessy M, et al. Major ABO-incompatible BMT: isohemagglutinin reduction with plasma exchange is safe and avoids graft manipulation. *Bone Marrow Transplant*. 2013;**48**(7): 953–957.

4. Eapen M, O'Donnell P, Brunstein CG, Wu J, Barowski K, Mendizabal A, et al. Mismatched related and unrelated donors for allogeneic hematopoietic cell transplantation for adults with hematologic malignancies. *Biol Blood Marrow Transplant*. 2014;**20**(10):1485–1492.

5. Gragert L, Eapen M, Williams E, Freeman J, Spellman S, Baitty R, et al. HLA match likelihoods for hematopoietic stem-cell grafts in the U.S. registry. *N Engl J Med*. 2014;**371**(4): 339–348.

6. Howard CA, Fernandez-Vina MA, Appelbaum FR, Confer DL, Devine SM, Horowitz MM, et al. Recommendations for donor human leukocyte antigen assessment and matching for allogeneic stem cell transplantation: consensus opinion of the Blood and Marrow Transplant Clinical Trials Network (BMT CTN). *Biol Blood Marrow Transplant*. 2015;**21**(1):4–7.

7. Pidala J, Lee SJ, Ahn KW, Spellman S, Wang HL, Aljurf M, et al. Nonpermissive HLA-DPB1 mismatch increases mortality after myeloablative unrelated allogeneic hematopoietic cell transplantation. *Blood*. 2014;**124**(16):2596–2606.

CHAPTER 2

HLA typing and implications

Bronwen E. Shaw[1] and Stephen R. Spellman[2]

[1] Center for International Blood and Marrow Transplant Research, Department of Medicine, Medical College of Wisconsin, Milwaukee, WI, USA

[2] Center for International Blood and Marrow Transplant Research, Minneapolis, MN, USA

Introduction

Allogeneic hematopoietic cell transplantation (HCT) offers the opportunity for a durable cure for a myriad of malignant and non-malignant diseases. The optimal allogeneic donor choice is an HLA identical sibling donor, however, the majority of patients (~70%) will not have a suitable match within their family. Patients without an optimal related donor can turn to alternative sources of allogeneic grafts including volunteer unrelated donors and cryopreserved umbilical cord blood units (UCB). Unrelated donor selection has evolved over time with the advent of DNA-based HLA testing technologies and studies that have demonstrated the importance of specific HLA loci for optimal HCT outcomes. This chapter provides an overview of HLA typing methodologies and concentrates on matching for unrelated donors.

HLA nomenclature and tissue typing techniques

HLA testing technologies and matching strategies have evolved significantly since the first use of unrelated donors in the late 1980s. The advent of DNA-based typing technologies and enhanced databases of well characterized HLA allele sequences have increased the precision and accuracy of typing leading to improved matching. Table 2.1 lists the commonly used tissue typing techniques and gives an example of the resulting resolution that would be seen on the tissue typing report. Figure 2.1 graphically displays the resolution as it relates to the structure of the HLA molecule.

Polymorphism

The HLA system is recognized to be the most polymorphic gene system known today. As the tissue typing technologies mentioned above developed, and greater accuracy could be achieved, this enormous degree of polymorphism became apparent and even today hundreds of new alleles are discovered, confirmed, named and added to the dictionary each year. The IMGT/HLA database currently contains 13,023 allele sequences (www.ebi.ac.uk/ipd/imgt/hla/intro.html/accessed June 2015). The classical HLA genes that are considered important for clinical transplantation are the Class I genes: HLA-A, -B, and -C and the Class II genes: HLA-DRB1, -DQB1, and -DPB1. Other HLA genes are less important either because they have low levels of polymorphism, because they are pseudogenes or they are not expressed (or expressed at a low level). The human MHC (where HLA genes are found) displays an important phenomenon called "linkage disequilibrium" (LD) where certain alleles are inherited together more frequently than would occur by chance – that is, the inheritance pattern is not random. In fact, in many cases all the HLA genes are inherited as a "package" or haplotype. These two phenomena make it possible to find donors despite the huge number of alleles that exist.

Unrelated donor search and tools for donor search and selection

HLA typing for donor search

Patients should be typed using high-resolution techniques at the HLA-A, -B, -C, and -DRB1 loci to facilitate an effective unrelated donor search. In addition, HLA-DQB1, DPB1, and DRB3/4/5 may be added to prioritize donors with minimal or permissive (discussed later) mismatching at these loci. Prospective donors should have high-resolution verification typing performed on a *newly drawn blood sample* for a minimum of HLA-A, -B, -C, and -DRB1. Additional loci including HLA-DQB1, DPB1 and DRB3/4/5 may be added if considering a 10/10 or 12/12 match, TCE permissive matching or overall match at the low-expression HLA loci, respectively. If the patient has been sensitized to HLA and carries anti-HLA antibodies, it is recommended that

Clinical Manual of Blood and Bone Marrow Transplantation, First Edition. Edited by Syed A. Abutalib and Parameswaran Hari.

Table 2.1 HLA typing techniques and resulting resolution.

Methodology	Approach	Interpretation	Resolution	Application	Results
Serology	Cellular assay based on complement fixation by HLA specific antibodies	Cell death – yes/no	Low	Family screening Null allele confirmation	A2, A24
Sequence-specific primers (PCR-SSP)	HLA sequence-specific PCR primers	Amplification – yes/no	Low to high, dependent on DNA sequence coverage	Family screening Verification typing	Low – A*02:XX, A*24:XX or A*02AB, A*24:BC High – A*0201 g, A*24:02 g
Sequence-specific oligonucleotide probes (PCR-SSOP)	HLA sequence-specific oligonucleotide probes that bind to polymorphic sequences of amplified DNA	Probe binding – yes/no	Low to high depending on DNA sequence coverage	Family screening Verification typing	Low – A*02:XX, A*24:XX or A*02AB, A*24:BC High – A*02:01G, A*24:02G
Sanger sequence-based typing (SBT)	HLA amplicon sequencing using base termination	Base pair reads and consensus alignment	High to allele level depending on coverage	All	High – A*02:01G, A*24:02G Allele – A*02:01:01:03, A*24:02:01:01
Next-generation sequencing (NGS)	Multiple platforms, based on massive parallel sequencing reactions	Base pair calling and consensus alignment	High to allele level depending on coverage	All	High – A*02:01G, A*24:02G Allele – A*02:01:01:03, A*24:02:01:01

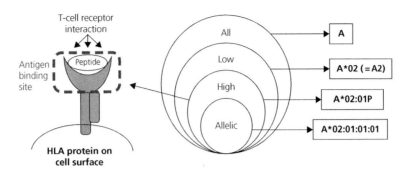

Figure 2.1 HLA nomenclature. HLA typing resolution. The Venn diagram illustrates increasing levels of HLA typing resolution. The figure on the left shows the antigen binding site of an HLA Class I molecule. High-resolution HLA typing defines the specific DNA sequence of the antigen binding site. Allelic resolution defines a single allele as defined by a unique DNA sequence for the HLA gene; in certain instances, the allele name may include synonymous DNA substitutions within the coding region, differences in the noncoding region, and changes in expression. An example of allelic resolution is A*01:01:01:01 for which synonymous DNA substitutions and differences in the noncoding region have been defined. A*02:07 is also an example of allelic resolution; this allele has not been found to have synonymous DNA substitutions or differences in the noncoding region to date. Source: Adapted from Nunes 2011 (Nunes E et al., Definitions of histocompatibility typing terms. Blood. 2011 Dec 1;**118**(23):e180-3. doi:10.1182/blood-2011-05-353490. Epub 2011 Oct 14. PubMed PMID: 22001389).

donors be typed for all sensitized loci to avoid selection of a donor with an anti-HLA antibody target and minimize the risk of primary graft failure.

The donor search

There are currently >25 million volunteer unrelated donors and UCB units listed on Bone Marrow Donors Worldwide (www.bmdw.org/accessed June 2015). This centralized database of donors allows clinicians, and other professionals involved in donor selection, to search for donors in their own country (registry) and donors all over the world simultaneously.

The probability of finding a suitably HLA-matched unrelated donor or UCB unit varies based on the racial/ethnic background of the searching patient. A recent study by the NMDP led by Gragert et al. evaluated the likelihood of finding a HLA-match among 21 distinct racial/ethnic subgroups in the United States population (Figure 2.2). The likelihood of finding an optimally HLA-matched (8/8 match at HLA-A, -B, -C, and -DRB1) ranged from 75% for patients of European descent down to 16% for Blacks of South or Central American descent. When other suitably matched donors (7/8 HLA-match) or UCB units (≥4/6 HLA-match), the likelihoods increase to over 90% for adult (>20 years old) and over 95% for pediatric (<20 years old) patients. The Global access to such a large number of donors ensures that most patients in need of an unrelated graft source will find a suitable HLA-match. Patients with common HLA phenotypes will often identify a donor on the first search of a registry. Those patients with less common phenotypes may not immediately find a suitable donor upon the first search. In those instances,

it is best to seek the support of a histocompatibility specialist to assist with the identification of the best potential donors. Prolonging a search and waiting for an optimally HLA-matched donor to be recruited to the worldwide registries is highly unlikely to result in a better match and increases the risk that the patient's disease will progress.

Once the search report generates a list of potential donors, health care professionals will usually need to contact individual registries directly to obtain more information on the donors (such as secondary donor characteristics, e.g., CMV status) and availability. They will need to request the verification typing mentioned previously, which also serves as an opportunity to confirm the commitment of the donor to donate their hematopoietic "stem" cells. The search report can be complicated and daunting to review for untrained people. One reason for this is that the tissue typing reported will vary greatly based on when the donor joined the registry and what typing techniques were used at that time (as described before). This means that a very well HLA-matched donor may not be found right at the top of the report if the available typing is low or medium resolution and thus could represent several different alleles when higher resolution typing is done. Several algorithms have been developed to try and assist health care professionals who are looking at these reports by assigning probabilities (based on what is known about the frequency of particular tissue types in their population) that the donor will have a particular allele and be matched with the patient. Figure 2.3 shows an example of the output of the search tool Traxis™ developed by the National Marrow Donor Program, which

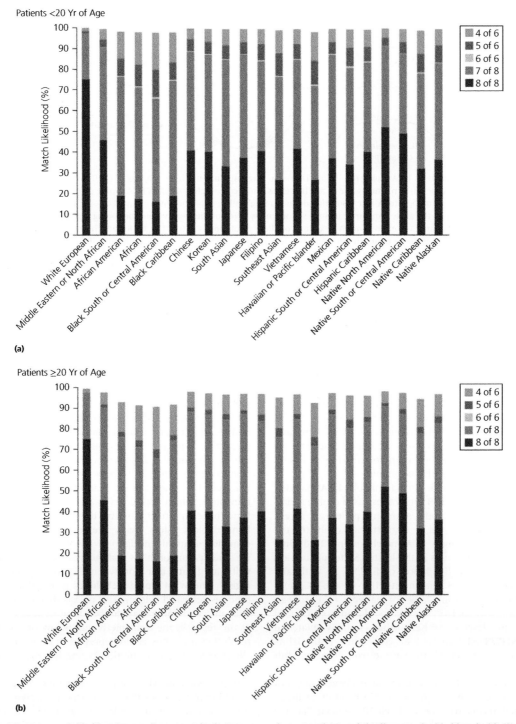

Figure 2.2 HLA-match likelihoods according to racial/ethnic group and age. Panel (a) and (b) illustrate the likelihood of finding a suitable match (defined as an 8/8 or 7/8 adult unrelated donor or ≥4/6 single or double UCB unit(s) with a minimum cell dose of 2.5×10^7/kg) for a pediatric patient (<20 years of age) and an adult patient (>20 years of age), respectively. Source: Adapted from Gragert 2014.

Date: National Marrow Donor Program®   Page:
Time: Donor List Report   Report: TC:

Recipient:	Original Search:	Diagnosis:	ALL - ACUTE LYMPHOBLASTIC LEUKEMIA
NMDP RID:	Date Formalized:	Race (Ethnicity): White - Unspecified (NHIS)	
Local ID:	Date of Search:	Transfer:	

TC Code:	Phen Seq	A	B	C	DRB1	DQB1	DRB3/4/5
Birth Date:		01:01	38:01	03:04	04:04	03:02	5*01:02
ABO:	1	31:01	40:01	12:03	15:02	06:01	
CMV:							

Donor

ID Number			CMV Sts - Date	S/I = Sample at Repository/International Indicator							
S/I	Age	Sex/Pg	Status - Date								
M Cat	ABO	Prev Don	Release Code		HLA Typing/Match Grade/Calculation					Composite Predictions	
Race (Ethnicity)				A	B	C	DRB1	DQB1	DRB3/4/5	Pr(n) of 10	Pr(n) of 8
0827-0438-8			U	01:EJTH	38:AF	03:EAKC	04:ZX			10/10 = 99%	8/8 = 99%
Y/-	21	F/0	AV	31:EJTU	40:EAPA	12:AUCW	15:02			9/10 = 99%	7/8 = 99%
10/10	0		-	P	P	P	P			8/10 = 99%	6/8 = 99%
White - Middle Eastern (NHIS)				P	P	P	A				
				99%	99%	99%	99%	99%			
0238-2782-7			U	s1	s38		04:YK		5*01:BMK	10/10 = 1%	8/8 = 1%
Y/-	48	F	AV	s31	s60		15:DEW			9/10 = 2%	7/8 = 93%
10/10	0		-	P	P		P			8/10 = 94%	6/8 = 99%
White - North American or European				P	P		P				
				99%	99%	95%	1%	1%			

Figure 2.3 An example of a search report from Traxis. Source: Spellman 2012. Reproduced with permission of Elsevier.

includes match probabilities calculated using the search algorithm Haplogic® (https://network.bethematchc linical.org/transplant-centers/materials-catalog/ haplogic-search-report-guide/accessed June 2015). HapLogic predicts the probability of high-resolution matches at the individual HLA-A, -B, -C, -DRB1, and -DQB1 loci and an overall match at the 8/8 and 10/10 level for the patient and each potential donor included on the search. This can provide guidance for donor selection when there are multiple potential donors typed at varying levels of resolution. Other tools that are commonly used are OptiMatch (www.zkrd.de/de/accessed June 2015) and Prometheus (www.hlasoft.com/index. php/prometheus-software/accessed June 2015).

Classical HLA alleles: Impact of mismatching

Table 2.2 shows the major international studies that have been performed to analyze the impact of HLA matching on unrelated donor transplantation outcome. Since the mid to late 1990s it was shown in several studies that high-resolution typing is essential to ensure a good match between the patient and the donor. Studies generally show that survival is worse after HLA mismatched transplantation and that this effect is incremental with increasing numbers of mismatches. GvHD and transplant-related mortality are inevitably shown to be increased in the HLA mismatched setting. Although primary graft failure (PGF) is not universally reported in these studies; however, when such studies are reported the incidence of PGF is higher compared to HLA-matched transplants. Interestingly HLA-match status has not been shown to impact upon disease in a reproducible manner, the exception being two studies from the Japan Marrow Donor Program that show that HLA-C mismatching may be protective against disease relapse. More differences between studies are found when the impacts of individual loci on outcomes are assessed. Reasons for this are likely to include: differing numbers of individual mismatches between studies, transplant center preferences (which may differ by country) for avoiding specific mismatches, genetic and ethnic differences in the specific mismatches that may be prevalent within a population and different time periods over which the studies were performed. When reviewing study results it should also be stressed the transplant population, conditioning regimens and GvHD prophylaxis differ and that this may impact the outcome of a mismatch in various ways – for example, *in-vivo* TCD (alemtuzumab or ATG) is shown to significantly reduce GvHD and thus the effect of HLA mismatches may be diminished. It should also be recognized that

Table 2.2 Major studies examining the outcome of unrelated donor transplantation when using high-resolution typing for all loci listed.

Study	Locus/gene	Numbers	Patient and transplant characteristics	Era	Outcomes
Petersdorf et al., 1998 (Blood. 15;92(10):3515–3520)	HLA-A, -B, -C, DRB1, -DQB1	300	CML MA T-cell replete	1985–1998	Multiple Class I MM: decreased engraftment, increased aGvHD, worse OS Class II MM: increased aGvHD Class I and II MM: decreased engraftment, increased aGvHD, worse OS
Sasazuki et al., 1998 (N Engl J Med. 22;339(17):1177–1785. Erratum in: N Engl J Med 1999 Feb 4;340(5):402)	HLA-A, -B, -C, DRB1, -DQB1	440			Class I MM: increased aGvHD –A and –C, worse OS with –A, reduced relapse -C
Morishima et al., 2002 (Blood. 2002 Jun 1;99(11):4200–4206)	HLA-A, -B, -C, DRB1, -DQB1	1298	Various diseases MA	1993–1998	Class I MM: decreased engraftment, increased aGvHD and cGvHD, worse OS, increase TRM with –A and –B mm Class II MM: increased aGvHD with –DRB1 MM Class I and II MM: decreased engraftment, increased aGvHD and cGvHD, increased TRM, worse OS
Flomenberg et al., 2004 (Blood. 2004 Oct 1;104(7):1923–1930)	HLA-A, -B, -C, DRB1, -DQB1	1874	Various diseases MA	1988–1996	Class I MM: decrease engraftment with -C MM, increased aGvHD and cGvHD with –A MM, worse OS Class II MM: Increased aGvHD and worse survival with -DRB1 MM
Lee et al., 2007	HLA-A, -B, -C, DRB1, -DQB1	3857	Various diseases MA	1988–2003	Single mm: increased aGvHD, increased TRM, decreased OS and DFS Specific locus: MM at –A and –DRB1 decreased OS Multiple MM: decrease OS Single DQB1 MM not associated with any adverse outcomes
Crocchiolo et al., 2009 (Blood. 2009 Aug 13;114(7):1437–1444)	HLA-A, -B, -C, DRB1, -DQB1	805	Various Disease MA, RIC	1999–2006	Single mm: decreased engraftment –DQB1 MM, increased aGvHD –B MM Multiple mm: increased aGvHD, increased TRM decrease OS
Shaw et al., 2010 (Leukemia. 2010 Jan;24(1):58–65)	HLA-A, -B, -C, DRB1, -DQB1	488	AML, ALL, CML MA, RIC TCD	1996–2006	MM: increase aGvHD and cGvHD, increased TRM (multiple MM), decreased OS (multiple MM)
Woolfrey et al., 2011 (Biol Blood Marrow Transplant. 2011 Jun;17(6):885–892)	HLA-A, -B, -C, DRB1, -DQB1	1933	AML, ALL, CML, MDS MA/RIC	1996–2006	Single MM: decreased OS Specific Locus: Increased aGvHD, increased TRM, decreased LFS, decreased OS with -C antigen (not allele) MM Single DQB1 MM not associated with any adverse outcomes
Kanda et al., 2013 (Br J Haematol. 2013 May;161(4):566–577)	HLA-A, -B, -C, DRB1	3003	AML, ALL, CML, MDS	1993–2009	Single MM: decreased engraftment –B, increased aGvHD, decreased TRM and OS
Pidala et al., 2014	HLA-A, -B, -C, DRB1, -DQB1	8003	AML, ALL, CML, MDS MA TC-replete/TCD	1999–2011	Single or multiple Class I MM: increased aGvHD and cGvHD, increased TRM, decreased overall survival
Morishima et al., 2015 (Blood. 2015 Feb 12;125(7):1189–1197)	HLA-A, -B, -C, DRB1, -DQB1	7898	Various diseases MA/RIC	1993–2010	Single MM: increase aGvHD with –A, –B, –C, –DRB1, decreased relapse -C, increased cGvHD -C, decrease OS with any Class I MM

aGvHD = acute Graft versus Host Disease, cGvHD = chronic GvHD, OS = overall survival, AML = Acute myeloid leukemia, ALL = acute lymphoblastic leukemia, CML = chronic myeloid leukemia, MA = myeloablative conditioning, MDS = myelodysplasia, MM = mismatch, RIC = reduced intensity conditioning, TCD = T-cell depleted, TRM = transplant-related mortality.

due to the enormous diversity of the HLA system, very large datasets are necessary to be able to adequately control for other important patient and transplant factors within the study.

The majority of the studies listed in Table 2.2 have also considered the impact of DQB1 matching status on transplant outcome. Two large studies in the USA failed to show an individual impact of DQB1 on survival and it is therefore common practice in the USA to consider an 8/8 matched donor as "fully matched." There are, however, other studies that have shown a lower survival with DQB1 mismatching, in particular, if this mismatch is added to a mismatch at HLA-A, B, C, and DRB1. This therefore remains an area of continued research and donor selection practices are frequently based on the data generated locally in the transplant center.

Non-classical HLA alleles and matching techniques: Impact on outcomes

Traditionally HLA matching has most commonly been considered at the allele level; however, there are several other methodologies for considering matching that may have clear functional relevance and therefore a significant impact on outcomes.

A good example of a locus where there have been different methodologies for assessing match status is HLA-DPB1 (see Table 2.3a). Unlike the "classical" HLA loci, DPB1 is most often not in LD with the rest of the HLA haplotype and thus the probability of finding an allele level match is greatly reduced for patients (<20%). Early transplantation studies examined the impact of allele level matching on outcomes and found that a DPB1 mismatch was associated with a significant increase in GvHD, but a corresponding decrease (protective effect) against disease relapse. The majority of these studies did not find an effect on overall survival, thought to be due to the balance of GvHD and relapse. Later studies began to investigate the impact of matching for T-cell epitopes (TCE) in DPB1. The rationale for this matching technique was based on a finding from Fleischhauer's group that patient's T-cells directed at a donor's single DPB1 mismatch were associated with

graft rejection in a patient. T-cell clones derived from that patient were able to produce varying degrees of allogenic response against different DPB1 alleles, allowing the group to classify DPB1 matching into three groups based on their immunogenicity (strong, medium, weak). Several clinical studies using this method of matching have validated that those with strongly immunogenic mismatches (termed "non-permissive") have a lower survival than those with weakly immunogenic mismatches (termed "permissive") or allele level matched pairs. This is a clinically very helpful method of considering matching status as it means that only 20–30% of donors will have a non-permissive mismatch and therefore the donor pool of ideal donors is significantly higher than would be seen if only allele level matching was considered. Thus approximately 50% of additional patients will have a survival benefit from the inclusion of HLA-DPB1 typing and matching when their donor is being selected. In order to assist clinicians and other search staff in make these selections a freely available online tool has been developed (Figure 2.4) (see www.ebi.ac.uk/ipd/imgt/hla/dpb.html).

There are several other examples of transplant studies that consider the impact of HLA matching in a "non-traditional" manner (Table 2.3b). Some studies have considered the specific allele mismatch and found that certain combinations are permissive (e.g., HLA-C*03:03 vs *03:04), in other words that patients do not have increased complications with a particular combination of HLA alleles within a locus, whilst they do with others. Some of this may be explained by the frequency of certain allelic mismatches within different populations. Other interesting work has looked at the expression levels of the HLA molecules on the cell surface. High levels of expression are associated with worse outcomes, but even the loci that are expressed at a low level have a "cumulative effect," so that more mismatches within these loci are associated with increased mortality after transplant. Several studies have addressed the issue of mismatching at an amino acid level. This is similar to the type of analysis done at DPB1 (where an "epitope" or group of amino acid changes has a greater impact on outcomes), but even more specific, where the impact of a single amino acid change was considered on transplant outcome. Certain amino acid positions in any of

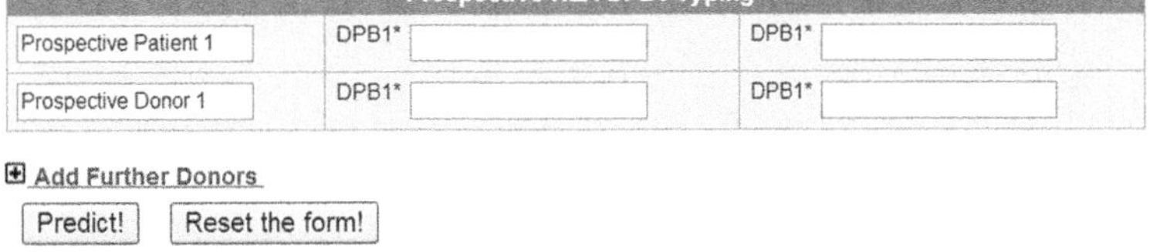

Prospective HLA-DPB1 Typing				
Prospective Patient 1	DPB1*		DPB1*	
Prospective Donor 1	DPB1*		DPB1*	

⊞ Add Further Donors

[Predict!]   [Reset the form!]

Figure 2.4 A screenshot of the HLA-DPB1 TCE prediction tool.

Table 2.3a Major studies examining the outcome of unrelated donor transplantation considering non-classical HLA HLA-DPB1 specific studies.

Study	Locus/gene	Numbers	Patient and transplant characteristics	Era	Outcomes
Shaw et al., 2003 (Bone Marrow Transplant. 2003 Jun;31(11):1001–1008)	-DPB1 allele	143	Various diseases MA TCD	1996–2001	DPB1 MM: increase aGvHD, decreased relapse
Shaw et al., 2006 (Blood. 2006 Feb 1;107(3):1220–1226)	-DPB1 allele	423	Various diseases MA TCD	1996–2003	DPB1 MM: increase aGvHD, decreased relapse, better OS in ALL
Shaw et al., 2007 (Blood. 2007 Dec 15;110(13):4560–4566)	-DPB1 allele	5929	Various diseases	1984–2005	DPB1 MM: increase aGvHD, decreased relapse
Shaw et al., 2010 (Leukemia. 2010 Jan;24(1):58–65)	-DPB1 allele	488	AML, ALL, CML MA/RIC TCD	1996–2006	DPB1 MM: decreased relapse, higher TRM (in 10/10 matched pairs), worse OS in early stage disease (in 10/10 matched pairs), better OS in late stage disease (in <10/10 matched pairs)
Morishima et al., 2015 (Blood. 2015 Feb 12;125(7):1189–1197)	-DPB1 allele	7898	Various diseases MA/RIC	1993–2010	DPB1 MM: increase aGvHD, decrease relapse
Zino et al., 2004 (Blood. 2004 Feb 15;103(4):1417–1424)	-DPB1 TCE	118	Various diseases MA TCD	1995–2002	TCE non-permissive MM: increased aGvHD, increased TRM
Crocchiolo et al., 2009 (Blood. 2009 Aug 13;114(7):1437–1444)	-DPB1 TCE	621	Various diseases MA/RIC	1999–2006	TCE non-permissive MM: increased aGvHD, increased TRM, worse OS
Fleischhauer et al., 2012	-DPB1 TCE	8539	AML, ALL, CML, MDS MA, RIC TC-replete/TCD	1993–2007	TCE non-permissive MM: increased aGvHD, TRM, decreased OS
Fleischhauer et al., 2014 (Bone Marrow Transplant. 2014 Sep;49(9):1176–1183)	-DPB1 TCE, -DPA1	1281	AML, ALL, CML, MDS MA TC-replete/TCD	1988–2003	TCE non-permissive MM: increased aGvHD, TRM, decreased OS, decreased relapse DPA1: NS
Pidala et al., 2014	-DPB1 TCE	8003	AML, ALL, CML, MDS MA TC-replete/TCD	1999–2011	TCE MM: increase aGvHD, decreased relapse TCE non-permissive MM: increased TRM, decreased OS
Petersdorf et al., 2015 (N Engl J Med. 2015 Aug 13;373(7):599–609)	-DPB1 expression	2029	AML, ALL, CML, MDS MA, RIC TC-replete/TCD	1988–2008	DPB1 MM: increased risk of aGvHD in recipients with high expression DPB1 alleles receiving grafts from donors with low-expression DPB1 alleles

aGvHD = acute Graft versus Host Disease, cGvHD = chronic GvHD, OS = overall survival, AML = Acute myeloid leukemia, ALL = acute lymphoblastic leukemia, CML = chronic myeloid leukemia, MA = myeloablative conditioning, MDS = myelodysplasia, MM = mismatch, NS = not significant, RIC = reduced intensity conditioning, TC = T-cell, TCD = T-cell depleted, TCE = T-cell epitope, TRM = transplant-related mortality

the Class I loci have been shown to be associated with a higher incidence of GvHD (e.g., 99 and 116). Another way of looking at matching is in the direction of the match – is this in the GvH direction (donor against patient), the HvG direction (patient against donor) or in both directions (bidirectional). Studies have consistently shown that bidirectional mismatches are associated with a worse OS, but the impact of GvH and HvG is not consistent.

Table 2.3b Major studies examining the outcome of unrelated donor transplantation considering non-classical HLA excluding HLA-DPB1 specific studies.

Study	Locus/gene	Numbers	Patient and transplant characteristics	Era	Outcomes
Ferrara et al., 2001 (Blood. 2001 Nov 15;98(10):3150–3155)	Amino acid	100	CML and other leukemia MA TC-replete marrow	1994-1999	Non-permissive amino acid MM: MM at position 116 in HLA Class I associated with increased risk of aGvHD and TRM.
Kawase et al., 2007 (Blood. 2007 Oct 1;110(7):2235–2241)	Allele combinations	5210	Various diseases MA/RIC (?) TC-replete marrow, <10% ATG	1993–2006	Non-permissive HLA MM: Identified 16 high-risk HLA allele combinations associated with aGvHD grades III–IV (4 – HLA-A, 1 – HLA-B, 7 – HLA-C, 1 – HLA-DRB1, 2 – HLA-DPB1 and 1 – HLA-DRB1-DQB1 combination). Non-permissive amino acid MM: Identified 6 HLA Class I amino acid MM associated with aGvHD grades III–IV.
Kawase et al., 2009 (Blood. 2009 Mar 19;113(12):2851–2858)	Amino acid	4643	ALL, AML, CML, Malignant Lymphoma, MM TC-replete marrow, <10% ATG	1993–2005	Relapse protection MM: 4 – HLA-C and 6-HLA-DPB1 MM combinations associated with a decreased risk of relapse and better OS than fully matched pairs. Specific amino acid MM in HLA-C, but not –DPB1 associated with less relapse.
Morishima et al., 2010 (Blood. 2010 Jun 10;115(23):4664–4670)	Conserved haplotypes	1810	Various diseases MA TC-replete marrow	1993–2006	Conserved extended Japanese haplotypes (HLA-A to HLA-DP) have variable associations with aGvHD grades II–IV in 12/12 matched transplantation.
Pidala et al., 2013 (Blood. 2013 Nov 21;122(22):3651–3658)	Amino acid	7313	ALL, AML, CML and MDS MA/RIC TC-replete/TCD	1988–2009	Non-permissive amino acid MM: HLA-C AAS 99 associated with increased TRM. HLA-C AAS 116 associated with increased aGvHD III–V. HLA-B AAS 9 associated with increased cGvHD.
Hurley et al., 2013. (Blood. 2013 Jun 6;121(23):4800–4806)	Mismatched direction	2687	ALL, AML, CML and MDS MA TC-replete/TCD	1988–2009	HvG only mismatches associated with comparable rates of aGvHD compared 8/8 matched. HvG, GvH and bidirectional mismatches associated with worse OS, TRM and DFS compared to 8/8. No influence of directionality on engraftment.
Petersdorf et al., 2014. (Blood. 2014 Dec 18;124(26):3996–4003)	HLA-C expression levels	1975	Various diseases MA/RIC TC-replete/TCD	1983–2011	Non-permissive HLA MM: Recipient HLA-C expression levels associated with increased risk of acute GvHD and mortality. MM at high expression HLA-C allotypes should be avoided.
Pidala et al., 2014	Permissive MM	7349	ALL, AML, CML and MDS MA/RIC TC-replete/TCD	1988–2009	Permissive HLA MM: HLA-C*03:03 vs *03:04 MM were not significantly different for OS, DFS, TRM, relapse, aGvHD, cGvHD or neutrophil engraftment compared to 8/8 matched cases. Other 7/8 matched cases were significantly worse than 8/8.
Fernández-Viña et al., 2013. (Blood. 2013 May 30;121(22):4603–4610)	Low-expression loci	3853	ALL, AML, CML and MDS MA TC-replete/TCD	1988–2003	>2 mismatches in low-expression loci (HLA-DRB3/4/5, DQA1, DQB1, DPA1 and DPB1) was associated with increased TRM in 7/8 matched transplantation.
Kanda et al., 2015 (Biol Blood Marrow Transplant. 2015 Feb;21(2):305–311)	Mismatched direction	3756	ALL, AML, CML and MDS MA/RIC T replete	2000–2011	Bidirectional HLA mismatches were associated with increased risk of aGvHD and worse OS and TRM compared to fully matched. GvH vector only MM were associated with increased aGvHD risk, but did not differ from the 0 MM group for OS or TRM. HvG vector only MM did not differ from the 0 MM group for any outcomes.

AAS=amino acid substitution, aGvHD=acute Graft versus Host Disease, cGvHD=chronic GvHD, OS=overall survival, AML=Acute myeloid leukemia, ALL=acute lymphoblastic leukemia, CML=chronic myeloid leukemia, DFS=disease free survival, HvG=Host versus graft, GvH=graft versus host, MA=myeloablative conditioning, MDS=myelodysplasia, MM=mismatch, NS=not significant, RIC=reduced intensity conditioning, TC=T-cell, TCD=T-cell depleted, TRM=transplant-related mortality

SUMMARY

- High-resolution methods should always be used when typing patients and donors/UCB for transplantation.
- Donor search can be simplified by the use of predictive algorithms and online tools.
- Transplant outcomes are improved when using donors/UCB well matched for the classical HLA loci.
- Non-traditional "matching" methods can define mismatches that are "permissive" or "non-permissive" and impact transplant outcomes.

Selected reading

1. Lee SJ, Klein J, Haagenson M, Baxter-Lowe LA, Confer DL, Eapen M, et al. High-resolution donor-recipient HLA matching contributes to the success of unrelated donor marrow transplantation. *Blood*. 2007 Dec 15;**110**(13):4576–4583. Epub 2007 Sep 4.
2. Fleischhauer K, Shaw BE, Gooley T, Malkki M, Bardy P, Bignon JD, et al. International Histocompatibility Working Group in Hematopoietic Cell Transplantation. Effect of T-cell-epitope matching at HLA-DPB1 in recipients of unrelated-donor haemopoietic-cell transplantation: a retrospective study. *Lancet Oncol*. 2012 Apr;**13**(4):366–374. doi: 10.1016/S1470-2045(12)70004-9. Epub 2012 Feb 15.
3. Spellman SR, Eapen M, Logan BR, Mueller C, Rubinstein P, Setterholm MI, et al. National Marrow Donor Program; Center for International Blood and Marrow Transplant Research. A perspective on the selection of unrelated donors and cord blood units for transplantation. *Blood*. 2012 Jul 12;**120**(2):259–265. doi: 10.1182/blood-2012-03-379032. Epub 2012 May 17.
4. Gragert L, Eapen M, Williams E, Freeman J, Spellman S, Baitty R, et al. HLA match likelihoods for hematopoietic stem-cell grafts in the U.S. registry. *N Engl J Med*. 2014 Jul 24;**371**(4):339–348. doi: 10.1056/NEJMsa1311707.
5. Pidala J, Lee SJ, Ahn KW, Spellman S, Wang HL, Aljurf M, et al. Nonpermissive HLA-DPB1 mismatch increases mortality after myeloablative unrelated allogeneic hematopoietic cell transplantation. *Blood*. 2014 Oct 16;**124**(16):2596–2606. doi: 10.1182/blood-2014-05-576041. Epub 2014 Aug 26. PubMed PMID: 25161269; PubMed Central PMCID: PMC4199961.
6. Tiercy JM. How to select the best available related or unrelated donor of hematopoietic stem cells? *Haematologica*. 2016;**101**:680–687.
7. Fernandez-Viña MA, et al. Identification of a permissible HLA mismatch in hematopoietic stem cell transplantation. *Blood*. 2014;**123**:1270–1278.
8. Fernández-Viña MA, et al. Multiple mismatches at the low expression HLA loci DP, DQ, and DRB3/4/5 associate with adverse outcomes in hematopoietic stem cell transplantation. *Blood*. 2013;**121**:4603–4610.
9. Hamdi A, et al. Are changes in HLA Ags responsible for leukaemia relapse after HLA-matched allogeneic hematopoietic SCT? *Bone Marrow Transplant*. 2015;**50**:411–413.

CHAPTER 3

Risk-benefit assessment in allogeneic hematopoietic transplant: Factors, scores, and models

Mahmoud Elsawy[1,3] and Mohamed L. Sorror[1,2]

[1] Clinical Research Division, Fred Hutchinson Cancer Research Center, University of Washington School of Medicine, Seattle, WA, USA

[2] Division of Medical Oncology, Department of Medicine, University of Washington School of Medicine, Seattle, WA, USA

[3] Department of Medical Oncology, National Cancer Institute, Cairo University, Egypt

Introduction

Hematopoietic cell transplantation (HCT) carries potential risks of subsequent relapse and non-relapse mortality (NRM). Several models were designed to estimate these risks and weigh them against the survival benefit in an effort to optimize decisions about a patient's suitability for HCT. This became specifically more important since the advent of reduced-intensity conditioning (RIC) regimens that extended the use of HCT to treat older and medically infirm patients who otherwise were previously denied the procedure. Here, we discuss different risk factors and models that need to be assessed prior to allogeneic HCT and how these factors and models could be used in evaluating mortality risks after allogeneic HCT.

What are the factors to consider prior to HCT?

Whether a patient should be offered a transplant or not relies on several factors, which are discussed next.

Age

Historically, an arbitrary cut-off of 50–60 years was the limit to consider patients eligible for HCT. The development of RIC regimens that are more tolerable with a better toxicity profile has allowed older and medically infirm patients to become potential candidates for HCT. However, this comes at the price of potentially higher rates of relapse. The percentage of older patients being considered for allogeneic HCT for treatment of malignant diseases continues to rise. Seventeen percent of allogeneic HCT recipients in 2006–2012 were older than 60 (Figure 3.1).

Recent studies have shown a limited impact of chronological age on outcomes of HCT. That impact was equivalent to the impact of a single comorbidity with a weight of 1 within the HCT-CI. In another study, patients aged 60–75 years old given nonmyeloablative (NMA) conditioning and allogeneic HCT had similar outcomes.

Thus, chronological age alone should not be the main determinant of transplant eligibility but should be considered (age 60–75) for conditioning intensity selection. It has to be used within the context of assessment of organ comorbidities to guide conditioning regimen selection.

Performance status

Karnofsky performance status (KPS) is the most widely used tool by physicians to assess a patient's functional status. However, this tool is highly subjective and physician dependent; hence its accuracy may be doubtful. For these reasons, there is no ideal cut-off KPS score to consider a patient eligible for HCT. Generally, a KPS score of ≥70–80% is required to consider a patient eligible for high-dose allogeneic HCT.

Socioeconomic status

Allogeneic HCT might require long-term post-transplant follow-up. As such, careful evaluation of the patient's social situation, particularly the availability of a caregiver, is crucial for the success of the procedure. Additionally, the financial burden should be discussed with the patient and family in order to consider potential financial hardships that may develop throughout the process.

Clinical Manual of Blood and Bone Marrow Transplantation, First Edition. Edited by Syed A. Abutalib and Parameswaran Hari.
© 2017 John Wiley & Sons Ltd. Published 2017 by John Wiley & Sons Ltd.

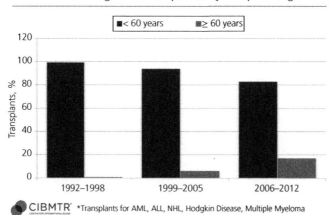

Figure 3.1 Changes in ages of allogeneic hematopoietic cell transplant recipients over time. Source: Pasquini MC, Zhu X. Current uses and outcomes of hematopoietic stem cell transplantation: 2015 CIBMTR Summary Slides.

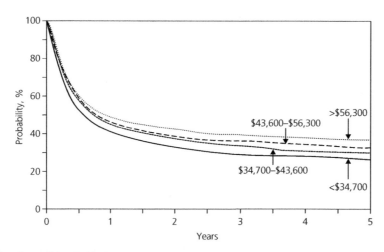

Figure 3.2 Probabilities of overall survival by income.

Allogeneic HCT is associated with significant post-transplant immunosuppression with a high incidence of infectious complications. Therefore, patients who lack access to essential post-transplant care might be at a higher risk for transplant-related mortality. Also, patients living in rural areas might not be referred to transplant centers, thus limiting their chances for cure of their hematological diseases.

Low socioeconomic status has been shown to correlate with poor HCT outcomes (Figures 3.2 and 3.3). This could be potentially attributed to inability to secure adequate health insurance coverage and, hence, the need to postpone transplant with risk of subsequent disease progression. Additionally, most insurance contracts have a lifetime maximum coverage. It is not uncommon

for the cost of for allogeneic HCT and subsequent medical care to exceed that maximum. Thus, patients will experience major out-of-pocket expenses.

Race

Some reports suggest that a patient's race could have an impact on HCT. Being African-American (AA), for example, has been shown in some reports to be associated with lower survival rates following allogeneic HCT. In a large study (n=2,221), mortality risks were significantly higher in AA patients compared to white patients (hazard ratio (HR)=1.65). However, other studies did not confirm these observations. One possibility that needs further investigation could be the higher prevalence of certain comorbidities in patients with darker

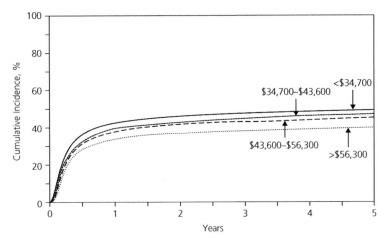

Figure 3.3 Cumulative incidence of treatment-related mortality by income.

skin color. Also, dark skin may potentially limit precise grading of severity of graft-versus-host disease (GvHD). Interpretation of the results of such studies should account for the fact that race is not just a biological factor; rather, it could dictate other social, economic, and cultural variabilities.

In another analysis of data from 6,207 allogeneic HCT recipients, AA patients had inferior OS (RR = 1.47) compared to whites. Additionally, NRM was higher in AAs (RR = 1.56) and Hispanics (RR = 1.30). Across all racial groups, patients with lower incomes had worse OS (RR = 1.15) and high NRM (RR = 1.21) than those with higher incomes. Thus, inferior outcomes in AAs cannot be fully explained by socioeconomic status; other factors such as genetic polymorphism and health behavior may contribute.

Organ function

Proper quantification of organ reserve is mandatory to individualize treatment plans and provide preemptive measures aiming to lessen post HCT complications. Thorough assessment of vital organ functions must be conducted using both laboratory tests and imaging studies.

1 *Pulmonary functions assessment*
Historically, a corrected diffusion capacity of the lung for carbon monoxide (DLco) of ≥60% was a requirement for eligibility for HCT. In a large study including 1,297 recipients of HCT (82% allogeneic and 12% autologous), DLco values less than 60% were associated with a 1.5-fold increase in hazards of post-transplant mortality. A subsequent study has shown DLco values of <70% to be associated with a 2.5-fold increase in the incidence of severe post-transplant hepatic sinusoidal obstructive syndrome (SOS) indicative of pre-existing systemic endothelial cell damage.

However, a subset of patients with a corrected DLco of <60% could still benefit from allogeneic HCT. Those are typically patients with autoimmune diseases that frequently involve the lungs, for example, scleroderma. However, in this subset of patients, certain agents should be avoided in conditioning regimens selected, such as BCNU (carmustine), busulfan, and total-body irradiation (TBI), given their potential effect of impairing lung diffusion capacity.

2 *Cardiac assessment*
The fluids and chemotherapy administration related to a particular conditioning regimen is likely to be well tolerated with no life-threatening complications in patients with adequate cardiac reserve. However, patients with borderline cardiac functions are suggested to experience greater complications. Generally, a left ventricular ejection fraction (LVEF) of more than 40% is chosen as an indicator of satisfactory cardiac reserve. Nevertheless, determination of an allowed degree of cardiac impairment remains largely dependent on the underlying disease, previous therapy, and the intensity of a selected conditioning regimen. All candidate of allogeneic HCT must have a 12-lead electrocardiogram (ECG). Rhythm abnormalities, particularly QT-interval prolongation or QT-interval dispersion, on an electrocardiogram is a predictor of a higher risk of post-transplant acute heart failure.

3 *Liver reserve assessment*
An adequate liver function is essential to ensure proper metabolism and detoxification of various chemotherapeutic agents. A substantial proportion of patients with hematological disorders have pretransplantion liver function abnormalities attributed to iron overload from frequent blood transfusions, previous therapy-related liver injury, or other common factors, for

example hepatitis, alcohol abuse. A diminished liver reserve significantly increases the risk of developing severe complications such as SOS. All patients undergoing assessment for HCT must have a baseline liver function assessment. Any abnormalities should be thoroughly investigated for an etiology.

4 *Renal reserve assessment*
Patients are exposed to several nephrotoxic or renal excreted agents throughout HCT, e.g. cyclosporine, tacrolimus, vancomycin, and aminoglycosides. Thus, an adequate renal function is essential to maintain therapeutic levels of these agents. A pretransplantion low glomerular filtration rate (GFR) has been shown to be an independent predictor of developing post-transplant chronic renal impairment. A combination of both low GFR and high serum creatinine are associated with a higher risk of developing acute renal failure following HCT.

5 *Nutritional assessment*
Nutritional assessment by a nutritionist prior to HCT is required for two main reasons. First, the dosage of most drugs is largely dependent on a patient's body weight. Second, a body mass index measurement is required for evaluation of nutritional needs before, during, and after HCT. Diabetic patients are particularly in need for close nutritional status monitoring to maintain proper glycemic control to lessen the risk of infectious complications.

Models used for risk-benefit measurement

Decision-making for allogeneic HCT relies on two major parameters. First, the patient's risk of NRM, which is largely dependent on the patient's overall health status. Second, the underlying disease risk of relapse, which is determined by diagnosis, disease status, and chromosomal/genetic abnormalities. Success of HCT relies on limiting both NRM and relapse after HCT.

Models estimating incidences of NRM

1 *Hematopoietic cell transplantation-specific comorbidity index (HCT-CI)*
The advent of RIC has expanded the use of potentially curative HCT to include previously ineligible patients, typically older patients and those with comorbidities. This expansion necessitated the need for a tool to measure the burden of comorbidities and provide a better estimate of transplant risk-benefit ratio. An HCT-CI was developed by modifying the Charlson comorbidity index to suit the HCT setting. The study included 1,055 recipients of allogeneic HCT after nonmyeloablative- (n=294) or high-dose- (n=761) conditioning regimens. The

index was derived from Cox proportional hazard models of NRM in the training set (n=708) and tested in the validation set (n=347). Investigators identified 17 different comorbid conditions to be significantly associated with the incidence of NRM. Comorbidities were assigned scores of 0, 1, 2, or 3 according to their respective HRs that could be summated into a total score for each patient (Table 3.1). The HCT-CI scores of 0, 1–2, ≥3 correlated with 2-year NRM incidences of 14, 21, and 41%, respectively, and 2-year survival rates of 71, 60, and 34%, respectively (Figure 3.4). The validity of the HCT-CI in estimating risks of NRM was shown in several large retrospective and prospective multi-center studies.

The HCT-CI scores were used to guide decision-making on treatment selection for certain hematological disorders (Table 3.2). One study investigated outcomes of allogeneic HCT recipients following non-myeloablative- (n=125) or high-dose- (n=452) conditioning regimens for treatment of acute myeloid leukemia (AML) (n=391) and myelodysplastic syndromes (MDS) (n=186). Higher HCT-CI scores and disease risk status were the two significant prognosticators for outcomes. Accordingly, patients were stratified into four risk groups with distinct outcomes based on their HCT-CI scores and disease risk (Table 3.2 and Figure 3.5).

The HCT-CI could successfully stratify outcomes of 220 recipients of allogeneic HCT for lymphomas including chronic lymphocytic leukemia (CLL) following nonmyeloablative (n=152) or high-dose conditioning (n=68) conditioning regimens (Table 3.2). In another study, outcomes of 82 patients with CLL were classified into four risk groups based on their HCT-CI scores and lymph node (LN) sizes. Rates of 4-year OS ranged between 74% for patients with HCT-CI scores of 0 and LN sizes<5cm, to 27% for those with comorbidities and LN sizes ≥5cm (Table 3.2).

In another study, a combination of HCT-CI scores and C-reactive protein (CRP) levels could successfully predict outcomes among 271 recipients of allogeneic HCT for chronic myeloid leukemia patients (CML) who failed first generation tyrosine kinase inhibitors (TKIs). Patients with low HCT-CI scores and low CRP levels had the best outcomes following allogeneic HCT with OS rates of 69.9 and 70%, respectively (Table 3.2).

The HCT-CI scores have been shown recently to correlate with risk of development of certain post-transplant morbidities. In a large analysis of data from 2,985 allogeneic HCT recipients from five different US institutions, higher HCT-CI scores correlated with development of grade III-IV acute GvHD (Table 3.3)

Table 3.1 Definitions of comorbidities included in the HCT-CI* and the augmented HCT-CI** and their corresponding scores.

The HCT-CI*		
Comorbidity	Definition	Score
Arrhythmia	Any type of arrhythmia that has necessitated the delivery of a specific anti-arrhythmia treatment at any time point in the patient's past medical history.	1
Cardiac	Coronary artery disease,§ congestive heart failure, myocardial infarction, or EF ≤50%	1
Inflammatory bowel disease	Crohn's disease or ulcerative colitis requiring treatment at any time point in patient's past medical history.	1
Diabetes	Requiring treatment with insulin or oral hypoglycemic agents continuously for 4 weeks before start of conditioning	1
Cerebrovascular disease	Transient ischemic attack or cerebrovascular accident	1
Psychiatric disturbance	Any disorder requiring continuous treatments for 4 weeks before start of conditioning	1
Hepatic, mild	Chronic hepatitis, bilirubin > ULN to 1.5 × ULN, or AST/ALT > ULN to 2.5 × ULN; at least two values of each within 2 or 4 weeks before start of conditioning.	1
Obesity	Patients with a body mass index >35 kg/m² for patients older than 18 years or a BMI-for-age of ≥95th percentile for patients of ≤18 years of age	1
Infection	Requiring antimicrobial treatment starting from before conditioning and continued beyond day 0	1
Rheumatologic	Requiring specific treatment at any time point in the patient's past medical history	2
Peptic ulcer	Based on prior endoscopic or radiologic diagnosis	2
Moderate/severe renal	Serum creatinine > 2 mg/dl (at least two values of each within 2 or 4 weeks before start of conditioning), on dialysis, or prior renal transplantation	2
Moderate pulmonary	Corrected DLco (via Dinakara equation) and/or FEV1 of 66–80% or dyspnea on slight activity	2
Prior malignancy	Treated at any time point in the patient's past history, excluding non-melanoma skin cancer	3
Heart valve disease	Of at least moderate severity, prosthetic valve, or symptomatic mitral valve prolapse as detected by echocardiogram	3
Severe pulmonary	Corrected DLco (via Dinakara equation) and/or FEV1 ≤65% or dyspnea at rest or requiring oxygen	3
Moderate/severe hepatic	Liver cirrhosis, bilirubin > 1.5 × ULN, or AST/ALT > 2.5 × ULN; at least two values of each within 2 or 4 weeks before start of conditioning	3
Augmented HCT-CI**: all of the above +		
High ferritin	Values of ≥2500 as measured the closest prior to start of conditioning	1
Mild Hypoalbuminemia	Values of <3.5–3.0 as measured the closest prior to start of conditioning	1
Thrombocytopenia	Values of <100,000 as measured the closest prior to start of conditioning	1
Moderate Hypoalbuminemia	Values of <3.0 as measured the closest prior to start of conditioning	2

Adapted from * Sorror ML et al. *Blood* **106**(8): 2912–2919, 2005.
** Vaughn JE et al. *Biol Blood Marrow Transplant* **21**(8): 1418–1424, 2015.
Abbreviations: DLco = diffusion capacity of carbon monoxide: EF = ejection fraction; FEV1 = forced expiratory volume in 1 second; ULN = upper limit of normal.
§ One or more vessel-coronary artery stenosis requiring medical treatment, stent, or bypass graft.

and subsequent mortality following diagnosis of grade II (HR = 1.24, p < 0.0001) or grade III-VI acute GvHD (HR = 1.19, p < 0.0001).

The calculation of a total HCT-CI score for an individual patient has been recently facilitated with the introduction of a training program for data acquisition

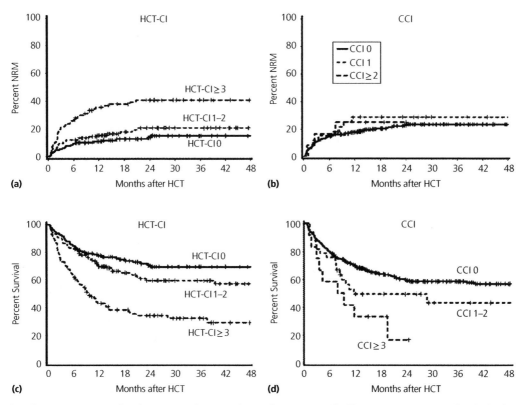

Figure 3.4 The HCT-CI compared with CCI. Cumulative incidence of NRM as stratified by (a) HCT-CI compared with (b) the original CCI and Kaplan–Meier estimates of survival as stratified by (c) the HCT-CI compared with (d) the original CCI. CCI, Charlson comorbidity index; HCT-CI, hematopoietic cell transplantation-specific comorbidity index; NRM, non-relapse mortality. Source: Sorror 2005. Reproduced with permission of American Society of Hematology.

from medical records and a web base calculator (www.hctci.org) (Figure 3.6).

More recently, the prognostic capacity of the HCT-CI was further augmented by addition of age to build a composite comorbidity/age index using a large dataset of 3,033 allogeneic HCT recipients. In multivariate models, an age of more than 40 years has been shown to impact NRM as equivalent to a single comorbidity with a score of 1. The composite comorbidity/age index could provide more accurate estimates of biological age. The predictive capacity of the HCT-CI was further augmented by the addition of some relevant biological markers, namely low platelets count, low serum albumin, and high ferritin (Table 3.1).

The HCT-CI was successfully combined with other risk assessment models to provide more prognostic information for HCT outcomes (Table 3.4). For example, a model combining the HCT-CI and KPS was successful to stratify risk outcome for 341 recipients of allogeneic HCT following nonmyeloablative conditioning. Similarly, a composite comorbidity/relapse model has been shown to stratify 5-year OS

for recipients of nonmyeloablative allogeneic HCT who were 60 years or older into nine distinct groups. Another composite model combined both the HCT-CI and the European Society for Blood and Marrow Transplantation (EBMT) score (discussed under the EBMT score). Finally, the HCT-CI in combination with the geriatric tool, Instrumental Activities of Daily Living (IADL), could stratify outcomes for HCT recipients 50 years or older into three risk groups for overall mortality.

2 *Comprehensive geriatric assessment (CGA)*

Median age of diagnosis for most adult related hematological malignancies is 65–70 years. With the advent of RIC regimens, increasing numbers of older patients are being considered for allogeneic HCT. Older patients might experience additional age-specific health limitations than encountered in younger adults. Unfortunately, available health status assessment tools such as KPS and European Cooperative Oncology Group performance status (ECOG) do not provide comprehensive overview of their health status. CGA could provide useful

Table 3.2 Role of HCT-CI scores in optimizing treatment selection for specific hematological disorders.

Study	Number of Patients	Disease Category	Conditioning Intensity	Risk Stratification		Outcomes				Comments
Sorror et al., 2007	577	AML (n=391) MDS (n=186)	MA (n=452) NMA (n=125)	HCT-CI score	Disease risk	2-yr NRM and OS (%)				Combined HCT-CI score and disease risk status stratified patients into four groups with distinct outcomes
						MA		NMA		
						NRM	OS	NRM	OS	
				0–2	low	11	78	4	70	
				0–2	Intermediate and high	24	51	3	57	
				≥3	low	32	45	27	41	
				≥3	Intermediate and high	46	24	29	29	
Sorror et al., 2008	82	CLL	2-Gy TBI (n=13) 2-Gy TBI+fludarabine (n=69)	HCT-CI score	LN size	5-yr OS (%)				Combined HCT-CI scores and LN size were the two most predictive factors of outcomes.
				0	<5cm	78				
				0	≥5cm	43				
				≥1	<5cm	60				
				≥1	≥5cm	27				
Sorror et al., 2008	220	CLL and lymphoma	MA (n=68) NMA (n=152)	HCT-CI score	Conditioning intensity	3-yr NRM (%)	3-yr OS (%)			Patients with HCT-CI score=0 had no statistically significant differences in outcomes, while patients with HCT-CI scores ≥1 had statistically significant better outcomes with NMA versus MA conditioning regimens, respectively.
				0	NMA	18	68			
				0	MA	15	60			
				≥1	NMA	28	47			
				≥1	MA	50	35			
Pavlu et al., 2010	271	Imatinib resistant CML	MA	HCT-CI score		5-yr NRM (%)	5-year OS (%)			CML Patients with low HCT-CI scores and low CRP values are better candidates for early MA HCT after imatinib failure
				0		5.3	69.6			
				≥1		18.5	55.5			
				CRP (ml/L)		5-yr OS (%)				
				≤9		70				
				>9		40				

Abbreviations: AML=acute myeloid leukemia, CLL=chronic lymphocytic leukemia, CML=chronic myeloid leukemia, CRP=C-reactive protein, HCT-CI=hematopoietic cell transplantation-specific comorbidity index, LN=lymph node, MA=myeloblative, MDS=myelodysplastic syndromes, NMA=non-myeloabalative, NRM=non-relapse mortality, OS=overall survival, RIC=reduced-intensity conditioning, yr=year.

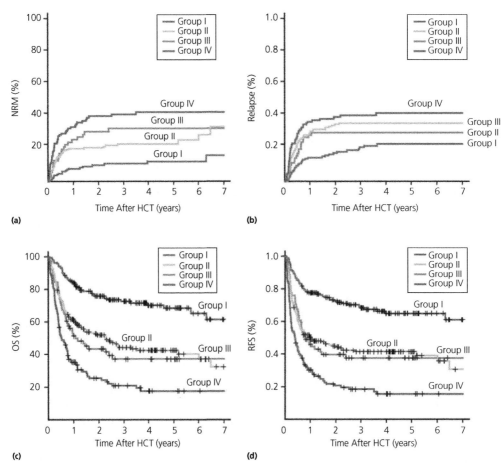

Figure 3.5 Risk stratification of patients with acute myeloid leukemia/myelodysplasia and receiving allogeneic hematopoietic cell transplantation (HCT). Group I included HCT-CI scores 0 to 2 plus low disease risk; group II included HCT-CI scores 0 to 2 plus intermediate and high disease risks; group III included HCT-CI scores ≥3 plus low disease risks; and group IV included HCT-CI scores ≥3 plus intermediate and high disease risks. HCT-CI, hematopoietic cell transplantation-specific comorbidity index; NRM, non-relapse mortality; OS, overall survival; RFS, relapse-free survival. Source: Sorror 2007. Reproduced with permission of American Society of Clinical Oncology.

information on additional factors that could be potential targets for peri-transplant modification to improve outcomes for this group of patients.

In an analysis of data from 203 recipients of allogeneic HCT who were between 50 and 73 years (median = 57 years), multivariate analysis could identify limitations of IADL as the most significant component of CGA to influence OS (HR = 2.28, $p < 0.001$). The hazard was even higher among patients older than 60 years (HR = 3.25, p < 0.001). Therefore, limitations of IADL was combined with HCT-CI scores to create a single three-point model (Table 3.4). Interestingly, none of patients with a combined score of 3 who were ≥60 years of age survived beyond 2 years following allogeneic HCT. Additional data are needed before widespread use of these tools since

Table 3.3 Association between HCT-CI scores and development of acute GvHD.

HCT-CI score	Incidence of grades III-IV acute GvHD*
0	13%
1–4	18%
≥5	24%

* $p < 0.0001$
Adapted from Sorror ML et al. *Blood* **124**(2): 287–295, 2014.

only 2% of the study population was >70 years of age. Moreover, another study of 126 (median age 74 years) recipients of allogeneic HCT for treatment of newly diagnosed AML showed self-reported cardiac

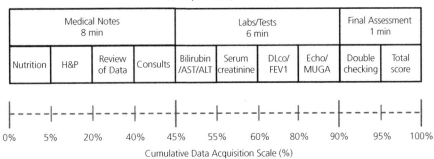

Three-Step Process (15 minutes)

Medical Notes 8 min				Labs/Tests 6 min				Final Assessment 1 min	
Nutrition	H&P	Review of Data	Consults	Bilirubin /AST/ALT	Serum creatinine	DLco/ FEV1	Echo/ MUGA	Double checking	Total score

0%   5%   20%   40%   45%   55%   60%   80%   90%   95%   100%

Cumulative Data Acquisition Scale (%)

Figure 3.6 Three-step methodology for comorbidity coding. Source: Sorror 2013. Reproduced with permission of American Society of Hematology.

Table 3.4 Augmentation of HCT-CI predictability by combining with other models.

Composite Model	Risk Groups		Outcomes at 2 Years		Outcomes at 4 or 5 Years	
	HCT-CI	KPS	NRM, %	OS, %	NRM, %	OS, %
Comorbidity/PS (Sorror et al. 2008)	0–2	>80%	16	68		
	0–2	≤80%	17	58		
	≥3	>80%	30	41		
	≥3	≤80%	39	32		
	HCT-CI/age					
Comorbidity/age score (nonmyeloablative vs RIC) (Sorror et al. 2014)	0		5–12	81–87		
	1–2		9–18	66–67		
	3–4		17–36	47–54		
	≥5		35–41	34–35		
Comorbidity/relapse score (patients ≥60 years old) (Sorror et al. 2011)	HCT-CI	Relapse risk score				
	0	Low				69
	0	Standard				45
	0	High				41
	1–2	Low				56
	1–2	Standard				44
	1–2	High				15
	≥3	Low				56
	≥3	Standard				23
	≥3	High				23
HCT-CI/EBMT (Elsawy et al. 2014)	HCT-CI	EBMT				
	0	<4			11	72
	0	≥4			19	61
	1–2	<4			16	63
	1–2	≥4			28	48

(Continued)

Table 3.4 (Continued)

Composite Model	Risk Groups		Outcomes at 2 Years		Outcomes at 4 or 5 Years	
	HCT-CI	KPS	NRM, %	OS, %	NRM, %	OS, %
	≥3	<4			31	40
	≥3	≥4			41	30
HCT-CI/IADL (Muffly et al. 2014) *HCT-CI score of ≥3 or IADL score <14 acquire a score of 1. Both abnormalities get a score of 2*	Scores					
	0			62		
	1			44		
	2			13		

Abbreviations: EBMT, European bone marrow transplant; HCT-CI, hematopoietic cell transplantation comorbidity index; NRM, non-relapse mortality; OS, overall survival; PS, performance status; RIC, reduced-intensity conditioning

history to be an independent prognostic factor for survival (HR = 2.290) while other CGA domains were not. More validation studies are still needed before introduction of CGA into transplant practice.

Given the contradicting results above and the relatively small number of patients, large studies are still needed to validate the usefulness of CGA in the HCT setting and to better identify which components are most relevant for outcome prediction.

Models estimating relapse risk

1 *Disease Risk Index (DRI)*

Investigators from Dana Farber Cancer Institute and the Fred Hutchinson Cancer Research Center (Fred Hutch) devised and validated a tool to estimate the impacts of the underlying disease and disease status on the success of HCT. The model was developed by utilizing data collected from 1,539 patients who received allogeneic HCT following nonmyeloablative/ RIC- (n = 727) or high-dose- (n = 812) conditioning regimens. In multivariate models, the DRI was built based on hazards of OS for each diagnosis and disease status.

DRI is composed of three disease risk categories and two status risk categories, together leading to six possible disease/status combinations which are further collapsed into four different risk groups (Table 3.5). In the Dana Farber/Fred Hutch study, rates of 4-year OS ranged between 56 and 6% and 4-year progression free survival (PFS) between 64% and 6% for low and very high risk groups, respectively (p < 0.001 for all) (Figure 3.7). Overall, mortality was attributed to relapse with cumulative incidences of relapse ranging between 19 and 63% for the low and very high groups, respectively (p < 0.001). Incidences of NRM were not statistically significantly different between all risk groups (p = 0.11). The DRI was then validated in an independent cohort of 672 patients form Fred Hutch. In the validation

cohort, the DRI successfully stratified patients for rates of OS and PFS (p < 0.001 for both) (Figure 3.8).

Recently, the DRI was validated and assignments of some disease/status categories were refined utilizing data from 13,131 allogeneic HCT recipients reported to Center for International Blood and Marrow Transplant Research (CIBMTR) (Table 3.6). The refined DRI has been shown to have a better predictive capacity compared to the original DRI (c-statistics 0.643 versus 0.637, respectively, no *p* value was reported). Further, the risk stratification ability of the DRI could be augmented in the future by the addition of relevant disease-specific features, for example molecular markers and minimal residual disease status.

Models estimating all-cause mortality

1 *EBMT score*

The EBMT score is a global model that aims to estimate risks of all-cause mortality for allogeneic HCT recipients. The model incorporates a mix of disease-specific and patient-specific variables, namely, age, disease stage, time interval between diagnosis and transplant, donor recipient sex combination, HLA- disparity, and donor gender. These variables were utilized to build a five-component model with a total score ranging from 0 to 7 (Table 3.7).

The EBMT score was first developed to guide the decision-making process of utilizing transplantation for patients with CML before the era of TKIs. The model was then tested in a large registry dataset of 56,505 patients with different hematological disorders who received their first allogeneic HCT at different centers in Europe. Rates of 5-year OS ranged from 71% to 24% for risk scores from 0 to 7, respectively. These results led to extending the applicability of EBMT score to include other hematological disorders than CML.

The EBMT score has undergone several modifications over time to improve its predictive capacity and

Table 3.5 DRI for patients undergoing allogeneic HCT.

Disease	Disease Risk
AML favorable cytogenetics	Low
CLL	
CML	
Indolent B-cell NHL	
ALL	Intermediate
AML intermediate cytogenetics	
MDS intermediate cytogenetics	
MPN	
Multiple myeloma	
HL	
DLBCL/transformed indolent B-cell NHL	
Mantle cell lymphoma	
T-cell lymphoma, nodal	
AML adverse cytogenetics	High
MDS adverse cytogenetics	
T-cell lymphoma, extranodal	

Stage	Stage risk
Any CR	Low
1st PR	
Untreated	
Chronic phase CML	
2nd or subsequent PR (if RIC)	
2nd or subsequent PR (if MAC)	High
Induction failure	
Active relapse	
Accelerated or blast phase CML	

Overall assignment		
Disease risk	Stage risk	DRI
Low	Low	Low
Low	High	intermediate
Intermediate	Low	
Intermediate	High	High
High	Low	
High	high	Very high

Adapted from Armand P, et al. *Blood* **120**(4): 905–913, 2012

Abbreviations: AML = acute myeloid leukemia, CLL = chronic lymphocytic leukemia, CML = chronic myeloid leukemia, CR = complete remission, DLBCL = diffuse large B-cell lymphoma, HL = Hodgkin lymphoma, MAC = myeloablative conditioning, MDS = myelodysplastic syndromes, MPN = myeloproliferative neoplasms, NHL = non-Hodgkin lymphoma, PR = partial remission, and RIC = reduced-intensity conditioning.

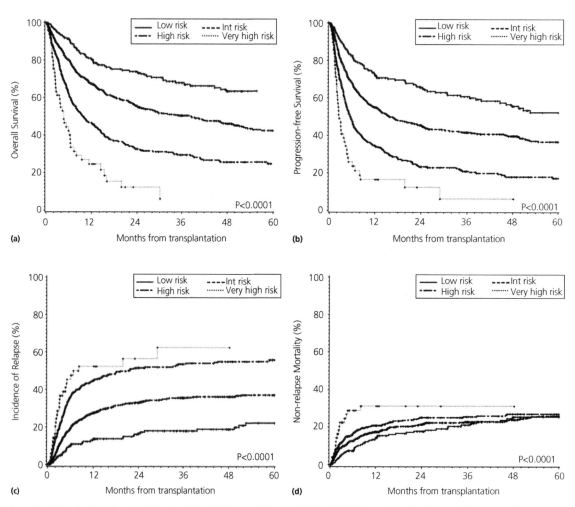

Figure 3.7 Risk stratification by DRI categories for (a) Overall survival, (b) PFS, (c) Cumulative incidence of relapse, and (d) Cumulative incidence of NRM. Source: Sorror 2012. Reproduced with permission of American Society of Hematology.

to accommodate recent changes in the practice of allogeneic HCT. A modified EBMT (mEBMT) score was developed in which an extra point was assigned to patients older than 60 years. Also, the time interval between diagnosis and HCT was omitted given its strong association with disease stage. The mEBMT demonstrated a higher predictive capacity for 4-year OS compared to the original model in a cohort of 306 RIC HCT recipients, $p = 0.001$ versus 0.06, respectively. In another study of 502 recipients of HLA-haploidentical grafts, authors modified the donor type component. A score of 0, 1, or 2 was assigned to recipients of one, two, or three human leukocyte antigen (HLA) mismatched grafts; these scores were then added to the total score of EBMT.

Recently, a composite model of EBMT and HCT-CI scores was tested in a cohort of 1,616 allogeneic HCT recipients. The predictive capacity of the composite model was better compared to either model alone (c-statistics of 0.63 for OS compared to 0.61 for the HCT-CI and 0.55 for the EBMT score; $p < 0.001$ for both) (Table 3.4 and Figure 3.9).

2 *Pretransplantation Assessment of Mortality (PAM) score*
The PAM score was developed and validated using a dataset of 2,802 patients who received their allogeneic HCT between 1990 and 2002 at Fred Hutch. The cohort was equally divided at random into a development cohort and a validation cohort. The validation cohort underwent further subdivision into an early subgroup (n = 853) for patients receiving their HCT before January 1, 1998, and a late subgroup (n = 548) for patients receiving their HCT on or after January 1, 1998. The model was designed to provide estimates of all-cause mortality in the immediate

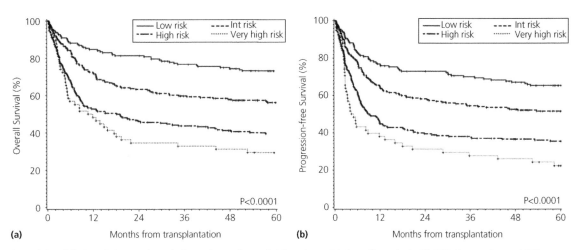

Figure 3.8 Validation of the DRI in an independent cohort of 672 patients. (a) Overall survival; (b) PFS. Source: Sorror 2012. Reproduced with permission of American Society of Hematology.

Table 3.6 Differences in diseases risk assignments between original and "Refined DRI" for patients undergoing allogeneic HCT.

Disease	Original DRI risk category	Refined DRI* risk category
HL in CR	Intermediate	Low
MCL in CR	Intermediate	Low
Advanced stage AML with favorable CG	Intermediate	High
Advanced stage high- risk MDS with Int CG	Intermediate	High
ALL in 2nd CR	Intermediate	High
ALL in 3rd CR	Intermediate	High
CML in blast phase	Intermediate	Very high
Early stage low-risk MDS with adverse CG	High	Intermediate
Advanced stage ALL	High	Very high
Advanced stage aggressive NHL	High	Very high
Advanced stage high- risk MDS with adverse CG	Very high	High
Advanced stage low- risk MDS with adverse CG	Very high	High

Potential limitations of DRI and "Refined DRI":
- Lack data on prognostic molecular markers, e.g. FLT3-ITD for AML
- They were developed utilizing data from a large cohort of patients with heterogeneous diseases and disease status combinations; this might limit their risk stratification ability within single disease studies.

* The "refined DRI" index still needs further studies to validate the modified risk assignments for various diseases.
Adapted from Armand P, et al. *Blood* **123**(23): 3664–3671, 2014.
Abbreviations: ALL, acute lymphoblastic leukemia HL; AML, acute myeloid leukemia; CG, cytogenetics; CML, chronic myeloid leukemia; CR, complete remission; Hodgkin's lymphoma; MCL, mantle cell lymphoma; MDS, myelodysplastic syndromes; NHL, non-Hodgkin lymphoma.

2-year period following allogeneic HCT. In multivariate models, eight risk factors could be identified as predictors of outcome, creating a 50-point model (Table 3.8). The index could successfully stratify outcomes into four different risk categories with risks of mortality ranging from 16 to 81% and from 8 to 82% for scores from 8 to 50 in the early and late validation cohorts, respectively.

Table 3.7 Components of EBMT risk score.

Risk factor	Score
Patient age, years	
>20	0
20–40	1
>40	2
Disease stage*	
Early	0
Intermediate	1
Late	2
Time interval from diagnosis to transplant, months⁺	
<12	0
>12	1
Donor type‡	
HLA-identical sibling	0
Unrelated, other	1
Donor recipient sex combination	
All other	0
Female donor, male recipient	1

Adopted from Gratwohl A, 1998. Reproduced with permission of Elsevier.
* Early diseases stage includes: acute leukemia (AL) transplanted in first complete remission (CR), myelodysplastic syndromes (MDS) untreated or in first CR, chronic myeloid leukemia (CML) in first chronic phase, and lymphoma and myeloma transplanted either untreated or in first CR. Intermediate disease stage includes: AL in second CR, CML at all other stages than first chronic phase or blast crisis, MDS in second CR or in partial remission (PR), lymphoma and myeloma in second CR, in PR or in stable disease. Late disease stage includes: AL in all other disease stages and lymphoma and myeloma in all disease stages other than defined as early or intermediate. No applicable stage for aplastic anemia (score 0)
⁺ Does not apply for patients transplanted in first CR (score 0)
‡ Does not apply for autologous transplantation.

The PAM score collects data on some comorbidities as well as disease-specific features. This global nature of its variables allows for estimation of both NRM and relapse. However, subsequent validation studies have been unable to confirm the prognostic power of the model. In a study of 276, patients were unevenly distributed into the four risk categories with most of patients assigned to categories 2 and 3, 16 and 66%, respectively. Authors modified cut-off values between different categories to allow for more homogenous distribution of patients (Table 3.8). In the modified model, categories 2 and 3 had 29% and 47% of patients, respectively. Overall, the c-statistic estimate was slightly higher in favor of the modified model compared to the original one (0.74 vs 0.70, respectively).

Recently, authors of the original model developed a revised version of the PAM score in a cohort of 1,549 allogeneic HCT recipients. Investigators omitted some variables, namely DLco, serum alanine amino transferase (ALT), and serum creatinine, due to loss of their associations with outcomes in multivariate models. Meanwhile, patient-donor cytomegalovirus (CMV) status was introduced as a new variable. Authors adapted DRI for disease risk stratification. The revised index has higher predictive power among recipients of high-dose conditioning rather recipients of RIC. The use of revised PAM score has been facilitated by introducing a web based calculator (www.pamscore.org).

How to evaluate a patient for fitness for HCT

Guidelines on pretransplantation data gathering

A thorough evaluation must be conducted for patients referred for HCT to identify suitable candidates as well as the most suitable transplant protocol. This evaluation consists of detailed history taking, physical exams, and laboratory and imaging studies.

1 *History taking*
   Includes:
   a History of underlying disease, disease stage at diagnosis, prior treatments received, date of the last cycle of chemotherapy, complications during previous courses of treatment, response to treatment, and the most recent staging results.
   b History of infectious complications, especially fungal infections.
   c Drug allergies with special focus on antibiotics.
   d Past medical conditions.
   e History of blood products transfusion.
   f Social and psychological status including caregiver availability, psychiatric disorders, financial situation analysis, smoking, alcohol, and illicit drug use.
2 *Physical examination*
   a KPS.
   b ECOG.
   c Dental examination.
3 *Laboratory studies*
   a ABO/Rh Blood grouping.
   b HLA typing.
   c Complete blood counts with differential counts.
   d Blood urea nitrogen/serum creatinine and creatinine clearance (CrCl).
   e Electrolytes.
   f Liver function tests (LFTs).
   g Pregnancy test for females in childbearing period.

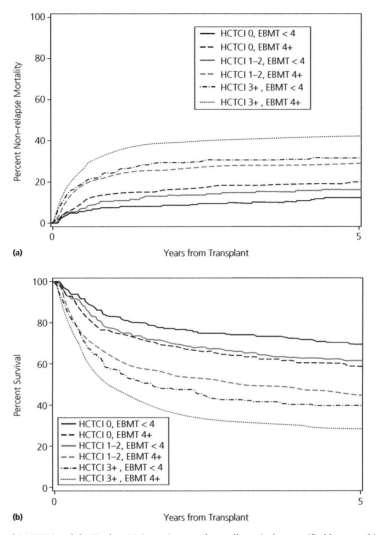

Figure 3.9 Probabilities of (a) NRM and (b) Kaplan–Meier estimates of overall survival as stratified by a combined model comprising the hematopoietic cell transplantation comorbidity index (HCT-CI) and the European Group for Blood and Marrow Transplantation (EBMT). Source: Elsawy 2014. Reproduced with permission of Elsevier.

h Lumber puncture and cerebrospinal (CSF) analysis in cases with previous CSF involvement.

i Bone marrow aspirate and biopsy for leukemia and myeloma.

j Virology screening for human immunodeficiency viruses 1 and 2, hepatitis B and C viruses, and CMV.

4 *Imaging studies*

  a Chest radiograph.

  b Echocardiography or multi-gated acquisition (MUGA) scan to measure LVEF and ECG.

  c Disease staging studies, for example, computed tomography (CT).

5 *Pulmonary function tests with corrected DLco*

Summary and practice points for eligibility for HCT

1 All patients undergoing pretransplantation assessment should have a full history taking, physical exam, and laboratory and imaging studies as discussed previously.

2 The availability of a caregiver and adequate insurance coverage must be addressed before proceeding with HCT.

3 Chronological age should not be the sole factor to determine eligibility for HCT; however, patients >65 years could be better considered for nonmyeloablative or RIC regimens.

Table 3.8 Components and categories of PAM score.

Age (years)	Score	
<20	1	
20–30	1	
30–40	1	
40–50	1	
50–60	3	
>60	5	
Donor type		
Matched related	1	
Unrelated	3	
Mismatched related	4	
Disease risk This model was developed before the DRI, hence it did not adapt DRI or Refined DRI The modified PAM score did adapt the DRI for disease risk classification (see text)		
Low	1	
Intermediate	8	
High	12	
Conditioning regimen		
Nonmyeloablative	1	
Non-TBI	4	
TBI with ≤12 Gy	8	
TBI with >12 Gy	9	
Serum creatinine level		
≤1.2 mg/dl	1	
>1.2 mg/dl	8	
Serum ALT level		
≤49 U/L	1	
>49 U/L	2	
FEV1		
>80%	1	
70%–80%	3	
<70%	6	
Corrected DL$_{CO}$		
>80%	1	
70%–80%	1	
<70%	4	
Category	Original Score	Modified score
1	9–16	8–19
2	17–23	20–25
3	24–30	26–30
4	31–44	31–50

Source: Mori 2012. Reproduced with permission of Nature Publishing group.
Abbreviations: ALT = alanine aminotransferase, DL$_{CO}$ = diffusion capacity of the lung for carbon monoxide, and FEV1 = forced expiratory volume in one second.
Low-risk diseases included: chronic myeloid leukemia (CML) in chronic phase, refractory anemia, aplastic anemia, and the Blackfan-Diamond syndrome.
Intermediate risk diseases included: CML in accelerated phase or chronic phase after blastic phase, acute leukemia or lymphoma in remission, refractory anemia with excess blasts, chronic lymphocytic leukemia, and paroxysmal nocturnal hemoglobinuria. High risk diseases included: CML in blastic phase, juvenile CML, acute leukemia or lymphoma in relapse, refractory anemia with excess blasts in transformation, myeloma, solid tumors, and non-hematologic diseases.

4 KPS of ≥70–80% or ECOG 0–1 is required for patients undergoing high-dose allogeneic HCT.

5 Patients with HCT-CI scores of ≥3 should not receive high-dose conditioning.

6 Patients older than 55 years should be assessed for limitations of IADL.

7 Recommended adequate organ functions before allogeneic HCT[6] (these parameters apply only for recipients of reduced intensity or nonmyeloablative conditioning and may vary according to individual centers' guidelines).

a LVEF of ≥35%

b DLco of >40%

c CrCl of >40 ml/min or serum Cr <2 mg/dL

d Absence of liver cirrhosis.

8 Recommended adequate organ functions before allogeneic HCT (only for recipients of high-dose conditioning and may vary according to individual centers guidelines):

a LVEF of ≥45%

b DLCO of ≥60%

c CrCl of ≥50 ml/min or serum Cr ≤1.5 mg/dL

d LFTs (total bilirubin and liver transaminases) < twice upper limit of normal. Patients with elevated LFTs that are attributable to Gilbert's syndrome or reversible drug-induced transaminitis with no other LFTs abnormalities could receive high-dose conditioning. Patients with LFTs ≥ twice upper limit of normal should receive a consult from a hepatologist to decide on their eligibility to receive high-dose conditioning.

Acknowledgments

The authors are grateful to the help by Bonnie Larson and Helen Crawford in manuscript preparation. They are also grateful for research support by grants HL088021, CA018029, HL036444, and CA078902 from the National Institutes of Health; Research Scholar Grant #RSG-13–084–01-CPHPS from the American Cancer Society, and a Patient-Centered Outcome Research Institute contract #CE-1304–7451 (for M.L.S.) and for grant JS2865 from the Egyptian Ministry of Higher Education (for M.E.).

Conflict of interest

No conflict of interest relevant to this work to be reported by either of the two authors.

Selected reading

1. Sorror ML, Storb RF, Sandmaier BM, Maziarz RT, Pulsipher MA, Maris MB, et al. Comorbidity-age index: a clinical measure of biological age before allogeneic hematopoietic cell transplantation. *J Clin Oncol* **32**(29): 3249–3256, 2014.

2. Baker KS, Davies SM, Majhail NS, Hassebroek A, Klein JP, Ballen KK, et al. Race and socioeconomic status influence outcomes of unrelated donor hematopoietic cell transplantation. *Biol Blood Marrow Transplant* **15**(12): 1543–1554, 2009.

3. Gyurkocza B, Sandmaier BM. Conditioning regimens for hematopoietic cell transplantation: one size does not fit all. *Blood* **124**(3): 344–353, 2014.

4. Sorror ML, Maris MB, Storb R, Baron F, Sandmaier BM, Maloney DG, et al. Hematopoietic cell transplantation (HCT)-specific comorbidity index: a new tool for risk assessment before allogeneic HCT. *Blood* **106**(8): 2912–2919, 2005.

5. Elsawy M, Storer BE, Pulsipher MA, Maziarz RT, Bhatia S, Maris MB, et al. Multi-centre validation of the prognostic value of the haematopoietic cell transplantation-specific comorbidity index among recipients of allogeneic haematopoietic cell transplantation. *Br J Haematol* **170**(4): 574–583, 2015.

6. Sorror ML, Sandmaier BM, Storer BE, Maris MB, Baron F, Maloney DG, et al. Comorbidity and disease status-based risk stratification of outcomes among patients with acute myeloid leukemia or myelodysplasia receiving allogeneic hematopoietic cell transplantation. *J Clin Oncol* **25**(27):4246–4254, 2007.

7. Sorror ML, Storer BE, Sandmaier BM, Maris M, Shizuru J, Maziarz R, et al. Five-year follow-up of patients with advanced chronic lymphocytic leukemia treated with allogeneic hematopoietic cell transplantation after nonmyeloablative conditioning. *J Clin Oncol* **26**(30): 4912–4920, 2008.

8. Pavlu J, Kew AK, Taylor-Roberts B, Auner HW, Marin D, Olavarria E, et al. Optimizing patient selection for myeloablative allogeneic hematopoietic cell transplantation in chronic myeloid leukemia in chronic phase. *Blood* **115**(20): 4018–4020, 2010.

9. Sorror ML, Martin PJ, Storb R, Bhatia S, Maziarz RT, Pulsipher MA, et al. Pretransplant comorbidities predict severity of acute graft-versus-host disease and subsequent mortality. *Blood* **124**(2): 287–295, 2014.

10. Sorror M. How I assess comorbidities prior to hematopoietic cell transplantation. *Blood* **121**(15): 2854–2863, 2013.

11. Sorror M, Storer B, Sandmaier BM, Maloney DG, Chauncey TR, Langston A, et al. Hematopoietic cell transplantation-comorbidity index and Karnofsky performance status are independent predictors of morbidity and mortality after allogeneic nonmyeloablative hematopoietic cell transplantation. *Cancer* **112**: 1992–2001, 2008.

12. Muffly LS, Kocherginsky M, Stock W, Chu Q, Bishop MR, Godley LA, et al. Geriatric assessment to predict survival in older allogeneic hematopoietic cell transplantation recipients. *Haematologica* **99**(8): 1373–1379, 2014.

13. Armand P, Gibson CJ, Cutler C, Ho VT, Koreth J, Alyea EP, et al. A disease risk index for patients undergoing allogeneic stem cell transplantation. *Blood* **120**(4): 905–9013, 2012.

14. Armand P, Kim HT, Logan BR, Wang Z, Alyea EP, Kalaycio ME, et al. Validation and refinement of the Disease Risk Index for allogeneic stem cell transplantation. *Blood* **123**(23): 3664–3671, 2014.

15. Au BK, Gooley TA, Armand P, Fang M, Madtes DK, Sorror ML, et al. Reevaluation of the pretransplant assessment of mortality score after allogeneic hematopoietic transplantation. Biol Blood Marrow Transplant: [Epub ahead of print 2015 Jan 30-doi: 10.1016/j.bbmt.2015.01.011], 2015.

CHAPTER 4

Donor and recipient pre-transplant evaluation

Shuang Fu[1] and Navneet S. Majhail[1,2]

[1] Blood & Marrow Transplant Program, Cleveland Clinic, Cleveland, OH, USA
[2] Cleveland Clinic Lerner College of Medicine, Cleveland Clinic, Cleveland, OH, USA

Introduction

Appropriate donor and recipient selection is a critical component of the transplantation procedure. Hence, donors require evaluations to ensure the safety of the donation process, and the integrity and quality of the collected HPC product (donor suitability), and to assess and minimize risk of transmission of infectious agents (donor eligibility). They can also assist with the selection of the best donor when several donor options are available. At the same time, recipients require evaluations to ascertain that they can undergo the transplantation process with an acceptable risk of morbidity and mortality and a reasonable probability of success. Finally, they are also required for regulatory purposes (e.g., by the Food and Drug Administration [FDA]) to facilitate collection and infusion of a high quality HPC product. The type of evaluations for regulatory purposes differ based on the type of transplant (autologous vs allogeneic) and the donor/graft source (related vs unrelated vs umbilical cord blood [UCB] and bone marrow vs peripheral blood hematopoietic cells [PBHC]).

Based on infectious and non-infectious evaluations, a donor may be:

1 Completely deferred and not allowed to donate as the risk of the donation process is not acceptable or there is a high probability of an adverse event in the recipient (e.g., transmission of a life-threatening infection),
2 Temporarily deferred to allow for treatment and resolution of an underlying medical condition or to allow for additional work-up to determine their suitability and eligibility, or
3 Found to be a suitable donor.
   A suitable donor may be:

1 Eligible if there are no risk factors for transmission of relevant communicable disease agents and diseases,
2 Ineligible if risk factors for infectious disease transmission are present, or
3 Determined to have incomplete eligibility if risk factors cannot be completely assessed (e.g., international donors where some infectious disease testing mandated by the US FDA is not routinely performed).

The decision to use a donor who is suitable but ineligible or with incomplete eligibility depends on the availability of other donor options and the risks to the recipient associated with possible transmission of an infectious disease.

Donor infectious evaluation

HPC products may transmit bacterial, viral, parasitic, and prion diseases, including human immunodeficiency virus (HIV), human T-cell lymphotropic virus (HTLV-I and HTLV-II), hepatitis B virus (HBV), hepatitis C virus (HCV), cytomegalovirus (CMV), West Nile virus (WNV), syphilis, and Chagas disease. Donor eligibility assessment evaluates the risk of transmitting infectious disease to the recipient (Table 4.1). Donor infectious evaluation includes:

History
- Presence of active infection
- Prior infectious disease history
- Recent infectious disease exposure
- Medical history: transfusions, hepatitis, toxoplasmosis, tuberculosis
- Social history: sexual activity, illicit drug use, tattoos, body piercing, immunizations, travel
- Vaccination history.

Table 4.1 Hematopoietic Progenitor Cell Donor History Questionnaire (DHQ-HPC).

Donor History Questionnaire-HPC, Apheresis and HPC, Marrow	Yes	No
Are you		
1. Currently taking an antibiotic?		
2. Currently taking any other medication for an infection?		
Please read the Medication Deferral List.		
3. Are you now taking or have you ever taken any medications on the Medication List?		
4. Have you read the educational materials?		
In the past **12 weeks** have you		
5. Had any vaccinations or other shots?		
6. Had contact with someone who had a smallpox vaccination?		
In the past **12 months** have you		
7. Been told by a healthcare professional that you have West Nile Virus infection or any positive test for West Nile Virus?		
8. Had a blood transfusion?		
9. Come into contact with someone else's blood?		
10. Had an accidental needle-stick?		
11. Had a transplant or graft from someone other than yourself, such as organ, bone marrow, stem cell, cornea, sclera, bone, skin or other tissue?		
12. Had sexual contact with anyone who has HIV/AIDS or has had a positive test for the HIV/AIDS virus?		
13. Had sexual contact with a prostitute or anyone else who takes money or drugs or other payment for sex?		
14. Had sexual contact with anyone who has ever used needles to take drugs or steroids, or anything not prescribed by their doctor?		
15. Had sexual contact with anyone who has hemophilia or has used clotting factor concentrates?		
16. Female donors: Had sexual contact with a male who has ever had sexual contact with another male? (Males: check "I am male.")	I am male ☐	
17. Had sexual contact with a person who has hepatitis?		
18. Lived with a person who has hepatitis?		
19. Had a tattoo?		
20. Had ear or body piercing?		
21. Had or been treated for syphilis or other sexually transmitted infections?		
22. Been in juvenile detention, lockup, jail, or prison for more than 72 hours?		
In the past **3 years** have you		
23. Been outside the United States or Canada?		
In the past **5 years**, have you		
24. Received money, drugs, or other payment for sex?		
25. Male donors: Had sexual contact with another male, even once? (Females: check "I am female.")	I am female ☐	
26. Used needles to take drugs, steroids, or anything not prescribed by your doctor?		
27. Used clotting factor concentrates?		

(Continued)

Table 4.1 (Continued)

Donor History Questionnaire-HPC, Apheresis and HPC, Marrow	Yes	No
From **1980 through 1996,**		
28. Did you spend time that adds up to three (3) months or more in the United Kingdom? (Review list of countries in the UK)		
29. Were you a member of the U.S. military, a civilian military employee, or a dependent of either a member of the U.S. military or civilian military employee?		
From **1980 to the present**, did you		
30. Spend time that adds up to five (5) years or more in Europe? (Review list of countries in Europe.)		
31. Receive a transfusion of blood or blood components in the United Kingdom or France? (Review list of countries in the UK.)		
Have you **EVER**		
32. Had a positive test for the HIV/AIDS virus?		
33. Had hepatitis or any positive test for hepatitis?		
34. Had malaria?		
35. Had Chagas disease and/or a positive test for *T. cruzi*?		
36. Had babesiosis?		
37. Tested positive for HTLV, had adult T-cell leukemia, or had unexplained paraparesis (partial paralysis affecting the lower limbs)?		
38. Received a dura mater (or brain covering) graft?		
39. Had sexual contact with anyone who was born in or lived in Africa?		
40. Been in Africa?		
41. Been diagnosed with any neurological disease?		
42. Had a transplant or other medical procedure that involved being exposed to live cells, tissues, or organs from an animal?		
43. Has your sexual partner or a member of your household ever had a transplant or other medical procedure that involved being exposed to live cells, tissues, or organs from an animal?		
44. Have any of your relatives had Creutzfeldt–Jakob disease?		

Source: Courtesy of The Foundation for the Accreditation of Cellular Therapy and Advancing Transfusion and Cellular Therapies Worldwide.

The Donor History Questionnaire (DHQ) developed by the AABB task force can be used as a checklist (Table 4.1).

Physical examination
- Skin: rash, ulcer, needle track, tattoo, body piercing, jaundice
- HEENT: icterus, oral thrush
- Lymphadenopathy, hepatomegaly
- Genital lesions.

Laboratory testing
- For lymphocyte and UCB donations, a specimen for testing must be obtained within 7 days before or after the donation. For PBHC and bone marrow donations, the specimen may be obtained up to 30 days before donation.
- Standard panel of infectious disease markers, including screening tests for HIV, HTLV, HBV, HCV, CMV, Epstein–Barr virus (EBV), varicella zoster virus (VZV), WNV, syphilis, and *Toxoplasma gondii*. Donors with a positive test may require additional confirmatory testing to determine whether the donor has a true infection or a false positive screening test.
- Donors who have resided in or traveled to endemic areas, need testing for endemic pathogens: *Strongyloides stercoralis*, *Trypanosoma cruzi*, and malaria.

Management

- Donors with HIV should be deferred.
- Donors with some active infections may be treated prior to donation (e.g., acute hepatitis A, acute CMV infection, acute EBV infection and acute toxoplasmosis).
- Donors who reside in or have traveled to endemic areas and who are suspected of having an acute infection should be temporarily deferred until infection with these pathogens is excluded (e.g., malaria, acute tick-borne infection such as Rocky Mountain spotted fever, Colorado tick fever, and acute ehrlichiosis).
- Donors with a past history of Q fever, babesiosis, Chagas disease should be deferred, because these parasites can persist despite therapy.
- Donors with antibodies to hepatitis B or C are eligible to donate. If PCR testing demonstrates hepatitis B or C viremia, viremic donors are not eligible to donate for unrelated recipients. However, viremic donors may be acceptable for related recipients, depending on the serology of the recipient and the ability of the donor and the recipient to receive antiviral therapy (see later for the rationale).
- Donors with latent TB are eligible to donate. Donors with signs or symptoms of active TB should be tested and treated prior to donating cells.

Special consideration for potentially unsafe products

- The use of unrelated donor who is at risk for or who has an infectious disease transmissible by HCT is generally precluded.
- The use of related donor who is at risk for or who has an infectious disease transmissible by HCT is determined by the HCT physician, especially when the donor at risk is the only possible donor and the patient is likely to succumb rapidly from the disease if an HCT is not received.
- If the physician weighs the risks and benefits of using potentially unsafe product and decides to proceed, the recipient must be informed of the potential risks.

Donor non-infectious evaluation

We also need to ensure that the HPC harvest/collection is safe for the donor and the donor is willing and able to donate. Donor medical suitability evaluates donor's health condition, and prevents the potential adverse events to the donor associated with HPC donation. Donor non-infectious evaluation includes:

History

For bone marrow donors, pay special attention to:
- Prior surgical history
- Any problems or contraindications for anesthesia, for example, severe cardiovascular disease, severe respiratory disease, neurological disorders (in particular, epilepsy)
- Neck, back or leg pain (patient cannot lie flat and be safely positioned during harvest).

For PBHC donors, pay special attention to:
- Prior blood donation history.
- Donors with the following conditions can increase the risk of reactions or serious complications with G-CSF administration (decision to donate to be made on a case by case basis):
  - Autoimmune diseases, which can be exacerbated by filgrastim administration
  - Inflammatory or immunological disorders
  - Thrombotic disorders or possible predisposition conditions
  - Sickle cell disease or trait, with increased risk for splenic rupture
  - Splenic disorders, with increased risk for splenic rupture
  - Liver disease
  - Previous history of cancers treated with chemo-radio-therapy, with increased risk for treatment-related MDS or leukemia.

Physical examination

For bone marrow donors, special attention to:
- Oral airway
- Spine
- Posterior iliac crests

For PBHC donors, special attention to:
- Venous access
- Splenomegaly

Laboratory testing

- General labs, including complete blood count with white cell differential, chemistry with liver and renal function and electrolytes, urine analysis
- Hemoglobin electrophoresis for screening for sickle cell trait or thalassemia, if donor is suspected to be a carrier
- ABO and Rh typing

Instrumental investigations

- Chest X-ray
- Electrocardiogram

Special consideration for female donors of child-bearing age group

- Serological pregnancy test is required for female donors less than 55 years, unless the donor is postmenopausal or is surgically infertile
- Pregnant donors cannot donate PBHC, because the safety of filgrastim administration on the fetus has not been determined

- Pregnant donors may donate bone marrow in the second or third trimester. However, they are not preferred and may only be considered in the setting of related recipients who need an urgent transplant and do not have any other donor options
- Pregnant donors are deferred from donating to unrelated recipients until after delivery

Recipient infectious evaluation

Infection is a common cause of morbidity and non-relapse mortality after HCT. Patients are at risk of developing bacterial, fungal, viral and/or parasitic infections. Therefore, it is important to prevent infections, including careful pre-transplant recipient evaluation, careful donor selection, and use of prophylactic and preemptive antimicrobial therapy.

History
- Presence of active infection and prior infectious disease history and exposures
- Medical history: transfusions, hepatitis, toxoplasmosis, tuberculosis, dental procedures
- Social history: sexual activity, illicit drug use, tattoos, body piercing, travel
- Vaccination history
- Prosthetic biomaterials

Physical examination
- Complete physical examination
- Dental evaluation

Laboratory testing
- Standard panel of infectious disease markers: HIV, HTLV-I/II, HBV, HCV, CMV, EBV, VZV, WNV, syphilis, *Toxoplasma gondii*
- TB screening using tuberculin skin test or interferon-gamma release assays is recommended for HCT candidates with risk factors for TB
- Appropriate HCT candidates with upper respiratory tract infection should be tested for Influenza, Respiratory Syncytial Virus (RSV), and Parainfluenza Virus
- Recipients who have resided in or traveled to endemic areas, may need testing for endemic pathogens, especially if they have appropriate signs and symptoms: *Strongyloides stercoralis*, *Trypanosoma cruzi*, malaria, *Coccidioides immitis*, and *Histoplasma capsulatum*
- Additional infectious disease work-up if clinically indicated in patients with risk factors and exposures: HSV serology, *Staphylococcus aureus* nasal culture, Vancomycin-resistant Enterococcus rectal culture

Management
- HIV: For HIV patients on HAART therapy with excellent disease control, HCT may be considered
- Hepatitis A: Acute hepatitis A is associated with increased risk of sinusoidal obstruction syndrome (SOS) following myeloablative conditioning regimens; HCT should be postponed for patients who are positive for hepatitis A virus IgM
- Hepatitis B:
  ○ Hepatitis B vaccine is recommended for HBV-seronegative HCT candidates prior to transplantation.
  ○ In general, HBV-seronegative HCT candidates should not receive transplant from HBV-positive donors, if another equally suitable donor is available; if no other donor is available or there is an urgent need to proceed with transplant, HBV-seronegative patients receiving a transplant from HBV-positive donors should be vaccinated against hepatitis B pre-transplant; hepatitis B immune globulin can be considered in recipients with low post-vaccination anti-HBs titers.
  ○ For HCT recipients who are anti-HBc and anti-HBs positive, prophylactic antiviral treatment with lamivudine may be considered in consultation with a hepatologist or infectious disease physician.
  ○ For HCT candidates with evidence of active HBV replication (HBsAg positive and/or HBV DNA positive), liver biopsy should be performed prior to HCT, and antiviral therapy with lamivudine should be initiated prior to conditioning. If HCT is not urgent, antiviral treatment should be administered for 3–6 months prior to conditioning.
- Hepatitis C:
  ○ HCT candidates with HCV infection should be assessed for evidence of chronic liver disease, especially for patients with iron overload, excessive alcohol intake, hepatitis C for >10 years and clinical evidence of chronic liver disease.
  ○ Patients with evidence of cirrhosis or hepatic fibrosis have significant increased risk of fatal SOS after conventional myeloablative conditioning therapy. If a transplant is indicated, conditioning regimens that do not contain cyclophosphamide or total body irradiation should be considered.
  ○ If transplant can be delayed, patients should receive treatment for chronic HCV infection in consultation with a hepatologist or infectious disease physician.
- CMV:
  ○ For CMV-seronegative allogeneic HCT recipients, blood products from CMV-seronegative donors or leukocyte-depleted blood products should be used to reduce the risk of CMV transmission.
  ○ For CMV-seropositive allogeneic HCT recipients and CMV-seronegative recipients with a CMV-seropositive donor, the risk of developing post-transplant CMV

disease is high, and these recipients should receive CMV prophylaxis from engraftment to at least 100 days after allo-HCT. Alternatively, these patients should be closely monitored and treated preemptively at the earliest sign of CMV reactivation.
o For patients with active CMV viremia, the risk of developing CMV disease is particularly high. These recipients should receive CMV directed antiviral treatment (ganciclovir, valganciclovir, or foscarnet), and the transplantation should be delayed until the CMV infection is controlled.
• EBV:
o For recipients with profound T-cell cytopenia (e.g., T-cell-depletion, anti-T-cell antibodies, UCB transplants, HLA-haploidentical transplants), the risk of developing post-transplant lymphoproliferative disorder (PTLD) is high.
o EBV prophylaxis using antiviral agents is not recommended because of lack of efficacy.
o EBV DNA can be monitored post-transplant in high-risk patients and in case of EBV reactivation or increase in DNA load, preemptive reduction in immunosuppression or treatment with rituximab can be considered.
• HSV:
o For HSV-seronegative HCT recipients, acyclovir prophylaxis is not indicated, even if the donor is HSV seropositive.
o For HSV-seropositive HCT recipients, acyclovir prophylaxis is recommended during the early post-transplant period (from conditioning to day 30 after HCT), to prevent HSV reactivation.
• VZV:
o For VZV-seronegative HCT recipients, passive immunization with varicella-zoster immunoglobulin is recommended after exposure to chickenpox or herpes zoster; acyclovir or valacyclovir may be used if VZIG is not available.
o For VZV-seropositive HCT recipients, long-term acyclovir prophylaxis is recommended for the first year after HCT to prevent VZV reactivation, and may be continued beyond 1 year for patients with chronic GvHD or on systemic immunosuppression therapy.
• TB:
o Isoniazid (INH) prophylaxis should be administered to HCT recipients who have recent exposure, or positive tuberculin skin tests, or positive interferon-gamma release assays.
o INH prophylaxis may be considered for recipients who live in an area with a high prevalence of TB.
• Community respiratory viruses:
o Upper respiratory tract infection with influenza or parainfluenza viruses or RSV may progress to lower respiratory tract infection in immune-compromised patients.

o If a patient has confirmed infection with these viruses, the transplant should be postponed until symptoms resolve.
o Zanamivir or oseltamivir can be prescribed to patients with confirmed influenza infection within 48 hours after symptom onset.
• Fungal infection:
o Patients with candidemia or invasive candidiasis (e.g., hepatosplenic candidiasis) need to be treated aggressively with anti-Candida therapy prior to transplantation.
o Patients with a history of invasive fungal infection, especially *Aspergillus* spp. infection, are at high-risk for recurrence following HCT. Mold specific antifungal prophylaxis is recommended (e.g., with voriconazole or posaconazole).

Recipient non-infectious evaluation

Type and status of the underlying disease and recipient's organ function and comorbidities are the major factors that determine whether the transplant is indicated and if the recipient can tolerate the procedure. Therefore, HCT recipients require comprehensive pre-transplant evaluations, including assessment of disease status, functional status and comorbidities, and to identify and address any psychosocial, financial and caregiver issues.

Assessment of disease type and status
Disease specific staging studies are tailored to underlying disease, and may include:
• Complete blood count
• Bone marrow aspiration and biopsy
• Imaging studies (e.g., CT scan, MRI scan, PET scan)
• Cerebrospinal fluid evaluation
• Additional investigations (e.g., cytogenetic and molecular studies).
    A Disease Risk Index (DRI) has been developed to assess the prognostic significance of disease status at transplantation (Table 4.2). Patients are stratified into four risk groups: low, intermediate, high and very high, with estimated 2-year overall survival (OS) ranging from 66 to 23%.

Assessment of functional status and comorbidities
The outcome of HCT is significantly impacted by recipient health condition and comorbidities. Recipients need a comprehensive pre-transplant evaluation, including detailed history, physical examination, routine blood work and infectious disease work-up, CXR, EKG, echocardiogram, or MUGA, and pulmonary function test (including DLCO). Based on age and these evaluations, a decision is also made

Table 4.2 DRI for assessing prognosis of patients prior to transplantation.

Disease	Stage	DRI Group	2-Year OS (%)
Hodgkin lymphoma CR		Low	66
CLL CR		Low	
Mantle cell lymphoma CR		Low	
Indolent NHL CR		Low	
AML favorable cytogenetics CR		Low	
Indolent NHL PR		Low	
CLL PR		Low	
CML chronic phase 1/2		Low	
CML advanced phase		Intermediate	51
Mantle cell lymphoma PR		Intermediate	
Myeloproliferative neoplasm	Any	Intermediate	
AML intermediate cytogenetics CR		Intermediate	
ALL CR1		Intermediate	
T-cell NHL CR		Intermediate	
Multiple myeloma CR/VGPR/PR		Intermediate	
Aggressive NHL CR		Intermediate	
Low-risk MDS adverse cytogenetics	Early	Intermediate	
T-cell NHL PR		Intermediate	
Low-risk MDS intermediate cytogenetics	Early	Intermediate	
Hodgkin lymphoma PR		Intermediate	
Low-risk MDS intermediate cytogenetics	Advanced[†]	Intermediate	
Indolent NHL	Advanced[†]	Intermediate	
CLL	Advanced	Intermediate	
High-risk MDS intermediate cytogenetics	Early	Intermediate	
Aggressive NHL PR		Intermediate	
T-cell NHL	Advanced[†]	High	33
AML favorable cytogenetics	Advanced[†]	High	
Hodgkin lymphoma	Advanced[†]	High	
High-risk MDS intermediate cytogenetics	Advanced[†]	High	
High-risk MDS adverse cytogenetics	Early	High	
ALL CR2		High	
AML adverse cytogenetics CR		High	
Mantle cell lymphoma	Advanced[†]	High	
High-risk MDS adverse cytogenetics	Advanced[†]	High	
Burkitt's lymphoma CR		High	
Multiple myeloma	Advanced[†]	High	
ALL CR3		High	
Low-risk MDS adverse cytogenetics	Advanced[†]	High	
AML intermediate cytogenetics	Advanced	High	

Table 4.2 (Continued)

Disease	Stage	DRI Group	2-Year OS (%)
CML blast phase		Very high	23
ALL	Advanced[†]	Very high	
Aggressive NHL	Advanced[†]	Very high	
AML adverse cytogenetics	Advanced[†]	Very high	
Burkitt's lymphoma PR	Advanced[†]	Very high	

Source: Adapted from Armand P, Kim HT, Logan BR, et al. *Blood.* 2014;**123**(23):3664–3671.
CR – complete remission; CLL – chronic lymphocytic leukemia; NHL – non-Hodgkin lymphoma; PR – partial remission; CML – chronic myeloid leukemia; AML – acute myeloid leukemia; ALL – acute lymphoblastic leukemia; VGPR – very good partial remission; MDS – myelodysplastic syndromes
[†] Advanced stage refers to induction failure or active relapse, including stable or progressive disease for non-Hodgkin lymphoma, Hodgkin lymphoma, and chronic lymphocytic leukemia

Table 4.3 Composite risk score of HCT specific comorbidities and age.

Comorbidity	Definitions of Comorbidities	HCT-CI Score
Age	Age ≥ 40 years	1
Arrhythmia	Atrial fibrillation or flutter, sick sinus syndrome, or ventricular arrhythmias	1
Cardiac	Coronary artery disease, congestive heart failure, myocardial infarction, or ejection fraction ≤ 50%	1
Inflammatory bowel disease	Crohn's disease or ulcerative colitis	1
Diabetes	Requiring treatment with insulin or oral hypoglycemics but not diet alone	1
Cerebrovascular disease	Transient ischemic attack or cerebrovascular accident	1
Psychiatric disturbance	Depression or anxiety requiring psychiatric consult or treatment	1
Hepatic, mild	Chronic hepatitis, bilirubin > ULN to 1.5 × ULN, or AST/ALT > ULN to 2.5 × ULN	1
Obesity	Patients with a body mass index > 35 kg/m^2	1
Infection	Requiring continuation of antimicrobial treatment after day 0	1
Rheumatologic	SLE, rheumatoid arthritis, polymyositis, mixed connective tissue disorder, or polymyalgia rheumatica	2
Peptic ulcer	Requiring treatment	2
Moderate/severe renal	Serum creatinine > 2 mg/dL, on dialysis, or prior renal transplantation	2
Moderate pulmonary	DLCO and/or FEV$_1$ 66–80% or dyspnea on slight activity	2
Prior solid tumor	Treated at any time point in the patient's past history, excluding non-melanoma skin cancer	3
Heart valve disease	Except mitral valve prolapse	3
Severe pulmonary	DLCO and/or FEV$_1$ ≤ 65% or dyspnea at rest or requiring oxygen	3
Moderate/severe hepatic	Liver cirrhosis, bilirubin > 1.5 × ULN, or AST/ALT > 2.5 × ULN	3
HCT-CI/Age Composite Score	**Regimen Intensity**	**2-Year OS (%)**
0	Myeloablative	79
	Reduced intensity	87
	Non-myeloablative	81

(Continued)

Table 4.3 (Continued)

HCT-CI/Age Composite Score	Regimen Intensity	2-Year OS (%)
1-2	Myeloablative	66
	Reduced intensity	66
	Non-myeloablative	67
3-4	Myeloablative	45
	Reduced intensity	47
	Non-myeloablative	54
≥5	Myeloablative	29
	Reduced intensity	34
	Non-myeloablative	35

Source: Adapted from Sorror ML, Storb RF, Sandmaier BM, et al. *J Clin Oncol.* 2014;**32**(29):3249–3256.

regarding the intensity of conditioning regimen to be pursued.

A number of scoring systems have been developed to estimate the mortality risk related to comorbidities in HCT recipients. The Hematopoietic Cell Transplantation-specific Comorbidity Index (HCT-CI) is most commonly used (Table 4.3). It weighs 17 possible comorbidities for a score ranging from 0 to 29. An age-specific HCT-CI score has also been developed (also see chapter 3).

Assessment of psychosocial, financial, and caregiver issues

HCT is a complex procedure that can have a major psychological impact on patients and their caregivers and requires patient compliance and care coordination. Pre-transplant assessments usually include an evaluation by a social worker or psychosocial clinicians to identify and address any psychological issues, determine a robust caregiving plan and to assist with any financial needs post-transplantation.

SUMMARY

HCT is a life-saving but potentially high-risk procedure. Both recipients and the donors need work-up before transplantation to determine the benefit versus risk of this procedure for individual patients and to assist with medical decision making.

Selected reading

1. Tomblyn M, Chiller T, Einsele H, et al. Guidelines for preventing infectious complications among hematopoietic cell transplantation recipients: a global perspective. *Biol Blood Marrow Transplant.* 2009;**15**(10):1143–1238.
2. Armand P, Kim HT, Logan BR, et al. Validation and refinement of the disease risk index for allogeneic stem cell transplantation. *Blood.* 2014;**123**(23):3664–3671.
3. Sorror ML, Maris MB, Storb RF, et al. Hematopoietic cell transplantation (HCT) – specific comorbidity index: a new tool for risk assessment before allogeneic HCT. *Blood.* 2005; **106**(8):2912–2919.
4. Sorror ML, Storb RF, Sandmaier BM, et al. Comorbidity-age index: A clinical measure of biologic age before allogeneic hematopoietic cell transplantation. *J Clin Oncol.* 2014; **32**(29):3249–3256.

CHAPTER 5

Autologous and allogeneic progenitor cell mobilization

Racquel D. Innis-Shelton and Luciano J. Costa

Division of Hematology and Oncology, Department of Medicine, University of Alabama at Birmingham, Birmingham, AL, USA

Introduction

Since the 1990s, the use of mobilized peripheral blood hematopoietic progenitor cells (PB-HPCs; CD34$^+$ cells are referred to as HPCs) to support hematopoietic recovery after high dose chemotherapy (HDT) has revolutionized transplantation for a variety of hematologic malignancies (see Chapters 6 and 7). PB-HPCs have, for the most part, replaced marrow graft source in the majority of the 10,000 autologous hematopoietic cell transplants (auto-HCT) performed yearly in the United States. PB-HPC have become the preferred graft source for approximately 65% of allogeneic hematopoietic cell transplants (allo-HCT).

There are several options on how to mobilize HPCs from the bone marrow to the peripheral blood for successful apheresis. Autologous and allogeneic hematopoietic cell mobilization have different challenges and priorities:

Autologous CD34$^+$ cell mobilization and collection:

1 How to avoid mobilization failures?
2 How to obtain the desired number of HPC in fewer apheresis sessions?
3 Can we spare cost and toxicity without compromising on the number of HPCs collected?

Allogeneic donor CD34$^+$ cell mobilization and collection:

1 How to optimize safety of volunteer donors?
2 Can we mobilize and collect products that would improve anti-malignancy effect and/or reduce the risk of graft-*versus*-host disease in the recipient?

Autologous mobilization
Who needs chemotherapy to mobilize CD34$^+$ cells?

Historically, there have been two basic modalities to mobilize HPC in autologous donors: growth factor (GF) alone or chemotherapy followed by growth factor (C + GF).

The administration of filgrastim (or GM-CSF) will cause expansion of the granulocytic population in the bone marrow and the release of proteases in the marrow environment that will disrupt several "anchors" keeping HPC (identified by the antigenic expression of CD34$^+$) within the marrow compartment, including the binding of CXCR4 in the HPC to SDF1 in the marrow stroma. Typically, after 4 days of GF administration there is substantial increase in the number of circulating CD34$^+$ and leukapheresis optimized for collection of mononuclear cells (MNC) will yield a product rich in CD34$^+$ cells (see Chapters 3, 6, and 7). GF administration and daily leukapheresis can continue until the desired number of CD34$^+$ cells are obtained, but typically (for practical reasons) not for longer than 4 days.

Chemotherapy agents at specific doses will cause significant bone marrow suppression. It has long been recognized that during the recovery from marrow suppression, there is a substantial increase in the number of circulating CD34$^+$ cells, an effect that can be magnified by the administration of GFs. This approach will lead to a sharp increase in circulating CD34$^+$ cells, typically 9–11 days from the administration of chemotherapy, an ideal time to proceed with leukapheresis. This strategy is

Clinical Manual of Blood and Bone Marrow Transplantation, First Edition. Edited by Syed A. Abutalib and Parameswaran Hari.
© 2017 John Wiley & Sons Ltd. Published 2017 by John Wiley & Sons Ltd.

not infrequent for autologous CD34+ cell collection especially in patients who are already on chemotherapy cycles, that is, lymphoma patients, and collection of HPC can occur on the "rebound" of the last intended chemotherapy cycle. Many centers opt for the administration of chemotherapy (typically cyclophosphamide or etoposide) with the exclusive intent to mobilize HPC, this strategy is falling out of favor.

There are no large randomized trials comparing GF with C+GF. However, there are several recognized advantages and disadvantages of each approach (Table 5.1). Importantly, even though more CD34+ cells are often obtained with C+GF, there is no definitive evidence that the rate of mobilization failure is different between the two methods.

How many CD34+ cells are needed for optimal hematopoietic engraftment?

The number of CD34+ cells/weight of intended recipient has been traditionally used to characterize cellular products intended to restore hematopoiesis. Table 5.2 summarizes the consensus recommendations and implications of different CD34+ cell doses.

It is common, particularly for patients with plasma cell dyscrasias, to collect enough cells to support two auto-HCT. Such intention evidently needs to be taken in account when planning the number of CD34+ cells to be collected.

Is there a better growth factor or better chemotherapy for CD34+ cell mobilization?

Three different growth factors, filgrastim (G-CSF), sargramostim (GM-CSF), and pegfilgrastim have been used to mobilized HPC, either alone or in combination with chemotherapy. Their doses and characteristics are displayed in Table 5.3.

The type of GF to be used will often depend on institution formulary, experience, and price. There is very little data supporting combinations of different GFs.

> **PRACTICE POINTS**
>
> Often times, C+GF is employed when the patient is already receiving chemotherapy for treatment of underlying disease. Regimens such as ICE, DHAP, ESHAP, DT-PACE, mini-BEAM, are routinely used as platforms for HPC mobilization.

Some centers will administer chemotherapy for HPC mobilization. The agent most routinely used is cyclophosphamide in doses of 1.5–7 g/m². The optimal dose of cyclophosphamide is unknown but higher doses are associated with more toxicity without any obvious gain in mobilization so doses higher than 4 g/m² are discouraged. There is also robust literature supporting the use of etoposide in doses of 750–2000 mg/m², but there are no prospective studies showing superiority of one mobilizing chemotherapy agent over another.

Table 5.4 displays some of the published experience with different CD34+ cell mobilization strategies.

When to use plerixafor

Plerixafor is a reversible partial antagonist of CXCR4 that competes with SDF-1 disrupting its interaction with CXCR4 in CD34+ cells (HPC). Unattached HPC are then released to enter the PB stream. In patients receiving GF for HPC mobilization, the subcutaneous administration of plerixafor leads to a sharp, 3–5-fold increase in circulating CD34+ cells that peaks at approximately 10 h allowing for a more effective collection.

The demonstration of superiority of growth factor + plerixafor (GF+P) over GF came from two randomized trials performed in multiple myeloma (MM) and non-Hodgkin lymphoma (NHL) patients. In the MM trial, 302 patients were randomized to receive

Table 5.1 Advantages and disadvantages of GF and C+GF mobilization and collection of CD34+ cells.

	Advantages	Disadvantages
Growth factor mobilization	• Shorter time from start of mobilization to transplant • Fewer days of GF administration • Onset of collection is more predictable	• No anti-tumor activity (hypothetical loss) • Fewer CD34+ collected than with C+GF
Chemotherapy + growth factor mobilization	• More CD34+ cells collected than with GF alone • Hypothetical gain in disease control	• Longer stay of intravascular catheter • Higher risk of infection • Neutropenia • Thrombocytopenia • Higher risk of complications requiring hospitalization • Higher cost

Table 5.2 Clinical consequences and recommendations for different CD34$^+$ cell doses.

Cell Dose	Implications	Recommendation
<1.5 × 10^6 CD34$^+$/kg	Delayed neutrophil and platelet recovery, increased transfusion requirement, higher risk of engraftment failure	Contraindicated especially in myeloablative setting
1.5–3.0 × 10^6 CD34$^+$/kg	Delay in platelet recovery	Discouraged but not contraindication
3.0–5.0 × 10^6 CD34$^+$/kg	Adequate neutrophil and platelet recovery	Adequate cell dose (comfort zone)
>5.0 × 10^6 CD34$^+$/kg	Possible minimal gain in earlier platelet and neutrophil engraftment. Possible improvement in long term platelet recovery, fewer transfusions	Uncertain benefit

Table 5.3 Growth factors utilized for mobilization of CD34$^+$ cells for transplantation.

Growth Factor	Dose	Comments
Filgrastim	Alone: 10–16 µg/kg/day After chemotherapy: 5–10 µg/kg/day	Most established GF. Superior to sargramostim when used after chemotherapy mobilization. Cost can be high in heavier patients and/or patients requiring many days of collection.
Sargramostim	8 µg/kg/day or 250 µg/m^2/day	Inferior to filgrastim when used after chemotherapy mobilization. Limited data on use without chemotherapy. Likely more side effects than filgrastim.
Pegfilgrastim	Alone: 6–12 mg single dose After chemotherapy: 6 mg single dose	No proper prospective comparison with filgrastim. Superior to filgrastim in retrospective analysis. More convenient to patients since single injection. Cost is high, particularly if 12 mg used.

placebo or plerixafor 240 µg/kg on the evening of the fourth day of filgrastim administration, continuing daily until completion of collection. The primary efficacy endpoint, the collection of 6 × 10^6 CD34$^+$/kg in ≤2 leukapheresis sessions was achieved in 71.6% of patients mobilizing with GF + P versus 34.4% of patients with GF + placebo. The median number of days required to collect 6 × 10^6 CD34$^+$/kg was 1 day in patients receiving plerixafor versus 4 days in the control group.

The NHL trial had near identical design and included 298 patients. Fifty-nine percent of patients receiving plerixafor and only 20% of the patients receiving placebo met the primary efficacy endpoint of collecting 5 × 10^6 CD34$^+$/kg in up to apheresis sessions resulting in 90% of the patients in the plerixafor group versus 55% in the control group being able to undergo auto-HCT.

Plerixafor has a very favorable side effect profile with the main toxicity being mild to moderate diarrhea. The greatest caveat to broader adoption of plerixafor has been cost. In fact, many patients will successfully collect an adequate number of HPC in few apheresis sessions with GF alone. Some centers have adopted the practice of utilizing plerixafor for patients who are at perceived high risk of mobilization failure. However, this approach has important limitations due to the lack of reliable tools to precisely predict poor mobilization (see next). We believe that "just in time" is a more effective strategy to utilize plerixafor. With this approach, plerixafor is added to an ongoing mobilization cycle according to the number of CD34$^+$ in the PB after 4 days of GF administration. This way, only patients who are actual (as opposed to predicted) poor mobilizers receive plerixafor. This approach has reduced the risk of mobilization failure to <5% while preventing "unnecessary" use of plerixafor in 40–60% of patients. Figure 5.1 displays an example of one algorithm for "just in time" use of plerixafor.

Although C + GF and GF + P are both strategies to increase yield of HPC collected (over GF alone), there has not been any prospective comparison between the two methods. Retrospective comparisons indicate similar cost with more toxicities and, in some studies, less collection success with C + GF over GF + P.

Table 5.4 Published experience with different CD34+ cell mobilization strategies.

Author	N Total	Trial Setting	Mobilization Tool	Median CD34+/kg Yield	p Value	Mobilization Success of Meeting CD34+/kg Target	Toxicities	Comments and Practice Implications
	Disease							
Tuchman	167 MM	Single Center Retrospective Analysis	Cy 3–4 g/m² + G-CSF 10 µg/kg/d vs G-CSF 10 µg/kg/d	12×10^6 vs 5.8×10^6	<0.01	NS	14% hospitalized vs 0	Higher yield of stem cells offset by cost of toxicities to patient
Herbert	52 Lymphoma, MM	Single Center Retrospective analysis	pegfilgrastim 12 mg or 6 mg vs G-CSF 10 µg/kg/d	4.78×10^6 vs 3.70×10^6	NS	91% vs 80%	0 vs 0	Similarity in yield deserves further exploration
Costa	131 Lymphoma, MM	Single Center Retrospective Analysis	pegfilgrastim 1 2 mg +/- plerixafor (240 µg/kg) vs G-CSF 10 µg/kg +/- plerixafor (240 µg/kg)	Day 4: 28.7×10^6 vs 18.1×10^6	NS	52/57 vs 68/74	NS	Similarity in yield deserves further exploration
Simona	64 Lymphoma	Single Center Retrospective	ESHAP + G-CSF 5 µg/kg/d vs ESHAP + Pegfilagrastim 6 mg	12.3×10^6 vs 9.4×10^6	NS	25/26 vs 36/38	Neutropenia (grade 4) In both groups	Toxicities to be considered in chemo-mobilization strategies
Hosing	84 NHL	Single Center Retrospective	R + IE + G-CSF 6 µg/kg/d vs R + IE + G-CSF + GM-CSF 250 µg/kg	10.34×10^6 vs 7.5×10^6	0.65	39/43 (90.7%) vs 35/41 (85.4%)	Neutropenia (grade 3 = 6) vs Neutropenia (grade 3 = 7)	Addition of additional GF may not be clinically advantageous
Kopf	103 Lymphoma, MM	Single Center Prospective Randomized	Cyclophosphamide, VIP, or vinblastine + G-CSF 5 µg/kg/d vs lenograstim 5 µg/kg/d vs molgramostatim 5 µg/kg/d	8.4×10^6 vs 5.8×10^6 vs 4.0×10^6	0.1	29/38 (76.3%) vs 29/36 (80.5%) vs 24/29 (82.7%)	Transfusions of PRBC (25%), platelets (19%) Grade 4 Neutropenia (70%)	Hematologic toxicities and additional blood utilization to be considered in chemo-mobilization strategies
Narayanasami	47 Lymphoma	Single Center Randomized	Cyclophosphamide 5 g/m² + G-CSF 10 µg/kg/d vs G-CSF 10 µg/kg/d	7.2×10^6 vs 2.5×10^6	0.004	NS	Transfusion of PRBC (14), platelets (16), and, hospitalizations (7) vs PRBC (5), platelets (5), and hospitalization (1)	Chemo-mobilization associated with higher yield that G only, but at the cost of more toxicity and resource utilization

Study	n / Disease	Study type	Regimen	CD34+ yield	p	Target achieved	Adverse events	p	Conclusion
Costa	89 MM	Single Center Retrospective	G-CSF 10 µg/kg/d or pegfilgrastim 12 mg +/- preemptive plerixafor (240 µg/kg dosed per institutional decision algorithm) A: no prior lenalidomide (n=40) B: 1–4 cycles lenalidomide (n=30) C: >4 cycles lenalidomide (n=19)	A: 8.1×10^6 B: 7.4×10^6 C: 7.0×10^6	NS	A: 100% B: 90% C: 79%		NS	Preemptive plerixafor overcomes negative impact of lenalidomide exposure
Antar	83 MM	Single Center Retrospective	Cyclophosphamide 5 g/m² + G-CSF (n=56) vs G-CSF+ preemptive plerixafor 240 µg/kg (n=27)	15.5×10^6 vs 7.5×10^6	0.005	100% both groups	Febrile neutropenia (60%), Transfusion of PRBCs (27%), platelets (27%), hospitalizations (64%) vs 0	NS	Chemo-mobilization associated with higher yield that G only, but at the cost of more toxicity and resource utilization
DiPersio	298 NHL	Multicenter Phase III Randomized Double-blind Placebo Controlled	G-CSF 10 µg/kg/d + placebo vs G-CSF 10 µg/kg/d + plerixafor	1.98×10^6 vs 5.69×10^6	NS	Target: $\geq 2 \times 10^6$ 47.3% vs 86.7% Target: $\geq 5 \times 10^6$ 19.6% vs 59.3%		NS	Pivotal trial evidences safety and efficacy of plerixafor

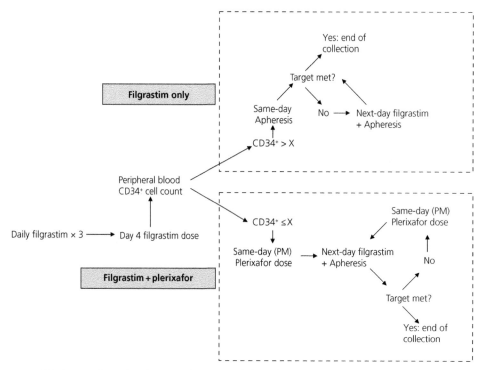

Figure 5.1 Proposed decision making algorithm to guide the use of plerixafor during autologous mobilization. Source: Costa 2012. Reproduced with permission of Nature Publishing Group.

What if CD34+ cell mobilization fails?

Mobilization failure can be defined as the failure to obtain sufficient HPC to proceed with transplantation, but the definition varies across different reports. Mobilization failure rates depend not only from the mobilization strategy utilized but also from the characteristics of individuals studied (see risk factors for poor mobilization next). Most patients who fail CD34+ cell mobilization and are still adequate candidates for auto-HCT will be able to proceed to transplant after remobilization. Some key points on planning remobilization are:[1,13]

- GF alone is not an adequate strategy for remobilization.
- C + GF can successfully remobilize a minority of patients failing GF alone.
- GF + P is successful remobilization in >70% of patients failing GF alone or C + GF.
- There is very little information on appropriate remobilization for patients who fail upfront GF + P. Some of these patients will successfully collect after C + GF with the addition of plerixafor.

Some practical aspects of autologous CD34+ cell mobilization

- Even though several clinical features are associated with poor mobilization (age, lymphoma diagnosis, multiple chemotherapy regimens, prolonged exposure to lenalidomide, prior exposure to melphalan, prior pelvic or spinal radiation, low platelet count, etc.) they are insufficient to effectively assign patients to one mobilization strategy over another. Strategies based on the patient's actual mobilization performance (e.g., "just in time" plerixafor) are preferable.
- Most transplant centers will assess one or more objective parameters prior to initiation of HPC collection. Monitoring of CD34+ in PB is preferable and most centers will not initiate leukapheresis unless CD34+ cell count > 10/μL (with variations ranging from 5 to 20 μL).
- There is no consensus on the volume of blood to be processed during a leukapheresis session (see Chapters 6 and 7). Many centers will process three total blood volumes. Large volume leukapheresis may improve collection yields but also lead to more side effects.

Allogeneic CD34⁺ cell mobilization
HPC graft: Bone marrow or peripheral blood?

Allogeneic HPC was primarily performed utilizing harvest bone marrow products. The establishment of safe methods of mobilization and collection of HPC from PB created the opportunity for more convenient procurement of a graft that produces faster engraftment. However, PB-HPC products have much higher lymphocyte content than bone marrow with possible implications in the risk of recurrence of the underlying hematologic malignancy and GvHD.

A meta-analysis of trials comparing bone marrow to PB-HPC as grafts for related donor transplantation found improved survival with PB-HPC among patients with more advanced hematologic malignancies at the cost of higher risk of severe acute and chronic GvHD.

Only more recently, bone marrow and PB-HPC as grafts for HLA-matched unrelated donor transplant were directly compared on a large randomized trial. There was no significant difference in survival, but with higher risk of graft failure and lower risk of chronic GvHD in the bone marrow arm. Adoption of PB-HPC for allo-HCT remains highly variable among centers and transplant physicians.

What is the best CD34⁺ cell mobilization regimen for allogeneic healthy volunteer donors?

There is far less variation in strategies for allogeneic mobilization than there is for autologous mobilization. Filgrastim, typically at doses of 10 μg/kg/day, is the near ubiquitous mobilizing agent and mobilization failures are rare. Figure 5.2 displays a proposed algorithm for allogeneic mobilization.

Plerixafor is not an approved agent for allogeneic mobilization. However, it has been tested as an alternative to filgrastim as a potentially more convenient and less toxic agent. However, grafts obtained with filgrastim and plerixafor mobilization have different cellular composition and lymphocyte cytokine profile and the effects of plerixafor mobilization on GvHD and risk of disease recurrence need to be better understood.

What is the optimal PB CD34⁺ cell dose for allogeneic hematopoietic cell transplantation?

Cell doses $<1.5 \times 10^6$ CD34⁺/kg are considered inadequate, may cause engraftment failure *or* delayed neutrophil and platelet recovery. Higher doses are associated

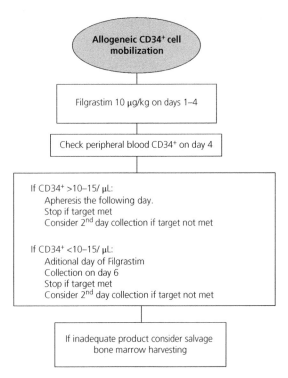

Figure 5.2 Proposed algorithm for allogeneic CD34⁺ mobilization.

with faster engraftment and, in some studies, reduced risk of leukemia relapse. The great concern, however, is that an excessively high cell dose would increase the risk of GvHD and some evidence exist that this may be the case for doses$>8\times10^6$ CD34⁺/kg. Therefore, cell doses of $4–5 \times 10^6$ CD34⁺/kg are considered optimal.

High yield points

1 CD34⁺ cell mobilization failures are costly and should be avoided.
2 Autologous mobilization should aim at collecting $3–5\times10^6$ CD34⁺/kg for each planned transplant procedure.
3 Autologous mobilization with GF alone is safe, but has lower CD34⁺ yields and higher risk of failure.
4 Autologous mobilization with C + GF yields more cells than GF alone, but with more cost and toxicity.
5 GF + P has lower risk of failure and yields more CD34⁺ cells than GF alone.
6 There are no prospective data directly comparing C + GF and GF + P. C + GF is likely more toxic and has higher risk of failure.
7 "Just in time" use of plerixafor can be a cost-saving alternative for "planned" plerixafor.

8 Autologous remobilization regimens should incorporate plerixafor, particularly if plerixafor is used in the initial mobilization.

9 Allogeneic mobilization strategies should prioritize donor safety and comfort.

10 Filgrastim is the near ubiquitous agent for allogeneic mobilization.

Selected reading

1. Giralt S, Costa L, Schriber J, Dipersio J, Maziarz R, McCarty J, et al. Optimizing autologous stem cell mobilization strategies to improve patient outcomes: consensus guidelines and recommendations. *Biology of Blood and Marrow Transplantation: Journal of the American Society for Blood and Marrow Transplantation.* 2014 Mar;**20**(3):295–308. PubMed PMID: 24141007.

2. Tuchman SA, Bacon WA, Huang LW, Long G, Rizzieri D, Horwitz M, et al. Cyclophosphamide-based hematopoietic stem cell mobilization before autologous stem cell transplantation in newly diagnosed multiple myeloma. *J Clin Apher.* 2015 Jun;**30**(3):176–182. PubMed PMID: 25293363.

3. Herbert KE, Gambell P, Link EK, Mouminoglu A, Wall DM, Harrison SJ, et al. Pegfilgrastim compared with filgrastim for cytokine-alone mobilization of autologous haematopoietic stem and progenitor cells. *Bone Marrow Transplantation.* 2013 Mar;**48**(3):351–356. PubMed PMID: 22858510.

4. Costa LJ, Kramer C, Hogan KR, Butcher CD, Littleton AL, Shoptaw KB, et al. Pegfilgrastim-versus filgrastim-based autologous hematopoietic stem cell mobilization in the setting of preemptive use of plerixafor: efficacy and cost analysis. *Transfusion.* 2012 Nov;**52**(11):2375–2381. PubMed PMID: 22404694.

5. Simona B, Cristina R, Luca N, Sara S, Aleksandra B, Paola B, et al. A single dose of Pegfilgrastim versus daily Filgrastim to evaluate the mobilization and the engraftment of autologous peripheral hematopoietic progenitors in malignant lymphoma patients candidate for high-dose chemotherapy. *Transfus Apher Sci.* 2010 Dec;**43**(3):321–326. PubMed PMID: 21036667.

6. Hosing C, Munsell MF, Reuben JM, Popat U, Lee BN, Gao H, et al. A randomized study comparing chemotherapy followed by G-CSF alone or in combination with GM-CSF for mobilization of peripheral blood stem cells in patients with non-Hodgkin's lymphomas. *J Blood Med.* 2010;**1**:49–55. PubMed PMID: 22282683. Pubmed Central PMCID: 3262333.

7. Kopf B, De Giorgi U, Vertogen B, Monti G, Molinari A, Turci D, et al. A randomized study comparing filgrastim versus lenograstim versus molgramostim plus chemotherapy for peripheral blood progenitor cell mobilization. *Bone Marrow Transplantation.* 2006 Sep;**38**(6):407–412. PubMed PMID: 16951690.

8. Narayanasami U, Kanteti R, Morelli J, Klekar A, Al-Olama A, Keating C, et al. Randomized trial of filgrastim versus chemotherapy and filgrastim mobilization of hematopoietic progenitor cells for rescue in autologous transplantation. *Blood.* 2001 Oct 1;**98**(7):2059–2064. PubMed PMID: 11567990.

9. Costa LJ, Abbas J, Hogan KR, Kramer C, McDonald K, Butcher CD, et al. Growth factor plus preemptive ('just-in-time') plerixafor successfully mobilizes hematopoietic stem cells in multiple myeloma patients despite prior lenalidomide exposure. *Bone Marrow Transplantation.* 2012 Nov;**47**(11): 1403–1408. PubMed PMID: 22484324.

10. Antar A, Otrock ZK, Kharfan-Dabaja MA, Ghaddara HA, Kreidieh N, Mahfouz R, et al. G-CSF plus preemptive plerixafor vs hyperfractionated CY plus G-CSF for autologous stem cell mobilization in multiple myeloma: effectiveness, safety and cost analysis. *Bone Marrow Transplantation.* 2015 Jun;**50**(6):813–817. PubMed PMID: 25751646.

11. DiPersio JF, Micallef IN, Stiff PJ, Bolwell BJ, Maziarz RT, Jacobsen E, et al. Phase III prospective randomized double-blind placebo-controlled trial of plerixafor plus granulocyte colony-stimulating factor compared with placebo plus granulocyte colony-stimulating factor for autologous stem-cell mobilization and transplantation for patients with non-Hodgkin's lymphoma. *Journal of Clinical Oncology: Official Journal of the American Society of Clinical Oncology.* 2009 Oct 1;**27**(28):4767–4773. PubMed PMID: 19720922.

12. DiPersio JF, Stadtmauer EA, Nademanee A, Micallef IN, Stiff PJ, Kaufman JL, et al. Plerixafor and G-CSF versus placebo and G-CSF to mobilize hematopoietic stem cells for autologous stem cell transplantation in patients with multiple myeloma. *Blood.* 2009 Jun 4;**113**(23):5720–5726. PubMed PMID: 19363221.

13. Duong HK, Savani BN, Copelan E, Devine S, Costa LJ, Wingard JR, et al. Peripheral blood progenitor cell mobilization for autologous and allogeneic hematopoietic cell transplantation: guidelines from the American Society for Blood and Marrow Transplantation. *Biology of Blood and Marrow Transplantation: Journal of the American Society for Blood and Marrow Transplantation.* 2014 Sep;**20**(9):1262–1673. PubMed PMID: 24816581.

14. Stem Cell Trialists' Collaborative G. Allogeneic peripheral blood stem-cell compared with bone marrow transplantation in the management of hematologic malignancies: an individual patient data meta-analysis of nine randomized trials. *Journal of Clinical Oncology: Official Journal of the American Society of Clinical Oncology.* 2005 Aug 1;**23**(22):5074–5087. PubMed PMID: 16051954. Pubmed Central PMCID: 1475795.

15. Anasetti C, Logan BR, Lee SJ, Waller EK, Weisdorf DJ, Wingard JR, et al. Peripheral-blood stem cells versus bone marrow from unrelated donors. *The New England Journal of Medicine.* 2012 Oct 18;**367**(16):1487–1496. PubMed PMID: 23075175. Pubmed Central PMCID: 3816375.

CHAPTER 6

Hematopoietic stem and progenitor cell collection by apheresis: Techniques and tricks

Anand Padmanabhan

Blood Center of Wisconsin & Medical College of Wisconsin, Milwaukee, WI, USA

Introduction

Hematopoietic progenitor cells (HPCs) are known to circulate in the blood of normal individuals, however, their low levels at steady state (i.e., without "mobilization") preclude harvesting of these cells from non-mobilized donors/patients. Over the last several years, blood-derived HPCs have been increasingly used for transplantation as mobilization regimens that are safe, reliable, and effective have been developed, and techniques for collection of mononuclear cells (MNCs) have evolved. HPC collection by apheresis, designated HPC (A), is now the most frequently used technique to obtain CD34+ cells for the purpose of hematopoietic cell transplantation (HCT). Given the frequent use of apheresis to collect HPCs, there is a critical need for HCT caregivers to understand the process, techniques, quality parameters and adverse events associated with this procedure. This chapter will focus on the following topics:

1 Techniques and devices used
2 Technical and clinical aspects of HPC (A) collections
3 Evaluating efficiency of HPC (A) collection
4 Optimizing timing of leukapheresis and determining when to terminate collections
5 Adverse events associated with HPC (A) collections
6 Quality indicators

Collection techniques and devices used

HPC (A) collection involves the extracorporeal separation and collection of white blood cells from whole blood using centrifugation-based techniques. The devices used either collect cells continuously, or discontinuously during multiple cycles of collection over the duration of the procedure. Separation and collection of white blood cells are optimized such that MNCs (of which CD34+ cells are a subset) are enriched, however, this enrichment is not absolute and variable levels of granulocytes are found in the product. Thus, the process of HPC collection results in a product that is heterogeneous from a cellular standpoint, with the cell of interest being defined by expression of the CD34+ receptor.

Apheresis devices used to collect HPCs differ somewhat in their hardware specifications, separation technologies and extracorporeal volume requirements. Commonly used devices referenced here include the *COBE Spectra* (Terumo BCT, Lakewood, CO), *Amicus* (Fresenius-Kabi, Lake Zurich, IL), and *Spectra Optia* (Terumo BCT, Lakewood, CO). The COBE Spectra and a recently approved protocol ("cMNC") on the *Spectra Optia* continually collect MNCs after separation in the centrifuge (Figure 6.1a). The *Amicus* collects MNCs intermittently during multiple cycles over the duration of the procedure (although flow of blood from the patient into the device and back to the patient is continuous; Figure 6.1b). Several clinical studies have detailed performance characteristics of these different apheresis instruments and systems. In general, the devices are viewed as similar/equivalent in their ability to collect HPCs. Differences, however, have been noted with respect to extent of platelet depletion induced by HPC (A) collections using these devices, with the *Amicus* being the most platelet sparing.

Clinical Manual of Blood and Bone Marrow Transplantation, First Edition. Edited by Syed A. Abutalib and Parameswaran Hari.
© 2017 John Wiley & Sons Ltd. Published 2017 by John Wiley & Sons Ltd.

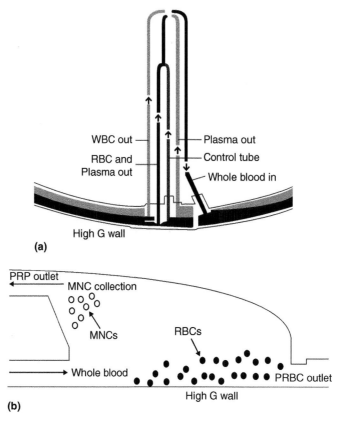

Figure 6.1 MNC Collection methodology for continuous collection (**a**; COBE Spectra, Terumo BCT, Lakewood, CO) and cyclical harvest (**b**; Amicus, Fresenius-Kabi, Lake Zurich, IL) is depicted below. In (**a**), whole blood entering the centrifuge is subject to a soft spin resulting of packing of red blood cells along the high-G wall, on top of which is the WBC layer (buffy coat), platelets and plasma. The buffy coat is continuously removed. In (**b**), during a cycle, whole blood enters the separation chamber and red cells reside along the high-G wall, while platelets are returned to the patients via the platelet-rich plasma (PRP) outlet. To trigger harvest of MNCs, the packed RBC (PRBC) outlet closes and a small volume of red blood cells is pumped into the chamber to lift and transfer MNCs through the PRP outlet into a collection bag. This cycle is repeated several times during the HPC (**a**) collection procedure. (**a**) Source: Reproduced with permission of Terumo BCT (Lakewood, CO).

Technical/clinical aspects of HPC (A) collections

Vascular access
HPC (A) procedures require high blood flow rates. In patients with adequate peripheral venous access, large bore needles (16/17 gauge) are utilized for draw and return of blood to the patient/donor. However, in instances where peripheral access is deemed inadequate, a large bore, rigid, double/triple lumen central venous catheter (CVC) is used to enable the rapid flow of blood (often >100 mL/min) into the apheresis device and return of blood to the patient. CVCs are usually placed in the subclavian or internal jugular veins, with femoral access being less frequently used due to higher risk of infection, particularly in autologous donors. In

patients undergoing HPC (A) collection for autologous HCT, placement of a semi-permanent (tunneled) CVC is commonly performed and is used for both HPC (A) collection and for long-term intravenous fluid/medication administration during the transplant process.

Large volume leukapheresis (LVL)
LVL for HPC collection involves processing 3-5 donor blood volumes (BV) (up to 15–25 l in a 70-kg adult) in a single session, and is frequently performed in both pediatric and adult patients. LVL has advantages over conventional collections (smaller volumes: 2–3 BV collections) in that it allows for collection of a greater number of HPCs. This may be particularly important in patients who are not well mobilized. In these patients, LVL gets them closer to the desired CD34+ cell collection

goal in fewer days. LVL procedures are long (4–7 h) and entail risks as detailed in the adverse effects section later in this chapter. It is critically important that the patient/donor has good venous access or a CVC to support rapid flow rates over several hours.

Anticoagulation during HPC (A) collection

The choice of anticoagulation used to facilitate HPC (A) collections varies and is often tailored to patient need. Heparin, anticoagulant citrate dextrose formula A (ACD-A), or a combination of the two have been used in HPC (A) collections, each with its own benefits and limitations. ACD-A is rapidly metabolized by the liver and therefore anticoagulation effects cease rapidly upon completion of the procedure. This may be particularly helpful in patients who are at a higher risk for bleeding due to factors such as thrombocytopenia or treatment with antiplatelet agents/anticoagulants. The key disadvantages of ACD-A include toxicities related to hypocalcemia (due to calcium chelation by citrate), and fluid overload. Use of heparin, on the other hand, does not alter calcium homeostasis but results in sustained anticoagulation for several hours after completion of the procedure, possibly putting the donor at a higher bleeding risk, and carries a risk, albeit small, of heparin-induced thrombocytopenia (HIT). In a typical, ACD-A based HPC (A) collection one part of anticoagulant solution is mixed with 12–15 parts of whole blood as it is drawn into the apheresis device. With heparin-based HPC (A) collection, the volume of anticoagulant used can be 2–3 times smaller relative to the volume of ACD-A used, thereby decreasing risk of volume overload in the donor. *At the author's institution, ACD-A-based anticoagulation is more commonly used while heparin-based anticoagulation is used on a case-by-case basis, particularly in patients with limited ability to tolerate additional intravascular volume.*

Special considerations for pediatric HPC donors/patients

HPC collection by LVL may be performed in children after considering pediatric-specific factors. Special considerations for pediatric donors include the ethical and legal aspects of informed consent; the frequent need for CVC access and use of sedation/anesthesia both for CVC placement and for keeping small children calm during the HPC (A) procedure. In children with low body weight (particularly <25 kg), the volume of the apheresis extracorporeal circuit may exceed 10–15% of the total blood volume (TBV) of the patient. In such situations, the apheresis tubing may be "primed" with packed RBCs to ensure that anemia/hypovolemia-related symptoms are not precipitated. As in adult collections, close attention should be paid to symptoms of hypocalcemia and the use of point of care ionized calcium

testing may be considered. At the author's institution, an HPC(A) collection algorithm is in place whereby information on pre-collection peripheral blood CD34$^+$ cell counts, recipient/donor size and HPC collection target is utilized to determine if procedure truncation is possible (see next and Figure 6.2). Decreased HPC (A) collection time is particularly desirable in small children who may need to be sedated for the duration of this lengthy procedure.

Efficiency of CD34$^+$ cell collection

The efficiency with which HPCs are collected by apheresis is often defined by the CD34$^+$ (or MNC) collection efficiency (CE). At the author's institution, evaluation of the CD34$^+$ CE with every procedure is an important aspect of the HPC (A) collection quality program. The CD34$^+$ CE is calculated by one of two formulae detailed in Table 6.1. Outside the context of a clinical trial, the CE2 is typically used for assessment of CE given the somewhat limited cost effectiveness of performing an additional post-procedure peripheral blood CD34$^+$ cell count that is needed to calculate CE1. Several programs set a CD34$^+$ CE2 collection threshold of 30–35%, below which a detailed evaluation of the technical and clinical aspects of the collection are performed to identify causative factors that led to the suboptimal collection. Some factors that may adversely impact CE include high CD34$^+$ or WBC counts, technical challenges in performance of the procedure due to poor vascular access or other factors, and not drawing cells from the appropriate depth in the buffy coat layer during the collection. Proactive steps may be taken to minimize the impact of high peripheral blood white counts on CE by making appropriate adjustments to the collect pump speed. Experienced operators working in conjunction with the apheresis physician is a critical component of this optimization process. For example, in patients with high MNC counts or high inlet speeds, optimal collection is achieved by increasing the collect pump rate using a formula that takes both these variables into account.

Prediction by pre-collection CD34$^+$ count and its impact on HPC (A) collection

Institutions vary in their practice on when to commence HPC (A) collections, with some centers measuring peripheral blood CD34$^+$ cell levels prior to collection in each patient, and others using this approach only in patients with known risk factors of mobilization failure. In programs that do utilize a CD34$^+$ cell count threshold, a count of >5–10 CD34$^+$ cells/uL is typically used as the collection trigger. An alternative approach that is somewhat infrequently used to optimize initiation of leukapheresis is evaluation of levels of "progenitor" cells by commercially

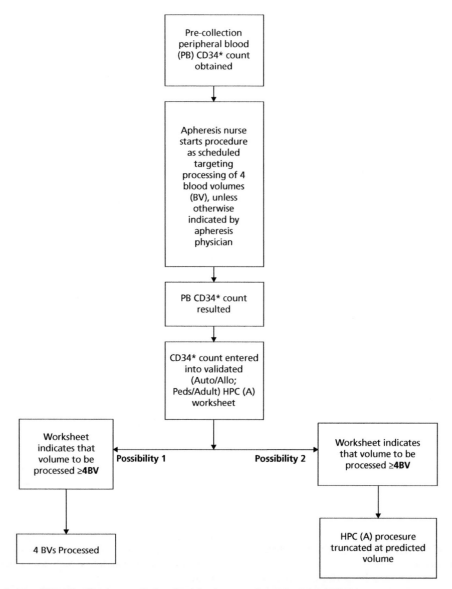

Figure 6.2 Optimizing HPC (A) collection: prediction algorithm in use at the author's institution.

available simple-to-use hematology analyzers (e.g., the *hematology analyzer XE-2100*, Sysmex, Mundelein, IL).

The blood CD34+ cell count may remain relatively constant, increase or decrease during HPC (A) collections. Despite these differences in kinetics of CD34+ cell recruitment from the bone marrow during the procedure, the pre-collection peripheral blood CD34+ cell count is generally a very reliable predictor of HPC yield. Some studies have utilized mid-procedure product sampling to determine if LVL may be truncated in the event that the desired CD34+ cell yield is collected prior to processing of a predesignated blood volume. An alternative method used by some centers for prediction of *BV to process* (BVP) to attain HPC target yield involves back-calculating BVP (from the formula in Table 6.1) assuming a "low" CD34+ CE2. The CE chosen is typically in the lowest fifth percentile of CD34+ CE2s. Such an approach is risk-averse and ensures that

Table 6.1 Evaluation of collection efficiency.

Collection Efficiency 1 (CE1)=CD34⁺ cells collected/[(Mean of pre- and post-collection PB CD34⁺ cell count) × BVP] × 100

Collection Efficiency 2 (CE2)=CD34⁺ cells collected/[(Pre-collection PB CD34⁺ cell count) × BVP] × 100

Example for CE2 calculation: 20 Liters of whole blood was processed to collect 350 million CD34⁺ cells in a patient/donor. The precollection peripheral blood CD34⁺ count was 50 cells/microliter. **CE2** = 350 million/[50 × 10⁶ cells/L × 20 L] × 100 = 35%

PB = Peripheral Blood; BVP = Blood Volume Processed (i.e., volume of patient/donor whole blood processed for the collection)

Table 6.2 Blood volume processing recommendations for matched unrelated allogeneic HPC (A) collections (NMDP).

Recipient	Donor
Total Body Weight (kg)	**Apheresis Procedures and Blood Volume Processed**
≤35	Single 12 L Apheresis
36–45	Single 15 L Apheresis
46–55	Single 18 L Apheresis or Two 12 L Apheresis
56–65	Single 22 L Apheresis or Two 12 L Apheresis
>65	Single 24 L Apheresis or Two 12 L Apheresis

the yield of HPCs will almost always be at or above the desired target. It is critically important to evaluate a large number of HPC (A) collections to define this "low" CD34⁺ CE2, and these analyses should be performed separately on adult, pediatric, autologous and allogeneic donors given that the intraprocedure kinetics of mobilization of CD34⁺ cells may likely vary between these patient populations. After this CE2 is defined, a calculation worksheet should be developed and validated. Figure 6.2 details this process of optimizing HPC (A) collections at the author's institution, which routinely results in truncation of procedures in autologous and allogeneic settings for both adult and pediatric patients. A specific "low" CD34⁺ CE2 value is not provided in Figure 6.2 since this value varies depending upon the patient/donor population undergoing HPC (A) collection.

For unrelated allogeneic collections often facilitated by registries such as the National Marrow Donor Program (NMDP), HPC (A) collections are based either on use of prediction algorithms (as discussed above) or on protocols based on recipient size. An example of a weight-based HPC (A) procedural recommendation is presented in Table 6.2.

Adverse effects associated with HPC (A) collections

This section discusses the most frequent adverse effects associated with HPC (A) collections, with mobilization-related effects discussed elsewhere. With ACD-A based LVL, citrate toxicity is very commonly seen. Symptoms may include perioral paresthesia, tingling in fingers/toes, and may proceed to chest tightness, nausea/vomiting, and further to tetany and cardiac arrhythmias, if not promptly addressed. Calcium supplementation may be either in the form of prophylaxis, or in response to symptoms of hypocalcemia. Prophylactic calcium infusions, especially in the setting of LVL with ACD-A anticoagulation is generally very effective at preventing moderate/severe symptoms of citrate toxicity and minimizes occurrence of mild symptoms. If symptoms of hypocalcemia occur, blood inlet flow rate should be decreased immediately and calcium should be administered. If providing calcium chloride intravenously, it should be noted that calcium chloride has three times the content of elemental calcium relative to calcium gluconate, and is not recommended for use via peripheral veins due to the risk of venous sclerosis. Alkalosis induced by large volume of citrate infused during the procedure can cause hypokalemia due to shifting of K+ into cells. Other adverse effects include fluid overload, which can be particularly problematic in patients sensitive to shifts in intravascular volume. One example would be amyloidosis patients with amyloid deposition in the heart. In such cases heparin-based anticoagulation may be more appropriate to minimize the volume of fluid given to the patient. LVL typically results in platelet loss of approximately 30–60% with the exception of the *Amicus device*, which is relatively platelet sparing. Platelet depletion can be particularly problematic in the poorly mobilized autologous transplant patient requiring multiple HPC (A) collection procedures to attain the required CD34⁺ cell dose. Platelet transfusions may be indicated for such patients in the setting of severe thrombocytopenia or bleeding.

Some adverse events associated with HPC (A) collection are related to CVCs. Subclavian and internal jugular CVCs have been associated with pneumo/hemothorax, cardiac perforation, and tamponade. Real-time sonographic visualization guided CVC placements are superior to blind puncture, and use of this technique significantly minimizes incidence of these risks. Femoral catheters are infrequently used in this setting due to higher risk of infection. Aseptic technique should be maintained to minimize risks of microbial contamination, which typically occur in a small number of collections. The incidence of culture-positive HPC (A) products reported in the literature ranges from 0 to 7.2%, but is typically <1–2%.

HPC (A) collection quality indicators

HCT programs should have a robust HPC (A) quality assurance program in place. These programs are typically accredited by various organizations such as the Foundation for the Accreditation of Cellular Therapy (FACT) and AABB. While HPC (A) collection quality indicators captured vary based on center, at the author's institution, key data captured and discussed at regularly scheduled HCT program quality meetings include:

1 CD34+ cell collection efficiency
2 BVP/Number of HPC (A) procedures needed to attain target CD34+ cell dose
3 Incidence, type and severity of adverse events
4 Product characteristics including volume, hematocrit and MNC content.

Citrate toxicity is typically the most common adverse event encountered in LVL. Hematocrit of the product is usually in the 2–4% range, with higher hematocrit products potentially being problematic in major ABO-incompatible allogeneic HCTs. It is desirable to attain high product MNC content while minimizing granulocyte content due to concerns of granulocyte-related infusion reactions. Tracking of these parameters assists with early detection of negative trends and helps ensure the safety and efficacy of HPC (A) collections.

SUMMARY

1. Peripheral blood is now the most commonly used source of hematopoietic stem and progenitor cells
2. HPC (A) collections typically involve processing large volumes of blood, a process referred to as large volume leukapheresis (LVL)
3. The choice of anticoagulant should be carefully made based on patient clinical status

4. Evaluation and monitoring of cellular collection efficiencies are an important component of assuring effective collections
5. Algorithms to optimize timing and duration of HPC (A) collections are increasingly being adopted
6. Adverse events associated with HPC (A) collections include but are not limited to citrate toxicity and fluid overload

Conflict of Interest

The author has received honoraria/research support from Terumo BCT, Lakewood, CO and Fenwal (now Fresenius-Kabi LLC), Lake Zurich, IL.

Selected reading

1. Schwartz J, Padmanabhan A, Francis RO, Linenberger ML. Mobilization and Collection of Peripheral Blood Hematopoietic Progenitor Cells. In: McLeod B, Szczepiorkowski ZM SZ, Weinstein R, Winters JL (eds). *Apheresis: Principles and Practice.* 3 ed: AABB Press; 2010.
2. Makar RS, Padmanabhan A, Kim HC, Anderson C, Sugrue MW, Linenberger M. Use of laboratory tests to guide initiation of autologous hematopoietic progenitor cell collection by apheresis: results from the multicenter hematopoietic progenitor cell collection by Apheresis Laboratory Trigger Survey. *Transfus Med Rev.* 2014 Oct;**28**(4): 198–204.
3. Rosenbaum ER, O'Connell B, Cottler-Fox M. Validation of a formula for predicting daily CD34(+) cell collection by leukapheresis. *Cytotherapy.* 2012 Apr;**14**(4):461–466.
4. Bolan CD, Cecco SA, Wesley RA, Horne M, Yau YY, Remaley AT, et al. Controlled study of citrate effects and response to i.v. calcium administration during allogeneic peripheral blood progenitor cell donation. *Transfusion.* 2002 Jul;**42**(7): 935–946.
5. Bolan CD, Yau YY, Cullis HC, Horwitz ME, Mackall CL, Barrett AJ, et al. Pediatric large-volume leukapheresis: a single institution experience with heparin versus citrate-based anticoagulant regimens. *Transfusion.* 2004 Feb;**44**(2): 229–238.
6. Ikeda K, Ohto H, Nemoto K, Yamamoto G, Kato K, Ogata T, et al. Collection of MNCs and progenitor cells by two separators for PBPC transplantation: a randomized crossover trial. *Transfusion.* 2003 Jun;**43**(6):814–819.

CHAPTER 7

Hematopoietic cell processing: From procurement to infusion

Jay S. Raval[1], Kathryn McKay[2], and Yara A. Park[1]

[1] *Department of Pathology and Laboratory Medicine, University of North Carolina at Chapel Hill, Chapel Hill, NC, USA*

[2] *Lineberger Comprehensive Cancer Center, University of North Carolina at Chapel Hill, Chapel Hill, NC, USA*

Introduction

Once hematopoietic progenitor cells (HPCs) are collected, many steps must occur to ensure the purity and potency of the product for transplant. The products need to have cell counts, flow cytometry analysis, sterility testing, viability analysis, and if needed, cryopreservation and storage. HPC products that will be used at a later date, which can range from days to years, must be stored in a manner that allows the cells to retain their viability and functionality to engraft once infused.

Regulations

HPC laboratories are highly regulated facilities. HPC products are considered biologics so laboratories must be registered or licensed with the Food and Drug Administration (FDA) in the U.S. In addition, the laboratories often are Clinical Laboratory Improvement Amendments (CLIA) certified, many using the College of American Pathologists (CAP) or a similar organization in other countries. Many HPC processing facilities are also accredited by AABB (formerly known as the American Association of Blood Banks) and the Foundation for the Accreditation of Cellular Therapy (FACT).

Regardless of the source of HPCs, many of these products require at least minimal manipulation and testing to ensure the product is not only effective, but also safe. In this chapter, we will address the issues and indications for cellular product manipulations of both autologous and allogeneic products, including cord blood products, peripheral blood hematopoietic cells (PBHC) obtained through apheresis collection, and bone marrow products.

Processing of autologous products

Autologous products do not pose the difficulties of ABO incompatibilities, but since patient and donor are the same the product often requires storage while the patient undergoes preparation for transplant. Currently, almost all autologous products are collected by apheresis. The product is aliquotted into storage bags based on the cell concentrations and then a cryoprotectant must be added prior to the freezing of the product. Sterility testing for bacterial and fungal contamination is typically performed immediately prior to cryopreservation but after the addition of cryoprotectant.

Optimizing cell concentrations during processing

The optimal total nucleated cell (TNC) concentration to use for cryopreservation of PBMC remains unknown. Poor mobilizers, typically defined as (1) not having achieved a circulating CD34+ count >20/μl up to 6 days after G-CSF at 10 μg/kg/day or 5 μg/kg/day after chemotherapy or (2) yielding <2.0 × 10^6 CD34+ cells/kg in ≥ 3 apheresis collections can be particularly challenging from a laboratory perspective. In these cases, the HPC product typically requires dilution prior to cryopreservation either with autologous donor plasma or an isotonic solution (Normosol-R, Plasmalyte-A) to reduce the total mononuclear cell concentration. From a laboratory standpoint, the need to freeze large product volumes is not only a resource-draining endeavor, it can also lead to volume overload in the patient (large volume shifts) and cryoprotectant-related toxicity upon infusion. Concerns have been raised in the past that a high cell concentration in the cryopreservative

Clinical Manual of Blood and Bone Marrow Transplantation, First Edition. Edited by Syed A. Abutalib and Parameswaran Hari.
© 2017 John Wiley & Sons Ltd. Published 2017 by John Wiley & Sons Ltd.

can also result in toxicity to the cells. However, the possibility of doubling the cell concentration without any loss of viability is a promising alternative to help reduce the amount of cryoprotectant that is infused. Volume reduction through centrifugation and removing excess plasma could benefit pediatric patients, patients with renal dysfunction, and poor mobilizers (high concentrations of TNC but low concentrations of CD34$^+$ cells). These smaller volume products would also require less storage space, laboratory materials and reagents, and result in shortened processing time.

PRACTICE POINT

While the optimal concentration of TNC in the HPC products prior to cryopreservation is unknown, the concentration can be adjusted with dilution or volume reduction. Autologous donors with high peripheral white blood cell counts and low circulating CD34$^+$ counts can have large volumes of product stored which can lead to large volume infusions at the time of transplant. These transplants require infusion over multiple days to ensure patient safety and limit adverse side-effects.

Cryopreservation: Storing HPC products for use at a later date

The cryopreservation process is of importance for all types of HPC collection being considered for later use (see Table 7.1). In these products cryopreservation allows the CD34$^+$ cells to remain viable and functional. Current strategies have been proven safe and not associated with significant adverse outcomes (i.e., failure to engraft, delayed engraftment); however, no single cryopreservation method has been universally adopted.

Variations in technique occur between different transplant centers and only slight changes have been observed over the last 15 years. Reinfusion of these cryopreserved cells has been associated with varying toxicities potentially attributed to total product volume, total cellular content, cell composition, and cryopreservatives in the solution. A commonly used cryoprotectant, such as dimethyl sulfoxide (DMSO), is necessary to prevent the formation of intracellular and extracellular ice crystals that could form during the freezing process. The ice crystals could ultimately lead to cell death, which is why addition, timing, and amount of cryoprotectant is a critical part of the process. Coupled with controlled rate freezing (CRF), DMSO at a standard concentration of 10% combined with electrolyte solution and albumin has been established to be a safe and effective cryopreservation agent.

Graft infusion: Wash or not to wash?

At the time of graft infusion, many centers thaw the HPC products at the patient's bedside and immediately infuse the cells. Some studies have shown DMSO to be toxic to cells at room temperature, so rapid thawing of the product in a 37 °C waterbath immediately before the infusion is advised. While some transplant centers will wash the products prior to the infusion, it is more common to infuse the product directly into the patient once thawed. Washing of the cells to remove DMSO and other additives risks loss of critical CD34$^+$ cells and lowering of the transplant dose.

DMSO associated adverse effects and prevention

DMSO is associated with many clinically significant side-effects that include nausea, vomiting, cardiovascular, respiratory, renal, and allergic presentations. Rare fatalities have been reported. Due to the potential adverse effects associated with DMSO, a maximum exposure of 1 g/kg/day is permitted. Depending on the TNC collected, the HPC product cell concentration in each bag, and the weight of the recipient, infusions of HPC products may have to occur over more than one day to prevent DMSO associated toxicity. Based on these observations, newer approaches have been tried. Lower doses of DMSO (typically 5%) in addition to

Table 7.1 HPC product storage and transport temperatures.

Product Storage	HPC, Apheresis	HPC, Marrow	HPC, Cord Blood
Fresh HPC product	RT or 1–6 °C up to 72 h	RT up to 48 h	RT or 1–6 °C up to 48 h
Frozen HPC product in vapor phase LN2	≤−150 °C	≤−150 °C	≤−150 °C
Frozen HPC product in liquid phase LN2	−196 °C	−196 °C	−196 °C

*RT-room temperature or ambient temperature, LN2 = liquid nitrogen
+Some facilities store for longer periods of time and/or at 1–6 °C

extracellular protectants like hydroxyethyl starch (HES) have been used with success in cryopreserving peripheral blood, marrow, and UCB grafts. Initial data shows improved viability with HES (3%) and DMSO (5%) versus DMSO (10%) alone. The issue is long-term storage with such solution combination and the limited availability of data on products cryopreserved in this manner. Although HES can be a useful supplement to DMSO, the most common ratio of HES and DMSO in cryoprotectant solutions has been established by simple trial and error and requires further investigation and optimization.

Freezing process

Controlled rate versus uncontrolled rate

If cryopreservation is planned, cryoprotectant containing 10% DMSO is added slowly, followed by freezing and storage in liquid nitrogen (LN2). The freezing process can occur in one of two ways: CRF and uncontrolled freezing (i.e., dump freezing). In CRF, the product is cooled at a computer controlled rate and the temperatures of the product and freezer are carefully monitored and documented. An advantage with CRF is the ability to shorten the latent heat of fusion phase. For example, cooling is temporarily accelerated to accommodate the increased energy released into the system. Uncontrolled freezing, or dump freezing, is a simple transfer of the HPC product from a −80 °C freezer to a LN2 storage freezer (<−150 °C). This process also cools at a general rate of 1–3 °C/min but does not mitigate the heat of fusion. The actual cooling rate is difficult to document and the freezer should be left undisturbed, which can be a potential problem for centers with multiple products in a day. In general, CRF is utilized more frequently by HPC laboratories.

Vapor phase LN2 versus liquid phase LN2

At a temperature of −80–−100 °C, the product can be stored long-term in one of two ways: in vapor phase (VP) LN2 or liquid phase (LP) LN2. Although LP freezers maintain fewer temperature fluctuations, newer jacketed VP freezers minimize temperature gradients and, importantly, negate the risks associated with potential viral and bacterial contamination between products. Storage within the gaseous phase of LN2 abrogates the theoretical risk of potential contamination of other HPC products within the same freezer (i.e., the likelihood of a potential infectious agent within a cryopreserved HPC product contaminating adjacent HPC units is virtually nil if cryopreservation is maintained by avoiding a liquid medium in favor of a gaseous medium). There is currently no defined expiration of frozen HPC products, and components frozen for over 10 years have been successfully transplanted.

> **PRACTICE POINT**
>
> Autologous HPC products are almost always cryopreserved. DMSO is the most commonly used cryopreservation agent at this time. Cell concentration in HPC product bags as well as the %DMSO used in cryopreservation are two laboratory variables that directly impact how much DMSO a patient will receive at the time of transplant. Regardless of freezing method, great care is taken to safely cryopreserve HPC products and maintain cellular viability and functionality. Viability of the cells is absolutely critical to patient engraftment; therefore, the time from addition of cryopreservation media to start of CRF (our preferred method) must be minimized. Regulatory and accrediting agencies require the validation and monitoring (stability programs) of a cryopreservation method and storage that preserves cellular viability both post-processing (pre-cryopreservation) and at infusion (post-thaw). Post-processing (pre-cryopreserving) total cell viability release criteria is typically >90% with post-thaw viabilities of at least 70%.

Processing allogeneic products

Unlike autologous products, allogeneic products harbor the attendant risks similar to any routine blood component from the blood bank, which can include but not limited to risks of infectious disease, allergic reactions, immunologic reactions, hemolytic reactions, and graft-versus-host-disease. Additionally, unlike in solid organ transplantation, infusion of ABO incompatible HPC components is routinely performed. However, many donor and product factors which would make a routine blood donor ineligible and unsuitable for donation may not automatically make the same individual unsuitable for donation of HPC products; these potentially detrimental factors are weighed against the benefit of transplantation of the impacted HPC product for a given recipient.

A donor-recipient pair is considered a major ABO mismatch if the recipient has isohemagglutinins that are incompatible with the donor's red blood cells (RBCs) (example: A donor and an O recipient). Conversely, the donor-recipient pair is considered a minor ABO mismatch if the donor's plasma contains isohemagglutinins against the recipient's RBC (example: O donor and a B recipient). Certain donor-recipient pairs can be both major and minor ABO mismatches (e.g., A donor and B recipient-bidirectional ABO mismatch).

HPC, apheresis allogeneic products

HPC, apheresis products collected from the peripheral blood usually have hematocrits of <5%; thus, major ABO incompatibilities due to incompatible RBCs are rarely of concern. The apheresis instruments are excellent at isolating the buffy coat and limiting the red cell contamination of the HPC product. However, since these products can have HPC immersed in up to several hundred milliliters of plasma, minor ABO incompatibility can occur which would require plasma reduction as a HPC processing manipulation to prevent a possible acute hemolytic reaction at the time of infusion (see Tables 7.2 and 7.3). The FACT Standards require that the transplant clinician specify the modifications that should occur to the product based on the ABO incompatibilities.

Plasma reduction to remove incompatible isohemagglutinins can be achieved by centrifugal separation. This can be done via manual centrifugation of the product bag and expressing off excess plasma or using an automated apheresis instrument to remove plasma in cases with minor ABO incompatibility. However, the benefits of plasma reduction must be weighed against the risk of CD34+ cell losses that may occur during the separation. HPC, apheresis products may be infused either fresh or after freezing (see Table 7.1). If they are cryopreserved, the same steps that were discussed in the autologous sections of the chapter apply.

PRACTICE POINT

Unlike autologous HPCs, allogeneic HPCs may be ABO incompatible. The ordering Bone marrow Transplant team member must indicate type of ABO incompatibility and steps needed to circumvent complications.

HPC, marrow allogeneic products

HPC, Marrow products collected in the operative suite from an anesthetized individual can routinely have volumes of up to 2000 ml with hematocrits of up to 35%; thus, major ABO incompatibility is a clinical concern (see Table 7.2). Most institutions set their own limit for the allowable quantity of incompatible RBCs, with up to 20–30 mL of incompatible cells being deemed acceptable. However, if this is exceeded, further RBC reduction is performed (also see Chapter 1).

All methodologies for RBC reduction are based upon densitometric separation of RBCs (specific gravity = 1.08–1.09) from mononuclear cells (MNCs; specific gravity 1.06–1.07). These methods include

procedures previously discussed such as centrifugation and automated apheresis separation, as well as two additional methods: HES-mediated densitometric separation and densitometric gradient separation.

When HES is combined with RBCs, rouleaux of the red cells occurs and the specific gravity of the RBC components increases. This results in a better densitometric separation between the RBCs (which sediment) and the MNCs (which remain afloat in the bag). RBCs can then be drained out, leaving behind a leukocyte (MNC)-rich product.

Densitometric gradient separations utilize agents, one example being hypaque-ficoll, to create a density barrier. After a centrifugation step, RBCs and polymorphonuclear cells (i.e., granulocytes) have a higher specific gravity and, following a centrifugation step, ultimately end up below the density gradient barrier. Cellular elements with a lower specific gravity, such as the MNCs (which contain the HPCs), remain above the

Table 7.3 Needed modifications depending on ABO mismatches. Red cell reductions are needed on HPC, Marrow products only. Plasma reductions are needed on HPC, Marrow and HPC, Apheresis products.

Donor	Recipient	Manipulation in the Product
O	O	None
O	A, B, AB	Plasma Reduction
A	A	None
A	O	Red cell reduction
A	B	Red cell and plasma reduction
A	AB	Plasma reduction
B	B	None
B	A	Red cell and plasma reduction
B	O	Red cell reduction
B	AB	Plasma reduction
AB	AB	None
AB	O, A, B	Red cell reduction

Table 7.2 ABO mismatches in HPC transplant.

	O Donor	A Donor	B Donor	AB Donor
O Recipient	compatible	major	major	major
A Recipient	minor	compatible	major and minor	major
B Recipient	minor	major and minor	compatible	major
AB Recipient	minor	minor	minor	compatible

gradient and can be subsequently isolated. As with plasma reduction, the benefits of any RBC reduction strategy versus the risks of HPC losses must be considered. HPC, Marrow products may be infused either fresh or after freezing (see Table 7.1).

HPC, Marrow products also contain a large volume of plasma. If there is minor ABO incompatibility between the donor and the recipient, the product would require a plasma reduction as described in the HPC, Apheresis section.

> **PRACTICE POINT**
>
> Unlike autologous HPCs, allogeneic HPCs may be ABO incompatible. The ordering Bone Marrow Transplant team member must indicate whether RBC reduction is needed for the removal of incompatible RBCs or a plasma reduction is needed to remove incompatible plasma in the donor HPC product.

HPC, cord blood allogeneic products

Cord blood collection is usually performed by trained staff with documented appropriate experience and technique. Use of a closed or semi-closed system (bag or syringe) by venipuncture of the umbilical vein after delivery of the placenta under aseptic conditions is required. At the completion of collection, the primary container is labeled, at a minimum, with product identification, source and destination, donor and recipient (if known), recommended conditions for storage and transportation (see Table 7.1), and product additives. Processing typically involves a series of steps to remove excess plasma and RBCs resulting in a final volume of 20 ml. Methods vary between manual and automated with a goal of a final product recovery of 90% MNCs.

Cryoprotectant containing 10% DMSO is added slowly, followed by CRF. Sterility testing for bacterial and fungal contamination is typically performed after the addition of cryoprotectant. Results are evaluated as a component of quality control for the procedure and specific release criteria. Cells are cryopreserved in various vessels including vials, bags, or other containers approved for cryopreservation and validated by the cord blood bank to maintain viability. Storage temperature requirements after cryopreservation should be less than or equal to −150 °C and continuously monitored in a LN2 tank equipped with an audible alarm system. At this time, there are no expiration dates assigned to stored UCB as there is no evidence at present that they lose viability or biological activity when stored at this manner. After thawing, UCB products must undergo additional HPC laboratory processing. If these products have not been RBC reduced prior to cryopreservation,

they must be washed; however, if they have been RBC reduced prior to cryopreservation, then these products can be either washed or diluted.

Regulation of handling UCB

In the US, current FDA regulations consider cord blood to be a "biological" product. Facilities that perform any of the manufacturing steps for UCB must register with the FDA and list their products and each of the steps they perform. Cord blood units stored for potential use by a patient *unrelated* to the donor must meet all the prescribed FDA current good manufacturing practice (cGMP) criteria and requirements and be licensed under a biologics license application (BLA). Unlicensed cord blood units (collected and stored prior to 2011) and non-licensed units are considered "investigational" and can only be used for transplantation under an active FDA IND (investigational new drug). This use requires review by an Institutional Review Board (IRB) and patient and physician approval.

> **PRACTICE POINT**
>
> Unlike autologous HPCs, allogeneic HPCs may be ABO incompatible. HPC, Cord Blood units are typically plasma and RBC reduced prior to cryopreservation. In contrast to other products, HPC, Cord units are thawed in the laboratory and either washed or diluted in preparation for infusion.

Potency of the HPC product

HPC laboratory standards require processes and protocols to confirm product identity, trace the product from donor to recipient, and product integrity or characterization of the product for quality and quantity. Release criteria are established for total cell count, viability, sterility, donor eligibility, and CD34+ cell dose, and acceptable values and ranges must be defined. There is a need for some variability in what is "acceptable" since the nature of these products, which are derived from and for individual patients, make them unique. Equipment, reagents, and supplies used in these processes should be qualified, there should be written definitions of the type and volume of samples to be obtained, and the time-points during production for sampling must be determined. It should be clearly defined whether quality control is an in-process control or whether it is a control of the final product. Minor manipulations, such as wash steps, volume reduction steps, or even cryopreservation require quality tests regarding cell numbers and bacterial and fungal contamination. Manipulations or processing steps involving culture or activation of cells are considered major manipulations. The same quality tests apply to minimal manipulations as well as evaluation for mycoplasma, viruses, and functionality. Allogeneic and autologous HPC products have a well-established proven clinical benefit for the patients and can be released despite quality control parameters being out of specification. The final decision to release a HPC product that does not meet specifications should be guided by the consideration that the benefits outweigh potential risks for the recipient.

Infectious disease testing

Testing must be performed per manufacturer's instructions using FDA-licensed and approved donor screening tests (see Table 7.4). Testing is not required on autologous donors; however, products must be labeled as "Not Evaluated for Infectious Substances" and stored appropriately.

The FDA also defines requirements for the use of biohazard specific warning labels for products that fall under the 21 CFR 1271 regulations. Donors are screened for eligibility based both on donor screening questions which determine potential risks to recipients as well as by infectious disease testing. Cellular therapy products require "incomplete" or "ineligible" donor evaluation and determination if the screening and/or testing is not finished for "incomplete" or if the screening and/or testing demonstrates risk for "ineligible". Donor criteria including screening, testing, and product labeling is designed to minimize the potential risk of disease transmission, but do not totally eliminate the risk of transmitting these agents. Some allogeneic donors may not meet all the requirements, but can still be approved for donation. In these situations,

a summary of records that contains information regarding why those requirements have not been met is provided to the transplant center prior to product procurement. A recipient's physician has the ability to authorize use of the product if the recipient has been advised and the product is labeled appropriately and released under urgent medical need.

Cell selection

A typical hematopoietic cell collection contains unmodified red cells, white cells, and CD34$^+$ progenitor cells when it is processed and stored. There is some belief that the removal of unneeded cells and possibly malignant cells (if identified) from these products may improve patient outcomes. However, cells pertinent to hematopoietic recovery must remain present, viable, and functional.

Purging – Monoclonal antibodies can recognize and adhere to antigens on malignant cells. The adherent antibodies are attached to microparticles containing the heavy metal nickel. These complexes settle out of the lighter fraction composed of stem cells leaving it virtually free of malignant cells.

CD34$^+$ selection – Mechanical selection techniques have existed since the early 1990s. These processes remove or select only HPCs leaving malignant cells and other immune cells to be discarded. In order for this to work, HPCs have to be reliably identified. One of the main markers that exists on the surface of a HPC is the CD34$^+$ antigen. In a positive selection, a device uses magnetic beads to bind the CD34$^+$ cells and remove them. These devices have been evaluated in

Table 7.4 US minimal requirements for testing for transmissible agents in cellular therapy products.

	Donors of HPC, M and HPC, A	Donors of HPC, C	Donors of Other Hematopoietic Cell-Derived Products Such as Lymphocytes
Timing of specimen collection	Up to 30 days before collection	Up to 7 days before or after collection	Up to 7 days before or after collection
Human immunodeficiency virus, type 1 and 2 (HIV-1, HIV-2)	X	X-Maternal Sample	X
Hepatitis B Virus (HBV)	X	X-Maternal Sample	X
Hepatitis C Virus (HCV)	X	X-Maternal Sample	X
Human T-cell lymphotrophic virus, types I and II (HTLV-I, II)	X	X-Maternal Sample	X
Cytomegalovirus (CMV) (if allogeneic)	X	X-Maternal Sample	X
Treponema pallidum (syphilis)	X	X-Maternal Sample	X

clinical trials and are able to exclude large numbers of malignant cells, but may also exclude other important immune cells.

PRACTICE POINT

It is technically possible to isolate specific cells in the HPC laboratory and either retain or remove them. Selection of cells for retention or removal may result in losses of other cell populations which might be important for prompt, full engraftment. At this time, cell selection for the removal of malignant cells or the inclusion of CD34+ cells has not been routinely recommended; thus, its use must be determined on a case-by-case basis.

Selected reading

1. Areman E.M., K. Loper. *Cellular Therapy: Principles, Methods, and Regulations.* AABB Press: Bethesda, MD. 2009.
2. Broxmeyer H.E. *Cord Blood: Biology, Transplantation, Banking, and Regulation.* AABB Press: Bethesda, MD. 2011.
3. Fung M.K., B.J. Grossman, C.D. Hillyer, C.M. Westhoff. *Technical Manual.* 18th Edn. AABB Press: Bethesda, MD. 2014.
4. FACT-JACIE *International Standards for Hematopoietic Cellular Therapy Product Collection, Processing, and Administration,* 6th Edn, 2015.
5. www.aabb.org
6. www.apheresis.org
7. www.factwebsite.org

CHAPTER 8

Graft manipulation: T-cell depletion and beyond

Christina Cho and Miguel-Angel Perales

Adult Bone Marrow Transplantation Service, Memorial Sloan Kettering Cancer Center, and Weill Cornell Medical College, New York, NY, USA

Introduction

Graft-versus-host disease (GvHD) is a potentially devastating complication of allogeneic hematopoietic cell transplantation (allo-HCT). The use of *ex vivo* T-cell depletion (TCD) of hematopoietic cell grafts has significantly reduced the risk of GvHD. Additional benefits include the decreased duration or need for post-transplant immunosuppression, avoidance of toxicities associated with standard agents utilized for GvHD prophylaxis and treatment, and the ability to employ myeloablative conditioning regimens (MAC) in older patients in whom the combination of ablative conditioning and GvHD prophylaxis would otherwise be prohibitively toxic.

Acute and chronic GvHD: Scope of the problem

GvHD contributes significantly to transplant-related morbidity and transplant-related mortality (TRM) with rates of 10–25% after allo-HCT. The risk of grade II–IV acute GvHD (aGvHD) in recipients of HLA-matched sibling donor (MSD) and unrelated donor (MUD) grafts approaches 35–50% and 40–70%, respectively, with the use of current immunosuppressive regimens. The combination of a calcineurin inhibitor (CNI) with methotrexate is the most common GvHD prophylaxis used. Implemented more than three decades ago, such regimens have demonstrated better control of aGvHD but are ineffective in preventing chronic GvHD (cGvHD).

Management of cGvHD remains a challenge, and it has become a significant health problem in transplant survivors especially with abundant use of mobilized peripheral blood hematopoietic cells. Current regimens for GvHD prophylaxis and treatment are limited by well-established issues including but not limited to potentiation of oral mucositis (methotrexate), renal toxicity (methotrexate and tacrolimus), variable risk of transplant-associated thrombotic microangiopathy (tacrolimus and sirolimus), constant serum monitoring, (tacrolimus and sirolimus), non-compliance (tacrolimus, sirolimus, and MMF), and the necessity of chronic persistent immunosuppression (tacrolimus). In our opinion, the anticipated toxicity of combined intervention with MAC and protracted GvHD prophylaxis may preclude the use of ablative conditioning in some older adults; as a result, transplant-eligible older adults frequently receive non-myeloablative or reduced-intensity conditioning regimen despite the potential of increased risk of relapse with such intervention.

Concepts and methods of TCD

The recognition that GvHD is mediated by donor-derived T-cells led to preclinical and clinical exploration of TCD as a strategy to reduce the risk of GvHD. Techniques used for TCD have varied over time, and the specific approach used should be noted when analyzing data in this regard. Several factors may impact the effectiveness and degree of TCD, including the type of cells depleted (T-cell only vs other populations such as B-cells, NK-cells, etc.), the graft source, HLA-matching, and the use of post-transplant immunosuppression. TCD of the graft can be performed by either *positive* or *negative* selection of CD34$^+$ cells.

Clinical Manual of Blood and Bone Marrow Transplantation, First Edition. Edited by Syed A. Abutalib and Parameswaran Hari.
© 2017 John Wiley & Sons Ltd. Published 2017 by John Wiley & Sons Ltd.

Negative selection

Negative selection by extraction of donor lymphocytes has been achieved through physical methods such as soybean lectin agglutination (SBA) followed by sheep red blood cell (sRBC)-rosette depletion (E-rosetting), or counterflow elution. Immunologic approaches to TCD have also been harnessed through the use of monoclonal antibodies, such as anti-CD6 monoclonal antibody-conjugated immunomagnetic beads. *Negative* depletion techniques retain a larger number of effector lymphocytes, such as NK-cells, in the allogeneic peripheral blood hematopoietic cell (PBHC) grafts compared with *positive* selection.

Positive selection

At present, *positive* selection by extraction of CD34$^+$ cells from the graft is the most common technique in clinical use to achieve TCD of the graft. In earlier studies, CD34$^+$ selection of PBHCs was performed on the ISOLEX 300i magnetic cell selection system (Baxter, Deerfield, IL), followed by E-rosetting. Current studies utilize super-paramagnetic particle-conjugated antibodies with the CliniMACS® CD34$^+$ Reagent System (Miltenyi Biotec, Bergisch Gladbach, Germany). Conventional T-cell replete marrow grafts typically contain 5×10^7 CD3$^+$ T-cells/kg, whereas mobilized peripheral blood grafts contain 3×10^8 T-cells/kg.

In recipients of TCD *marrow* grafts from HLA-MSD, the risk of GvHD has been demonstrated to increase if the graft contained $>1 \times 10^5$ T-cells/kg, and the risk of both acute and cGvHD decreases significantly when the degree of TCD is 3-log using marrow, or 4–5 log using PBHCs. While formal analysis of T-cell dose in MUD grafts is pending, the rates of aGvHD reported with *ex vivo* TCD have been similar with grafts from MSD and MUD.

The CliniMACS® CD34$^+$ Reagent System can achieve a 5-log reduction in T-cells, whereas the ISOLEX 300i system (no longer available in the US) achieved a 3.5–5-log reduction, depending on the settings, and required additional TCD through E-rosetting in the case of the lower log reduction. Lower degrees of TCD, on the order of 1–2 logs, do not result in a significant reduction in the incidence of GvHD and typically require post-transplant GvHD prophylaxis.

> **PRACTICE POINT**
>
> TCD by 3-log using bone marrow or 4–5 log using PBHC in MSD or MUD grafts is recommended to achieve adequate reduction of GvHD.

Impact of T-cell depletion on engraftment

One of the potential consequences of CD34$^+$ cell selection of the allograft is a higher rate of graft failure. Initial studies of TCD grafts demonstrated a higher risk of graft failure compared with conventional T-cell replete transplants, which negatively impact on disease-free survival (DFS) and overall survival (OS). It has been postulated that, in unmodified transplants, donor T-cells in the graft marrow may help to sustain engraftment by eliminating host cells that could mediate graft rejection. In order to overcome this immunologic barrier in TCD HCT, modifications of the conditioning regimen, and in particular the incorporation of antithymocyte globulin (ATG), has shown to promote engraftment with rates of graft failures similar to the rates observed with unmanipulated grafts. In addition, the available data for the use of CD34$^+$ cell selected grafts includes only MAC regimens. It is thought that reduced-intensity conditioning (RIC) regimens did not provide adequate myelo- and immunosuppression and would result in higher rates of rejection; therefore TCD is not performed in patients receiving RIC or non-myeloablative regimen for allo-HCT.

> **PRACTICE POINT**
>
> The use of ATG with CD34$^+$-selected grafts promotes engraftment and ensures a low rejection rate comparable to conventional transplants. The use of CD34$^+$ cells selected grafts requires an ablative conditioning regimen, which may exclude patients with significant co-morbidities or advanced age.

Impact of TCD on GvHD

The use of *ex vivo* TCD grafts has significantly reduced the risk of GvHD in a variety of hematologic malignancies (summarized in Table 8.1). The principal benefit of TCD is a significant decrease in both acute and chronic GvHD compared with conventional transplants. Studies of TCD-HCT at Memorial Sloan Kettering Cancer Center (MSKCC) have reported incidences of aGvHD (limited to grade II) of 8% and cGvHD of 9% in recipients of matched related grafts and incidences of acute and chronic GvHD of 9 and 29%, respectively, in recipients of HLA-MUD grafts.

These single-center experiences were validated in a single-arm, phase II multicenter trial performed by the Blood and Marrow Transplant Clinical Trials Network (BMT CTN 0303). Among 44 patients with AML in CR1 or CR2 who received TCD PBHC grafts from HLA-identical siblings, the incidence of grade II–IV acute GvHD was 22.7%, and the incidence of extensive cGvHD limited to 6.8% at 24 months.

> **PRACTICE POINT**
>
> The use of TCD or CD34$^+$ selected allografts results in a significant reduction in both acute and chronic GvHD.

Table 8.1 Single-center studies of T-cell depletion allo-HCT in hematologic malignancies.

Author, Publication/ Date	N	Disease(s)	Conditioning Regimen	Graft Source and Method of TCD Depletion	GvHD	Survival
Papadopoulos, 1998	39	AML	TBI, thiotepa, cyclophosphamide	• MRD • BM grafts, SBA-sRBC	• aGvHD: Grade I 5%, no grade II-IV • Extensive cGvHD: 1/35 evaluable patients	• Estimated probability of 4-year DFS 77% (CR1) or 50% (CR2)
Jakubowski, 2007	52	Multiple	TBI, thiotepa, fludarabine	• MRD • PBHC grafts, ISOLEX-sRBC	• aGvHD: Grade II 8%, no grade III-IV • cGvHD: 9%	• Estimated probability of 3-year DFS 61%, OS 62%
Castro-Malaspina, 2008	49	MDS, AML evolved from MDS	TBI- or busulfan-based	• MRD • BM grafts, SBA-sRBC or PBHC grafts, ISOLEX-sRBC	• aGvHD: Grade I-III 7% in patients surviving after 28 days, no grade IV • cGvHD: 2% in patients surviving after 100 days	• 3-year DFS 36.7%, OS 30.6% • Among patients who received chemotherapy prior to conditioning 3-year DFS and OS were 50% and 54% in patients who had achieved CR or second refractory cytopenia phase
Perales, 2010	61	NHL	TBI, thiotepa, cyclophosphamide or TBI, thiotepa, fludarabine	• MRD (42/61), MUD, MMRD, MMUD • BM grafts, SBA-sRBC or PBHC grafts, ISOLEX-sRBC	• aGvHD: Grade II-III 18%, no grade IV • cGvHD: 12%	• 10-year EFS 43%, OS 50%
Jakubowski, 2011	35	Multiple	TBI, thiotepa, fludarabine, ATG	• MUD • BM grafts, SBA-sRBC or PBHC grafts, ISOLEX-sRBC	• aGvHD: Grade II-III 9%, no grade IV • cGvHD: 29%	• Estimated probability of 4-year DFS 57%, OS 59%
Goldberg, 2013	56	ALL	TBI, thiotepa, cyclophosphamide or TBI, thiotepa, fludarabine	• MRD (22/56), MUD, MMRD, MMUD • BM grafts, SBA-sRBC or PBHC grafts, ISOLEX-sRBC	• aGvHD: Grade II-III 20%, no grade IV • cGvHD: 15%, extensive cGvHD 5%	• 2-year DFS 38%, 5-year DFS 38%; 2-year OS 39%, 5-year OS 38%

TBI: Total body irradiation
BM: Bone marrow
PBHC: Peripheral blood hematopoietic cell
MRD: Matched related donor
MUD: Matched unrelated donor
MMRD: Mismatched related donor
MMUD: Mismatched unrelated donor
SBA-sRBC: Soybean lectin agglutination (SBA) followed by sheep red blood cell (sRBC)-rosette depletion
ISOLEX-sRBC: ISOLEX 300i magnetic cell selection followed by sheep RBC-rosette depletion

Impact of TCD on GvHD: Comparisons with conventional allo-HCT

Multiple studies have compared outcomes in patients undergoing TCD allo-HCT with those who receive unmodified grafts (Table 8.2):

- In a 2012 analysis, Pasquini et al. compared patients treated on the phase 2 BMT CTN 0303 study with a similar subset of patients on BMT CTN 0101 who had received conventional T-cell replete grafts from HLA-MSD and pharmacological immune suppression as GvHD prophylaxis for AML in CR1 or CR2. There were comparatively lower rates of cGvHD at 2 years with TCD grafts (19 vs 50%, p<0.001), and TCD was associated with enhanced GvHD-free survival at 2 years (41 vs 19%, p<0.006).
- A retrospective analysis by Bayraktar et al. compared 115 patients with AML in CR1 who received TCD grafts after MAC at MSKCC with a cohort of 181 similar patients who received unmodified grafts after conditioning with busulfan/fludarabine and GvHD prophylaxis with tacrolimus/methotrexate at MD Anderson Cancer Center (MDACC). This analysis demonstrated a significant reduction in the incidence of grade II-IV a GvHD (5 vs 18%, p=0.005) and cGvHD at 3 years (13 vs 53%, p<0.001) with TCD, though with similar RFS and OS in the two cohorts.
- A similar analysis by Hobbs et al. comparing 52 patients with ALL in CR1 or CR2 treated with TCD allo-HCT at MSKCC with 115 patients who underwent unmodified transplant at MDACC demonstrated decreased grade II-IV aGvHD (17.3 vs 42.6%, p=0.001) as well as cGvHD (13.5 vs 33.4% at 3 years, p=0.006) with the use of TCD (10). Again, no significant difference in relapse free survival or OS was seen.

The results of the BMT CTN 0303 study led to the FDA approval of the CliniMACS® CD34⁺ reagent system as a humanitarian device for CD34⁺-selection of PBHC from an allogeneic, HLA-MSD in patients with AML in CR1 undergoing a MAC transplant. An international phase III trial (in the US and Germany) is currently comparing TCD with the CliniMACS® CD34⁺ reagent system to post-transplant cyclophosphamide and a control arm (tacrolimus and methotrexate) in patients with acute leukemias and MDS who are eligible for MAC transplant from HLA-matched related or unrelated donors (BMT CTN 1301, NCT02345850).

> **PRACTICE POINT**
>
> The use of CD34⁺ selected allografts using the CliniMACS® CD34⁺ reagent system is currently FDA approved in patients with AML in CR1 undergoing a MAC PB-HCT from an HLA-MSD.

Impact of TCD on malignant relapse

A significant potential limitation of TCD is the elimination of the recognition of the tumor by donor-derived T-cells, the so-called graft-versus-leukemia (GvL) effect, which may raise concern that TCD places recipients of allo-HCT at increased risk of disease relapse. In chronic myelogenous leukemia (CML), GvL indeed plays a significant role in preventing disease relapse, and CML patients who receive a TCD transplant have been shown to have up to a 2.5-fold increase in relapse compared with patients receiving unmodified grafts. It should be noted that, in such cases of relapsed disease, complete remission was attained after donor lymphocyte infusion (DLI) in the majority of patients with subsequent similar OS. Ultimately, however, CD34⁺-selected transplants are not routinely recommended for these patients.

While the CML experience clearly supports the critical role of GvL in allo-HCT, patients with AML or ALL appear to have similar rates of disease relapse and survival whether they receive TCD or unmodified allografts:

- In the analysis by Pasquini et al, patients with AML saw an overall relapse rate of 24% at 36 months if they received TCD grafts on BMT CTN 0303, versus 27% with conventional grafts and pharmacologic immunosuppressive therapy on BMT CTN 0101 (p=0.6).
- In the retrospective evaluation by Bayraktar et al. comparing clinical outcomes in patients with AML in CR1 who received TCD transplant at MSKCC versus recipients of unmodified transplants at MDACC, there was no significant difference in the relapse rate between the TCD and unmodified transplant groups at 1 year (17 vs 21%, p=0.4) and 3 years (18 vs 25%, p=0.9).
- Similarly, Hobbs et al. noted a cumulative incidence of relapse of 23% in patients receiving TCD allografts for ALL, with 2- and 5-year OS and DFS that were comparable to those reported in conventional transplants.

Thus, we conclude that CD34⁺-selected transplants do not appear to place patients with ALL or AML at increased risk for relapse.

> **PRACTICE POINT**
>
> Consider TCD in patients undergoing allo-HCT for MDS, AML, ALL, or high-grade NHL. TCD is generally not recommended in CML.

Impact of TCD on immune recovery

Immune recovery following allo-HCT is dependent on the conditioning regimen, the allograft, and the thymic activity of the recipient, which decreases with age. TCD is associated with delayed recovery of thymic function, and in turn delayed recovery of total and naïve CD4⁺

Table 8.2 Studies comparing TCD with conventional allo-HCT.

Author, Date	Study Populations	Disease	Graft Source and Method of TCD Depletion	GvHD	Survival
Pasquini, 2012	• TCD graft, n=44 (BMT CTN 0303) • T-cell replete graft and IST, n=84 (BMT CTN 0101)	AML	• MRD • PBHC grafts, CliniMACS	• aGvHD: Grade II–IV 23% (TCD) vs 39% (IST) • cGvHD: 19% (TCD) vs 50% (IST)	• No significant difference in survival • Estimated probability of 2-year DFS 54% (TCD) vs 55% (IST); OS 65% (TCD) vs 59% (IST)
Bayraktar, 2013	• TCD graft, n=115 (MSKCC) • T-cell replete graft and IST, n=181 (MDACC)	AML	• MRD, MUD, MMRD, MMUD • BM grafts, SBA-sRBC or PBSC grafts, ISOLEX-sRBC or CliniMACS	• aGvHD: Grade II–IV 5% (TCD) vs 18% (IST) • cGvHD: 13% (TCD) vs 53% (IST)	• No significant difference in survival • 3-year DFS 58% (TCD) vs 60% (IST); OS 57% (TCD) vs 66% (IST)
Hobbs, 2015	• TCD graft, n=52 (MSKCC) • T-cell replete graft and IST, n=115 (MDACC)	ALL	• MRD, MUD, MMRD, MMUD • BM grafts, SBA-sRBC or PBHC grafts, ISOLEX-sRBC or CliniMACS	• aGvHD: Grade II–IV 17.3% (TCD) vs 42.6% (IST) • cGvHD: 13.5% (TCD) vs 33.4% (IST)	• No significant difference in survival • 3-year DFS 42.8% (TCD) vs 35.9% (IST); OS 42.6% (TCD) vs 43.0% (IST)

T-cells, prolonged inversion of the CD4$^+$/CD8$^+$ ratio, and delayed recovery of T-cell mitogen responses, which places patients at increased risk of opportunistic infections, including Epstein-Barr virus (EBV)-associated lymphoproliferative disorders, particularly in the first year post-transplant (also see Chapters 35 & 41).

In the analysis by Bayraktar et al. comparing TCD with conventional transplants performed in patients with AML at MSKCC and MDACC, respectively, 6 (5%) vs 2 (1%) patients died of infectious complications in the first 100 days post-transplant (p=0.04). However, as noted above, despite this difference in the rate of deaths from infection, there were ultimately no differences in RFS or OS. It is also important to remember that GvHD itself has a significant impact on immune recovery, including direct effects on the thymus, and because of the need for immunosuppressive agents to treat GvHD once it occurs.

Nevertheless, strategies to enhance post-transplant immune recovery represent a critical unmet need in both TCD and unmodified allo-HCT. A number of approaches are currently under active investigation. These include the use of keratinocyte growth factor (KGF), which promotes epithelial cell proliferation and differentiation in the thymus; sex steroid ablation, which may enhance thymic and peripheral T-cell reconstitution; interleukin-7 (IL-7), which plays a central role in T-cell development and survival; and adoptive transfer of T-cells specific for viruses such as CMV and EBV. In particular, recombinant human IL-7 (rhIL-7, CYT107, Revimmune) has demonstrated safety as well as efficacy in a phase I trial in recipients of a TCD-HCT, with observed increases in CD4$^+$ and CD8$^+$ T-cells, evidence of thymic output, and generation of functional T-cells.

PRACTICE POINT

The use of TCD-HCT results in delayed immune recovery compared with conventional grafts. Patients should be monitored closely for viral reactivation (CMV, EBV, and adenovirus) and receive anti-infectious prophylaxis until immune recovery is demonstrated.

Optimal patient selection for TCD allografts

Any decision regarding the use of a TCD versus an unmodified graft should take into account the individual patient, including the underlying disease, donor and degree of HLA matching, and preexisting comorbidities. As a general guideline, the following patients should be considered for CD34$^+$-selected grafts:

- Patients at elevated risk of post-transplant GvHD, such as those who will receive mismatched related or unrelated donor transplants.

- Patients with nonmalignant conditions such as sickle cell anemia and severe combined immunodeficiency, who do not benefit from GvL effects.
- Patients with MDS, AML, ALL, and high-grade NHL. These individuals are optimal candidates for CD34$^+$-selected transplants given the similar rates of survival and relapse compared with unmodified transplants.
- Patients who are able to tolerate a MAC regimen but are limited by the risk of GvHD or nephrotoxicity.

Future directions: Other approaches to TCD

As noted previously, the current approach for TCD relies on positive selection of CD34$^+$ cells. However ongoing studies are also investigating negative selection through CD3, CD3/CD19, and TCRαβ$^+$/CD19$^+$ depletion strategies. In particular, recent studies with the CliniMACS system have investigated the depletion of TCRαβ$^+$ and CD19$^+$ cells. This approach yields comparable numbers of CD34$^+$ cells compared with CD34 positive selection and CD3/CD19 depletion approaches. A study in 29 patients who received CD3/CD19 depleted grafts from HLA-haploidentical related donors showed rapid count recovery and full donor chimerism within 2–4 weeks. Finally, results of a randomized trial comparing CD3/CD19 depleted PB-HCT and CD34$^+$ positive selected grafts form matched sibling or matched unrelated donors showed faster recovery of NK-cells in the CD3/CD19 depleted group, which may aid in the anti-tumor response early after transplant.

Summary

Please also see Table 8.3.
- Despite continued improvements in outcomes and survival, the success of allo-HCT continues to be limited by GvHD and related complications including medication-related toxicities and infectious complications.
- TCD significantly reduces risk of acute and chronic GvHD after allo-HCT.
- In many hematologic malignancies, including AML, ALL, MDS, and NHL, TCD has not been demonstrated to increase risk of disease relapse. TCD is generally not recommended for patients with CML.
- Limitations of TCD include potential impairment of engraftment, which has been resolved though addition of ATG, the requirement for an MAC regimen, and delayed immune recovery compared with unmodified grafts. These limitations can be attenuated to some extent by advanced strategies to promote immune recovery, which remain an important area of investigation.

Table 8.3 Advantages and disadvantages of T-cell-depleted allo-HCT.

Outcome	Advantages	Disadvantages
GvHD	Decrease in acute and chronic GvHD	
Regimen		No data in reduced intensity conditioning
Toxicity	Reduced mucositis related to methotrexate, reduced renal toxicity due to calcineurin inhibitors	
Immune complications	Decreased need for chronic immunosuppression	Delay in immune recovery
Engraftment		Potential increase in risk of graft failure
Relapse	Survival and relapse comparable to conventional grafts in patients with ALL, AML, MDS, and NHL	Increased risk of relapse in patients with CML
Quality of life (QoL)	Decreased morbidity associated with chronic GvHD	

Selected reading

1. Papadopoulos EB, Carabasi MH, Castro-Malaspina H, Childs BH, Mackinnon S, Boulad F, et al. T-cell-depleted allogeneic bone marrow transplantation as postremission therapy for acute myelogenous leukemia: freedom from relapse in the absence of graft-versus-host disease. *Blood*. 1998;**91**(3): 1083–1090.
2. Jakubowski AA, Small TN, Young JW, Kernan NA, Castro-Malaspina H, Hsu KC, et al. T-cell-depleted stem-cell transplantation for adults with hematologic malignancies: sustained engraftment of HLA-matched related donor grafts without the use of antithymocyte globulin. *Blood*. 2007;**110**(13):4552–4559.
3. Castro-Malaspina H, Jabubowski AA, Papadopoulos EB, Boulad F, Young JW, Kernan NA, et al. Transplantation in remission improves the disease-free survival of patients with advanced myelodysplastic syndromes treated with myeloablative T-cell-depleted stem cell transplants from HLA-identical siblings. *Biol Blood Marrow Transplant*. 2008;**14**(4): 458–4568.
4. Perales MA, Jenq R, Goldberg JD, Wilton AS, Lee SS, Castro-Malaspina HR, et al. Second-line age-adjusted International Prognostic Index in patients with advanced non-Hodgkin lymphoma after T-cell-depleted allogeneic hematopoietic SCT. *Bone Marrow Transplant*. 2010;**45**(9):1408–1416. Epub 2010/01/12.
5. Jakubowski AA, Small TN, Kernan NA, Castro-Malaspina H, Collins N, Koehne G, et al. T-cell-depleted unrelated donor stem cell transplantation provides favorable disease-free survival for adults with hematologic malignancies. *Biol Blood Marrow Transplant*. 2011;**17**(9):1335–1342. Epub 2011/01/15.
6. Goldberg JD, Linker A, Kuk D, Ratan R, Jurcic J, Barker JN, et al. T-cell-depleted stem cell transplantation for adults with high-risk acute lymphoblastic leukemia: long-term survival for patients in first complete remission with a decreased risk of graft-versus-host disease. *Biol Blood Marrow Transplant*. 2013;**19**(2):208–213. Epub 2012/09/18.
7. Devine SM, Carter S, Soiffer RJ, Pasquini MC, Hari PN, Stein A, et al. Low risk of chronic graft-versus-host disease and relapse associated with T-cell-depleted peripheral blood stem cell transplantation for acute myelogenous leukemia in first remission: results of the blood and marrow transplant clinical trials network protocol 0303. *Biol Blood Marrow Transplant*. 2011;**17**(9):1343–1351. Epub 2011/02/16.
8. Pasquini MC, Devine S, Mendizabal A, Baden LR, Wingard JR, Lazarus HM, et al. Comparative outcomes of donor graft CD34+ selection and immune suppressive therapy as graft-versus-host disease prophylaxis for patients with acute myeloid leukemia in complete remission undergoing HLA-matched sibling allogeneic hematopoietic cell transplantation. *J Clin Oncol*. 2012;**30**(26): 3194–3201. Epub 2012/08/08.
9. Bayraktar UD, de Lima M, Saliba RM, Maloy M, Castro-Malaspina HR, Chen J, et al. Ex vivo T-cell-depleted versus unmodified allografts in patients with acute myeloid leukemia in first complete remission. *Biol Blood Marrow Transplant*. 2013;**19**(6):898–903. Epub 2013/03/08.
10. Hobbs GS, Hamdi A, Hilden PD, Goldberg JD, Poon ML, Ledesma C, et al. Comparison of outcomes at two institutions of patients with ALL receiving ex vivo T-cell-depleted or unmodified allografts. *Bone Marrow Transplant*. 2015;**50**(4):493–498. Epub 2015/01/27.
11. Perales MA, Goldberg JD, Yuan J, Koehne G, Lechner L, Papadopoulos EB, et al. Recombinant human interleukin-7 (CYT107) promotes T-cell recovery after allogeneic stem cell transplantation. *Blood*. 2012;**120**(24):4882–4891. Epub 2012/09/27.

CHAPTER 9

Graft-versus-host disease prophylaxis

Melhem Solh and Asad Bashey

The Blood and Marrow Transplant Group of Georgia at Northside Hospital, Atlanta, GA, USA

Historic perspective

Starting with experimental models in early 1950s, murine GvHD was recognized as an immunological phenomenon mediated by donor derived T lympho-cytes. The first allogeneic human marrow transplants were complicated by signs of GvHD similar to those described among animal models and immune deficient children receiving blood products. The manifestations of human GvHD include inflammation, organ dysfunction, and immune deficiency. GvHD remains the major factor underlying transplant-induced morbidity and mortality among recipients of allogeneic HCT today.

However, GvHD has been historically difficult to separate from anti-neoplastic alloreactivity (graft-versus-tumor effect, GvT) and thus attempts to prevent problematic GvHD have been moderated by the risk of collateral loss of curative GvT.

Donor selection

The most powerful predictor of acute GvHD is human leukocyte antigen (HLA) disparity between the donor hematopoietic cells and the recipient. The impact of mismatched HLA class I and II alleles have been well documented in recent literature among related and unrelated donors. When analyzing mismatches at HLA-A, B, C, DRB1, and DQ, a high-resolution mismatch at HLA-A, B, C, and DRB1 was associated with increased mortality and GvHD after marrow unrelated HCT. Among 8/8 matched unrelated HCT recipients, Pidala and colleagues reported increased risk of GvHD with HLA-DPB1 and –DQB1. Nonpermissive HLA-DPB1 mismatches were also associated with increased transplant related mortality compared to those with matched

or permissive mismatch at HLA-DPB1 locus. Minor histocompatibility antigen disparities are also associated with increased GvHD risk among recipients of matched donor grafts. Please see Chapter 2 (HLA Typing and Implications).

Other factors that have been shown to increase the risk of GvHD include donor gender and parity. Sex mismatch and, in particular, female to male transplant as well as previously parous donors, were shown to increase the risk of GvHD. Age of the donor has also been linked to GvHD in some studies but not in a recent Center for International Blood and Marrow Transplant Research (CIBMTR) retrospective analysis. CD34+ cell source (peripheral blood versus bone marrow), total CD34+ cell dose in the graft, intensity of conditioning and use of total body irradiation may increase the risk of acute GvHD and PB grafts that generally deliver a higher donor T-cell dose than marrow grafts appear to increase the risk of chronic GvHD. Thus, when a choice exists, selecting the best donor may help decrease the risk of GvHD and the need for more aggressive regimens to prevent GvHD. Please see Chapter 1 (Donor and Graft Selection Strategy).

Pharmacological prophylaxis for GvHD

Prevention of GvHD has been reliant on *in-vivo* suppression of donor T-cell activity or depletion of T-cell numbers through pharmacological methods or *ex-vivo* depletion of T-cells from the graft before infusion using pharmacologic or physical means. In this chapter, we will focus on the pharmacologic prevention of GvHD. Organizations tasked with accreditation of transplant programs (JACIE and FACT) have mandated that centers develop and use guidelines for GvHD prevention

---

Clinical Manual of Blood and Bone Marrow Transplantation, First Edition. Edited by Syed A. Abutalib and Parameswaran Hari.
© 2017 John Wiley & Sons Ltd. Published 2017 by John Wiley & Sons Ltd.

Table 9.1 The European Group for Blood and Marrow Transplantation and the European Leukemia Net Working Group consensus recommendations for GvHD prophylaxis in adult patients receiving a HLA-matched sibling or unrelated donor transplantation.

GvHD prophylaxis: myeloablative conditioning
The standard prophylaxis is CsA+ MTX. Tacrolimus + MTX is regarded as equivalent.
CsA
The initial dose is 3 mg/kg/day starting day −1.
The drug is given as short i.v. bolus infusion in two daily doses.
The administration is changed to oral route when oral intake is possible.
The first oral dose is twice the i.v. dose, administered in two daily doses.
The CsA target concentration is 200–300 µg/L during the first 3–4 weeks, then 100– 200 µg/L until 3 months after transplantation if there is no GvHD or toxicity.
The duration of CsA prophylaxis is 6 months in the absence of GvHD.
The dose is tapered from 3 months onwards if no GvHD is present. The dose is not tapered as long as there are signs of acute GvHD or signs of chronic GvHD exceeding mild skin disease.
MTX
The initial dose is 15 mg/m² given on day +1.
Three additional doses of 10 mg/m² are given, on days +3, +6, and +11.
The drug is given as bolus i.v. injection.
Leucovorin rescue is given to all patients.
GvHD prophylaxis: reduced-intensity conditioning
The standard prophylaxis is CsA + MMF.
MMF
The dose is 30 mg/kg/day, given p.o. in two doses.
The administration is started on day +1.
The duration of MMF prophylaxis is 1 month in sibling transplantations, 3 months in transplantations from unrelated or mismatched donor. In case of persistent disease or relapse (sub-population chimerism or other sensitive method) prevention should be reduced earlier.
ATG
ATG has been shown to reduce chronic GvHD and improve the quality of life in transplantations from an unrelated donor. Therefore, ATG can be included in the regimen for unrelated donor transplantations. Institutions using ATG should follow the EBMT/ELN recommendations or establish institutional guidelines and follow them.
The brand is ATG-F or Thymoglobulin.
The dose of ATG-F is 10 mg/kg on 3 days (total 30 mg/kg) and that of Thymoglobulin is 2.5 mg/kg on 3 days (total 7.5 mg/kg).
ATG is administered on days −3, −2, and −1.

CsA: Cyclosporin; MTX: methotrexate; ATG: anti-thymocyte globulin

and treatment. Guidelines for GvHD prophylaxis were recently published by the European group for Bone Marrow Transplant (EBMT) (Table 9.1). These guidelines differ somewhat from established practice in the United States where tacrolimus is typically used instead of cyclosporine.

Combinations using calcineurin inhibitors

The calcineurin inhibitors (CNI) cyclosporine and tacrolimus are considered the backbone of most GvHD prophylaxis regimens. Both medications have similar mechanism of action and toxicity profile. Cyclosporine is a cyclic peptide that was originally extracted from two strains of fungi is soil samples in 1969. Tacrolimus (FK506) is a macrolide antibiotic extracted from the soil fungus Streptomyces tsukubaensis. They share a similar mechanism of action. T-cell-receptor engagement results in calmodulin binding to calcium leading to binding of calcineurin. The activated calcineurin dephosphorylates nuclear factor of activated T-cells (NFAT) allowing its translocation into the nucleus to form a transcriptional activator of the IL-2 gene. Both cyclosporine and tacrolimus bind cytosolic proteins cyclophilin and tacrolimus binding protein (FKBP) leading to interruption of dephosphorylation of NFAT and preventing it from translocating to the nucleus to activate IL-2.

1-Cyclosporine plus methotrexate

Methotrexate is an antimetabolite, folic acid antagonist that is believed to cause immune suppression by inhibiting cellular growth and division in activated T-cells.

The earliest studies for GvHD prevention employed single agent prophylaxis with cyclosporine alone or a short course of methotrexate on days +1, +3, +6, and +11 post-transplant. However, in a randomized comparison, the combination of methotrexate and cyclosporine was found superior to either drug alone in preventing GvHD. The cumulative incidence of grade II–IV acute GvHD was reported to be in the range of 34% among leukemia patients receiving methotrexate plus cyclosporin compared to 54% among those receiving cyclosporine alone. These studies established the two-drug combination as the standard prophylaxis for some time.

Since the regimen of cyclosporine plus methotrexate regimen was developed in Seattle it has undergone some modifications. Cyclosporine is typically given on day 2 or 1 intravenously for several days till the patient can tolerate oral intake with adequate absorption. Methotrexate is given as a short intravenous course on days +1, +3, +6, and +11 with or without leucovorin rescue based on institutional guidelines. Although there are limited data to demonstrate direct correlation between the trough blood level of cyclosporine and clinical outcomes, it is routinely administered to achieve a therapeutic level that is determined by institutional guidelines. A trough level of 200–400 ng/ml in the first 90 days is what we follow at our institution. The EBMT group recommends a target of 200–300 ng/ml in the first 3–4 weeks then 100–200 ng/ml until 3 months post HCT if there is no evidence of GvHD. These levels are used to increase the dose if the level is below the therapeutic threshold. For levels that are above the target, the dose does not need to be reduced unless the patient is experiencing side effects or the level is 1.5–2 times higher than the upper limit of the therapeutic range.

The dose of methotrexate is 15 mg/m^2 on day +1 and 10 mg/m^2 on Days +3, +6, and +11. The alternative regimen of methotrexate especially when combined with tacrolimus (see later) labeled as "mini-dose methotrexate" includes a reduced dose of 5 mg/m^2 given on days +1, +3, +6, and +15. A comparison between both methotrexate schedules showed similar overall prevention of GvHD with lower toxicities among patients receiving the mini-methotrexate dose.

2-Tacrolimus (FK 506) plus methotrexte

Tacrolimus has been evaluated in combination with methotrexate and was compared to cyclosporine/methotrexate combination. Among recipients of HLA-identical marrow transplants, tacrolimus with methotrexate had a lower incidence of grade II–IV acute GvHD (41 vs 50%) compared to cyclosporine plus methotrexate. The difference was mostly in grade II acute GvHD. The tacrolimus group in this study had a higher incidence of regimen related toxicity, in particular, renal failure and hemodialysis that were seen in 19% of the tacrolimus group versus 8% of the cyclosporine group at 8 weeks post post-transplant. Other studies have shown at least equivalent results for tacrolimus plus methotrexate compared to cyclosporine plus methotrexate among recipients of unrelated donor transplantation. Based on these results, both tacrolimus and cyclosporine are in routine use for prevention of GvHD. The dose used in most of the clinical trials is 0.03–0.04 mg/kg/day as a continuous infusion and switched to oral once the patients can tolerate. The oral dose is 0.15 mg/kg/day divided in two daily dosages. Trough level monitoring is necessary with dose adjustment to maintain target levels. The exact target level has varied and ranges of 5–15 ng/ml and 10–20 ng/ml are commonly used.

3-Calcineurin inhibitors plus mycophenolate mofetil (MMF)

MMF is de-esterified to mycophenolic acid (MPA) *in vivo*. MPA inhibits the enzyme inosine monophosphate dehydrogenase, a critical enzyme in the *de novo* biosynthesis of purine nucleotides specifically guanosine monophosphate (GMP) resulting in inhibition of T-cell activation.

The combination of MMF with either CNI has been used following both reduced-intensity and myeloablative condition with apparently similar efficacy to methotrexate-based regimens. However, a recent retrospective analysis suggested an increased risk of grade III–IV acute GvHD among patients receiving cyclosporine plus MMF versus cyclosporine plus methotrexate after a myeloablative HLA-identical sibling transplantation. The drug is typically administered at 15 mg/kg/day in bid or tid dosing without monitoring of levels. Toxicity is mostly hematologic and gastrointestinal. In current practice, MMF plus CNI is mostly used in the reduced-intensity and non-ablative settings whereas methotrexate-based combinations are used in the myeloablative settings.

Sirolimus (rapamycin)

Sirolimus is a macrolide that is produced by a strain of Streptomyces hygroscopicus that binds to the same family of intracellular receptors as tacrolimus, called tacrolimus binding proteins or FKBPs. Sirolimus exhibits its immunosuppressive effects through different mechanisms: it inhibits the progression of cells from G_1 into the S phase and hence inhibiting cell proliferation, it affects signal transduction pathways that mediate cytokine responses, affects the CD28 signaling pathway that is required for T-cell activation and expands CD4+ CD25+ Foxp3+ regulatory T-cells.

Sirolimus has been used in the prevention of GvHD in combination with tacrolimus and methotrexate in the HLA-mismatched setting and with tacolimus alone in HLA-matched recipients. The data from these and other studies showed a low rate of grade II–IV GvHD (26% for HLA-mismatch and 10% for matched sibling recipients) suggesting that sirolimus is a promising alternative to methotrexate for GvHD propylaxis. The main concern of combining sirolimus plus calcineurin inhibitors is the increased risk of thrombotic microangiopathy. The use of sirolimus plus tacrolimus in the setting of myeloablative conditioning regimen using busulfan/cyclophosphamide was associated with a very high risk (55%) of thrombotic microangiopathy.

Pharmacologic T-cell depletion

1-Antithymocyte globulin (ATG)

ATG is a polyclonal immunoglobulin against the human T-cells. The efficacy and safety of ATG for the prevention of GvHD have been investigated through multiple studies with mixed results. A 2012 Cochrane meta-analysis investigating ATG use for GvHD prophylaxis included 568 patients and showed that ATG did not impact overall survival, incidence of relapse, and non-relapse mortality. The use of ATG had a lower incidence of grade II–IV acute GvHD (RR 0.68; 95% CI 0.55–0.85). This and many other studies fail to demonstrate a survival benefit of using ATG in this setting.

The impact of ATG and the dose was evaluated in two randomized trials (7.5 mg/kg/day and 15 mg/kg/day for 3 days). The higher dose of ATG was shown to have reduced GvHD incidence but with the cost of increased risk of lethal infections. Different preparations of ATG have been examined most commonly including rabbit ATG. The addition of rabbit ATG to a GvHD prophylaxis regimen of cyclosporine and methotrexate among recipients of matched unrelated donors resulted in lower incidence and severity of chronic GvHD without affecting relapse, survival, and grade III–IV acute GvHD. ATG in the reduced-intensity setting was investigated in a retrospective analysis among 1676 adults and was found to result in a similar rate of acute GvHD, lower rate of chronic GvHD, higher rates of relapse, and worse overall survival at three years. The exact role of ATG in allogeneic HCT remains unclear. The EBMT group recommends using ATG in the unrelated donor recipients in addition to the standard GvHD prophylaxis of calcineurin inhibitor plus MMF or methotrexate where it was shown to decrease the incidence of chronic GvHD.

2-Alemtuzumab (campath-1H)

Alemtuzumab is a humanized monoclonal antibody against CD52. CD52 is a protein on the surface of mature lymphocytes but not on lymphoid progenitors. Alemtuzumab binds CD52 and leads to an antibody-dependent cell mediated cytotoxicity leading to killing of the lymphocytes. Campath-1H has been used in reduced-intensity conditioning as well as haploidentical transplantation and was shown to enable durable engraftment and low incidence of GvHD. In the mismatched unrelated setting, campath was also associated with a low incidence of GvHD and similar overall survival despite a higher rate of graft rejections (8 vs 0%) when compared to match unrelated recipients. It is not universally used as part of GvHD prophylaxis due to concerns with infections and increased relapses. It has a longer half-life than ATG, is severely immunosuppressive at conventional doses and may require frequent donor lymphocyte infusions post transplantation to maintain chimerism and remission status.

Investigational therapies

Several newer approaches to GvHD prophylaxis are currently being investigated. *Regulatory T-cells* (CD4+ CD25+) T-cells are important modulators of self-tolerance and are critical in developing tolerance to alloantigens, hence decreasing incidence of GvHD. Several studies have established the feasibility of Tregs in GvHD prevention, however major challenges remain in manufacturing and purifying these cells on a large scale.

Mesenchymal stem cells (MSCs) are a heterogenous population of multipotent stromal cells that can differentiate into bone, cartilage, and fat cells. Recent studies showed that infusing third party MSCs may reduce high grade GvHD among recipients of mismatched unrelated HCT. MSCs were also tested among matched related recipients and was found to be associated with reduced GvHD but increased risk of relapse.

CTLA4-Ig also known as abatacept is a fusion protein of the Fc portion of human IgG1 fused with CTLA4 is approved for rheumatoid arthritis. The feasibility of abatacept in addition to methotrexate/cyclosporine was investigated among 10 patients receiving MUD HCT. A phase II randomized study is underway to assess GvHD prevention post HLA-MUD HCT.

Rituximab: The role of B-cells in the pathogenesis chronic GvHD and possibly also acute GvHD has become increasingly evident. Based on encouraging trials in the treatment of GvHD, the chimeric anti-CD20 monoclonal antibody rituximab has aroused interest as a prevention strategy. In a recent report from the CIBMTR, prior exposure to rituximab among 435 lymphoma patients was associated with a lower incidence of acute GvHD. The role of rituximab in GvHD prevention still warrants further evaluation.

Maraviroc is a chemokine receptor 5 (CCR5) antagonist that is approved for treatment of multi-drug resistant CCR5-tropic HIV-1. CCR5 also facilitates lymphocyte migration to target tissues and therefore, using a CCR5 inhibitor can potentially help decrease incidence of visceral GvHD. Maraviroc was combined with tacrolimus/methotrexate among 38 patients with reduced-intensity conditioning and yielded a low acute GvHD rate of 14.7% in the first 100 days.

Bortezomib is a proteasome inhibitor approved for the treatment of multiple myeloma. It blocks NF-Kappa β activation leading to blockage of T-cell activation, proliferation, and survival within alloreactive T-cells. Its use for GvHD prophylaxis with tacrolimus/methotrexate among HLA-mismatched unrelated recipients yielded a low incidence of grade 2–4 acute GvHD (22% at day 180), low chronic GvHD (29% at 1 year), and a 64% 2-year overall survival. The BMT Clinical trials network (BMTCTN) is evaluating maraviroc versus bortezomib versus a post-transplant cyclophosphamide based approach in a randomized phase II trial after reduced-intensity matched sibling or unrelated donor transplantation.

Histone deacetylase inhibitors (HDAC) modulate indoleamine-2,3-dioxygenase dependent innate immune and allo-stimulating function of antigen presenting cells in STAT-3 dependent manner and enhance Treg function. These mechanisms lead to inhibition of proinflammatory cytokines and prevention of GvHD. Vorinostat was combined with tacrolimus-MMF among adult patients receiving reduced-intensity conditioning from a matched related sibling. This prospective study showed a 22% incidence of acute GvHD and a low risk of relapse. Further studies to evaluate HDAC inhibitors are underway to delineate the role of these drugs in GvHD prevention.

Use of post-transplant cyclophosphamide (ptCy) to prevent GvHD

Administration of high-dose cyclophosphamide in the early post-transplant period (ptCy) has recently emerged as an effective strategy to prevent both acute and chronic GvHD following allografting. Initially developed clinically as a tool to control bidirectional alloreactivity following HLA-haploidentical donor transplants (HIDT), it has also been explored either alone or in combination with other agents as a GvHD prevention strategy following HLA-matched related and unrelated donor allografts.

Work in animal models first established that ptCy could induce tolerance to donor but not third party antigens when administer post allografting. Following pre-clinical work at Johns Hopkins University Luznik et al. developed a regimen for clinical HLA-haploidentical donor bone marrow transplantation using pre-transplant fludarabine and low dose TBI followed by bone marrow grafts and post-transplant high-dose cyclophosphamide administered on day 3 and 4 (ptCy) combined with tacrolimus and mycophenolate. The regimen appeared to effectively control alloreactivity following HIDT without the need for *ex-vivo* T-cell depletion or *in-vivo* serotherapy directed against T-cells. This approach appears to selectively target highly activated and proliferative alloreactive T-cells in the early post-transplant period while effector memory T-cells that are important for anti-infection immunity and Treg cells are spared unlike the case with non-selective strategies of ex-vivo or in-vivo T-depletion that rely on anti-T-cell antibodies. Consistent with the concept of selective depletion of alloreactive T-cells and sparing of effector memory cells targeting infection, a single center retrospective comparison from the M.D. Anderson Cancer Center demonstrated that rates of opportunistic infections and non-relapse mortality following T-replete haploidentical donor allografts using ptCy appears to be much lower than following haploidentical allografts using ex-vivo and in-vivo non-selective T-depletion. This resulted resulting in better rates of overall and progression-free survival following HIDT using ptCy. Furthermore, although randomized comparisons have not yet been reported, retrospective comparisons suggest that outcomes of haploidentical transplants using ptCy may not be inferior to those seen following conventional matched donor allografts. For example, a study of contemporaneous patients transplanted at a single center demonstrated that rates of acute and chronic GvHD, NRM, relapse, disease-free, and overall survival were similar in patients undergoing T-replete HIDT using ptCy when compared to patients who underwent conventional matched related and unrelated donor transplants. A study by the CIBMTR focusing on AML has also shown that HIDT-ptCy is associated with similar long term outcomes than 8 of 8 HLA allele matched unrelated donor transplants. Chronic GvHD appears significantly lower following HIDT-ptCy.

The degree of HLA-mismatch on the non-shared haplotype also does not appear to affect outcomes following HIDT-ptCy. While the original approach to HIDT-ptCy developed in Baltimore utilized a bone marrow graft with non-myeloablative conditioning, other investigators have shown that ptCy can also be used to effectively prevent GvHD following HIDT using PB graft and myeloablative regimens. The simplicity and efficacy of HIDT-ptCy has made it perhaps the most easily disseminated method for HIDT in comparison to the other approaches discussed previously. Furthermore, it appears to be the most economically viable. It is therefore likely that HIDT-ptCy will be significantly more popular than other approached to HIDT in the foreseeable future.

The successful use of ptCy for prevention of alloreactivity following HIDT has raised interest in using this approach for prevention of GvHD following conventional (HLA-identical sibling and matched unrelated) donor transplants. Luznik and colleagues reported on 117 patients treated with myeloablative doses of busulfan and cyclophosphamide who underwent allogeneic BMT from HLA-matched related or unrelated donors and received single agent high-dose post-transplant cyclophosphamide only for GvHD prophylaxis. Cumulative incidence of non-relapse mortality at two years was 17% and the maximum cumulative incidences of acute GvHD grade II–IV, grade III–IV, and chronic GvHD were 43, 10, and 10%, respectively, and did not different between related and unrelated donor transplants. These rates of GvHD were confirmed in a later analysis of 209 patients which also demonstrated that 43% of patients required no additional treatment for GvHD beyond the prophylaxis and that overall survival at 3 years was 58%. Similar outcomes were reported in a study of single agent ptCy for GvHD prophylaxis using myeloablative busulfan and fludarabine conditioning. Bone marrow was used almost exclusively as the graft source in these studies originating Johns Hopkins University. Other investigators have studied the use of ptCy as GvHD prophylaxis following PB allografts from matched related and unrelated donors. While studies using ptCy in combination with other immunosuppressive agents following PBSC grafts from matched donors have generally reported favorable rates of GvHD and post-transplant outcomes, some investigators have reported high rates of GvHD following PB grafts when ptCy alone was used as GvHD prophylaxis, for example high rates of acute and chronic GvHD were also reported in a trial of reduced-intensity busulfan and fludarabine and single agent ptCy for GvHD prophylaxis despite bone marrow being the predominant graft source. The authors implied that the ptCy as single agent may be insufficient for GvHD prophylaxis after reduced-intensity conditioning in matched donor allografts.

ptCy is well tolerated although both neutrophil and platelet engraftment are delayed by a few days when compared to conventional CNI and methotrexate GvHD prophylaxis even when a PB graft is used. Furthermore, BK virus associated cystitis that can manifest as bladder spasms, urinary frequency, and hemorrhage is more frequent particularly when high-dose busulfan is also used in the preparative regimen.

The simplicity, tolerability, and relative inexpensiveness of ptCy makes it an attractive option for GvHD prophylaxis. The available data suggest that ptCy in combination with tacrolimus and mycophenolate mofetil is highly effective at preventing severe detrimental post-transplant alloreactivity following HIDT. Indeed, the use of ptCy and T-replete grafts has proved revolutionary for HIDT making this type of donor usable for allografting as never before. Following matched donor transplants, single agent ptCy appears effective for GvHD prophylaxis when using myeloablative conditioning and bone marrow grafts. However, its adequacy as a single agent for GvHD prophylaxis when using PB grafts and/or reduced-intensity condition remains unclear and will be clarified by future studies. Combination GvHD prophylaxis of which ptCy is a part appears to be an effective strategy with all regimen intensities and graft sources.

Selected reading

1. Pidala J, Lee SJ, Ahn KW, Spellman S, Wang HL, Aljurf M, et al. Nonpermissive HLA-DPB1 mismatch increases mortality after myeloablative unrelated allogeneic hematopoietic cell transplantation. *Blood*. 2014 Oct 16;**124**(16): 2596–2606.

2. Rezvani AR, Storer BE, Guthrie KA, Schoch HG, Maloney DG, Sandmaier BM, et al. Impact of donor age on outcome after allogeneic hematopoietic cell transplantation. *Biology of Blood and Marrow Transplantation: Journal of the American Society for Blood and Marrow Transplantation*. 2015 Jan;**21**(1): 105–112.

3. Ruutu T, Gratwohl A, de Witte T, Afanasyev B, Apperley J, Bacigalupo A, et al. Prophylaxis and treatment of GvHD: EBMT-ELN working group recommendations for a standardized practice. *Bone Marrow Transplantation*. 2014 Feb;**49**(2): 168–173.

4. Ratanatharathorn V, Nash RA, Przepiorka D, Devine SM, Klein JL, Weisdorf D, et al. Phase III study comparing methotrexate and tacrolimus (prograf, FK506) with methotrexate and cyclosporine for graft-versus-host disease prophylaxis after HLA-identical sibling bone marrow transplantation. *Blood*. 1998 Oct 1;**92**(7):2303–2314.

5. Hamilton BK, Rybicki L, Dean R, Majhail NS, Haddad H, Abounader D, et al. Cyclosporine in combination with mycophenolate mofetil versus methotrexate for graft versus host disease prevention in myeloablative HLA-identical sibling donor allogeneic hematopoietic cell transplantation. *Am J Hematol*. 2015 Feb;**90**(2):144–148.

6. Rodriguez R, Nakamura R, Palmer JM, Parker P, Shayani S, Nademanee A, et al. A phase II pilot study of tacrolimus/ sirolimus GvHD prophylaxis for sibling donor hematopoietic stem cell transplantation using 3 conditioning regimens. *Blood*. 2010 Feb 4;**115**(5):1098–1105.

7. Solomon SR, Sizemore CA, Zhang X, Brown S, Holland HK, Morris LE, et al. Preemptive DLI without withdrawal of immunosuppression to promote complete donor T-cell chimerism results in favorable outcomes for high-risk older recipients of alemtuzumab-containing reduced-intensity unrelated donor allogeneic transplant: a prospective phase II trial. *Bone Marrow Transplantation*. 2014 May;**49**(5): 616–621.

8. Koura DT, Horan JT, Langston AA, Qayed M, Mehta A, Khoury HJ, et al. In vivo T-cell costimulation blockade with abatacept for acute graft-versus-host disease prevention: a first-in-disease trial. *Biology of Blood and Marrow Transplantation: Journal of the American Society for Blood and Marrow Transplantation*. 2013 Nov;**19**(11): 1638–1649.

9. Luznik L, O'Donnell PV, Symons HJ, Chen AR, Leffell MS, Zahurak M, et al. HLA-haploidentical bone marrow transplantation for hematologic malignancies using nonmyeloablative conditioning and high-dose, posttransplantation cyclophosphamide. *Biol Blood Marrow Transplant*. 2008 Jun;**14**(6):641–650.

10. Bashey A, Zhang X, Sizemore CA, Manion K, Brown S, Holland HK, et al. T-cell-replete HLA-haploidentical hematopoietic transplantation for hematologic malignancies using posttransplantation cyclophosphamide results in outcomes equivalent to those of contemporaneous HLA-matched related and unrelated donor transplantation. *J Clin Oncol*. 2013 Apr 1;**31**(10):1310–1316.

CHAPTER 10

Acute lymphoblastic leukemia

Ghada Zakout[1] and Adele K. Fielding[2]

[1] *Royal Free London NHS Foundation Trust, London, UK*

[2] *UCL Cancer Institute, London, UK*

Introduction

Current therapeutic modalities for acute lymphoblastic leukemia (ALL) in adults have resulted in a steady improvement in outcomes over the past two decades such that almost 90% of patients achieve complete remission (CR) with first-line therapy. However, the event-free survival (EFS) rates in adults are lower compared to those in children with relapse occurring in approximately 25–50%. Allogeneic hematopoietic cell transplantation (allo-HCT) is a frequent treatment modality in adults with ALL in their first remission (CR1) or subsequent remission and is recommended if an advantage in the projected disease-free survival (DFS) can be deduced from the patient's disease-related risk without being compromised by the transplant-related mortality (TRM). This requires disease-specific risk assessment including incorporation of time-dependent risk factors and identifying a "suitable" donor upon diagnosis, all within the context of an integrated, patient-tailored management approach (Figure 10.1).

ALL risk stratification – an evolving paradigm

Recent and emerging data from comprehensive genomic profiling of ALL has provided significant insights into leukemic heterogeneity thus allowing better understanding of its genetic basis through identifying key cellular leukemogenic permutations that has succinctly redefined the "standard-risk" subtype. It has also enabled the characterization of the relationship between inherited genetic variants, clonal heterogeneity, risk of relapse, and therapeutic targets. Nevertheless, the best way to of integrate these newly identified genomic profiles in the risk stratification is unclear. Many current risk stratifications and therapeutic algorithms incorporate several conventional pre-therapeutic risk factors that were originally based on retrospective large patient cohort analyses (Table 10.1). Their prognostic impact is very well established through a multitude of clinical trials. However, this is not the case for newly identified genomic features such as *IKZF1* alteration and the potentially-actionable Philadelphia chromosome (Ph)-like ALL mutations (see Roberts et al. review). These have been associated with poor prognosis in several studies, although their utility in refining prognosis in studies that employ intensive therapy and minimal residual disease (MRD)-driven risk stratification has varied among studies and cohorts.

A recent ad-hoc analysis by Dhédin et al. demonstrated that adult Ph-negative (Ph⁻) ALL patients with *IKZF1* focal deletion treated prospectively with pediatric-inspired induction therapy benefited from allo-HCT (HR: 0.42 (95% CI: 0.19–0.89); p = 0.025). However, analysis was confounded by exclusion of MRD responders (MRD negative) with the *IKZF1* deletion. Thus, new genomic information will require careful prospective evaluation in age-specific clinical algorithms that incorporate monitoring response by MRD for risk assignment.

Has MRD refined the risk-directed strategy for adult ALL?

MRD in ALL can be measured by PCR-based quantification of immunoglobulin/T-cell receptor rearrangements (Ig/TCR), flow cytometry using a leukemia-specific phenotype or more recently using next-generation sequencing to quantify patient-specific Ig/TCR. The association between MRD and disease relapse is well established using the first

Clinical Manual of Blood and Bone Marrow Transplantation, First Edition. Edited by Syed A. Abutalib and Parameswaran Hari.

© 2017 John Wiley & Sons Ltd. Published 2017 by John Wiley & Sons Ltd.

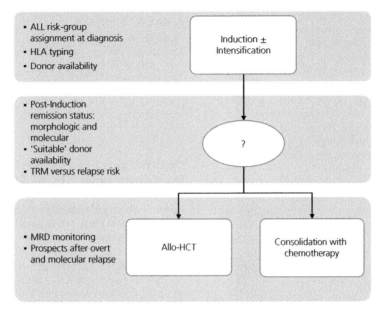

Figure 10.1 Variables for decision making prior to allo-HCT in adult ALL patients in CR1.

Table 10.1 Basic ALL prognostic parameters currently used in various protocols to define "high-risk."

	Clinical	"Genetic"
Adverse risk factors used to determine who might have "upfront" allo-HCT	Advancing age	*BCR-ABL1* translocation
	High Presenting WBC: B-cell phenotype; >30 × 10⁹/L T-cell phenotype; >100 × 10⁹/L	*MLL-AF4* translocation
	Persistence of MRD at a protocol-relevant timepoint	Complex (≥5 unrelated chromosomal abnormalities without other established abnormality)
		Low-hypodiploid (30–39 chromosomes)/near-triploid (60 to 78 chromosomes)

two methods in both pediatric and adult ALL settings, which allowed for risk assignment. It is widely perceived as the strongest independent risk parameter for relapse. There are no clinical trials to-date that have examined applicability of allo-HCT based solely on MRD status, though this is subject to investigation in the next French Group for Research on Adult ALL (GRAALL)-2014 trial. So, what can be inferred from currently available evidence regarding the role of MRD pre-allo-HCT?

Philadelphia chromosome-negative (Ph⁻) ALL

Gökbuget et al. for the German Multicenter Adult ALL Study Group (GMALL) used polymerase chain reaction (PCR) of patient-specific immunoglobulin heavy chain/T-cell receptor (Ig/TCR) gene rearrangements to detect MRD to identify patients with MRD levels of $>10^{-4}$ or $>5 \times 10^{-4}$ at protocol-relevant timepoints as "poor MRD responders" with particularly poor prognosis. A potential benefit from allo-HCT was demonstrated. Two other prospective nonrandomized trials; Northern Italy Leukemia Group (NILG) and GRAALL had similar findings. Conversely, Ribera et al. did not observe superiority of allo-HCT over chemotherapy in poor early cytological/MRD responders (using multicolor flow cytometry (MFC)), likely attributed to a lower 5-year DFS (32%) post-allo-HCT than expected. Bassan et al. correlated quantitative post-induction Ig/TCR-MRD and allo-HCT outcome. Patients with MRD from 10^{-4} to $<10^{-3}$ had superior overall survival (OS) (60% versus 27%) and DFS (60% *vs* 18%) and lower relapse (23%

versus 64%) compared with those with level $\geq 10^{-3}$ despite all MRD-positive patients benefiting from allo-HCT (6-year OS: 42% vs 18% with auto-HCT). Dhédin et al. reported superior relapse free survival (RFS) in Ph⁻ patients with Ig/TCR-MRD level $\geq 10^{-3}$ post pediatric-inspired induction therapy who underwent allo-HCT. However, patients with a level $<10^{-3}$ had equivalent outcomes whether transplanted or treated with chemotherapy. Ribera et al. did not offer allo-HCT to Ph⁻ "high-risk" patients with MRD levels $<5 \times 10^{-4}$ at week +17 and good early morphologic response. These two studies challenged the long-standing precept in some centers of allo-HCT as the "definitive" post-remission therapy in adults and suggest that allo-HCT can be avoided in good MRD responders. The United States Children's Oncology Group (COG) showed that next-generation sequencing (NGS)-MRD predicted early post-allo-HCT relapse and survival more accurately than MFC-MRD in 56 Ph⁻ ALL patients aged up to 21 years, especially the MRD-negative cohort. Logan et al. showed the predictive power of NGS-MRD for post-allo-HCT relapse with pre-allo-HCT levels $\geq 10^{-4}$ and post-allo-HCT levels $\geq 10^{-6}$ in 29 adult patients. This technique is yet to be evaluated in larger prospective cohorts.

Philadelphia chromosome-positive (Ph⁺) ALL

Prior to tyrosine kinase inhibitor (TKI)-era, several studies demonstrated good correlation between *BCR-ABL1* status post-induction therapy and outcome but the levels differed in their discriminative value at different time-points. With TKIs, this correlation was more consistent. Lee et al. used CML criteria for assessing MRD response kinetics and identified that a ≥ 3-log reduction in *BCR-ABL1* transcript level following 4-week imatinib therapy strongly predicted superior 4-year OS and DFS. GRAALL showed imatinib-related improved molecular remission rates pre-transplant was associated with improved outcome.

However, the correlation between MRD status pre-allo-HCT and outcome has not been universally noted. In two successive studies by Mortuza et al. PCR-MRD was not predictive of post-allo-HCT relapse. Patel et al. reported similar finding in 36 B-ALL allo-HCT recipients; 5-year EFS was 52% for PCR-MRD-positive patients versus 50%. Several factors account for such discrepancy including heterogeneity of studied cohort, pre-transplant chemotherapy, conditioning regimen, and donor source.

Optimal post-remission therapy for adults with ALL in CR1

Data with myeloablative conditioning regimen and HLA-MSD and HLA-matched Urelated Donor
Ph⁻ ALL

Despite significant progress in adult ALL management, the optimal post-remission therapy including the role of allo-HCT remains unresolved. The fact that each study has used subtly different factors to define "high-risk" (and hence which patients should receive allo-HCT) has also been a complicating factor in interpretation of data. Several prospective trials – including a meta-analysis and a Cochrane Collaborative Review – have confirmed the survival advantage in having a HLA-matched sibling donor over no-donor where the latter received chemotherapy or autologous HCT (auto-HCT) (Table 10.2). The largest trial, UKALLXII/Eastern Cooperative Oncology Group (ECOG) E2993 reported a superior 5-year OS of patients with Ph⁻ ALL with a sibling donor compared to those with no donor and lower relapse rate risk across all adult age group. In this study "adult" was defined as 15–65 years, although in modern practice, 15 years old would no longer be considered an adult. In a sub-group analysis, the lack of benefit for the high-risk group was clearly attributed to high non-relapse mortality (NRM) in older patients. Similar results were reported by Cornelissen et al. from two prospective studies for the Hemato-Oncologie voor Volwassenen Nederland (HOVON) group.

Philadelphia chromosome-positive (Ph⁺) ALL

In the pre-TKI era treatment outcomes for adult Ph⁺ ALL patients were dismal and allo-HCT was considered the optimal post-remission therapy. This has been demonstrated by two large prospective trials – UKALLXII/ECOG E2993 and LALA-94, which reported superior outcomes in allo-HCT recipients over chemotherapy. Several phase II studies incorporating TKI to treatment regimens showed substantial improvement in outcomes

Table 10.2 Summary of select published trials in Adult ALL.

Author	N Total / N allo	Trial Setting	Conditioning	cGvHD allo-HCT	TRM	OS	DFS	Comments and Practice Implications
(A) Donor vs No-Donor Studies								
Goldstone et al.	1031/72	Post-induction allo-HCT assignment based on donor availability	13.2Gy TBI/Etoposide	N/R	@2 y: high-risk: 36% donor, 14% no-donor; standard-risk: 20% donor, 7% no-donor	@5 y: high-risk: 41% donor, 35% no-donor; standard-risk: 62% donor, 52% no-donor	N/R	Survival benefit with allo-HCT in the standard-risk but not high-risk group
Cornelisson et al.	257/96	As above	12Gy TBI/Cy	N/R	@5 y: 16% donor; 3% no-donor	@5 y: high-risk: 53% donor vs 41% no-donor; standard-risk: 69% donor vs 49% no-donor	Donor 60% vs no-donor 42% (p = 0.01)	Standard-risk patients with sibling donor had favorable survival with allo-HCT due to reduced relapse and NRM
Ribera et al.	156/72	As above	12Gy TBI/Cy	N/R	10% donor; 2% no-donor	44% donor, 35% no-donor	39% donor, 35% no-donor	No survival benefit with matched sibling donor allo-HCT or chemotherapy in high-risk patients
Kako et al.	649/408	decision analysis of ALL93 and ALL97 trials to identify the optimal strategy in adult Ph+ ALL patients in CR1	N/R	N/R	N/R	@10y: standard-risk: allo-HCT, 54%; chemotherapy, 40%; high-risk: allo-HCT 38%; chemotherapy 25%	Ph+ patients @6y: allo-HCT (n = 8) 44%; chemotherapy (n = 14) 7%	Allo-HCT was superior to other therapies for 10-year survival probability
(B) RIC vs MAC								
Mohty et al.	NA/449 MAC, 127 RIC	Retrospective comparative analysis of RIC vs MAC allo-HCT outcomes	MAC: Cy/high-dose TBI or high-dose chemotherapy RIC: low-dose TBI or chemotherapy alone (other chemotherapy±flu)	34%; comparable between MAC and RIC (p = 0.37)	@2 y: MAC 29%, RIC 21%; p = 0.03	@2 y: MAC 45%, RIC 48% (p = 0.56)	@2 y: MAC 38%, RIC 32%; p = 0.07	RIC allo-HCT is a potential option for patients not eligible for MAC
Marks et al.	NA/1428 FI, 93 RIC	Compared RIC outcomes with FI allo-HCT in Ph-ALL in CR1 or CR2	FI: Cy/TBI or Cy/high-dose bu RIC: busulfan, melphalan, low-dose TBI or flu/2Gy TBI	@3 y: FI 42%, RIC 34% (p = 0.16)	@3 y: 33% FI, 33% RIC	@3 y: 51% FI, 45% RIC	@3 y: FI 49%, RIC 36%	conditioning intensity didn't affect TRM or relapse risk
Nishiwaki et al.	NA/81 MAC, 26 RIC	Comparative retrospective analysis of RIC vs MAC in adult Ph- ALL in CR outcomes	N/R	N/R	@2 y: MAC 40%, RIC 36%	@2 y: MAC 58%, RIC 63%	@2 y: MAC 58%, RIC 63%; p = 0.90	RIC allo-HCT is a viable therapeutic option for Ph- ALL

Abbreviations: Cy – Cyclophosphamide, Flu – Fludarabine, Gy – Gray, TBI – Total body irradiation, FI – full-intensity, N/R – not reported, NA – not applicable

with CR rates often exceeding those attained in Ph⁻ ALL even when induction intensity was reduced. Chalandon et al. reported a randomized prospective study showing fewer induction deaths and higher CR rates in recipients of high-dose imatinib/reduced-intensity chemotherapy compared with standard imatinib/chemotherapy. There was no difference in major molecular response rate between the arms. Allo-HCT was associated with significant improvement in RFS and OS. With such improvement in outcomes conferred by TKI, is allo-HCT dispensable in Ph⁺ ALL? A report from the COG of Ph⁺ ALL patients aged up to 21 years showed similar 3-year EFS rate among patients who received imatinib/chemotherapy (88%) compared to allo-HCT from HLA-matched related (57%) or unrelated (72%) donor, without major toxicities with imatinib. A significant proportion of patients underwent off-protocol MUD allo-HCT which confounded data interpretation. However, these data have suggested that children and young persons up to 21 years of age may be spared allo-HCT. A subgroup analysis of 94 Ph⁺ ALL patients from NILG reported significantly higher 5-year OS (38 vs 23%; p = 0.009) and DFS (39% versus 25%; p = 0.005) rates in patients who received imatinib and underwent allo-HCT when compared to those who did not receive imatinib. An intent-to-treat analysis in UKALLXII/ECOG E2993 reported superior OS, EFS, and RFS in the imatinib versus historic non-imatinib cohort treated in the same trial; partly attributed to more patients achieving allo-HCT (46 vs 31%). Overwhelming evidence supports a survival advantage of TKI in combination with chemotherapy. There is insufficient evidence to support omission of allo-HCT in Ph⁺ ALL adults.

> **PRACTICE POINTS**
>
> Adult ALL patients and where applicable their sibling(s) should undergo HLA-typing upon diagnosis to facilitate later allo-HCT if needed, as some poor prognostic factors such as persistence of MRD will not be clear at diagnosis.

Transplant from an alternative donor using MAC/ regimen in CR1

The role of alternative donor allo-HCT in ALL is not well defined with most of the data from registries by and large included children, small sample sizes, collectively analyzed all acute leukemia patients, and/or being observational from single centers. However, approximately 25–30% of patients in the "transplantable" age group have an HLA-MSD, so there is an increasing need for expanding donor options. The likelihood of finding 8/8 HLA-MUD using high-resolution HLA-typing for

Caucasians, Hispanics, and Blacks is approximately 75, 35, and 18%, respectively, as per a population-based genetic model by the US donor registry. Seven on 8 HLA-MUD increases this to 90, 75, and 70%. When HLA-haploidentical or umbilical cord blood (UCB) transplants are considered a donor can be found for over 95% of the patients. However, this expansion, at present, is at the expense of potentially higher NRM, GvHD, and graft failure, which increases with age and increasing HLA disparities despite more resolute HLA-typing and improved supportive care. Therefore, careful considerations should be made when deciding to transplant using an alternative donor.

HLA-MUD transplants

Cornelissen et al. reviewed the National Marrow Donor Program (NMDP) experience pre-TKI era of HLA-MUD allo-HCT in 127 adults with poor-risk ALL (defined as having t(9;22), t(4;11), or t(1;19)). Independent predictors of better DFS included short interval between diagnosis and transplantation, transplantation in CR1, DRB1 locus match (10/10 HLA-match), t(9;22) and donor/recipient CMV negativity. Nishiwaki et al. reported comparable outcome in HLA-MSD (n=310) and HLA-MUD (n=331) allo-HCT Ph⁻ ALL recipients. Four-year relapse rates were significantly higher in HLA-MUD recipients (32 vs 22%; p = 0.03) but with lower NRM (14% vs 27%; p=0.0002) and grade II–IV aGvHD) (42 vs 30%). A retrospective observational analysis for Center for International Blood and Marrow Transplant Research (CIBMTR) by Marks et al. of 169 adult Ph⁻ ALL patients who received MAC HLA-MUD allo-HCT in CR1 reported 5-year TRM, relapse and OS rates of 42, 20, and 39%.

Cord blood transplants

Despite the low cell dose, the less stringent HLA-matching, rapid accessibility and lower acute and chronic GvHD (cGvHD) incidence makes UCB a more appealing choice though its utility in adults is principally based on pediatric experiences. A CIBMTR retrospective analysis by Eapen et al. reported comparable leukemia-free survival (LFS) rates for less well-matched UCB and 8/8 and 7/8 unrelated donor allele-matched allo-HCT recipients but with higher TRM. Ferrá et al. included higher-risk patients and reported comparable 5-year survival in UCB and MUD allo-HCT recipients though with slightly higher OS (33 vs 22%). Atsuta et al. reported similar 3-year OS and relapse rates in UCB and MUD bone marrow allo-HCT ALL recipients but with significantly lower TRM and aGvHD in the UCB recipients.

HLA-Haploidentical transplants

HLA-Haploidentical donor allo-HCT usually requires T-cell depletion of the graft or post-transplant cyclophosphamide "tolerization" to eliminate allo-reactive T-cells, thereby minimizing GvHD and allowing earlier immunologic recovery. This approach has shown promising results primarily in acute myeloid leukemia though remains investigational and requires further exploration in larger trials.

One antigen mismatch transplants

Valcárcel et al. for CIBMTR demonstrated no statistically significant difference in OS, DFS, TRM, or relapse between one antigen-mismatched related donor (MMRD) and MUD allo-HCT though cGvHD incidence was significantly lower in the former. Kanda et al. observed statistically significant higher overall mortality rates in single-antigen MMRD recipients when compared with 8/8 HLA-MUD recipients in standard-risk but not high-risk acute leukemia patients.

> **PRACTICE POINTS**
>
> Current evidence is insufficient to guide decisions on using HLA-MUD, UCB, haploidentical, or HLA-MMRD allo-HCT over HLA-MSD transplants. In the absence of a "suitable" HLA-matched (MSD and MUSH) donor, an alternative donor (haploidentical and/or UCB) search may be considered if very high-risk features are identified at diagnosis or post-induction therapy.

MAC allo-HCT beyond CR1

ALL following relapse is associated with second remission (CR2) rates from 31–44% following first salvage therapy and long-term OS of only 5–8%. Presently allo-HCT represents the only therapy capable of conferring long-term survival, although there is a higher TRM and relapse rates. Where applicable, participation in a clinical trial is recommended.

Refractory ALL has a dismal prognosis and the utility of allo-HCT remains controversial where CR cannot be achieved. CIBMTR evaluated the outcome of 582 ALL patients not in remission at the time of MAC allo-HCT. Three-year survival was 16% and day 100 mortality rate was 41%. Four adverse pre-transplantation variables influenced survival; refractory first or later relapse, ≥25% marrow blasts, CMV-positive donor and age > 10 years. Patients with ≤1 of these variables had a 3-year OS of 46% vs 10% in those with ≥3 thus delineating subgroups were allo-HCT may be a reasonable option.

> **PRACTICE POINTS**
>
> All fit patients of suitable age with relapsed ALL who achieve CR should be offered MAC allo-HCT with conventional or alternative donors.

Emerging role for RIC regimens in ALL

RIC allo-HCT, which relies principally on harnessing the putative graft-versus-leukemia (GvL) effect with the "theoretical" advantage of preserving T-cell reconstitution, has extended allo-HCT utility to "older" and/or "less fit" patients given its lower TRM. Data on its use in ALL is limited and difficult to interpret due to regimen and patient characteristics variability and are summarized in Table 10.2. The European Blood and Marrow Transplantation (EBMT) reported outcomes of 576 ALL adults who underwent allo-HCT in CR1 from HLA-MSD and showed a lower 2-year NRM but higher relapse incidence with RIC versus MAC allo-HCT. There was comparable LFS, although the numbers analyzed were insufficient to detect small differences. Marks et al. reported no difference in outcomes between recipients of RIC and MAC in Ph⁻ ALL patients who underwent HLA-MSD or -MUD allo-HCT in CR1 or CR2 in an IBMTR study. The British Society of Blood and Marrow Transplantation Registry (BSBMT) evaluated the feasibility of *in-vivo* TCD approach in high-risk Ph⁻ ALL patients to lower GvHD and reported a 5-year OS, DFS, and relapse mortality of 61, 59, and 13%. The incidences of grade II–IV aGvHD and extensive cGvHD were 27 and 22%. These encouraging results have made RIC transplantation in "older," less fit patients more plausible but require further scrutiny within prospective standardized setting, which is being undertaken in the ongoing United Kingdom multicenter trial, UKALL14 (NCT01085617).

> **PRACTICE POINTS**
>
> RIC allo-HCT can be considered when the higher risk for TRM such as age and/or comorbidities is prohibitive for MAC allo-HCT.

Does intensity of conditioning regimen matters in ALL?

Various studies comparing outcomes of RIC with MAC in ALL patients have already been discussed (see previous and Table 10.2). These studies have several limitations including significant heterogeneity in patient cohort and/or lack of details in comorbidities and decision-making process. Analysis is not uncommonly confounded by selection bias with patients at high risk of relapse being pragmatically selected for MAC and advanced age and/or comorbidities vindicating RIC. No study to-date has shown superiority of RIC over MAC in ALL. Although several investigators advocate a set age cutoff of 40 years for MAC allo-HCT it should be noted that chronologic age alone is not sufficient surrogate for defining fitness. Individual patient evaluation to determine conditioning choice should be undertaken.

How to evaluate MRD after allo-HCT and what action to take?

Zhao et al. evaluated the prognostic significance of post-allo-HCT MRD monitoring in 139 patients primarily by flow cytometry. MRD-positive patients had lower EFS (0.54 vs 0.80; p < 0.001) and higher relapse rates (0.54 vs 0.08; p < 0.001) compared with MRD-negative patients with post-allo-HCT MRD and this was an independent prognostic factor on multivariate analysis. Flow cytometrically determined-MRD correlated with PCR-determined-MRD. However, approximately 25% of patients lost their leukemia-associated phenotype post-allo-HCT so flow cytometrically determined MRD required cautious interpretation. Mortuza et al. reported that the presence of MRD post-allo-HCT was associated with increased relapse risk in patients with Ph⁻ ALL. Spinelli et al. used Ig/TCR MRD assessment and showed significantly lower 3-year relapse rate in high-risk patients with MRD PCR-negativity at day +100 post-allo-HCT; 7 versus 80% for those who were PCR-positive.

Whether MRD timing and/or kinetics facilitate decision making in the peri-transplant setting remains to be shown in unbiased large-scale prospective studies.

> **PRACTICE POINTS**
>
> Patients with measurable MRD post-allo-HCT should be considered for pre-emptive immunotherapy including rapid immunosuppression withdrawal and/or donor lymphocyte infusion (DLI) or other novel approaches where available in the window prior to overt relapse. Methods of measuring MRD and their standardization differ between countries and the relevance of MRD is strictly related to the protocol used, so no firm guidelines can be given in such a chapter. An excellent review of the topic and how it is evolving in ALL is provided by Van Dongen et al.

Is there evidence to merit chimerism monitoring in ALL?

Persistence or reappearance of recipient hematopoiesis measured primarily by fluorescence-based PCR amplification of short tandem repeat markers termed as mixed chimerism may signal a risk of disease relapse thereby providing a window for therapeutic intervention. Its utility in ALL for predicting relapse risk is not definitive with data mainly based on retrospective analyses from relatively small series, inconsistent timing and methodology, heterogeneity of patient cohort, and being primarily investigated in pediatric settings where distinct immunologic mechanisms may exist. A retrospective analysis of 101 MAC allo-HCT recipients by Tewrey et al. showed that increased recipient chimerism in any cell subset predicted relapse. Measurement of chimerism on bone marrow samples detected relapse risk 2–3 months earlier than peripheral blood though was less specific. Comparative subgroup analysis showed MRD being much more sensitive and specific in predicting relapse than chimerism. Unlike MRD studies chimerism analysis can predict isolated extramedullary relapse. There are no clear data to support the utility of lineage-specific chimerism in predicting relapse in ALL, despite its in-vitro sensitivity.

Despite scant evidence on the role of chimerism in adult ALL, the kinetics of chimerism, rather than a single timepoint analysis is likely to be a reasonable approach.

> **PRACTICE POINTS**
>
> Where a patient appears to show progressive loss of donor chimerism, intervention either by immunosuppression tapering and/or institution of DLI to promote conversion to full-donor chimerism should be considered. Administration of DLI in the situation of mixed T-cell chimerism following allo-HCT for ALL is currently being prospectively evaluated in the multicenter UK National Research Cancer Institute (NCRI) UKALL14 trial.

Does DLI post-allo-HCT for ALL work?

There is robust evidence for GvL effect in ALL, which is primarily driven by donor-derived T lymphocytes. A report by CIBMTR of 1132 ALL patients showed those with GvHD reduced relapse risk whether transplanted in CR1 or CR2 irrespective of their phenotype. Lee et al. reported significant anti-leukemic effect conferred by cGvHD on relapse risk in adult ALL MAC allo-HCT recipients. However, in a larger retrospective analysis from CIBMTR that included 1798 ALL MAC allo-HCT recipients cGvHD did not impact late relapses; 5-year relative risk: 1.09 (95% CI: 0.87–1.37) owing to significantly higher TRM and inferior outcomes. Despite the large sample size, lack of standardized GvHD definition and variability in GvHD treatment confounds data interpretation. Terwey et al. applied the NIH cGvHD grading consensus criteria and reported superior OS due to fewer relapses in patients who developed cGvHD of any grade, though this was not associated with improved NRM.

These studies demonstrate a GvL effect of allo-HCT in ALL and have led to DLI being used in three different scenarios: for treatment of hematological relapse, as prophylaxis in patients at high risk of post-allo-HCT relapse or to promote attainment of full-donor chimerism. The efficacy of DLI in relapsed in ALL is may be limited by ALL cells ability to evade immunologic attack through induction of T-cell anergy, inadequate co-stimulation, and insensitivity to donor NK-cell alloreactivity. Several groups have published small reports on DLI given post-allo-HCT for frank relapse and showed very limited success.

PRACTICE POINTS

DLI should be considered where there is evidence of molecular relapse and/or worsening donor chimerism, preferentially within a clinical trial. Since GvHD is the main complication of DLI, the benefit/risk ratio must be considered carefully as when given as prophylaxis or to promote full donor chimerism.

Post-allo-HCT TKI for Ph+ ALL

The need for TKI post-allo-HCT, under what circumstances, and for how long remains unclear. Pfeifer et al. prospectively randomized 55 patients to starting imatinib either 3 months post-allo-HCT versus only on *BCR-ABL1* positivity and showed no significant difference in outcome (5-year OS: 82 vs 78%) - but noted poor tolerability, resulting in early discontinuation. Ram et al. reported better tolerability with imatinib when given following RIC allo-HCT which was associated with reduced mortality, though its effect on relapse was not significant.

PRACTICE POINTS

Post-transplant TKI decisions can made upon individual patient assessment as long as *BCR-ABL1* is closely monitored and remains negative, but where patients remain or become *BCR-ABL1* positive after allo-HCT, addition of TKI and-or-consideration of other therapies is strictly necessary to prevent relapse.

Relapse post-allo-HCT

Relapse post-allo-HCT is associated with extremely poor prognosis. Treatment options vary from palliation to a second allo-HCT. Current data indicate limited efficacy of the latter. Duration of remission after first allo-HCT is the most relevant prognostic factor together with development of cGvHD following DLI, which is associated with highest rate of response. A retrospective analysis by EBMT of 465 adult patients who relapsed post-allo-HCT reported 5-year survival of 8% (median survival 5.5 months) with only six of 93 patients who underwent second allo-HCT remained alive. Several immunologic and oncogene-targeted approaches are being investigated/under development and could be considered preferentially within a clinical trial. Of these blinatumomab, inotuzumab and chimeric antigen receptor T-cells engineered to target CD19 have shown promising early results in post-transplant relapse.

See Table 10.3 for the authors' practice.

Table 10.3 Who, when, and how of allo-HCT for ALL.

Authors' practice:

A. PATIENT FACTORS:

Age:
We do not typically recommend allo-HCT for those over the age 70 years. We consider biological over chronological age with meticulous attention to performance status (PS), comorbidities, age-specific life expectancy and other disease-related high-risk features

PS and Comorbidity:
ECOG PS 0–1 and with no substantial comorbidities (see Chapters 3 and 4)

B. DISEASE FACTORS:

Newly diagnosed ALL:

ALL Risk Stratification:
See Table 10.1

Relapsed ALL:
Allo-HCT is offered only upon achieving morphologic CR in our center

C. DONOR EVALUATION:
Ideal: HLA-matched sibling donor followed by HLA-MUD

Alternative donor: If the above is not available:
Single-antigen HLA- mismatched or haploidentical donor in (the context of a clinical trial where available) is offered in our center

D. CONDITIONING THERAPY:
Where transplant forms part of a clinical trial, trial protocol will be followed. Otherwise patients aged ≤ 40 years receive TBI-based MAC regimen and those > 40 years RIC regimen. We consider MAC for high-risk patients aged up to 45 if fit, without co-morbidity and following rigorous pre-transplant organ function assessment

E. POST ALLOTRANSPLANT THERAPY:
RIC allo-HCT recipients receive 3-monthly prophylactic intrathecal methotrexate for 2 years post-transplant for CNS prophylaxis starting 3 months post-transplant. DLI may be given for mixed-chimera and/or MRD-positivity in the context of a clinical trial where available.

We do not routinely restart TKI post-allo-HCT for Ph+ ALL without evidence of molecular relapse. We test for *BCR-ABL1* domain-kinase mutations to exclude emerging resistance to TKI.

Selected reading

1. Roberts KG and Mullighan CG. Genomics in acute lymphoblastic leukaemia: insights and treatment implications. *Nat Rev Clin Oncol* 2015; **12**(6):344–357.
2. Dhedin N, Huynh A, Maury S, Tabrizi R, et al. and the GRAALL group. Role of allogeneic stem cell transplantation in adult patients with Ph-negative acute lymphoblastic leukemia. *Blood* 2015 Apr 16;**125**(16):2486–2496; quiz 2586.
3. Ribera JM, Oriol A, Morgades M, et al. Treatment of highrisk Philadelphia chromosome-negative acute lymphoblastic leukemia in adolescents and adults according to early cytologic response and minimal residual disease after consolidation assessed by flow cytometry: final results of the PETHEMA ALL-AR-03 trial. *J Clin Oncol.* 2014 May 20;**32**(15):1595–1604.
4. Mortuza FY, Papaioannou M, Moreira IM, et al. Minimal residual disease tests provide an independent predictor of clinical outcome in adult acute lymphoblastic leukemia. *J Clin Oncol.* 2002 Feb 15;**20**(4):1094–1104.
5. Patel B, Rai L, Buck G, et al. Minimal residual disease is a significant predictor of treatment failure in non T-lineage adult acute lymphoblastic leukaemia: final results of the international trial UKALL XII/ECOG2993. *Br J Haematol.* 2010 Jan;**148**(1):80–89.
6. Cornelissen JJ, van der Holt B, Verhoef GE, et al. Dutch-Belgian HOVON Cooperative Group. Myeloablative allogeneic versus autologous stem cell transplantation in adult patients with acute lymphoblastic leukemia in first remission: a prospective sibling donor versus no-donor comparison. *Blood.* 2009 Feb 5;**113**(6):1375–82. doi: 10.1182/blood-2008-07-168625.
7. Fielding AK. Philadelphia-positive acute lymphoblastic leukemia – is bone marrow transplant still necessary? *Biol Blood Marrow Transplant* 2011;**17**(1 Suppl):S84–88.
8. Dombret H, Gabert J, Boiron JM, et al. (GET-LALA Group). Outcome of treatment in adults with Philadelphia chromosome-positive acute lymphoblastic leukemia–results of the prospective multicenter LALA-94 trial. *Blood.* 2002 Oct 1; **100**(7):2357-66.PMID:12239143.
9. Cornelissen JJ, Carston M, Kollman C, et al. Unrelated marrow transplantation for adult patients with poor-risk acute lymphoblastic leukemia: strong graft-versus-leukemia effect and risk factors determining outcome. *Blood.* 2001 Mar 15;**97**(6):1572–1577.
10. Marks DI, Perez WS, He W, et al. Unrelated donor transplants in adults with Philadelphia-negative acute lymphoblastic leukemia in first complete remission. *Blood.* 2008 Jul 15;**112**(2):426–434.
11. Eapen M, Rubinstein P, Zhang MJ, et al. Comparable long-term survival after unrelated and HLA-matched sibling donor hematopoietic stem cell transplantations for acute leukemia in children younger than 18 months. *J Clin Oncol.* 2006 Jan 1;**24**(1):145–151.
12. Mohty M, Labopin M, Volin L, et al. and Acute Leukemia Working Party of EBMT. Reduced-intensity versus conventional myeloablative conditioning allogeneic stem cell transplantation for patients with acute lymphoblastic leukemia: a retrospective study from the European Group for Blood and Marrow Transplantation. *Blood.* 2010 Nov 25;**116**(22):4439–4443.
13. Zhao XS, Liu YR, Zhu HH, et al. Monitoring MRD with flow cytometry: an effective method to predict relapse for ALL patients after allogeneic hematopoietic stem cell transplantation. *Ann Hematol.* 2012 Feb;**91**(2):183–192.
14. Terwey TH, Hemmati PG, Nagy M, et al. Comparison of chimerism and minimal residual disease monitoring for relapse prediction after allogeneic stem cell transplantation for adult acute lymphoblastic leukemia. *Biol Blood Marrow Transplant.* 2014 Oct;**20**(10):1522–1529.
15. Ram R, Storb R, Sandmaier BM, et al. Non-myeloablative conditioning with allogeneic hematopoietic cell transplantation for the treatment of high-risk acute lymphoblastic leukemia. *Haematologica.* 2011 Aug;**96**(8):1113–1120.

CHAPTER 11

Acute myeloid leukemia

Hillard M. Lazarus[1] and Masumi Ueda[2]

[1] *Department of Medicine, University Hospitals Seidman Cancer Center, Case Western Reserve University, Cleveland, OH, USA*

[2] *Clinical Research Division, Fred Hutchinson Cancer Research Center, Seattle, WA, USA*

Introduction

Outcomes for persons with acute myeloid leukemia (AML) undergoing allogeneic hematopoietic cell transplantation (HCT) have improved in recent years as a result of progress in supportive care, graft-versus-host disease (GvHD) prevention and treatment, control and prevention of infections, modification of pre-transplant conditioning regimens, and better donor selection, among other factors. As such, an increasing number of transplants are being done for AML. Despite these advancements, relapse rates have not improved significantly and actually may have increased. A large number of patient-, disease-, and transplant-related factors influence survival and AML relapse after allogeneic HCT. The goal of allogeneic transplant in AML is to reduce long-term risk of disease relapse while minimizing treatment-related morbidity and mortality. Identifying the individual person in whom transplant will achieve this goal and knowing the best strategy for transplant remains a challenge. This chapter summarizes the currently available data, and we present recommendations regarding if and when to pursue a transplant for persons with AML, the optimal conditioning regimen, the graft type, and use of alternative donors.

Current results

Large international registries such the Center for International Blood and Marrow Transplant Research (CIBMTR) report that 58% (±1%) of AML patients undergoing HCT from an HLA-matched sibling donor in first remission and 49% (±1%) of those in second remission are alive at three years after transplant. Outcomes are less favorable in those transplanted in relapsed or refractory disease, with estimated 3–5 year survivals around 25% (Figure 11.1). Of course, these data do not imply that transplants are best done in early stage disease because such observational databases contain data only on subjects who received a transplant and not all who could have received a transplant. Furthermore, these data are not compared with outcomes after alternative therapies, such as chemotherapy.

Transplant versus chemotherapy for post-remission therapy

Several meta-analyses compared results of allogeneic HCT to chemotherapy alone or autologous HCT as post-remission therapy in AML. These trials compared outcomes based on donor availability, or "biologic randomization." Those patients with identified donors who underwent allogeneic HCT were compared to subjects treated with either chemotherapy alone or autologous transplant (donor *vs* no donor comparisons) (Table 11.1). These studies report lower relapse rates and better survival in persons <60 years old with AML in first remission in the allogeneic transplant cohort. In most studies the benefit appears limited to persons with intermediate-risk cytogenetics. Persons with favorable and high-risk features did not benefit from a transplant in all studies. The major limitations are selection biases operating in the absence of true randomization and dropout of subjects who have an identified donor but who never received a transplant. Despite such limitations, few data indicate worse survival after allogeneic transplant, so the key question is not whether to pursue transplant or not but to determine who will benefit from transplant and when to pursue it.

Clinical Manual of Blood and Bone Marrow Transplantation, First Edition. Edited by Syed A. Abutalib and Parameswaran Hari.

© 2017 John Wiley & Sons Ltd. Published 2017 by John Wiley & Sons Ltd.

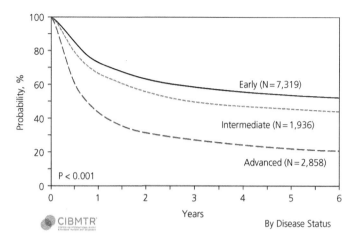

Figure 11.1 Survival after HLA-identical sibling donor transplants for AML, 2001–2011.

Table 11.1 Results of meta-analyses for donor versus no donor status on overall survival and DFS for persons with AML age <60 in CR1.

	# of patients	Pooled estimated HR for survival (95% CI)	Pooled estimate HR for DFS (95% CI)
Koreth et al. 2009*	>1700 donor vs >3000 no donor	0.9 (0.82–0.97); p<0.01	0.8 (0.74–0.86); p<0.01
Cornelissen et al. 2007*	>1100 donor vs >1900 no donor	0.87 (0.79–0.97); p=0.01	0.79 (0.72–0.88); p=0.001

* The results favor allogeneic HCT (see text)

Who should receive allogeneic transplant?

Determining candidacy for transplant should start with assessment of the individual's likelihood of tolerating the transplant chemotherapy regimen; such involves a combined assessment of existing co-morbidities and overall functional status. Chronologic age alone should not be a factor. Tools are available for objective quantification of these baseline patient-related factors associated with outcomes after allogeneic HCT. The transplant-specific co-morbidity index, a weighted scoring system for co-morbidities modeled for persons receiving diverse conditioning regimens, is a strong independent predictor of treatment-related mortality (TRM) and survival. The European Society for Blood and Marrow Transplantation (EBMT) risk score combines age, donor type, interval from diagnosis to transplant and donor-recipient gender combination to estimate survival. For older adults, there is growing evidence that a comprehensive geriatric assessment is an important indicator of outcomes after chemotherapy;

this approach likely can be extrapolated to the transplant setting. In addition, subjects deemed unfit for myeloablative conditioning (MAC) regimens increasingly undergo transplant using reduced-intensity conditioning (RIC) regimens; thus, the patient-specific factors determining candidacy for transplant are evolving.

Is allogeneic transplant needed?

Once a person is deemed physically fit for transplant, the next question is, should you proceed? For persons that do not achieve first remission with conventional chemotherapy, transplant typically is recommended assuming they have a compatible donor and acceptable baseline health that make them likely to survive the transplant. The decision is less straightforward in the larger percentage of persons who achieve first complete remission after standard chemotherapy. In such cases, the risk of relapse and probable likelihood of cure with conventional therapy are the key variables involved in making a decision to transplant an AML patient in first remission. Cytogenetic and genetic data can be used to

Table 11.2 European leukemia net risk groups.

Genetic Group	Subset
Favorable	t(8;21); *RUNX1-RUNX-1T1*, inv(16), t(16;16); *CBFB-MYH* Mutated *NPM1* without *FLT3-ITD* (normal karyotype) Mutated *CEBPA* (normal karyotype)
Intermediate I	Mutated *NPM1* with *FLT3-ITD* (normal karyotype) Wild-type *NPM1* with or without *FLT3-ITD* (normal karyotype)
Intermediate II	t(9;11); *MLLT3-MLL* Cytogenetic abnormalities not classified as favorable or adverse
Adverse	inv(3) or t(3;3); *RPN1-EVI1* t(6;9); *DEK-NUP214* t(v;11)*; *MLL* rearranged −5 or del (5q); −7; abnl (17p); complex karyotype**

Adapted from Dohner, H., et al., *Blood*, 2010. **115**(3): p. 453–474.

*v should not be chromosome 9

**Three or more chromosomal abnormalities

decide regarding proceeding with transplant or not. Many retrospective and a few prospective studies investigated the benefit of allogeneic transplant versus chemotherapy in various risk categories of AML. For example, the European LeukemiaNET panel divides AML into four prognostic risk groups (Table 11.2). Typically, persons in first complete remission with core-binding factor (CBF) leukemia (t(8;21); inv16, t(16;16)); mutated *NPM1* without *FLT3-ITD*; and bi-allelic *CEBPA* (CCAAT-enhancer-binding protein alpha) mutation with normal karyotype have a low risk of relapse and usually are not considered for transplant (until time of relapse) in CR1. In contrast, persons in first remission with adverse risk leukemia have a high relapse incidence after chemotherapy. The treating physicians often recommend to proceed with allogeneic HCT if a HLA-matched donor graft is available and the patient has an acceptable chance of surviving the transplant. It is important to remember, however, that such adverse risk factors in play after standard chemotherapy also may operate after allogeneic transplant. In other words, in the setting of adverse risk AML, use of transplant may not circumvent a poor outcome. The recommendation of transplant for patients with chromosome normal (CN)-AML with intermediate-risk features are unclear, and generally pursued if the transplant itself is deemed to be low- or intermediate-risk for adverse treatment-related outcomes. Although data from prospective trials are not yet available, allogeneic HCT should be considered in those with *FLT3-ITD* and deferred in those with favorable genotypes such as mutated *NPM1* without *FLT3-ITD* or homozygous mutated *CEBPA*. Such generalizations, however, are further complicated by increasing

knowledge of the interaction between cytogenetic risk and other genetic alterations. For example, although CBF leukemias are considered favorable, those with CBF-AML plus c-*KIT* mutation have higher rate of relapse, and outcomes with concomitant CBF-AML with adverse cytogenetics are largely unknown. *NPM-1* mutations also are considered favorable; however, concurrent mutations in *NPM1* in cytogenetically normal AML (CN-AML) and *IDH1 or IDH2* (isocitrate dehydrogenase) mutation have been associated with inferior relapse-free survival (5-year RFS 37 vs. 67%, p=0.02) and survival (5-year survival 41 vs 65%, p=0.03) compared to an isolated *NPM1* mutation in CN-AML. At this time, it is unknown whether persons with *NPM1* mutation without concomitant *IDH* mutation should undergo HCT. The negative impact of *FLT3-ITD* may not be overcome by allogeneic HCT, and *NPM1* mutation does not overcome *FLT3-ITD* unless the burden is low (*FLT-ITD/FLT*-wild-type ratio <0.5). Finally, while *CEBPA* mutations are traditionally accepted as favorable, recent studies have shown the benefit only in those who are homozygous for the mutation. Determining the benefit of allogeneic HCT in persons heterozygous for or homozygous for the *CEBPA* mutation needs further investigation.

Additional somatic mutations are increasingly identified as having clinical significance. For example, *TET2* mutations are associated with lower remission rates, disease-free survival (DFS), and survival in otherwise favorable risk AML. *IDH1* and *IDH2* mutations in CN-AML may confer poor outcomes. Other mutations associated with CN-AML and adverse outcomes, include mixed lineage leukemia (*MLL*), *RUNX1*, and *ASXL1*;

survival, may be improve with allogeneic HCT. The impact of these genetic mutations on prognosis further complicates the recommendations for which persons with AML are the best candidates for transplant.

PRACTICE POINT

The decision about whether an individual with AML should receive a transplant requires a risk-adapted approach that considers the chance of disease relapse without transplant, the patient's predicted tolerance of the transplant procedure, and availability of a suitable donor. This situation requires an individualized approach that must balance the predicted risk of relapse versus the predicted risk of mortality and morbidity related to the transplant.

Timing of allogeneic transplant

There is no consensus on the optimal timing of transplant for a person with AML (Figure 11.2). Recently, more first remission (CR1) AML patients are being considered for transplant. This trend may be related to the growing availability of alternative donors and use of RIC regimens. Additionally, there is seemingly better outcome of transplants in persons in first rather than second remission based on observational databases (as discussed above) and a perceived lower rate of second remission in those who relapse. One must exercise

caution, however, when considering such rationale for allotransplant in first remission. First, observational data indicating better outcomes for transplant in first versus second remission fail to account for the entire population of subjects who could have received a transplant in first or second remission but did not. Further, other factors affecting outcomes are not accounted for in observational studies. Better overall outcomes after first versus second remission does not mean that an individual should receive transplant in first rather than second remission. The second flawed argument is that the chance of achieving a second remission after relapse is so low that one should be transplanted in first remission. Some studies, in fact, report high second remission rates and long leukemia-free survival (LFS) in persons with AML who relapse and who have specific favorable prognostic variables such as young age, long first remission, and good-risk cytogenetics. Second, there are no convincing data proving that attempting to achieve a second remission (CR2) is better than immediate transplant for people who relapse. A recent analysis of >1200 subjects <50 years old with AML who relapsed reported a >50% second remission rate with approximately 20% of patients alive at 5 years. About two-thirds of persons achieving CR2 received a transplant; their 5-year survival was about 40%, indicating that a proportion of subjects relapsing after initial chemotherapy can be safely rescued. Better survival after a transplant was reported in subjects with intermediate-risk cytogenetics but not in those with good- or poor-risk cytogenetics.

PRACTICE POINTS

We are unable to predict on a subject level the relapse risk of an AML first remission patient. Most prognostic variables operate earlier on in the time course of AML treatment, before a transplant decision is made. Thus, the timing of allotransplant in AML is highly individualized and dependent on many factors including donor availability, patient preference, and treating physician bias. A general approach to the main variables considered in allogeneic HCT for AML is summarized in Table 11.3.

Transplant in relapsed or refractory AML

There are no data from intent-to treat analysis showing benefit to chemotherapy for recurrent AML prior to transplant *vs* proceeding with transplant in relapse. Any benefit may be offset by adversely impacted performance status or subjects becoming transplant-ineligible after chemotherapy and its related complications.

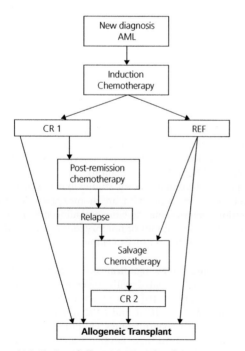

Figure 11.2 Timing of allogeneic transplant for AML.

Table 11.3 Who, when, and how of allogeneic HCT for AML.

A. PATIENT FACTORS

Age alone is not a factor in deciding candidacy for transplant.

Persons with adequate baseline functional status based on co-morbidity scoring are considered for transplant.

Patients not considered candidates for myeloablative transplants may be considered if using RIC regimens.

B. DISEASE FACTORS

In general, intermediate or poor-risk disease (based on cytogenetics and molecular testing, see Table 11.2) AML patients in 1st or 2nd remission are considered for transplant.

Those with favorable risk are usually not transplanted in first remission, until the time of relapse or if they have concurrent cytogenetic or genetic abnormalities such as c-*KIT*.

It is unclear whether transplant in first remission results in superior outcomes to transplant in second remission.

Transplants for refractory disease have poor outcomes.

C. DONOR EVALUATION

Ideal donor is a HLA- matched sibling or -matched unrelated donor matched at all HLA A, B, C, and DRB1 loci. Sibling donors are preferred.

No consensus on best alternative donor (HLA haplotype-matched vs. mismatched umbilical cord blood). Transplants using alternative donors should be pursued on a clinical trial.

Mismatched related or mismatched unrelated donor transplants have inferior outcomes.

D. CONDITIONING THERAPY

Busulfan and Cyclophosphamide vs Cyclophosphamide and Total Body Irradiation (TBI) have comparable outcomes.

RIC results in higher relapse rates but does not appear to reduce TRM.

E. POST ALLOTRANSPLANT THERAPY

No intervention has been proven to reduce relapse risk in randomized controlled trials. At this time, such interventions should only be investigated in the context of clinical trials.

Measurable residual disease (MRD)

MRD, sometimes referred to as "minimal residual disease," can be assessed in the patient by the testing of marrow samples using multi-parameter flow cytometry (MFC) or fluorescence in-situ hybridization (FISH) for a known genetic aberration. This tool is increasingly recognized as an important variable in the management of AML. Data from reports of MRD testing in first remission AML patients indicate a correlation with detecting MRD pre-transplant and relapse risk. For example, Terwijn et al. studied the validity of MRD testing by MFC as a predictor of relapse risk in adults with AML in a multi-center trial. MRD was tested after two cycles of induction chemotherapy. A positive MRD test was associated with increased relapse risk in multivariate analysis (HR 2.60; 95% CI 1.49–4.55). However, about 30% of subjects who were MRD-positive never relapsed, and about one-third of subjects who were MRD-negative relapsed. Analysis of the impact of positive post-transplant MRD by FISH or MFC in 287 subjects with AML showed more relapses in subjects with MRD detected up to 5 years post-transplant. Again, some subjects with MRD did not relapse and others without MRD did. In addition to such false-positive and negative results, there are many other challenges to be considered before MRD testing can reliably guide treatment decisions in AML allogeneic transplant. For example, given the genetic heterogeneity of AML with evidence of distinct sub-clones at diagnosis and relapse, MRD testing by MFC for leukemia-associated phenotypes (LAP) may not distinguish the presence or absence of residual leukemia. Although more definitive and prospective data are needed, MRD may be used in the future in a variety of settings, including (1) predicting outcomes in first remission AML patients; (2) selecting persons with AML in first remission who should receive a transplant; and (3) implementing post-transplant maintenance therapy based on presence or absence of post-transplant MRD.

Types of grafts

Bone marrow cells, blood cells, or umbilical cord blood cells are used for AML allotransplants. Grafts may be manipulated *in vitro* by techniques using monoclonal antibodies or physical methods to enrich for specific cell types such as CD34+ cells. Grafts can be depleted of some cell types such as T-cells by positive- or negative-selection methods. Also, sometimes there is manipulation of the donor before collecting the graft such as giving granulocyte- or granulocyte/macrophage colony-stimulating factor (G- and G/M-CSF).

Blood cell grafts, which are the result of the administration of agents to the donor in order to mobilize hematopoietic progenitors from the marrow into the

Table 11.4 Relative advantages/disadvantages of graft types.

	Blood	Marrow	Umbilical Cord
Blood count recovery	+++	++	+
Relapse risk	+	++	++ to +++
GvHD	+++	++	+

blood, also are referred to as mobilized blood cell grafts. This donor cell source is commonly used for allotransplants for AML. While these grafts are associated with faster hematopoietic cell recovery, the incidence of chronic GvHD also is higher compared to marrow grafts. A randomized trial reported more graft-failure with bone marrow grafts but more chronic GvHD with blood cell grafts. Other outcomes including survival were similar. Based on these data, some investigators believe that bone marrow grafts seem more favorable because of reduction in the incidence and severity of chronic GvHD, a syndrome associated with substantial morbidity. More than 80% of the grafts used today are mobilized blood, in part a result of the more practical issues, such as ease of collection and donor decision of which type of graft to use. Graft type is further confounded by the degree of donor-recipient HLA-matching such as umbilical cord blood cell grafts which are almost always HLA-mismatched with the recipient. Relative advantages and disadvantages of different graft types are summarized in Table 11.4.

Donor selection

An HLA-identical sibling is the best donor. Fewer than 30% of persons with AML, however, are considered to have an appropriate HLA-identical sibling donor. In such cases, transplants from alternative donors, including HLA-matched unrelated or mismatched unrelated donors, umbilical cord blood cells, and HLA-haplotype-matched related donors (sibling, parent, or child) are considered. Outcomes of transplants from HLA-matched unrelated donors are only slightly inferior to those of transplants from HLA-identical siblings. Transplants using HLA less well-matched unrelated donors have worse outcomes. Outcomes of HLA-matched or –mismatched umbilical cord blood cells in adults with AML is less well-known but are generally associated with slower bone marrow and immunologic recovery, less GvHD, more relapses, and worse LFS and survival compared with transplants from HLA-identical siblings or full HLA-matched unrelated donors. Finally, HLA-haplotype-matched transplants are available to most everyone with AML. Several series of

HLA-haplotype-matched donor transplants in AML recently have been reported. Several approaches to prevent GvHD in this setting are being studied. These strategies include *ex vivo* graft manipulation with CD3/CD19 selection combined with conventional post-transplant immunosuppression and use of unmanipulated grafts followed by post-transplant administration of cyclophosphamide, the latter given to eliminate alloreactive T-cells that arise soon after graft infusion.

PRACTICE POINTS

An HLA-matched sibling donor or fully matched unrelated donor is most favorable, and if neither are available, efforts should be made to enroll patients in randomized clinical trials using alternative donors. Choosing the *best* alternative donor for an AML patient who does not have an HLA-identical sibling donor or matched unrelated donor requires an individualized assessment of the risk-benefit ratio. Sometimes an otherwise acceptable subject may no longer be thought appropriate if use of an alternate donor is required; however, inferior outcomes using alternate donors are at times acceptable in light of the suboptimal outcomes of conventional therapy. The issue of alternative donors and donor selection is discussed in greater detail in Chapter 1.

Conditioning regimens

The ideal conditioning regimen for AML allogeneic transplantation should eliminate leukemia cells, provide enough immunosuppression to allow engraftment of donor cells and be minimally toxic to the recipient. A variety of preparative regimens exist; here we discuss the two most frequently encountered.

Myeloablative regimens

Cyclophosphamide (CY) combined with total body radiation (TBI), or busulfan in combination with CY, are the two most commonly used high-intensity (or myeloablative) conditioning regimens for AML allotransplant. A retrospective analysis of CIBMTR data with >1200 first remission AML subjects receiving HLA-identical sibling transplants or HLA-matched unrelated donor transplants compared outcomes with these two regimens.

Busulfan plus CY was associated with significantly less TRM, lower likelihood of relapse, and better 5-year survival in subjects compared with CY and TBI. A prospective cohort study involving >1400 mostly AML patients reported similar results. In contrast, an EBMT observational database study of >1600 AML subjects reported similar NRM and survival but slightly more relapses in the CY and intravenous busulfan cohort compared with CY and TBI.

> **PRACTICE POINT**
>
> In the absence of data from large well-designed prospective studies, one can conclude that CY and intravenous busulfan is at least as good as CY and TBI and may be better.

Reduced-intensity conditioning (RIC)

Older adults with AML and persons with co-morbidities are at increased risk of an adverse outcome when given an intensive pre-transplant conditioning regimen. Thus, conditioning regimens of reduced intensity, which still allowed for engraftment of donor cells, were developed. This approach is termed RIC or non-myeloablative (NMA) conditioning based on the relative intensity of bone marrow suppression. Less-intensive pre-transplant conditioning regimens rely more on the immune-mediate anti-leukemia effects associated with GvHD (although not leukemia specific, i.e., allogeneic effect) to reduce risk of relapse rather than intensity of the chemotherapy.

How do results of less intensive regimens compare with conventional regimens and do they decrease TRM? A CIBMTR observational database analysis of >3700 subjects with AML in various disease states receiving transplants from HLA-identical siblings, HLA-matched unrelated donors and HLA-partially or HLA-mismatched unrelated donors addressed this question. Appropriate adjustments were made to achieve comparability among subjects receiving less intensive regimens who were more likely older and with more co-morbidities. After adjustment, TRM was similar in the cohort receiving conventional, RIC, or NMA conditioning regimens at 3 and 5 years. Such findings indicate intensity of the pre-transplant conditioning regimen is not the sole determinant of TRM. However, subjects receiving less intensive regimens had a greater relapse risk. Adjusted 5-year survival was similar for the conventional and RIC cohorts and worse in the NMA cohort. An EBMT observational database study reported similar results. Recently, a prospective, randomized study conducted by the Blood and Marrow Transplant Clinical Trials Network (BMT CTN) comparing conventional and RIC conditioning was closed because of significantly inferior survival in the RIC cohort. The sum of these

data is in comparable subjects comparing conventional and RIC transplants result in similar outcomes including comparable TRM. However, some may interpret these data to favor RIC transplants since conditioning is less-intense and results seem comparable.

Post-transplant strategies to prevent relapse

Disease relapse occurs in about 10–40% of AML CR1 patients, 40–50% of those transplanted in or beyond CR2 and >50% in those transplanted without achieving a first remission or with more advanced AML. Other factors associated with relapse include poor-risk cytogenetics, older patient age, preceding myelodysplastic syndrome (MDS), *FLT3-ITD* mutation, donor-recipient gender match (female donor with male recipient), donor and graft type (mobilized blood vs marrow; matched-related vs unrelated matched; degree of disparity between host and recipient; and alternative donor grafts), and development of acute and/or chronic GvHD. Many interventions to decrease post-transplant relapse in persons with AML have been investigated, including interferon, interleukin-2, azacitidine, and tyrosine kinase-inhibitors such as sorafenib and midostaurin. Vaccines targeting leukemia-associated or leukemia-specific antigens also are being studied. Examples include vaccination against Wilm tumor (WT1) gene product peptide and HLA-A2 restricted leukemia-associated peptide PR1. No approach is convincingly-proved to prevent AML relapse in a randomized trial, and at this time interventions should only be done in the context of clinical trials.

> **PRACTICE POINTS**
>
> Allogeneic HCT can be an effective, sometimes curative treatment, for AML. However, it is a treatment approach encompassing many variables, each of which must be customized to a specific person with a unique disease and other factors that may affect the transplant outcome. Thus, on an individual subject level, it is often difficult to predict which persons should receive transplant, and if so, when and how? Although outcomes in recent years have improved after allogeneic transplant for AML, much of this effect stems from better supportive care rather than enhanced anti-leukemic activity of the various transplant modalities. Prevention of post-transplant complications such as GvHD and relapse after transplant remain active areas of investigation. As alternative donors and RIC regimens make transplant an option for a growing number of AML patients, knowing the best transplant approach for a specific individual with AML remains increasingly complex. Future progress will depend on the ability to more accurately predict the appropriate candidates for the therapies at hand.

Selected reading

1. Pasquini MC WZ. Current use and outcome of hematopoietic stem cell transplantation: CIBMTR Summary Slides. 2013.
2. Yanada M, Matsuo K, Emi N, Naoe T. Efficacy of allogeneic hematopoietic stem cell transplantation depends on cytogenetic risk for acute myeloid leukemia in first disease remission: a metaanalysis. *Cancer.* 2005;**103**(8):1652–1658.
3. Cornelissen JJ, van Putten WL, Verdonck LF, Theobald M, Jacky E, Daenen SM, et al. Results of a HOVON/SAKK donor versus no-donor analysis of myeloablative HLA-identical sibling stem cell transplantation in first remission acute myeloid leukemia in young and middle-aged adults: benefits for whom? *Blood.* 2007;**109**(9):3658–3666.
4. Koreth J, Schlenk R, Kopecky KJ, Honda S, Sierra J, Djulbegovic BJ, et al. Allogeneic stem cell transplantation for acute myeloid leukemia in first complete remission: systematic review and meta-analysis of prospective clinical trials. *JAMA: The Journal of the American Medical Association.* 2009;**301**(22):2349–2361.
5. Sorror ML, Sandmaier BM, Storer BE, Maris MB, Baron F, Maloney DG, et al. Comorbidity and disease status based risk stratification of outcomes among patients with acute myeloid leukemia or myelodysplasia receiving allogeneic hematopoietic cell transplantation. *Journal of Clinical Oncology: Official Journal of the American Society of Clinical Oncology.* 2007;**25**(27):4246–4254.
6. Dohner H, Estey EH, Amadori S, Appelbaum FR, Buchner T, Burnett AK, et al. Diagnosis and management of acute myeloid leukemia in adults: recommendations from an international expert panel, on behalf of the European LeukemiaNet. *Blood.* 2010;**115**(3):453–474.
7. Paschka P, Schlenk RF, Gaidzik VI, Habdank M, Kronke J, Bullinger L, et al. IDH1 and IDH2 mutations are frequent genetic alterations in acute myeloid leukemia and confer adverse prognosis in cytogenetically normal acute myeloid leukemia with NPM1 mutation without FLT3 internal tandem duplication. *Journal of Clinical Oncology: Official Journal of the American Society of Clinical Oncology.* 2010;**28**(22):3636–3643.
8. Burnett AK, Goldstone A, Hills RK, Milligan D, Prentice A, Yin J, et al. Curability of patients with acute myeloid leukemia who did not undergo transplantation in first remission. *Journal of Clinical Oncology: Official Journal of the American Society of Clinical Oncology.* 2013;**31**(10):1293–1301.
9. Terwijn M, van Putten WL, Kelder A, van der Velden VH, Brooimans RA, Pabst T, et al. High prognostic impact of flow cytometric minimal residual disease detection in acute myeloid leukemia: data from the HOVON/SAKK AML 42A study. *Journal of Clinical Oncology: Official Journal of the American Society of Clinical Oncology.* 2013;**31**(31):3889–3897.
10. Appelbaum FR. Pursuing the goal of a donor for everyone in need. *The New England Journal of Medicine.* 2012;**367**(16):1555–1556.
11. Walter RB, Pagel JM, Gooley TA, Petersdorf EW, Sorror ML, Woolfrey AE, et al. Comparison of matched unrelated and matched related donor myeloablative hematopoietic cell transplantation for adults with acute myeloid leukemia in first remission. *Leukemia.* 2010;**24**(7):1276–1282.
12. Eapen M, Klein JP, Sanz GF, Spellman S, Ruggeri A, Anasetti C, et al. Effect of donor-recipient HLA matching at HLA A, B, C, and DRB1 on outcomes after umbilical-cord blood transplantation for leukaemia and myelodysplastic syndrome: a retrospective analysis. *The Lancet Oncology.* 2011;**12**(13):1214–1221.

CHAPTER 12

Myelodysplastic syndromes

Melinda Biernacki and H. Joachim Deeg

Fred Hutchinson Cancer Research Center and the University of Washington, Seattle, WA, USA

Introduction

Myelodysplastic syndromes (MDS) comprise a varied group of clonal myeloid stem cell disorders with a broad spectrum of clinical presentations. The major morbidities of MDS are related to blood cytopenias and the evolution of MDS into acute myeloid leukemia. MDS are primarily disorders of older adults, with an incidence that rises sharply with age to a rate of 50 or more per 100,000 per year or higher among patients in their 70s. Treatment with high-dose chemotherapy may cure a small subset of patients, but the majority of patients will eventually show progressive disease, the median survival being in the range of 3–4 years.

Allogeneic hematopoietic cell transplantation (allo-HCT) is curative for 30–70% of patients with MDS. However, challenges of allo-HCT for MDS patients include: (1) identification of patients most likely to benefit from allo-HCT based on patient and disease characteristics, (2) optimization of the pre-HCT conditioning regimen, (3) prevention of graft-versus-host disease (GvHD) while promoting the graft-versus-MDS (GvM) effect, and (4) prevention and treatment of post-HCT relapse. Disease classification and risk scoring systems define the prognosis of MDS and allow clinicians to distinguish patients with high-risk disease who would benefit from HCT from patients with low-risk MDS who are likely to do well for extended periods of time without allo-HCT. Assessment of patient comorbidities is an integral part of transplant risk assessment. While HLA-matched relatives or unrelated donors remain the donors of choice, recent data suggest that HLA-haploidentical relatives or umbilical cord blood also provide excellent graft sources for transplantation. The optimal conditioning regimen for MDS patients remains to be determined, but the emphasis has shifted from high-intensity to reduced-intensity conditioning regimens, which are associated with lower transplant-related mortality, albeit with higher relapse rates. Post-HCT relapse remains a significant challenge. Pre-HCT bone marrow myeloblast percentage and cytogenetics are the strongest predictors of post-HCT relapse. Optimal therapies to treat patients who relapse remain to be developed, although current options include hypomethylating agents, induction chemotherapy, or second allo-HCT in select patients.

Disease classification, risk stratification, and allo-HCT

The spectrum of MDS is broad, and the prognosis varies greatly. While none of the available classification schemes are completely satisfactory, they have been prognostically useful and crucial in selecting appropriate treatment strategies for individual patients. The French-American-British (FAB) classification categorized patients on the basis of the presence of dysplasia in at least two of the three hematopoietic cell lineages and the proportion of myeloblasts in the marrow and peripheral blood. The 2001 World Health Organization (WHO) classification evolved from the FAB system and expanded the definition of MDS to include unilineage dysplasia provided the dysplasia persisted for ≥6 months and was not due to other causes. The 2008 revision of the WHO criteria further refined the diagnostic criteria for previously described MDS subtypes and incorporated additional clinical, cytogenetic, and molecular information into the classification scheme. Further, patients with 20–30% bone marrow myeloblasts, previously referred to as having refractory cytopenia with excess blasts in transformation (RAEB-T) were not

---

Clinical Manual of Blood and Bone Marrow Transplantation, First Edition. Edited by Syed A. Abutalib and Parameswaran Hari.
© 2017 John Wiley & Sons Ltd. Published 2017 by John Wiley & Sons Ltd.

considered as having AML. The 2008 WHO revision also distinguished subcategories of MDS with superior prognosis, such as patients with an isolated 5q31–33 deletion and <5% bone marrow blasts (5q deletion syndrome) (Table 12.1).

Risk stratification scoring systems provide another tool to define patient disease characteristics and determine the most appropriate therapeutic strategy (conservative vs aggressive). The International Prognostic Scoring System (IPSS) classified patients into four risk

Table 12.1 WHO classification of MDS.

Disease	Blood Findings	BM Findings
Refractory cytopenia with unilineage dysplasia (RCUD): (refractory anemia [RA]; refractory neutropenia [RN]; refractory thrombocytopenia [RT])	Unicytopenia or bicytopenia* No or rare blasts (<1%)[†]	Unilineage dysplasia ≥10% of the cells in one myeloid lineage <5% blasts <15% of erythroid precursors are ring sideroblasts
Refractory anemia with ring sideroblasts (RARS)	Anemia No blasts	≥15% of erythroid precursors are ring sideroblasts Erythroid dysplasia only <5% blasts
Refractory cytopenia with multilineage dysplasia (RCMD)	Cytopenia(s) No or rare blasts (<1%)[†] No Auer rods <1 × 10⁹/L monocytes	Dysplasia in ≥10% of the cells in ≥2 myeloid lineages Neutrophil and/or erythroid precursors and/or megakaryocytes <5% blasts in marrow No Auer rods ±15% ring sideroblasts
Refractory anemia with excess blasts-1 (RAEB-1)	Cytopenia(s) <5% blasts[†] No Auer rods <1 × 10⁹/L monocytes	Unilineage or multilineage dysplasia 5%–9% blasts[†] No Auer rods
Refractory anemia with excess blasts-2 (RAEB-2)	Cytopenia(s) 5%–19% blasts[‡] Auer rods ±[‡] <1 × 10⁹/L monocytes	Unilineage or multilineage dysplasia 10%–19% blasts[‡] Auer rods ±[‡]
Myelodysplastic syndrome–unclassified (MDS-U)	Cytopenias <1% blasts[†]	Unequivocal dysplasia in 10% of cells in one or more myeloid lineages when accompanied by a cytogenetic abnormality considered as presumptive evidence for a diagnosis of MDS <5% blasts
MDS associated with isolated del(5q)	Anemia Usually normal or increased platelet count No or rare blasts (<1%)	Normal to increased megakaryocytes with hypolobated nuclei <5% blasts Isolated del(5q) cytogenetic abnormality No Auer rods

* Bicytopenia may be present. Cases with pancytopenia should be classified as MDS-U.
[†] If marrow myeloblasts are <5% but 2–4% myeloblasts are present in the blood, the case qualifies as RAEB-1. Patients with RCUD or RCMD with 1% myeloblasts in the blood are classified as MDS-U.
[‡] If there are <5% myeloblasts in the blood and <10% in the marrow but Auer rods are present, the disease should be classified as RAEB-2. Similarly, cases of RAEB-2 may have <10% blasts in the marrow but may be diagnosed by the other two findings, Auer rod+ or 5–19% myeloblasts in the blood.

categories ("low," "intermediate-1," "intermediate-2," "high") based on the number of blood cytopenias, percentage of bone marrow myeloblasts, and cytogenetic features. The WHO classification-based prognostic scoring system (WPSS) incorporates the morphologic WHO classification, cytogenetics, and the need for red blood cell transfusions to categorize patients into five risk groups ("very low," "low," "intermediate," "high," "very high"). The Lower-Risk Prognostic Scoring System (LR-PSS) is a fourth prognostic model developed by investigators at MD Anderson Cancer Center to help identify patients with lower-risk disease (IPSS "low" or "intermediate-1") but with poor prognosis and incorporates clinical characteristics (age, performance status, transfusion need), hematologic parameters (cytopenias, leukocytosis), morphology (bone marrow myeloblast percentage), and cytogenetics. The recently revised IPSS (IPSS-R; Table 12.2) further refined patient risk categories from the original IPSS into five groups ("very low," "low," "intermediate," "high," "very high") by incorporating more detailed cytogenetic subgroups including monosomal karyotype, the depth of cytopenias, and further subdividing by percentage of marrow myeloblasts. The predictive value of the IPSS-R has been validated by multiple independent studies.

Other factors, currently not considered in any of the scoring systems, include morphologic and genetic features, or the presence of marrow fibrosis, which is independently associated with more rapid disease progression and shortened survival; it may also affect post-HCT outcomes. Patients with marrow fibrosis might, thus, be considered for allo-HCT even with otherwise lower-risk disease. More recently somatic DNA mutations with prognostic significance have been identified. In a study of 439 MDS patients, Bejar and coworkers identified mutations in six genes (ASXL1, RUNX1, TP53, EZH2, and ETV6) that were associated with poor prognosis. For patients with IPSS scores of "intermediate-2" or lower with any of those mutations, survival was similar to that of the next-higher IPSS risk group. Another study, aimed at validating the LR-PSS, identified the presence of mutations in EZH2 as an independent risk factor for decreased overall survival (OS).

MDS classification schemes, risk stratification scoring systems, and morphologic information on the presence or absence of bone marrow fibrosis are readily available tools to help clinicians determine an individual patient's risk related to MDS. Molecular testing to identify

Table 12.2 Revised International Prognostic Scoring System (IPSS-R).

A. Variables and scores

Variable	Score						
	0	0.5	1	1.5	2	3	4
Cytogenetics	Very Good		Good		Intermediate	Poor	Very Poor
Marrow Blasts (%)	≤2		>2–<5		5–10	>10	
Hemoglobin (g/dL)	≥10		8–<10	<8			
Platelets (x10⁹/L)	≥100	50–<100	<50				
Neutrophils (x10⁹/L)	≥0.8	<0.8					

B. IPSS-R scores and survival in non-transplanted patients

Patient Age (years)	IPSS-R Risk category/Score				
	Very low ≤1.5	*Low* >1.5–3	*Intermediate* >3–4.5	*High* >4.5–6	*Very High* >6
Any	8.8	5.3	3.0	1.6	0.8
<60	Not reached	8.8	5.2	2.1	0.9
>60	7.5	4.7	2.6	1.5	0.7

Cytogenetic categories:
Very low risk: −Y, del(11q)
Low risk: Normal, del(5q), del(20q), del(12p), double abnormalities that include del(5q)
Intermediate risk: del(7q), +8, i(17q), +19, any other single abnormality not included in other categories, any double abnormality that does not
    include either del(5q) or −7/del(7q)
Poor risk: −7, inv(3)/t(3q)/del(3q), double abnormalities including −7/del(7q), complex karyotype with three abnormalities
Very poor risk: Complex karyotype with >3 abnormalities

recurrent MDS-associated mutations are progressively being incorporated into scoring schemes. Patients with higher-risk disease (IPSS "intermediate-2" or "high;" IPSS-R "high" or "very high") should be considered for aggressive therapy including allo-HCT. HCT may also be considered in patients with lower-risk disease (by established criteria) but with other poor prognostic features such as marrow fibrosis or somatic mutations.

> **PRACTICE POINTS**
>
> Several classification and scoring systems have been developed. With the recognition of the role of somatic mutations for the prognosis of MDS it is important to incorporate those findings into the overall risk assessment for patients. With high-risk scores by scoring systems such as the Hematopoietic Cell Transplantation-Comorbidity Index (HCT-CI) patients may not be candidates for transplantation.

Indications for transplantation

Allo-HCT most clearly benefits patients with high-risk MDS, and consequently upfront allo-HCT is often indicated for fit patients with high-risk disease based on prognostic models. Patients with WPSS or IPSS-R high-risk or very high-risk scores, be it on the basis of cytogenetics, high blast count or transfusion dependence, are typically offered HCT. HCT can also be considered for patients with lower-risk disease but with other concerning features, including transfusion dependency despite growth factor support, disease refractory to hypomethylating agents (HMAs), or the presence of other clinical or pathologic features predicting poor prognosis such as marrow fibrosis. HCT may also be appropriate for younger patients with earlier stage disease as curative therapy; single-arm studies have shown high success rates with modest toxicity.

Transplant assessment

Patient characteristics

MDS is a disease of older adults, with a median age of >70 years in most series, an age bracket for which allo-HCT has generally not been considered. However, recent studies indicate that comorbidities rather than chronologic age exert a significantly higher negative impact on transplant outcome. The HCT-comorbidity index (HCT-CI) scores the presence (or absence) of multiple comorbidities such as hypertension, prior diagnosis of a solid tumor, organ dysfunction (e.g., pulmonary, hepatic, renal), obesity, and others. Patients with high HCT-CI scores have inferior post-HCT outcomes. A composite HCT-CI/age score includes

age ≥40 years as a single variable along with 15 comorbidities as additional variables, such that an otherwise healthy individual ≥65 years of age would have a lower score than a patient <40 years old with multiple medical problems and might, therefore, be a candidate for allo-HCT. Higher HCT-CI/age composite scores predict poor outcomes and increased non-relapse mortality (NRM) independent of transplant conditioning intensity (see Chapters 3 and 4).

The development of less intensive conditioning regimens ("non-myeloablative" and reduced-intensity [RIC]) now enables patients to undergo allo-HCT who are ineligible for high-intensity "myeloablative" conditioning because of older age and comorbidities. For example, Koreth and coworkers, using a Markov decision model, showed that that patients 60–70 years of age with high-risk (IPSS) MDS will benefit from allo-HCT after RIC by gaining a quality of life (QoL) adjusted survival advantage (Figure 12.1).

See Table 12.3 for pretransplant strategies and Table 12.4 for more about suitability for transplant.

> **PRACTICE POINT**
>
> The age of patients accepted for transplantation has risen progressively. The decision is often based on "biologic age," and no absolute limit has been established.

Optimal conditioning regimen: Do we know?

The optimal conditioning regimen for patients with MDS undergoing allo-HCT remains to be determined. Given the patient factors (i.e., median age of diagnosis) detailed before, emphasis has shifted from high-intensity conditioning regimens that rely on high-dose chemotherapy, radiation, or both for cytotoxic cell kill, to lower intensity/RIC regimens that rely heavily on the immunologic GvT effect for disease eradication. Treatment with low intensity regimens reduces the incidence and severity of treatment-related toxicity and has reduced day-100 treatment-related mortality (TRM) to <10% and even <5%. However, low intensity regimens are generally associated with a higher incidence of MDS relapse. In a multicenter retrospective analysis of 878 adults with high-risk (IPSS) MDS and AML who underwent allo-HCT from HLA-matched sibling donors (MSD), patients who received low intensity conditioning experienced a significantly higher incidence of relapse (in the first 12 months post-HCT, HR 3.9, p<0.01) and had inferior progression-free and overall survival in the reported 7-year follow-up compared to patients given high-intensity conditioning (OS was 29% with low intensity versus 53% for those treated with intermediate dose, 56% with "conventional" and 51%

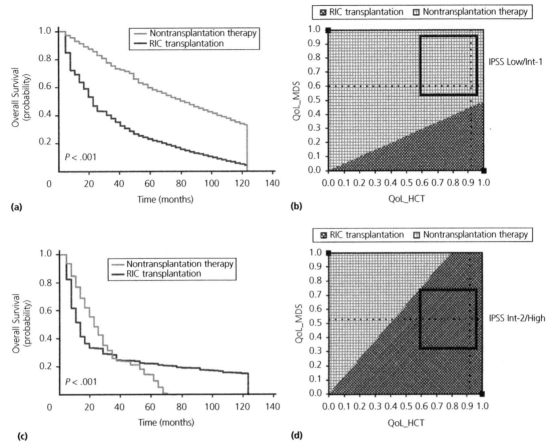

Figure 12.1 Benefit of allo-HCT after RIC in patients with low risk and high-risk MDS. Koreth and coworkers used a Markov decision model with quality-of-life utility estimates for different stages of MDS to evaluate the benefit of HCT in 514 patients aged 60–70 years with de novo MDS. Median life expectancy for patients with *higher-risk* MDS was 36 months with RIC transplantation versus 28 months with non-transplantation therapies **(c)**. For patients with lower risk MDS, the median life expectancy was 38 months with RIC HCT versus 77 months with non-transplant approaches **(a)**. The gain in quality-adjusted life years is illustrated in parts (**d** and **b**), respectively. These retrospective data strongly argue for conservative management in older patients with low-risk MDS. Patients with high-risk MDS are likely to benefit, although this benefit was apparent only with considerable delay after HCT. Reprinted with permission. © (Year of publication being used) American Society of Clinical Oncology. All rights reserved. Koreth, J. et al: *J Clin Oncol*, Role of reduced-intensity conditioning allogeneic hematopoietic cell transplantation in older patients with de novo myelodysplastic syndromes: An international collaborative decision analysis, 2013; **31**(21):2662–2670.

with high-dose regimens, p < 0.01). Similarly, in a retrospective registry analysis from the Center for International Bone Marrow Transplantation Research (CIBMTR) low intensity regimens were inferior with regards to relapse-free survival (RFS) (HR for relapse 1.73, p < 0.001) and OS (HR for mortality 1.20, p = 0.006). However, it may be possible to modify higher intensity regimens such that both NRM and probability of relapse are optimized. For example, Gyurkocza and coworkers transplanted patients with MDS or AML from HLA-matched sibling or unrelated donors after

conditioning with I.V. treosulfan, fludarabine, and low-dose total-body irradiation and reported OS of 72%, relapse incidence of 27%, and NRM of 8% at 2 years (Figure 12.2).

PRACTICE POINT

Multiple reduced-intensity regimens have been developed. Combinations of fludarabine with melphalan or fludarabine plus low to intermediated dose total-body irradiation are promising.

Table 12.3 Pretransplant strategies for patients with MDS.

Induction chemotherapy (ICT)	• Higher rate of CR than after HMAs; better outcomes after transplant, especially in patients undergoing NMA/RIC • Favorable cost-effectiveness ratio	• High toxicity (inappropriate for older patients and those with comorbidities) • Patient hospitalization required (not an outpatient procedure) • Ineffective for poor-risk cytogenetics; no benefit with low marrow blast percentage • High patient drop-out rate (not reaching transplantation) due to complications
HMAs	• Favorable cost-effectiveness ratio • Low-toxicity profile (appropriate for older patients and those with comorbidities) • Administration to outpatients • More effective than ICT in patients with unfavorable cytogenetics	• Cost of treatment • Lower CR rate • Long treatment duration: multiple cycles of treatment are needed before response can be assessed • Responses to treatment are of short duration in patients with unfavorable cytogenetics • High patient drop-out rate (not reaching transplantation) due to complications from pretransplant treatment or rapid progression to AML • Risk of transformation to AML before allo-HCT
Upfront allo-HCT	• No debulking-treatment-related toxicity • Allo-HCT can be performed as soon as a suitable donor is identified	• Post-transplant interventions may be necessary, especially in patients undergoing NMA/RIC • Increased risk of post-transplant relapse in patients transplanted with progressive disease

Table 12.4 Candidacy for allo-HCT: Decision algorithm based on disease characteristics, patient age, and comorbidities.

Patient Characteristics	Disease Characteristics		ICT	HMAs	Upfront HCT
	Marrow Blasts (%)	Cytogenetics*			
Age >60 yr or comorbidities	Any	Any	Possible[†]	BO	Possible
Age <60 yr and no comorbidities	<5	<High risk	NI	BO	Possible
	<5	High risk	NI	Possible	BO[‡]
	5–10	<High risk	Possible	BO	Possible
	5–10	High risk	NI	Possible	BO[‡]
	>10	<High risk	BO	Possible	Possible
	>10	High risk	Possible	Possible	BO[‡]

Abbreviations: HCT = hematopoietic cell transplantation; ICT = induction chemotherapy; HMA = hypomethylating therapy; BO = best option; NI, not indicated.

* As assessed by the International Prognostic Scoring System.

[†] Clearly, certain patients in this category will tolerate ICT and, particularly with high marrow blast counts, might benefit from intensive debulking efforts.

[‡] If the patient can undergo HCT rapidly; currently available data are not conclusive as to the benefit of chemotherapy debulking in patients with high-risk cytogenetic disease.

Donor-recipient immunity

One challenge with allo-HCT is the bidirectional immunologic reactivity of donor and host cells. Rejection of the donor cells by the host immune system is rare, but clinically significant donor versus host reactions in the form of GvHD are common. GvHD may occur with more acute or more chronic presentations, but there is considerable overlap, and mixed presentations occur. Reported incidence figures range from 15 to 50% for acute- and 30 to 60% for chronic GvHD. *In vitro* depletion of donor T-cells decreases the incidence, primarily of acute GvHD but may be associated with graft failure

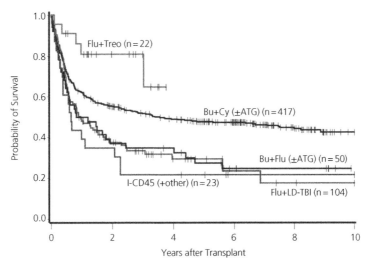

Figure 12.2 Probability of long-term post-HCT survival in patients with MDS by conditioning regimen.

and an increased incidence of disease relapse. *In vivo* prophylactic regimens use agents such as cyclosporine, tacrolimus, sirolimus, methotrexate, mycophenolate mofetil, or cyclophosphamide, among others.

> **PRACTICE POINTS**
>
> Multiple regimens are used. Cyclosporine plus methotrexate was the first effective combination. Currently, combinations of tacrolimus, MMF, and sirolimus are widely used.

Graft source

HLA-MSD remain the preferred hematopoietic graft source. However, with the selection of HLA-matched unrelated donors (MUD) on the basis of high-resolution HLA typing, outcomes of recipients of matched URD allo-HCT enjoy transplant outcomes basically comparable to those obtained with HLA-MSD, except for slightly higher rates of acute- and chronic-GvHD. Whether results with transplantation from an older sibling or a younger HLA-MUD yield superior outcomes remains controversial. An EBMT series of 719 MDS patients aged >50 years showed a survival advantage with allografts from HLA-MUD younger than 30 years when compared to older (>50 years) HLA-MRD or HLA-MSD.

> **PRACTICE POINT**
>
> We still prefer HLA-MSD. However, the field is in flux. Results with unrelated HLA-matched donors are excellent, and growing numbers of HLA-haploidentical transplants are carried out successfully.

Graft from peripheral blood or marrow?

G-CSF-mobilized peripheral blood hematopoietic cells (PBHC) offer several advantages over hematopoietic cells obtained by direct aspiration from the marrow. PBHC provide the most rapid engraftment of any allo-graft source, and exert a more potent GvT effect. The disadvantage are higher rates of chronic-GvHD than observed with bone marrow, with rates of 53 versus 41% with PBHC and marrow, respectively, in patients transplanted from HLA-MUD.

> **PRACTICE POINT**
>
> PBHC is the preferred hematopoietic progenitor source due to more rapid engraftment and decreased relapse rates compared to bone marrow, albeit with a higher incidence of chronic GvHD.

Beyond HLA-matched grafts: Is it reasonable approach?

Unrelated umbilical cord blood (UCB) cells or cells from HLA-haploidentical family members provide reasonable alternatives for patients for whom neither an HLA-matched related or URD can be identified. In a feasibility study of UCB transplants in 98 older (>55 years) MDS and AML patients, no significant difference in 3-year OS, relapse incidence, or TRM was observed between patients receiving UCB and those transplanted from

HLA-MSD. UCB cells tend to engraft slowly, with a consequent increase in the risk of infection and bleeding. Increasing the infused cell dose either by transplanting two cord blood units or after expanding a single unit *in vitro* (experimental) improves survival. UCB allografts appear to confer a lower post-HCT relapse risk compared with grafts from adult donor sources. The administration of post-HCT cyclophosphamide in patients receiving T-cell-replete HCT from HLA-haploidentical family members has yielded results similar to those in patients receiving allografts from HLA-matched related or URDs. The risk of graft rejection is higher with the use of HLA-haploidentical donors, but modification to conditioning regimens may reduce the rejection risk. Importantly, rates of GvHD in patients receiving HLA-haploidentical transplants are not higher than with fully HLA-matched allografts, presumably due to the effect of high-dose cyclophosphamide after HCT. Currently, there is insufficient experience in MDS to draw any conclusions regarding the effect of HLA-haploidentical HCT for these disorders.

> **PRACTICE POINTS**
>
> As MDS is primarily a disease of older individuals, other medical conditions may be present and must be considered when deciding upon transplantation and the design of the transplant conditioning regimen. Reduced intensity is generally more appropriate for older patients. Most transplant physicians use HLA-matched siblings as the first-choice donor. However, results with HLA-MUD have improved progressively, and even HLA-haploidentical donors are used with increasing success.

Role of therapy and disease burden prior to allo-HCT

High disease burden as reflected by marrow myeloblast percentage (>5%) increases the risk for post-HCT relapse, particularly with low intensity conditioning regimens. Administering induction chemotherapy to reduce pre-HCT disease burden may reduce relapse risk post-HCT in patients who achieved pre-HCT remission. However, there are no results from controlled prospective trials and induction chemotherapy can have significant toxicities that may delay or even preclude HCT. Even less convincing are the data of a beneficial impact of pre-HCT induction chemotherapy in patients with high-risk cytogenetics.

HMA such as azacitidine and decitabine represent an alternative to induction therapy with fewer treatment-related toxicities. However, multiple retrospective analyses have failed to show significant differences in post-HCT outcomes between patients who were treated with HMAs *vs* those given induction chemotherapy

pre-HCT (reviewed in). The role of allo-HCT in patients with progressive disease while on treatment with HMAs is not clear. Patients transplanted with disease progression while on azacitidine have longer median OS than those who do not undergo allo-HCT (19 months vs 3–9 months), but only patients who did not progress on HMA appeared to derive a lasting benefit from allo-HCT.

> **PRACTICE POINTS**
>
> The role of pretransplant therapy has not been well defined, and it is not clear whether "debulking" therapy improves post-transplant results. Ideally patients should be enrolled in ongoing (prospective) trials.

Post-transplant outcomes

Post-HCT outcomes depend upon two major factors: transplant-related toxicity (including TRM) and disease relapse. As discussed, comorbidities are major contributors to TRM. The most frequent problem, however, is GvHD and the profound immunosuppression associated with its treatment. Prevention and more effective therapy of GvHD remain active areas of investigation.

As described, "myeloablative" conditioning regimens carry a lower risk of post-HCT relapse than lower intensity regimens. Prognostic scoring systems used to assess disease risk in the non-transplant setting also predict post-HCT outcomes. Della Porta and coworkers identified significant differences in OS and rates of relapse between patients with lower risk (low or intermediate) and higher-risk (high or very high) IPSS-R scores. This and other studies have shown a strong association between the presence of high-risk cytogenetics, including monosomal karyotype, and increased risk of post-HCT relapse (Figure 12.3), and decreased OS. The effect of monosomal karyotype (MK) appears to be independent of IPSS-R score with a probability of 5-year OS of 0% in patients with very high-risk IPSS-R scores and MK compared to 27% in patients with the same IPSS-R risk but without MK. Evolution of cell subclones likely contributes to post-HCT relapse. In one analysis of post-HCT relapse of patients with MDS, 70% of patients with late post-HCT relapse on whom sequential cytogenetic data were available showed evolution of new clonal abnormalities either in addition to or replacing those present at pre-HCT. Mutations in individual genes also influence post-HCT outcomes independent of other factors, as shown in a study by Bejar and coworkers in which mutations in TP53, TET2, and DNMT3 were independently associated with shorter OS. Patients with mutations in any of the three genes had 3-year OS after allo-HCT of 19%.

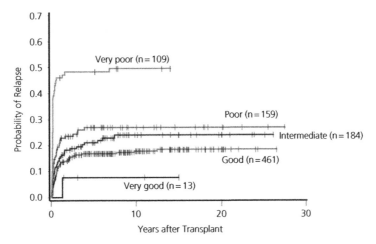

Figure 12.3 Stratification of patients into five cytogenetic risk groups discriminates more clearly among patients with the highest and lowest risk of post-HCT relapse than does the original three-group classification.

Treatment and prevention of post-HCT relapse

Relapse after allo-HCT remains a challenge, with cumulative incidence rates of 10–50% dependent primarily upon the patient's karyotype. Prognosis for patients who relapse after allo-HCT is poor, particularly with relapse early post-HCT (<100 days to <1 year in different studies). Treatment strategies include withdrawal of immunosuppression, donor lymphocyte infusion (DLI), treatment with HMAs, and, in select patients, second allo-HCT. The use of HMAs has been explored in several studies. A retrospective review by the German Cooperative Transplant Study Group investigated the outcomes of 154 patients receiving azacitidine combined with or without DLI for post-HCT relapses of AML and MDS and reported a 27% complete response rate (33% overall response rate) with the majority of patients responding after DLI rather than after azacitidine alone. The 2-year OS in MDS patients was 66%. Acute- and chronic GvHD occurred in about one-third of patients who received DLI after azacitidine; in patients who received azacitidine only, generally mild manifestations of GvHD occurred in 18%, and the majority of those patients had preexisting GvHD. A single-arm prospective multicenter phase II trial of azacitidine followed by DLI for AML and MDS patients with post-HCT relapse showed similar findings and reported greater likelihood of response in patients with MDS or AML with myelodysplasia-related changes. Azacitidine with or without DLI appears to be a safe and potentially effective strategy for treating post-HCT relapse of MDS.

HMAs have also been investigated as maintenance or pre-emptive therapy post-HCT. Azacitidine at doses of 32 mg/m² daily for 5 days and for four 40-day cycles was safe and appeared to delay relapse. Platzbecker and coworkers used a pre-emptive strategy in which patients whose CD34⁺ donor chimerism fell below 80%, signaling impending relapse, received azacitidine, 75 mg/m² for four cycles, and showed that this strategy increased donor chimerism and delayed or prevented relapse.

Lenalidomide, which provides highly effective therapy in patients with del(5q) MDS, has been tested as a prophylactic post-HCT strategy to prevent relapse, but was associated with an unacceptable increase in GvHD.

> **PRACTICE POINTS**
>
> Post-transplant relapse continues to be a challenging problem in MDS. Molecular monitoring and institution of therapy, for example with a hypomethylating agent, when only minimal residual disease is detected may be the most promising approach. Cellular therapies are being developed.

Limitations and future prospects

Allogeneic HCT remains the sole therapy for MDS with proven curative potential (Table 12.5). Advances in the understanding of the clinical and pathologic features that impact prognosis have led to the development of improved risk stratification scoring systems that allow clinicians to identify high-risk patients likely to benefit from HCT. Other factors, such as the presence of certain somatic mutations, are not yet included in any risk stratification scoring system but also help inform clinical

Table 12.5 The who, when, and how of allogeneic HCT for MDS.

A. PATIENT FACTORS

Age *alone* is not a factor in deciding candidacy for transplant.

Persons with adequate baseline functional status based on comorbidity scoring are considered for transplant.

Patients not considered candidates for high-intensity conditioning transplants may be considered if using reduced-intensity conditioning regimens are appropriate.

Allo-HCT may also be appropriate for younger patients with earlier stage ("very low or low-risk IPSS-R") disease as curative therapy

B. DISEASE FACTORS

Disease classification and risk scoring systems define the prognosis of MDS; however, none of the available classification schemes or prognostic models are completely satisfactory

Those with low-risk MDS are usually not transplanted upon diagnosis or at first remission

Patients with marrow fibrosis might be considered for allo-HCT even with otherwise low-risk ("very low or low IPSS-R") MDS

It is not known whether patients with low-risk ("very low or low IPSS-R") MDS and prognostically detrimental somatic DNA mutations fair better from upfront transplant compared to conservative therapy

Transplant may be considered in selected patients with intermediate risk (IPSS-R) MDS patients

Allo-HCT is an effective strategy for treating patients with high-risk ("high or very high IPSS-R") MDS

The role of pretransplant therapy (induction chemotherapy or HMA) has not been well defined, and it is not clear whether "debulking" therapy improves post-transplant results (refer to table-3)

Patients who achieve complete responses with HMAs pre-HCT have similar outcomes to those who achieved CR with induction chemotherapy (refer to Table 12.3).

C. DONOR EVALUATION

Ideal donor is an HLA- matched sibling or HLA-matched unrelated donor (matched at HLA A, B, C, and DRB1; DQ and DP matching may further enhance results). Sibling donors are preferred.

No consensus on best alternative donor (HLA-haploidentical vs mismatched UCB) for transplant has been achieved

Transplants using alternative donors should preferably be pursued on a clinical trial.

D. CONDITIONING THERAPY

Optimal conditioning regimen for patients with MDS undergoing allo-HCT remains to be determined

Reduced-intensity conditioning results in higher relapse rates

Novel "high-intensity/low-toxicity" regimens using, for example, a combination of treosulfan, fludarabine, and TBI, have shown promise

E. POST ALLOTRANSPLANT THERAPY

Pre-HCT bone marrow myeloblast percentage and cytogenetics are the strongest predictors of post-HCT relapse

No intervention has been proven to reduce relapse risk in randomized controlled trials.

HMAs, particularly azacitidine, hold some promise

decisions especially as sequencing data become more readily available. Incorporating other prognostic factors into clinical decision-making will also help to identify patients with lower-risk scores but poor prognosis, based on those factors, who might benefit from HCT.

Improvements in the field of transplantation have led to a better understanding of the role of comorbidities in TRM and post-HCT outcomes. The optimal conditioning regimen for patients with MDS remains to be determined. Low-intensity regimens have improved toxicity profiles and decreased TRM in comparison to high-intensity regimens, but the cost appears to be higher rates of relapse. The role of induction chemotherapy pre-HCT is not well defined. HMAs present a promising alternative to induction chemotherapy for cytoreduction pre-HCT, and post-HCT outcomes are poor and relapse rates are high for patients with progressive disease despite therapy, whether treated with HMAs or induction chemotherapy. Recent findings also indicate that emergence of new subclones and presence of certain mutations herald poor post-HCT outcomes. Optimal therapies to prevent or treat post-HCT relapse of MDS remain to be developed. The patients at highest risk for poor post-HCT outcomes are also those with the strongest indication for HCT. Future advances in MDS care will need to focus on improvements for this group of patients.

Selected reading

1. Malcovati L, Germing U, Kuendgen A, Della Porta MG, Pascutto C, Invernizzi R, et al. Time-dependent prognostic scoring system for predicting survival and leukemic evolution in myelodysplastic syndromes. *J Clin Oncol.* 2007;**25**(23): 3503–3510.

2. Greenberg PL, Tuechler H, Schanz J, Sanz G, Garcia-Manero G, Sole F, et al. Revised international prognostic scoring system for myelodysplastic syndromes. *Blood.* 2012;**120**(12): 2454–2465.

3. Bejar R, Stevenson KE, Caughey BA, Abdel-Wahab O, Steensma DP, Galili N, et al. Validation of a prognostic model and the impact of mutations in patients with lower-risk myelodysplastic syndromes. *J Clin Oncol.* 2012;**30**(27): 3376–3382.

4. Cutler CS, Lee SJ, Greenberg P, Deeg HJ, Perez WS, Anasetti C, et al. A decision analysis of allogeneic bone marrow transplantation for the myelodysplastic syndromes: delayed transplantation for low-risk myelodysplasia is associated with improved outcome. *Blood.* 2004;**104**(2):579–585.

5. Koreth J, Pidala J, Perez WS, Deeg HJ, Garcia-Manero G, Malcovati L, et al. Role of reduced-intensity conditioning allogeneic hematopoietic stem-cell transplantation in older patients with de novo myelodysplastic syndromes: an international collaborative decision analysis. *J Clin Oncol.* 2013;**31**(21):2662–2670.

6. Gyurkocza B, Gutman J, Nemecek ER, Bar M, Milano F, Ramakrishnan A, et al. Treosulfan, fludarabine, and 2-Gy total body irradiation followed by allogeneic hematopoietic cell transplantation in patients with myelodysplastic syndrome and acute myeloid leukemia. *Biol Blood Marrow Transplant.* 2014;**20**(4):549–555.

7. Mukherjee S, Boccaccio D, Sekeres MA, Copelan E. Allogeneic hematopoietic cell transplantation for myelodysplastic syndromes: lingering uncertainties and emerging possibilities. *Biol Blood Marrow Transplant.* 2015;**21**(3): 412–420.

8. Prebet T, Gore SD, Esterni B, Gardin C, Itzykson R, Thepot S, et al. Outcome of high-risk myelodysplastic syndrome after azacitidine treatment failure. *J Clin Oncol.* 2011;**29**(24): 3322–3327.

9. Della Porta MG, Alessandrino EP, Bacigalupo A, van Lint MT, Malcovati L, Pascutto C, et al. Predictive factors for the outcome of allogeneic transplantation in patients with MDS stratified according to the revised IPSS-R. *Blood.* 2014;**123**(15):2333–2342.

10. Deeg HJ, Scott BL, Fang M, Shulman HM, Gyurkocza B, Myerson D, et al. Five-group cytogenetic risk classification, monosomal karyotype, and outcome after hematopoietic cell transplantation for MDS or acute leukemia evolving from MDS. *Blood.* 2012;**120**(7):1398–1408.

11. Yeung CC, Gerds AT, Fang M, Scott BL, Flowers ME, Gooley T, et al. Relapse after allogeneic hematopoietic cell transplantation for myelodysplastic syndromes: analysis of late relapse using comparative karyotype and chromosome genome array testing. *Biol Blood Marrow Transplant.* 2015;**21**(9):1565–1575.

12. Bejar R, Stevenson KE, Caughey B, Lindsley RC, Mar BG, Stojanov P, et al. Somatic mutations predict poor outcome in patients with myelodysplastic syndrome after hematopoietic stem-cell transplantation. *J Clin Oncol.* 2014;**32**(25): 2691–268.

13. Schroeder T, Rachlis E, Bug G, Stelljes M, Klein S, Steckel NK, et al. Treatment of acute myeloid leukemia or myelodysplastic syndrome relapse after allogeneic stem cell transplantation with azacitidine and donor lymphocyte infusions – a retrospective multicenter analysis from the German Cooperative Transplant Study Group. *Biol Blood Marrow Transplant.* 2015;**21**(4):653–660.

14. de Lima M, Giralt S, Thall PF, de Padua Silva L, Jones RB, Komanduri K, et al. Maintenance therapy with low-dose azacitidine after allogeneic hematopoietic stem cell transplantation for recurrent acute myelogenous leukemia or myelodysplastic syndrome: a dose and schedule finding study. *Cancer.* 2010;**116**(23):5420–5431.

15. Yakoub-Agha I, Deeg J. Are hypomethylating agents replacing induction-type chemotherapy before allogeneic stem cell transplantation in patients with myelodysplastic syndrome? *Biol Blood Marrow Transplant.* 2014;**20**(12):1885–1890.

CHAPTER 13

Chronic myelogenous leukemia

Daniel Egan and Jerald Radich

Fred Hutchison Cancer Research Center, Seattle, WA, USA

The advent of tyrosine kinase inhibitor (TKI) therapy dramatically and irreversibly altered the treatment of chronic myeloid leukemia. However, often forgotten is that prior to the TKI era, the most common use of allogeneic stem cell transplantation (BMT*) was CML. Is there still a place for transplantation in the management of CML?

The past informs the present: lessons from the BMT era

Before discussing the current indications for BMT in the care of the CML patient, it is useful to quickly outline some relevant key points. Selected randomized trials are summarized in Table 13.1.

Does disease phase matter?
Yes, and hugely so. All therapies, be it interferon, BMT, or TKI work dramatically better in chronic phase compared to accelerated or blast phase. Data from the International Bone Marrow Transplant Registry showed 5-year overall survival (OS) for patients transplanted in chronic, accelerated or blast phase to be 75, 40, and 10%, respectively. Moreover, patients transplanted in accelerated phase patients by cytogenetic criteria only (normal blast counts) had roughly twice the 4-year survival compared accelerated phase cases with elevated blast counts.

After TKI therapy fails (either with resistance or progression to advanced phase disease), BMT can salvage cases and lead to long-term survival. The survival experience of these cohorts does not appear to differ significantly from the pre-TKI era, with OS for CP >80%, AP 40–50%, and BC 10–20%.

Time before transplant and outcome
In the pre-imatinib era, studies showed a clear correlation between worse outcomes and increased duration of time from diagnosis to transplant, including both relapse and non-relapse mortality, even for patients still in chronic phase at the time of transplant. While this was true for therapies such as busulfan, hydroxyurea, and interferon, the same does not seem to be true with TKI therapy, as treatment with TKIs prior to BMT does not seem to effect regimen related mortality or relapse rates.

Does the preparative regimen matter?
Yes. Early allogeneic transplants in the 1980s mainly utilized the preparative regimen of cyclophosphamide at 120 mg/kg followed by total body irradiation (TBI). A randomized controlled trial of higher dose TBI (15.75 Gy) versus conventional dose TBI (12.0 Gy) did not result in improved overall or disease-free survival, owing to the increased non-relapse mortality with the increased radiation. A subsequent randomized controlled trial of busulfan 16 mg/kg combined with 120 mg/kg cyclophosphamide (BU-CY) versus conventional CY-TBI showed a

---

*There are many acronyms for allogeneic transplantation. Many now revolve around some use of "hematopoietic cell" since peripheral blood hematopoietic cells have largely replaced bone marrow as the source of the allograft. However, we are going "old school" and using "BMT" to stand for blood and bone marrow transplantation.

Clinical Manual of Blood and Bone Marrow Transplantation, First Edition. Edited by Syed A. Abutalib and Parameswaran Hari.
© 2017 John Wiley & Sons Ltd. Published 2017 by John Wiley & Sons Ltd.

Table 13.1 Randomized and selected non-randomized trials in allogeneic hematopoietic cell transplant for CML.

Author	Trial Setting	Randomized?	N	Conditioning	cGvHD	NRM	OS	PFS	Comments
Clift (1991)	Prospective study comparing total body irradiation (TBI) dose in chronic phase CML	Randomized	57 TBI (12.0 Gy); 59 TBI (15.75 Gy)	Cyclophosphamide 120 mg/kg with TBI (12.0 Gy) versus (15.75 Gy)	Not reported	24% vs 34% at 4 years; p = 0.13	60% vs 66% at 4 years; p = 0.36	58% vs. 66% at 4 years (p value not reported)	No difference in overall survival with increased TBI dose compared to 12.0 Gy. Decrease risk of relapse with higher TBI dose offset by trend towards increased TRM.
Clift (1994)	Prospective study comparing two conditioning regimens	Randomized	73 Bu-Cy; 69 Cy-TBI	Busulfan 16 mg/kg and cyclophosphamide 120 mg/kg (Bu-Cy) versus cyclophosphamide 120 mg/kg and TBI 12.0 Gy (Cy-TBI)	Not reported	18% vs 24% at 4 years (p value not reported)	80% vs 80% at 3 years	71% vs 68% at 3 years (p = 0.43)	Doses exceeding 200 mg per day associated with reversible myelosuppression.
Oehler (2005)	Prospective, multicenter study comparing donor stem cell source in CML	Randomized	40 BM; 32 PBSC	Busulfan (oral, 16 mg/kg) and cyclophosphamide (120 mg/kg), n = 68; TBI (13.2 Gy) and etoposide (60 mg/kg), n = 4.	50% vs 59%, p = 0.46	20% vs 19% at 3 years; p = 0.86	72% vs 81% at 3 years; p = 0.42	65% vs. 81%, p=0.10	No statistically significant difference in acute or chronic GvHD, NRM, or OS between BM and PBSC recipients. A trend towards higher relapse with BM was noted (7% versus 0%, p = 0.10).
Hehlmann (2007)	Prospective, multicenter study comparing survival with HCT versus drug therapy, according to availability of related donor vs no related donor	Biologically "randomized" according to donor status	135 related donor (123 rec'd transplant); 219 no related donor (114 rec'd transplant)	Busulfan 16 mg/kg and cyclophosphamide 120 mg/kg, n = 110; cyclophosphamide plus TBI (12 Gy), n = 135; other drug combinations, n=2	Not reported	TRM 28.8% vs 17.8%; p = 0.003	76% vs. 89% at 2 years; 56% vs. 57% at 8 years (p values not reported)	Not reported	Improved short-term survival in patients receiving drug therapy compared to early HCT. Survival curves ultimately converge at 8 years follow-up. Note: Survival was analyzed according to "intention to treat" (related donor = HCT; no related donor = drug therapy), with censoring of patients without related donor who underwent MUD transplants. Drug therapy was primarily IFN or imatinib based.

(Continued)

Table 13.1 (Continued)

Author	Trial Setting	Randomized?	N	Conditioning	cGvHD	NRM	OS	PFS	Comments
Davies (2001)	Retrospective study comparing matched related and matched unrelated donors for HCT in first chronic phase	Nonrandomized	96 MRD 45 MUD	Cyclophosphamide (120 mg/k) plus TBI (13.2 Gy), n = 134; Other, n = 7	Not reported	TRM RR 1.1 (p = 0.7)	58% vs 53% at 5 years (p = 0.4)	44% vs 42% at 5 years (p = 0.6)	Matched related donor and matched unrelated donor HCT resulted in similar overall and disease-free survival.
Oehler (2007)	Retrospective study comparing HCT patients with prior imatinib exposure to historical cohort	Nonrandomized	145 treated with imatinib pre-HCT; 231 without prior imatinib	Busulfan 16 mg/kg and cyclophosphamide 120 mg/kg, n = 164; cyclophosphamide plus TBI (12 Gy), n = 168; TBI (13.2 Gy) and etoposide (60 mg/kg), n = 9; other drug combinations, n = 14	HR 0.65 favoring imatinib-treated patients (p = 0.03)	20% vs 19% at 1 year (p value not reported)	57% vs 59% at 3 years (p value not reported)	74% vs 78% (p value not reported)	Imatinib prior to HCT did not result in increased TRM or worse outcomes following HCT
Copelan (2015)	Retrospective study comparing myeloablative conditioning regimens for HCT in first chronic phase (both matched related and unrelated donors)	Nonrandomized	222 CyTBI; 354 oral BuCy; 97 i.v. BuCy	Cyclophosphamide (98–120 mg/k) plus TBI (12–13.2 Gy), n = 222; oral busulfan (10–25 mg/kg) and cyclophosphamide (105–120 mg/kg), n = 354; i.v. busulfan (9–17 mg/kg) and cyclophosphamide (98–120 mg/kg), n = 97	55% vs 62% vs 67% (p = 0.082)	25% vs 20% vs. 16% at 1 year (p = 0.142)	67% vs. 74% vs 77% at 3 years (p = -0.097)	55% vs 62% vs. 74% at 3 years (p = 0.006)	Cyclophosphamide in combination with i.v. busulfan was associated with less relapse than TBI or oral busulfan, in patients undergoing HCT in first chronic phase.

similar survival (~80%), relapse rate (~13%) and event-free survival (~70%) at 3 years, though by 10 years of follow-up there was an OS advantage with the BU-CY regimen, 78% versus 64%. Targeting a steady-state busulfan concentration at 900–1200 ng/mL over the 4-day administration period has resulted in encouraging outcomes with non-relapse mortality ~15%, relapse rate 8% and 3-year OS of ~85%. A recently published retrospective data from Copelan et al. compared outcomes in more than 650 patients in first chronic phase receiving myeloblative conditioning with either Cy/TBI, oral BuCy, or i.v. BuCy and showed that the risk of relapse was significantly decreased in those receiving i.v. busulfan versus oral busulfan or TBI.

Reduced-intensity conditioning (RIC) regimens would seem particularly well suited for chronic phase CML, given (1) the median age of diagnosis in CML is 67, and (2) the well described sensitivity of CML to the graft-*versus*-leukemia (GvL) effect (see next). Flu-TBI or low-dose TBI represent non-myeloablative regimens that have resulted in 2-year OS of 70% for a Seattle cohort of chronic or accelerated phase recipients of matched, related donors (median age 58 years). As demonstrated in a European Bone Marrow Transplant (EBMT) retrospective analysis, patients receiving bone marrow or peripheral blood stem cells, various donor types and across all stages of CML had a combined 62% complete cytogenetic response rate and a 3-year OS of 58%, DFS 37%. A retrospective analysis comparing patients ages 40–49, 50–59, or older than 60 years, receiving reduced-intensity or non-myeloablative transplants showed that treatment related mortality and OS were not adversely impacted by age. Importantly, overall relapse and disease-free survival outcomes were inferior in those receiving non-myeloablative conditioning, suggesting that reduced-intensity regimens should be considered even in older individuals.

PRACTICE POINTS

At our institution, we prefer to use a conditioning regimen of myeloablative intensity in younger patients with either TKI intolerance or failure. We prefer BU/CY regimen with either oral or Intravenous (IV) busulfan. BU is typically given orally at a dose of 1 mg/kg every 6 hours (total daily dose of 4 mg/kg/day) for 4 days (total BU dose over 4 days = 16 mg/kg). BU may be given at a once-daily IV dose of 3.2 mg/kg/day for 4 days as an alternative to oral BU. All patients have BU levels and doses adjusted to target a Concentration at Steady State (CSS) of at least 900 nng/ml. CY is given at a dose of 60 mg/kg/day for × 2 days (total dose = 120 mg/kg) with BU.

In cases of advanced phase CML, a fully ablative transplant will likely be needed given the high relapse rates.

Does donor type affect outcome?

Probably not. At experienced transplant centers, OS using matched related donors is similar to matched unrelated donors. In this setting, there are different competitive risks, with relapse being more of a problem with related donors, whereas non-relapse mortality (especially due to GvHD) is more an issue in the unrelated setting. In advanced stage disease, the 5-year OS and DFS was similar between umbilical cord and matched related donors, again due to the significantly higher regimen related mortality and lower relapse rate in the cord blood group.

Peripheral blood or bone marrow?

Pick 'em. Two large, randomized controlled trials of various hematologic malignancies compared HLA-matched, sibling bone marrow cells to granulocyte-colony stimulating factor (G-CSF)-mobilized peripheral hematopoietic cells (PBHC). Patients using PBHC had a more rapid myeloid and platelet engraftment, and improved OS compared to bone marrow. Unfortunately, studies were not adequately powered to investigate the impact of hematopoietic cell source for CML, specifically, though a trend toward improved survival in CML was seen. A randomized study comparing peripheral blood versus bone marrow in CML patients undergoing HLA-matched, related donor transplant did not find differences in outcomes overall, though among chronic phase patients there was a trend toward higher relapse in the bone marrow group and higher rate of chronic GvHD in the peripheral blood group. For all practical purposes, PBHC wins, since transplanters are loathe to return to the days of long, painful bone marrow harvests (for both patients and transplanters!).

Is there an established role for T-cell depletion?

Probably not. Depletion of T-cells from the allogeneic graft was initially explored in the 1980s as a means of preventing GvHD. While this was successful *per se*, there was also an increase in both graft failure and relapse.

Up-front allogeneic HCT for first chronic phase: Why or why not?

Reasons one might consider up-front allogeneic HCT include the fact that transplant is the only proven curative therapy for CML, and the knowledge that outcomes are considerably better if transplant is performed early in chronic phase. *However*:

1 There is considerable transplant-related morbidity and mortality with allogeneic transplant.
2 TKIs are associated with excellent response rates and favorable toxicity profiles.

3 Current molecular testing techniques allow for accurate, non-invasive monitoring of disease burden, allowing for early detection of disease progression.

There are no (and likely never will be any) randomized trials comparing BMT and TKI therapy (particularly for chronic phase disease). A "biologic" randomization of newly diagnosed chronic phase patients (comparing those with a matched, related donor versus those without an available donor) has been reported on. The comparison revealed a significant early survival benefit to those receiving drug therapy as opposed to transplant. The survival curves ultimately converge so that by 10 years of follow-up, there is no difference in survival (53 vs 52%, respectively). Importantly, when the trial began, many patients in the non-transplant group were treated with interferon as opposed to TKIs, so the observed non-transplant survival may underestimate that of modern TKI therapy. However, the no-donor group included patients who underwent an unrelated transplant, and the good survival of this group buoyed the no donor survival curve.

The long-held belief that BMT represents the only "curative" therapy is also being challenged. Recent clinical trials of TKI discontinuation in selected patients with a sustained deep molecular response suggest that a proportion (~40%) may have long-term disease-free survival even after stopping the TKI. In those who do relapse, the vast majority will respond when re-challenged with TKI therapy. Also, even in long-term BMT survivors, relapse does occur, albeit at low rates (<1%/y after 10 years).

It has also been shown that prior TKI therapy does not have an adverse effect on transplant outcomes, though there is some evidence to suggest that those intolerant to TKIs may have improved survival compared to those with TKI failure.

PRACTICE POINT

Chronic phase CML patients should always be started on TKI, and should not be considered for transplant.

OK, who should get a transplant?

In the modern era, indications for allogeneic HCT include (see Table 13.2):

1 *Intolerance of TKIs.* TKI agents tend to be "cross-tolerant," meaning that if a particular toxicity occurs (say, a rash) on TKI "A", it is unlikely to occur with agent "B." However, there are those rare patients who cannot seem to tolerate any TKI. For these patients, BMT is encouraged.

Table 13.2 Suggested indications for allogeneic hematopoietic cell transplantation in CML by disease phase.

Disease Phase	Indications for Transplant
Chronic phase	After second line failure of TKI therapy
	After first line failure of TKI therapy with T315I (if ponatinib not available)
	Intolerance of TKIs
Accelerated phase	In newly diagnosed patients, after failure of TKI therapy
	If accelerated phase develops while on TKI therapy
Blast crisis	Following treatment with chemotherapy and TKI (best outcomes if transplanted in 2nd chronic phase)

2 *Primary TKI failure* (e.g., failure to reach NCCN or ELN guidelines, such as lack of PCyR at 3–6 months, less than MCyR by 12 months or CCyR by 18 months). These patients should receive a trial of a different TKI, but it is prudent to make sure these patients see a transplant center, and start HLA typing. Failure of the second agent in this setting would be a reasonable indication for BMT.

3 *Secondary resistance.* Once patients become resistant to a front line agent, the probability of placing them into a CCyR with a second line agent is approximately 40%. In addition, the probability of such patients failing second line therapy and developing progression or a T315I mutation is greatly increased compared to TKI naïve patients. Thus, it is prudent to have the transplant discussion and look for a donor once a patient fails front line therapy. Of note is that several groups have found that cytogenetic response 3 months after beginning a second line therapy is a strong predictor of outcome. This is convenient since this lines up well with the time it takes to acquire a potential donor. Thus, a patient can be placed on a second line therapy and evaluated when a donor is found; if they have achieved a CCyR, one can continue TKI therapy, if not, move to transplant while still in chronic phase.

4 *Patients with T315I mutation.* Ponatinib is highly effective in chronic phase patients with the T315I mutation, and certainly most patients should initially be started on this agent. However there is considerable risk of venous and arterial occlusive disease, so patient with a high risk of vascular events, or who are young and might need to be on ponatinib for many years, should consider the transplant option.

5 *Accelerated or blast phase disease.* The rare patients who present with accelerated phase respond well to TKI therapy, and might not need a transplant (though it is worthwhile to begin looking for a donor early in these cases). Patients who present in blast crisis should get intensive therapy (often chemotherapy combined with a TKI), and move to transplant when a donor is identified. Patients who progress to advanced phase disease while on a TKI have a median survival of less a year, and need transplantation in short order.

6 *Clonal abnormalities with myelodysplasia.* Clonal changes in Ph-negative cells occur in ~5% of patients in CCyR. In the majority of cases, these do not seem to affect the natural history. However, in rare cases patients have a −5 or −7 abnormality, associated with features of MDS. These patients should consider BMT.

Management of post-transplant relapse

As many as 20% of patients with chronic phase CML and 40% of patients with advanced phase CML have disease relapse after transplant. Among patients with relapse, factors adversely affecting long-term survival include a short interval between transplant and relapse, prolonged time from diagnosis to transplant, having an unrelated donor, and advanced phase disease.

There are a variety of options to treat post-BMT relapse:

1 *TKIs.* Consistent with the efficacy profile in the pre-transplant setting, TKIs can induce hematologic and cytogenetic responses with an increased chance of response in chronic phase compared to accelerated or blast phase. Numerous case series describe the use of imatinib, second-generation, or others for treatment of relapse. Several retrospective and prospective studies aim to establish a potential role for TKI prophylaxis in the post-transplant setting.

While there is little evidence to guide the selection of which specific TKIs to administer post-transplant, it reasons to consider the presence of resistance mutations and toxicity profile. BCR-ABL mutation analysis of a cohort of CML and Ph + ALL patients who underwent allogeneic transplant demonstrated that baseline mutant clones often survive despite the different selection pressures associated with transplantation. In the analysis, 9 of 14 patients with pre-transplant resistance mutations also had the mutation detected after transplant. Furthermore, among the seven who relapsed after transplant, the majority (71%) had received a predictably ineffective TKI in the early post-transplant period.

2 *Donor leukocyte infusion (DLI).* CML provides perhaps the strongest evidence for a beneficial GvL effect with allogeneic stem cell transplantation. The considerable increase in relapse with T-cell depletion, compared to unmodified donor grafts, clearly illustrates the prominent role of T-cells in eradicating the abnormal CML clone. The identification of several minor histocompatibility antigens expressed solely on hematopoietic tissues might explain how some patients without GvHD may still benefit from a presumed GvL effect.

Donor lymphocytes, which may be infused for post-transplant relapse of a multitude of hematologic malignancies, consistently demonstrates the most favorable outcomes in patients with CML, with response rates in the range of 70% or higher. DLI are particularly effective in exploiting the apparent sensitivity of CML to immune-mediated clearance, as evidenced by the fact that CML has the *highest* response rates of any malignancy, with various series reporting roughly 70% of patients responding. Achieving molecular remission is associated with long-term OS.

Complications of DLI include bone marrow aplasia, GvHD, and increased infection risk.

The incidence of GvHD after DLI is in the range of 50%, and there is a very close, albeit not absolute, association between development of GvHD and achievement of a complete remission. An escalating dose approach has improved response outcomes (including improved survival) with less GvHD (see Chapter 36).

3 *Interferon (IFN).* Interferon has been shown to induce clinical and cytogenetic remissions in patients with post-transplant relapse, as well as molecular remissions in those with PCR positivity at 6–12 months post-transplant, though its use is becoming less frequent because of the availability of TKIs.

4 *Second transplant.* Second ablative transplants are possible, though they are fraught with a high regimen related toxicity, and probably only produce long-term survival in 20% of cases. In general, if transplantation is the only option after post-BMT relapse (i.e., no disease control with TKI, DLI, or IFN), a non-ablative preparative regimen is preferred, though if a patient is in advanced phase disease, a fully ablative regimen will likely be required for disease eradication.

The preference of which of the above therapies to use at relapse depends on several factors (see Table 13.3). What is the degree of relapse – molecular or cytogenetic versus chronic phase, or even accelerated/blast disease? Does the patient have GvHD? How healthy is the patient? Is there an available donor? In younger and/or "healthier" patients with less comorbidities, a preference might be made for second transplant, particularly if long-term TKI administration is limited by issues of cost or TKI intolerance. Conversely, the transplant-related mortality and morbidity often preclude a second transplant in older individuals or in those with significant

Table 13.3 Impact of clinical characteristics on selection of therapy for relapsed CML post-transplant.

		TKI	DLI	2nd Transplant
Age / Comorbidities	Younger / low CI	–	+	+ +
	Older / high CI	+ +	+	–
Graft-versus-host disease	Present	+	– –	~
Disease phase	Molecular / cytogenetic relapse	+ +	+	–
	Chronic phase	+	+ +	~
	Advanced phase	–	–	+ +

CI = Comorbidity Index; " ~ " denotes characteristic does not strongly favor or contraindicate treatment

Table 13.4 Who, when, and how of allogeneic HCT for CML.

Authors' practice:

A. *PATIENT FACTORS:*
Age:
The median age at diagnosis is 67 years for patients with CML. Reduced-intensity and non-myeloablative conditioning regimens have expanded the possibility of HCT to older patients with appropriate indications (e.g., TKI failure, advanced phase disease), though fully myeloablative regimens are preferred in younger patients.
Performance Status (PS) and Comorbidity:
HCT is generally restricted to those with excellent PS, in particular because of the availability of pharmaceutical (non-transplant) treatment options. Reduced-intensity regimens allow for HCT in those individuals with comorbidities or borderline PS.
Patients with CML (<65 years) who have indications for transplant and with good PS and low co-morbidity scores are considered for myeloablative HCT at our center. Older patients or those with comorbidities may alternatively be considered for reduced intensity or non-myeloablative regimens at our center. However, patients are only considered for transplant if TKI therapy has failed them (lack of efficacy or intolerance).

B. *DISEASE FACTORS:*
Phase of disease in newly diagnosed CML:
1 Blast phase: Patients presenting with blast phase disease should, if at all possible, be reverted back to second chronic phase followed by immediate HCT, given the very short duration of response in these high-risk patients.
2 Accelerated phase: Long-term TKI therapy may be considered in most patients presenting with *de novo* accelerated phase. However, patients who progress to accelerated phase while on TKI are rapid HCT candidates.
3 Chronic phase: Initial therapy with TKIs is standard of care.
*Note that in some resource-limited countries, the cost of indefinite ("lifelong") TKI may be prohibitive and, therefore, a preference for early HCT may be observed.
Primary or secondary TKI failure:
1 Switching to an alternative TKI may be considered in most situations.
2 Patients with T315I mutation should be considered for HCT.
3 Patients who develop accelerated phase disease while on TKI therapy should be referred for HCT.
We offer HCT consultation to eligible patients with any of the above criteria, as well as those with TKI intolerance.

C. *DONOR EVALUATION:*
Ideal donor: Matched sibling donor, or an unrelated donor matched at all A, B, C, DRB1 loci using high resolution typing.
If an ideal donor has been identified, HCT is offered either on a clinical trial protocol or as standard of care for patients defined above after risks and benefits have been discussed.
Alternative donor: Umbilical cord blood, HLA-haploidentical, or -antigen-mismatched donors may be considered in those without a matched-related or -unrelated donor.
We offer HCT using a cord, haploidentical or other mismatched donor only on a clinical trial protocol and only for those without an ideal donor.

D. *CONDITIONING THERAPY:*
Preference is made for myeloablative conditioning (typically a combination of targeted busulfan and cyclophosphamide) whenever possible. Fludarabine- or TBI-based non-myeloablative or other reduced-intensity regimens are considered on a case-by-case basis.

E. *POST ALLOTRANSPLANT THERAPY:*
For relapsed disease post-transplant, options include TKI, DLI, and interferon therapy. CML has the highest observed response rates to DLI (see Chapter 36). Prophylactic use of TKIs may also be considered in the early post-transplant period, particularly for those with persistent positive BCR-ABL.

comorbidities. Mutation analysis may help guide selection of TKI, versus preference for DLI or transplant if the T315I mutation is present. Clearly, the decision to transplant or administer DLI is limited by the availability of donor cells. The presence of active GvHD at baseline is a contra-indication to administering DLI. On the other hand, there is emerging evidence that immunomodulatory properties of TKI may be beneficial in patients with GvHD.

Monitoring disease post-transplant: Can relapse be prevented?

Early detection of relapse is important, given the fact that response to TKIs or DLI work better with less disease burden, and in chronic phase. Moreover, the detection of molecular relapse (or persistent PCR positivity), identifies patients at increased risk for hematologic relapse, though notably a proportion of patients with low levels of detectable disease may remain clinically stable for an extended period of time.

There are several clinical correlations with post-transplant PCR monitoring: (1) Molecular positivity at 6–12 months post-transplant is predictive of relapse (42 vs 3% in PCR positive and negative individuals, respectively); (2) The level of detectable BCR-ABL (by quantitative PCR) in the early (3–5 month) post-transplant period correlates with cumulative relapse rate; and (3) Significance of molecular positivity is less clear in the later (18 months+) post-transplant period. Note that with T-cell depleted transplants, any molecular positivity at any time point is associated with a high risk of relapse.

TKIs have been studied for prophylactic administration in patients with detectable BCR-ABL post-transplant. Several trials have investigated the safety and efficacy of imatinib, which has been shown to be safe in the early transplant period and compared against historical controls suggests a potential benefit in preventing relapse. Prospective, randomized controlled trials are needed to further establish their appropriate prophylactic use.

Is there a role for autologous transplantation?

Probably not. Initial studies using unmanipulated autologous stem cells derived from marrow or peripheral blood resulted in a cytogenetic response in a small number of chronic phase CML patients, though responses were often short-lived. Several randomized controlled trials investigating the utility of autologous HCT were initiated but closed prematurely due to poor accrual (because of the increasing frequency with which imatinib was prescribed). A meta-analysis of trials comparing autologous HCT versus interferon therapy showed no difference in survival, hematologic response or cytogenetic responses at 1 year (CML Autograft Trials Collaboration 2006). More recently, clinical research strategies have included: *ex vivo* graft manipulation to selectively depletion of Ph + progenitors; or *in vivo* cytoreduction of Ph + cells with high-dose chemotherapy prior to autologous hematopoietic cell collection. See Table 13.4.

Selected reading

1. Nair AP, Barnett MJ, Broady RC, et al. Allogeneic hematopoietic stem cell transplantation is an effective salvage therapy for patients with chronic myeloid leukemia presenting with advanced disease or failing treatment with tyrosine kinase inhibitors. *Biol Blood Marrow Transplant* 2015;**21**:1437–1444.
2. Deininger M, Schleuning M, Greinix H, et al. The effect of prior exposure to imatinib on transplant-related mortality. *Haematologica* 2006;**91**:452–459.
3. Clift RA, Buckner CD, Applebaum FR, et al. Allogeneic marrow transplantation in patients with chronic myeloid leukemia in chronic phase: a randomized trial of two irradiation regimens. *Blood* 1991;**77**:1660–1665.
4. Clift RA, Radich J, Appelbaum FR, et al. Long-term follow-up of a randomized study comparing cyclophosphamide and total body irradiation with busulfan and cyclophosphamide for patients receiving allogeneic marrow transplants during chronic phase of chronic myeloid leukemia. *Blood* 1999;**94**:3960–3962.
5. Slattery JT, Clift RA, Buckner CD, et al. Marrow transplantation for chronic myeloid leukemia: the influence of plasma busulfan levels on the outcome of transplantation. *Blood* 1997;**89**:3055–3060.
6. Copelan EA, Avalos BR, Ahn KW, et al. Comparison of outcomes of allogeneic transplantation for chronic myeloid leukemia with cyclophosphamide in combination with intravenous busulfan, or busulfan or total body irradiation. *Biol Blood Marrow Transplant* 2015;**21**:552–558.
7. Crawley C, Szydlo R, Lalancette M, et al. Outcomes of reduced-intensity transplantation for chronic myeloid leukemia: an analysis of prognostic factors from the Chronic Leukemia Working Party of the EBMT. *Blood* 2005;**106**:2969–2976.
8. Warlick E, Ahn KW, Pedersen TL, et al. Reduced intensity conditioning is superior to nonmyeloablative conditioning for older chronic myelogenous leukemia patients undergoing hematopoietic cell transplant during the tyrosine kinase inhibitor era. *Blood* 2012;**119**:4083–4090.
9. Davies SM, DeFor TE, McGlave PB, et al. Equivalent outcomes in patients with chronic myelogenous leukemia after early transplantation of phenotypically matched bone marrow from related or unrelated donors. *Am J Med* 2001;**110**:339–346.
10. Goldman JM, Majhail NS, Klein P, et al. Relapse and late mortality in 5-year survivors of myeloablative allogeneic hematopoietic cell transplantation for chronic myeloid leukemia in first chronic phase. *J Clin Oncol.* 2010;**28**:1888–1895.
11. Egan DN, Beppu L, Radich J. Patients with philadelphia-positive leukemia with BCR-ABL kinase mutations prior to allogeneic transplantation predominantly relapse with the same mutation. *Biol Blood Marrow Transplant.* 2015 Jan;**21**(1):184–189.

CHAPTER 14

Philadelphia chromosome negative myeloproliferative neoplasms

Nicolaus Kröger

Department of Stem Cell Transplantation, University Medical Center Hamburg-Eppendorf, Hamburg, Germany

Introduction

Primary or post ET/PV myelofibrosis is one of the Philadelphia-negative myeloproliferative neoplasms (MPN) with worst survival rates. Allogeneic hematopoietic cell transplantation (allo-HCT) can cure a substantial number of patients but is still not universally applicable due to toxicity that leads to therapy-related morbidity and mortality. In the more recent years, the outcome of allo-HCT has improved by less toxic conditioning regimens and optimization of relapse prevention strategies. The introduction of novel therapies such as JAK2 inhibitors may also be helpful in preparation of the transplant by reducing spleen size and constitutional symptoms. To reduce the risk of relapse, molecular monitoring and adoptive immunotherapy with donor lymphocytes have been introduced. The benefit/risk ratio should be considered in each patient taking also transplant- and patient-specific factors into account. This chapter will summarize available data and present recommendations that are mainly derived from an international expert panel from European Society of Blood and Marrow Transplantation (EBMT) and European Leukemia Net (ELN) with respect to indication and performing allogeneic hematopoietic cell transplantation in patients with myelofibrosis.

Prospective and retrospective studies of allo-HCT

In the late 1980s and the early 1990s, the feasibility of allo-HCT for myelofibrosis was shown in small reports. In the late 1990s, one multicenter European-American report described in a retrospective study a larger cohort in which allo-HCT was performed using myeloablative conditioning (MAC) in relatively young patients (median age 42 years). Non-relapse mortality (NRM) was 27% and the incidence of graft failure was 9%. The overall survival (OS) and progression-free survival (PFS) was 47 and 39%, respectively, at 5 years. Another study from the Fred Hutchinson Cancer Center in Seattle included 104 patients, most of whom received allo-HCT after MAC and NRM at 5 years of 34% and OS at 7 years of 61% were reported. A total body irradiation (TBI)-based study resulted in a high risk of NRM of 48% and a 2-year OS of 41%. Because median age at diagnosis of PMF is about 65 years there is a need to improve the tolerability of allo-HCT and enable more patients with advanced age to benefit from this treatment modality. Evidence of the graft-versus-myelofibrosis effect was already available through documented responses to donor lymphocyte infusion (DLI) after failure of allo-HCT. This resulted in the introduction of reduced-intensity conditioning (RIC) for PMF. Larger clinical trials were published but only two prospective studies with a large sample size are available so far. The EBMT published in 2009 after including 103 patients who received a busulfan/fludarabine based RIC regimen followed by HLA-matched related or unrelated HCT. The median age was 55 years and the NRM at 1 year was 16%. Cumulative incidence of relapse (CIR) was 22% at 3 years. The PFS and OS at 5 years were 51 and 67%, respectively. Advanced age and HLA-mismatched donor were independent predictive factors for reduced OS. An update of the study after a median follow-up of 60 months showed 8-year OS of 65% with stable plateau. Five-year DFS was 40% and 5-year cumulative incidence of relapse/progression was 28% with 3-year NRM of 21%. The Myeloproliferative

Clinical Manual of Blood and Bone Marrow Transplantation, First Edition. Edited by Syed A. Abutalib and Parameswaran Hari.
© 2017 John Wiley & Sons Ltd. Published 2017 by John Wiley & Sons Ltd.

Disorders Research Consortium performed a prospective phase II trial including 66 patients with primary or post ET/PV myelofibrosis investigating a RIC with melphalan and fludarabine. With a median follow-up of 25 months OS was 75% in the HLA-matched sibling group and only 32% in the HLA-matched unrelated group due to a higher NRM in the unrelated donor group (59 vs 22%).

What is the optimal conditioning regimen for PMF?

About 500 allo-HCT for patients with PMF or post ET/PV MF are performed yearly in Europe and reported to EBMT. Retrospective and prospective studies using RIC or MAC confirmed the curative effect of allo-HCT irrespectively of the intensity of the conditioning regimen. The majority of patients received a RIC regimen (76%) (EBMT data).

There is some concern regarding reduction of intensity by using RIC regimens which reduce NRM but the advantage may be offset by a higher risk of relapse. Currently, there is no prospective comparison between MAC and RIC in PMF. However, two retrospective comparisons did not show a statistically significant difference in relapse incidence or OS. Busulfan/fludarabine, melphalan/fludarabine, and thiotepa/fludarabine-based regimens are most frequently used as reduced conditioning regimen. The optimal conditioning regimen still needs to be determined.

> **PRACTICE POINT**
>
> The optimal intensity of the conditioning regimen still needs to be defined. For patients with older age or with comorbidities, or both, a lower intensity regimen is more appropriate, while for patients with advanced disease and good performance status a more intensive regimen should be selected. A spectrum of RIC regimens and protocols has shown acceptable TRM and OS. There is no direct evidence to recommend which of these regimens should be preferentially adopted.

Role of molecular markers

The detection of specific molecular aberration in patients with myelofibrosis such as JAK2V617F, calreticulin (CALR), and MPL allow monitoring patients post-transplant in order to detect or monitor minimal residual disease (MRD). Specific and sensitive assays to monitor JAK2V617F or MPLW515L/K mutation have been reported. These markers also can be used to guide adoptive immunotherapy with donor cell infusion. Recently, more mutations and molecular markers such as TET2, ASXL-1, IDH or EHZ2, and CALR could be discovered in Ph-negative MPN. The possibility to use those markers for MRD analysis in MF is currently under investigation. Apart of using molecular marker for MRD some of those such as CALR, ASXL1, EZH2, SRSF2, and IDH1/2 seem to influence also prognosis independently of International Prognostic Scoring System (IPSS) and may be a useful tool to select intermediate-1 patients for allo-HCT. One study showed improved outcomes for JAK2 positive patients in comparison to JAK wild-type patients and more recently CALR-mutated patients had the best outcome after allo-HCT followed by JAK2V617F and MPL-mutated patients while outcomes for "triple negative" patients were inferior.

> **PRACTICE POINTS**
>
> Although the use of molecular risk classification for the identification of candidates for allo-HCT among intermediate-1 risk patients deserves further clinical validation, patients in this risk category who are triple negative (i.e., JAKV617F, CALR, and MPL negative) or ASXL1 positive, or both, should be considered for allo-HCT.

Bone marrow fibrosis regression: Is it possible after allo-HCT?

Bone marrow fibrosis is a hallmark of the disease. The fibrogenesis is believed to be caused by cytokines such as platelet-derived growth factor (PDGF), beta-fibroblast-derived growth factor (β-FGF), or/transforming growth factor β (TGF-β) secreted from clonal megakaryocytes, and/or clonal monocyte/histiocyte proliferation. Bone marrow fibrosis regression after allo-HCT has been reported. In a small study including 22 patients a complete (MF-0) or nearly complete (MF-1) regression of bone marrow fibrosis was seen in 59% at day +100, in 90% at day +180, and in 100% at day +360 and no correlation between occurrence of acute graft-vs-host disease and fibrosis regression on day +180 was reported. In a larger cohort including 57 patients a complete or near complete resolution of bone marrow fibrosis at day +100 after RIC-HCT resulted in a favorable survival independently of IPSS risk score at transplantation and correlated with improved graft function and significantly less red blood cell and platelet transfusions. Regression of bone marrow fibrosis is determined by bone marrow histology but can be monitored also by whole body

MRI or more recently by PET-CT scan which is a promising technique for quantitation of bone marrow inflammation in myelofibrosis.

Selecting the optimal donor

The inferiority of the HLA-unrelated donor, especially in case of HLA-mismatch, has been reported by several investigators. Cord blood transplantation is associated with high risk of graft failure. More recently, use of HLA-haploidentical donors by preventing GvHD by post-transplant cyclophosphamide has been a more frequently used alternative donor source for hematological malignancies but systematic investigations for myelofibrosis are lacking so far. Currently, the HLA-identical sibling seems to be the preferred donor.

PRACTICE POINT

Patients with IPSS, DIPSS, or DIPSS plus intermediate-2, or high-risk disease lacking an HLA-matched sibling or - unrelated donor, should be enrolled in a protocol using HLA non-identical donors such as HLA-mismatched unrelated donors, cord blood, or HLA-haploidentical HCT. Alternative donor sources may be effective, but the actual success rates and the incidence of complications such as graft failure, and GvHD remain to be determined. Those patients should be enrolled in prospective clinical trials and data should be reported to registries.

Disease-specific risk scores and optimal timing of allo-HCT

The International Working Group for Myelofibrosis Research and Treatment (IWG-MRT) established the IPSS for PMF, which employs five prognostic variables: age > 65 years, constitutional symptoms, Hb < 100 g/L, leukocyte count > 2.5×10^9/L, and the presence of circulating blasts. Median survival (MS) in the low-risk category (no risk factor) was 135 months, intermediate-1 risk category (one risk factor) 95 months, intermediate-2 risk category (two risk factors) 48 months and high-risk category 27 months. IPSS is a powerful risk stratification tool to estimate the life expectancy of PMF patients at diagnosis. To track change of prognosis due to the acquisition of new risk factors over time, IWG-MRT introduced the dynamic IPSS (DIPSS), which includes the same variables used in IPSS but applies more weight on the acquisition of anemia. Several other IPSS independent risk factors such as unfavorable cytogenetics (+8, −7/7q-, i(17q), inv(3), −5/5q-, 12p-, or

11q23 rearrangement, MS approximately 40 months) and transfusion dependency (MS approximately 20 months) were identified recently and combined with DIPSS resulting in the DIPSS-plus stratification system. These systems are increasingly used in daily practice to advice PMF patients about their individualized risk status and guide therapy decisions. More recently, molecular mutation has proved useful as a prognostic model. Several risk scores were adapted or developed after allo-HCT. In a study including only RIC patients Lille score correlated significantly with OS but discriminated poorly between the intermediate and high-risk groups (5-year OS 56 and 51%, respectively). IPSS and DIPSS correlated with OS but differences between intermediate-1 and intermediate-2 groups were not significant (5-year OS 78 vs 78 and 70, 60%, respectively). Modified EBMT and Cervantes models did not predict OS post-HCT. Others found a good correlation between DIPSS score and outcome after transplantation.

Other reported risk models consisted of age, JAK2V617F-status, and constitutional symptoms spleen size, transfusion frequencies, and unrelated donor. A large retrospective comparison between allo-HCT and conventional therapy according to DIPSS in the pre-ruxolitinib era indicates that PMF patients 65 years of age or younger at diagnosis with intermediate-2 or high-risk disease are likely to benefit from allo-HCT, while for patients with low-risk disease, non-transplant approaches may be appropriate. Individual counseling is indicated for intermediate-1 risk patients. Apart from disease-specific risk factors also patient-specific factors has to be taken into account. Besides age as risk factor, the presence of comorbidities is a major risk factor for treatment-related complications including NRM. The Hematopoietic Cell Transplantation Comorbidity Index has been validated in MDS and AML but a formal validation in myelofibrosis patients is lacking so far.

PRACTICE POINT

All patients with intermediate-2 or high-risk disease according to IPSS, DIPSS, or DIPSS plus, and aged less than 70 years, should be considered potential candidates for allo-HCT. Patients with intermediate 1-risk disease and age less than 65 years should be considered candidates for allo-HCT if they present with either refractory, transfusion-dependent anemia, or a percentage of blasts in peripheral blood >2%, or adverse cytogenetics (as defined by the DIPSS-plus classification). Patients with low-risk disease should not undergo allo-HCT. They should be monitored and evaluated for transplant when disease progression occurs.

Individual transplant-specific prognostic factors should be considered in every patient candidate for allo-HCT to arrive at an individualized decision. Transplant-specific high-risk factors include: spleen extending more than 22 cm, having been transfused with more than 20 units of pRBC, being transplanted from an HLA non-identical donor, low PS (ECOG status >2), high comorbidity index (HCT-CI score >3), presence of portal hypertension. The decision regarding transplantation should involve the patient, whose propensity to risk-taking and motivation should be considered.

Role of spleen size and splenectomy in anticipation for allo-CT

A clear impact of splenectomy prior to allo-HCT for survival has not been shown so far. Faster engraftment of splenectomized patients has been reported but the mortality risk of the procedure is reported to be 7%. Also, splenic irradiation has been reported in some patients to reduce spleen size prior to allo-HCT. A large registry study of CIBMTR failed to show any benefit from splenectomy or splenic irradiation on survival after allo-HCT including patients with myelofibrosis. In a small series splenectomy, after allo-HCT has been reported as successful for patients with persistent splenectomy and poor graft function.

PRACTICE POINT

In patients with refractory, symptomatic splenomegaly, the evidence supporting improvement of transplant outcome with splenectomy is not sufficient to recommend splenectomy as a standard pre-transplant procedure. Pre-transplant splenectomy in patients with refractory splenomegaly should be decided on a case by case basis, considering clinical characteristics. It is recommended that if splenectomy is performed, it should be in a controlled setting of registries or clinical trials. Spleen irradiation before transplantation is frequently associated with development of severe cytopenia that can provoke complications (infections, hemorrhages) that could result in a delay of transplantation and therefore is not recommended.

Role of JAK inhibition prior to allo-HCT

The discovery of JAK2V617F mutation has led to the development of JAK inhibition in the treatment of myelofibrosis, which resulted in reduction of splenomegaly,

improvement of constitutional symptoms, and maybe also to a positive impact on survival. Because reduction of spleen size may positively influence engraftment, graft function, and reduction of constitutional symptoms could reduce transplant-related morbidity and mortality the drug may be used as bridge for patients with constitutional symptoms and/or splenomegaly prior to allo-HCT. The reduction of proinflammatory cytokines and the suppressive effect on T-cells and NK-cells may have some impact on the occurrence of GvHD after allo-HCT. Early data using ruxolitinib before allo-HCT to reduce spleen size and constitutional symptoms have shown feasibility and did not negatively affect outcomes of allo-HCT. Only one prospective French study reported on cardiac toxicity and tumor lysis syndrome. A more recent retrospective multicenter study including 93 patients who received ruxolitinib prior to allo-HCT did not report adverse effects on early transplant outcome and continuation of ruxolitinib treatment until day of conditioning reduced the risk of "withdrawal symptoms." Responding patients had a significant improved survival than relapsed or non-responding patients.

PRACTICE POINT

Pre-transplant JAK inhibitor therapy with ruxolitinib is indicated in patients with a symptomatic spleen and/or constitutional symptoms. The drug should be initiated at last 2 months before transplant and should be titrated to the maximum tolerated dose. A careful wean starting 5–7 days prior to conditioning should occur, in an attempt to avoid a rebound phenomenon, with the drug stopping the day before conditioning.

The problem of graft failure and poor graft function

Most likely due to the bone marrow fibrosis the incidence of graft failure is higher than in other diseases and ranged between 5 and 25%. The incidence was higher after unrelated or mismatch donors than after HLA-MSDs.

Another issue of post-transplant complications is the poor graft function which has been observed in 17% of patients. Poor graft function is defined as single, bi-, or trilineage cytopenia with full donor chimerism and absence of active GvHD and myelosuppressive medication.

Major risk factor for poor graft function is a persistent splenomegaly post transplantation. However, this complication can be treated successfully with CD34+ selected cell boost from the donor in selective cases also with post-transplant splenectomy.

PRACTICE POINT

In patients with poor graft function, use of growth factors (EPO, G-CSF) is recommended for anemia or neutropenia, respectively. The experience with the use of thrombopoietin analogs post allo-HCT is limited, and the drug should be used in a controlled setting (registries or clinical trials). In patients with late decline of graft function who have full donor chimerism and no evidence of active GvHD, the direct "booster" infusion (without prior re-conditioning) of donor hemopoietic selected cells (usually after CD34+ cell selection) is recommended. In that patient with persistent splenomegaly and complete donor cell chimerism, splenectomy may be an option, but it is not without risks. JAK inhibition in this setting has not been tested so far, and potential negative effects on hematopoiesis should be taken into consideration. In patients with graft failure and no autologous reconstitution, the only available option is a second allo-HCT.

Leukemic transformation

Transformed AML or blast phase in myelofibrosis is generally associated with a very poor outcome. In one study, MS of patients with blastic phase of myelofibrosis did not exceed 4.6 ± 5.5 months and no significant differences of survival were noted between patients with PV, ET, or PMF prior to transformation. In another study by the Mayo Clinic, MS of the treated patients was 3.3 months while for those who received supportive care MS was only 2.1 months. The EBMT reported a series of 47 patients who receievd allo-HCT for into AML transformed myelofibrosis. The OS and PFS at 3 years after HCT were 33 and 26%, respectively. In a univariate analysis only remission status prior to HCT complete remission versus no complete remission was significantly predictive for OS and PFS (69 vs 22%; p=0.008 for OS and 55 vs 19%; p=0.02 for PFS). The MD Anderson reported on 14 patients who received allo-HCT for transformed myelofibrosis and reported a 49% OS. PV that has transformed to acute leukemia can also be treated successfully by allo-HCT. The EBMT reported on 57 PV patients who transformed to AML and received allogeneic hematopoietic cell transplantation. The NRM was 29% and the OS 28%.

PRACTICE POINT

Patients in blast transformation (blasts in peripheral blood or in bone marrow or both equal to or greater than 20%) are not good candidates for allo-HCT. They should receive debulking therapy and be reconsidered for transplant after achieving a partial or complete remission of leukemia (consensus guidelines published in Leukemia 2015).

Treatment and prevention of relapse after allo-HCT

Depending of the risk score and time of transplantation between 10 and 18% of the patients with myelofibrosis will experience relapse after myeloablative and 29–43% after RIC. Molecular markers and deceasing donor cell chimerism can be used to detect MRD or imminent clinical relapse. A small study reported successful treatment of molecular relapse or residual molecular disease by DLIs in lower doses that resulted in no or less severe GvHD. In a two-step approach for 30 relapsed patients first DLI was given to 26 patients and 39% responded with 12% acute and 36% chronic GvHD. Thirteen did not respond and four patients with primary graft failure achieved a second allo-HCT procedure resulting in a 2-year relapse-free and OS of 67 and 70%, respectively.

PRACTICE POINT

Disease-specific markers such as karyotypic abnormality, JAK2V617F, CALR, and MPL mutations should be monitored to detect MRD after allo-HCT. Timing of analysis should be paired with chimerism determination. In patients with evidence of MRD or with decreasing donor cell chimerism after allo-HCT, discontinuation of immune-suppressive drugs, DLI, or both are appropriate strategies to avoid clinical relapse. To avoid severe GvHD an escalating dose scheme is recommended. No recommendation for prophylactic DLI can be provided.

In patients who relapse after allo-HCT and do not have severe GvHD, reduction of the doses of immuno-suppressive drugs or DLI are the treatment strategies of choice. In patients who failed to achieve complete remission after DLI, and who are deemed fit to undergo the procedure, a second allo-HCT may be considered. In patients relapsing with constitutional symptoms or splenomegaly, JAK inhibitor treatment is recommended, but remains experimental.

Regarding the decision for transplantation and a potential scenario, please see Figure 14.1 and 14.2 and Table 14.1.

Conflict of Interest Statements

No relevant disclosure.

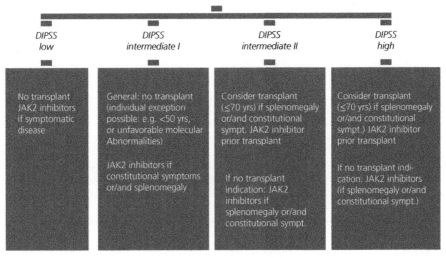

Figure 14.1 Decision for allogeneic HCT and JAK inhibitor treatment in myelofibrosis.

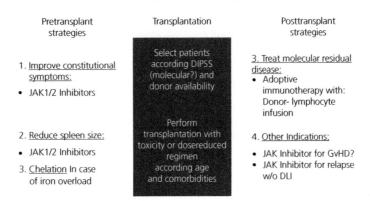

Figure 14.2 Scenario of allogeneic HCT in myelofibrosis.

Table 14.1 Who, when, and how of allo-HCT for PMF.

A. PATIENT FACTORS
1. Age alone is not a factor in deciding candidacy for transplant.
2. Comorbidities and functional status should be considered due to the higher NRM.
3. Any measure that improves the patient's PS and that reduces the individual transplant-specific risk should be considered in the pre-transplant phase (reduction of spleen size with JAK inhibitor or chelation in case of iron overload).
4. Portal hypertension is a risk factor for NRM.

B. DISEASE FACTORS
1. In general, intermediate-2 or high-risk according to DIPSS are considered for transplant.
2. Allo-HCT in blastic phase resulted in worse outcome.
3. Beside the risk factors included in dynamic IPSS (DIPSS), cytogenetic and thrombocytopenia are additional disease-specific factors that influence outcome and transplant decision.
4. The role of molecular marker is currently under investigation and may influence the transplant decision in near future.

(Continued)

Table 14.1 (Continued)

C. DONOR EVALUATION
1. HLA-identical sibling donors are preferred.
2. 10/10 HLA-matched unrelated donors are the second choice.
3. Mismatched unrelated donors have worse outcome.
4. Cord blood is associated with a high rate of graft failure.
5. The role of HLA-haploidentical donors is currently under investigation.

D. CONDITIONING THERAPY
1. For patients with older age or with comorbidities, or both, a lower intensity regimen is more appropriate, while for patients with advanced disease and good performance status a more intensive regimen should be selected.
2. A spectrum of RIC regimens and protocols has shown acceptable TRM and OS.
3. There is no direct evidence to recommend which of these regimens should be adopted preferentially.

E. POST ALLOTRANSPLANT THERAPY
1. Disease-specific markers such as JAK2V617F, CALR, and MPL mutations should be monitored to detect MRD after allo-HCT.
2. In patients with evidence of MRD or with decreasing donor cell chimerism after transplantation, discontinuation of immune-suppressive drugs, DLI, or both are appropriate strategies to avoid clinical relapse.
3. For patients with poor graft function a CD34+ selected cell boost should be considered.

Selected reading

1. Alchalby H, Badbaran A, Zabelina T, et al. Impact of JAK2V617F mutation status, allele burden, and clearance after allogeneic stem cell transplantation for myelofibrosis. *Blood*. 2010;**116**: 3572–3581.
2. Guardiola P, Anderson JE, Bandini G, et al. Allogeneic stem cell transplantation for agnogenic myeloid metaplasia: a European Group for Blood and Marrow Transplantation, Societe Francaise de Greffe de Moelle, Gruppo Italiano per il Trapianto del Midollo Osseo, and Fred Hutchinson Cancer Research Center Collaborative Study. *Blood*. 1999;**93**: 2831–2838.
3. Kröger N, Alchalby H, Klyuchnnikov E, et al. JAK2-V617F-triggered preemptive and salvage adoptive immunotherapy with donor-lymphocyte infusion in patients with myelofibrosis after allogeneic stem cell transplantation. *Blood*. 2009;**113**: 1866–1868.
4. Kröger N, Deeg J, Olavarria E et al. Indication and management of allogeneic stem cell transplantation in primary myelofibrosis: a consensus process by an EBMT/ELN International working Group. *Leukemia*. 2015 Nov;**29** (11):2126–2133.
5. Kröger N, Giorgino T, Scott BL, et al. Impact of allogeneic stem cell transplantation on survival of patients less than 65 years with primary myelofibrosis. *Blood*. 2015 May 21;**125** (21): 3347–3350.
6. Kröger N, Holler E, Kobbe G, et al. Allogeneic stem cell transplantation after reduced-intensity conditioning in patients with myelofibrosis: a prospective, multicenter study of the Chronic Leukemia Working Party of the European Group for Blood and Marrow Transplantation. *Blood*. 2009;**114**: 5264–5270.
7. Panagiota V, Thol F, Markus B, et al. Prognostic effect of calreticulin mutations in patients with myelofibrosis after allogeneic stem cell transplantation. *Leukemia*. 2014;**28**: 1552–1555.
8. Passamonti F, Cervantes F, Vannucchi AM, et al. A dynamic prognostic model to predict survival in primary myelofibrosis: a study by the IWG-MRT (International Working Group for Myeloproliferative Neoplasms Research and Treatment). *Blood*. 2010;**115**:1703–1708.
9. Rondelli D, Goldberg JD, Isola L, et al. MPD-RC 101 prospective study of reduced-intensity allogeneic hematopoietic stem cell transplantation in patients with myelofibrosis. *Blood*. 2014;**124**:1183–1189.
10. Scott BL, Gooley TA, Sorror ML, et al. The Dynamic International Prognostic Scoring System for myelofibrosis predicts outcomes after hematopoietic cell transplantation. *Blood*. 2012;**119**:2657–2664.
11. Stübig T, Alchalby H, Ditschkowski M, et al. JAK inhibition with ruxolitinib as pretreatment for allogeneic stem cell transplantation in primary or post-ET/PV myelofibrosis. *Leukemia*. 2014;**28**:1736–1738.
12. Thiele J, Kvasnicka HM, Dietrich H, et al. Dynamics of bone marrow changes in patients with chronic idiopathic myelofibrosis following allogeneic stem cell transplantation. *Histol Histopathol*. 2005;**20**:879–889.

CHAPTER 15

Chronic lymphocytic leukemia

Fabienne McClanahan Lucas[1] and John Gribben[2]

[1] The Ohio State University, Columbus, OH, USA

[2] Centre for Haemato-Oncology, Barts Cancer Institute, Queen Mary University of London, London, UK

Introduction

Most patients with chronic lymphocytic leukemia (CLL), will have an indolent course and when treatment is required, first-line immune-chemotherapy results in high overall response rates (ORR) and long progression-free survival (PFS). This approach is unsuitable or unsuccessful for patients with poor-risk features and allogeneic hematopoietic cell transplantation (allo-HCT) is a promising treatment option for selected patients. This, however, must always be considered in view of other, potentially less toxic therapies, many of which have only recently become available for the treatment of CLL. These include several new agents and cellular therapies, which demonstrate impressive and durable responses in patients who might have previously been candidates for transplant. As a result, allo-HCT in CLL faces the following challenges:

- to identify patients who benefit most from allo-HCT and in which novel approaches are unlikely to have long-term curative potential,
- to recognize the appropriate time when allo-HCT should be offered throughout the course of disease,
- to determine whether its full potential can be capitalized by intelligent combination approaches.

The aim of this chapter is to summarize the current knowledge on allo-HCT in CLL and to critically discuss its role in the era of novel treatment strategies.

Allogeneic transplant in CLL: Is this required in an indolent disease?

CLL is mostly a disease which follows an indolent course. In those patients whose disease progresses to the point of requiring therapy, a range of novel treatment options have been developed over the past decade. Older patients generally benefit from combinations of anti-CD20 antibodies with chlorambucil. In young patients without significant comorbidities, immune-chemotherapy with fludarabine, cyclophosphamide, and the anti-CD20 monoclonal antibody rituximab (FCR) is now established as the first-line standard treatment of choice. While this approach leads to high ORR and prolongs PFS, it is unsuitable or unsuccessful for patients with TP53 abnormalities and even without this poor-risk feature, some patients will relapse shortly after initial therapy. These subgroups have repeatedly been identified as having a poor long-term response to standard immunochemotherapy, and their clinical management has been extremely challenging.

What are prospectively validated negative predictors for response and survival?

Poor response to standard immune-chemotherapy and impaired survival are determined by deletion of the chromosome region 17p13.1 (del17p-):

- del17p-, determined by fluorescence in situ hybridization (FISH). This occurs in 5% of previously untreated CLL patients and in up to 30% in relapsed and refractory disease mainly in patients with unmutated immunoglobulin heavy chain variable ($IGHV_{mutated}$). Patients with del17p- typically require therapy within one year of diagnosis and have a median overall survival (OS) of just 32 months from the time of diagnosis.
- Within recent clinical trials of immune-chemotherapy, del17p- was the strongest negative predictive factor for response to therapy and survival, and clinical responses that were achieved were not durable.

Clinical Manual of Blood and Bone Marrow Transplantation, First Edition. Edited by Syed A. Abutalib and Parameswaran Hari.

- This lack of chemosensitivity is caused by the malfunction of the tumor suppressor protein TP53 – the TP53 gene locus is located on the short arm of chromosome 17, and deletion of 17p- leads to the inactivation of the TP53 gene.
- This is often accompanied by inactivating mutations of the second TP53 allele, which results in a complete loss of function, and TP53 mutations even in the absence of del17p- are associated with equally poor prognosis.

"High-risk CLL": What does this imply?

This is largely reflected by the currently available 2008 iwCLL guidelines:

- Patients with disease that is refractory to a purine analog-based therapy or to autologous hematopoietic cell transplantation (auto-HCT), a short time to progression, and del17p- should be considered "high-risk."
- Based on the predicted effectiveness of conventional immune-chemotherapy, it has also been proposed to consider specific subgroups as "highest-risk" patients. Features defining "highest-risk" include TP53 loss/mutation, purine analog-refractoriness, relapse within 24 months after FCR (or FCR-like) treatment, and failure to achieve complete response after FCR.
- Another population that is not included in these definitions but is very difficult to manage are those who have undergone Richter's transformation (RT), the development of an aggressive lymphoma, mostly diffuse large B-cell lymphoma or Hodgkin lymphoma, and occurs in up to 10% of CLL patients. Risk factors include advanced stage and poor prognostic markers such as CD38 positivity and ZAP-70 expression and del17p- and del11q-, as well as genetic mutations, but the exact pathological mechanisms are still poorly understood. As RS patients have dismal response rates and survival, there is an urgent need to identity patients at risk for transformation at an early time in the course of their disease.

> **PRACTICE POINT**
>
> High highest-risk and RT patients should be offered alternative approaches and investigative clinical protocols, including allo-HCT.

What is the evidence for the efficacy of allo-HCT in CLL?

The first myeloablative treatment based transplantation strategies in CLL were developed 30 years ago. Although demonstrating potent disease control, they were unsuitable for the vast majority of patients because of their substantial morbidity and mortality. However, it was soon recognized that toxicities could be reduced by the use of non-myeloablative reduced intensity conditioning (RIC) strategies without risking to compromise engraftment and antitumor activity. This has made HCT accessible to a larger cohort of CLL patients. Indeed, CLL is currently the most frequent indication for allo-HCT among lymphomas. Several large prospective studies have been conducted, some of which have now reached a median follow-up of up to 6 years. These long-term results indicate that RIC based allo-HCT provides long-term disease control in about 40% of patients, and also overcomes the negative prognostic effect of p53 abnormalities and fludarabine-refractoriness, as well as of recently identified adverse mutations such as SF3B1 and NOTCH1. The results from the largest reported prospective studies are summarized in Table 15.1. The efficacy of allo-HCT in CLL is largely owed to the GvL effect, which continuously mounts an antitumor immune response, likely directed at minor host antigenic variations as well as CLL associated antigens.

> **PRACTICE POINT**
>
> Allo-HCT provides long-term disease control in a considerable proportion of patients, including those with adverse prognostic markers and is mediated by a strong graft-versus-leukemia effect.

What are adverse events and risks associated with allo-HCT in CLL?

GvL activity in CLL seems to be closely correlated to graft-versus-host disease (GvHD), as patients with chronic GvHD (cGvHD) have a reduced risk of relapse and prolonged OS. Accordingly, several studies observed an increased relapse rate when donor T-cells were depleted. However, cGvHD remains a significant clinical problem. Across published large prospective studies, cGvHD affects almost 60% of patients and is the major cause for increased non-relapse mortality (NRM) rates (Table 15.1). In addition, it is the major determinant of quality of life after allo-HCT. Due to substantial improvements of supportive and anti-infective treatments and the availability of dedicated transplant units, acute side effects such as nausea, mucositis, and infections are considerably easier to manage than in the era of myeloablative allo-HCT. This is also reflected in very low early mortality rates in the first 100 days after allo-HCT. A summary of key adverse events reported in the largest prospective studies of RIC HCT in CLL is contained in Table 15.1.

Table 15.1 Results of selected phase II studies of RIC allogeneic hematopoietic cell transplants in CLL.

Author	N-allo	Trial Setting	RIC	Severe cGvHD	TRM	OS	PFS	Comments and Practice Implications
Sorror et al. 2008	82	Fred Hutchinson Cancer Center	Flu/low-dose TBI	53%	23%	50% (5yrs)	39% (5yrs)	Median follow-up 60 months Early mortality (<100 d) <10%
Dreger et al. 2010	90	German CLL Study Group	Flu/Cy ± ATG	55%	23%	58% (6yrs)	38% (6yrs)	Median follow-up 72 months Early mortality (<100 d) <3%
Khouri et al. 2011	86	MD Anderson Cancer Center	Flu/Cy ± R	56%	17%	51% (6yrs)	36% (6yrs)	Median follow-up 37 months Early mortality (<100 d) <3%
Brown et al. 2013	76	Dana Farber Cancer Institute	Flu/Bu (0.8 mg/ kg × 4 d)	48%	16%	63% (6yrs)	43% (6yrs)	Median follow-up 61 months Early mortality (<100 d) <3%

Abbreviations: Flu – fludarabine; TBI – total body irradiation; Cy – cyclophosphamide; ATG – antithymocyte globulin; R – rituximab; Bu – busulfan.
References: Sorror et al. (2008). Five-year follow-up of patients with advanced chronic lymphocytic leukemia treated with allogeneic hematopoietic cell transplantation after nonmyeloablative conditioning. *Journal of Clinical Oncology* **26**(40): 4912–4920.
Dreger et al. (2010). Allogeneic stem cell transplantation provides durable disease control in poor-risk chronic lymphocytic leukemia: long-term clinical and MRD results of the German CLL Study Group CLL3X trial. *Blood* **116**(14): 2438–2447.
Khouri et al. (2011). Nonmyeloablative allogeneic stem cell transplantation in relapsed/refractory chronic lymphocytic leukemia: long-term follow-up, prognostic factors, and effect of human leukocyte histocompatibility antigen subtype on outcome. *Cancer* **117**(20): 4679–4688.
Brown et al. (2013). Long-term follow-up of reduced-intensity allogeneic stem cell transplantation for chronic lymphocytic leukemia: prognostic model to predict outcome. *Leukemia* **27**(2): 362–369.

PRACTICE POINT

Chronic GvHD contributes significantly to treatment-related mortality and morbidity.

What determines the success of allo-HCT in CLL?

Allo-HCT seems particularly active in patients with complete or partial disease remission at the time of transplantation, that is in patients with chemo-sensitive disease. Here, the 5-year OS can be increased to up to 80%. Achieving a good remission state has been however challenging, especially in patients with p53 abnormalities and RT. Dose-intensified immune-chemotherapy and CD52 monoclonal antibody based regimens might help prepare patients for successful allo-HCT by improving their pre-transplant remission stage, but come to the cost of high toxicities. Other pre-transplant characteristics predictive of OS that can be modeled by specific risk scores such as the European Society of

Blood and Marrow Transplantation (EBMT) score include age, time from diagnosis to transplant, donor type (i.e., HLA-matched unrelated donors versus HLA-matched sibling donors), and donor–recipient gender combination. Novel agents are improving the outcome and response rates for chemo-resistant patients, but the management of RT remains a major challenge.

PRACTICE POINT

Remission status at the time of transplantation and pre-transplant characteristics are predictive of allo-HCT outcome.

Should MRD kinetics and GvL activity be monitored after allo-HCT?

For CLL, minimal residual disease (MRD) is defined as a presence of one CLL cell in 10,000 cells in the absence of clinical signs or symptoms of the disease. Patients showing less than one CLL cell in 10,000 benign leukocytes in peripheral blood or bone marrow are considered as being MRD negative. MRD levels have been demonstrated to be an independent predictor of PFS and OS after immune-chemotherapy, and add significantly to the prognostic power of known pre-treatment parameters. After transplant, MRD kinetics rather than levels seems to identify patients that are at risk of clinical relapse, long before clinical signs become apparent. This is most likely mediated by ongoing GvL activity of donor T lymphocytes and their continuous immunotherapeutic activity, which is highly sensitive to immunomodulation by immune suppression or donor lymphocyte infusions (DLI).

> **PRACTICE POINT**
>
> MRD kinetics aid in the assessment of response and indicate the level of ongoing GvL-mediated immunotherapeutic activity after allo-HCT.

What is the outcome of patients who relapse after allo-HCT?

To date, no standard treatment or guidelines exist for patients who failed allo-HCT and are unresponsive to post-HCT immunomodulation by immune suppression or DLI. However, with 2- and 5-year PFS rates of almost 70 and 40%, post-HCT relapses are sensitive to salvage therapy. Commonly used salvage treatment regimens are anti-CD20 monoclonal antibody, alemtuzumab-based immunochemotherapy, and novel agents, such as lenalidomide and ibrutinib.

> **PRACTICE POINT**
>
> Relapse after allo-HCT is challenging but seems to be sensitive to immune-chemotherapy treatment and may be improved by the use of novel agents.

Is there a role for autologous hematopoietic cell transplantation in CLL?

Several prospective trials have demonstrated that myeloablative therapy followed by autologous cell transplantation (auto-HCT) can prolong EFS and PFS if used as part of early front-line treatment, but fails to improve OS and lacks the potential to overcome the negative impact of biomarkers that confer resistance to chemotherapy or early relapse. In addition, it is associated with an increased risk of late adverse events such as secondary malignancies. Therefore, auto-HCT does currently not

play a role in the treatment of CLL, and patients that have benefited from this approach in the past are also most likely to be those patients who would respond to conventional immunochemotherapy.

> **PRACTICE POINT**
>
> Autologous HCT should no longer be considered an adequate CLL treatment outside the setting of a clinical trial.

Do alternative immunochemotherapy-based treatment options for patients with p53 abnormalities exist?

The only immunochemotherapy-based treatment option that existed that was able to overcome the negative prognostic value of p53 abnormalities was the anti-CD52 monoclonal antibody alemtuzumab and its combination with chlorambucil, high-dose corticosteroids, rituximab, and FCR. Although effective, these regimens are associated with a high rate of hematological and non-hematological toxicities and severe infectious complications. As alemtuzumab no longer has a license for CLL in the European and US market, identifying new strategies for the del17p- and TP53 mutated CLL patient subsets remains especially urgent. In relapsed CLL patients (without and with TP53 abnormalities), FCR, and combinations with high-dose corticosteroids, alemtuzumab or alternative regimens consisting of rituximab, oxaliplatin, cytarabine, and fludarabine have only limited and short-term efficacy and are associated with high toxicity rates. They might, however, serve as suitable (and in some instances the only available) strategies to prepare suitable patients for transplantation.

> **PRACTICE POINT**
>
> Alternative immune-chemotherapy-based treatment options for patients with p53 abnormalities exist but come at the cost of high toxicities.

Are novel treatments changing the standard of care in CLL?

The availability of novel treatments is dramatically changing the standard of care in CLL. These approaches include:

- *Monoclonal antibodies*, such as new anti-CD20 monoclonal antibodies, and monoclonal antibodies against receptor tyrosine kinase-like orphan receptor 1 (ROR-1) or CD44.

- *B-cell receptor signaling pathways inhibitors*, such as the Bruton's tyrosine kinase (BTK) inhibitor ibrutinib, and the PI3K regulatory subunit p110δ inhibitor idelalisib.
- *BCL-2 antagonists* such as navitoclax and GDC-0199, which mainly work by triggering apoptosis via modulating mitochondrial stability.
- *Chimeric antigen receptor (CAR) technology*, which allows specific targeting of malignant cells with precisely engineered T-cells.

Monoclonal antibodies are now integral components of CLL therapy, and agents inhibiting BCR signaling are well tolerated and very active. In a phase I/II study in 85 heavily pre-treated patients, the ORR of single-agent ibrutinib was 71%, with a PFS of 75% and an OS of 83% at 26 months. Importantly, these responses were independent of the presence of del17p-. Treatment was very well tolerated and toxicities included grade 1 or 2 transient diarrhea, fatigue, and upper respiratory tract infection. After a median follow-up 3 years, improved response qualities and durable responses in both treatment-naïve and relapsed/refractory CLL patients were reported, and higher grade adverse events diminished. Idelalisib has demonstrated ORR of 72% in a phase I study of 54 heavily pre-treated patients with relapsed/refractory CLL, including patients with del17p-. A randomized trial comparing idelalisib in combination with rituximab to rituximab plus placebo was interrupted after the first interim analysis due to overwhelming improvement in efficacy in the idelalisib arm. However, higher grade adverse events are frequent and include pneumonia, neutropenic fever, diarrhea, rash, and transaminitis. The major dose-limiting toxicity for BCL-2 antagonists is thrombocytopenia, but newer agents are more specific for BCL-2 and lack platelet-depleting activity. CAR technology uses the single chain variable fragment from an antibody molecule fused with an internal T-cell signaling domain to form a CAR, which is then transduced into T-cells. A major advantage of this approach is that it eliminates MHC restriction, and several clinical trials have reported impressive results with anti-CD19 CARs.

Are novel agents active in high-risk CLL patients?

In a single-arm phase II study of single-agent ibrutinib in patients with p53 aberrations, both the activity and safety profile supported the consideration of the drug as a treatment option for high-risk CLL patients in both first- and second-line settings. In combination with rituximab, ibrutinib is well tolerated, and active in patients with high-risk CLL. In a phase 3 randomized trial, compared to ofatumumab monotherapy, ibrutinib demonstrated significantly improved ORR, PFS and OS and was able to overcome the adverse effect of del17p- in relapsed/refractory CLL patients. Similarly, impressive results were obtained in a phase 3 trial with the combination of rituximab and idelalisib compared to rituximab plus placebo. Although both agents appear to be able to overcome the primary resistance of TP53 deleted or mutated cases, long-term disease control appears less and disease progression occurs more often in patients with del17p-, indicating that the natural dismal course associated with this cytogenetic alteration is simply prolonged. Based upon the impressive results of the front-line treatment with ibrutinib or idelalisib, allo-HCT is no longer the treatment of choice for TP53 deleted/mutated patients, and can be deferred until later in the disease course when these agents are available for patients.

Are there additional limitations to novel agents?

Although effective in the majority of patients, existing data on novel agents are not yet mature enough to allow any conclusions on their long-term efficacy. In addition, patients that have previously responded can become resistant because of mutations of drug binding sites within the BCR pathway or because of microenvironmental signals. Recent studies indicate that up to 25% of patients on ibrutinib have to discontinue treatment, mostly because of disease transformation, progressive CLL, and adverse events. Rescuing or re-treating these patients has proven to be extremely difficult, and median OS is currently just a few months. Several clinical trials exploring whether this can be overcome by intelligent combinations of conventional and novel substances are ongoing. Of note, all currently available novel agent treatments are associated with substantial individual out-of-pocket and societal costs.

What are the limitations of CAR T-cells?

CAR T-cell therapy can be associated with severe complications such as cytokine release syndrome and persisting normal B-cell depletion. Their long-term efficacy is potentially hampered by increased expression of inhibitory immune receptors such as PD-1 and the ongoing presence of an immune suppressive tumor microenvironment. Altogether, the success of CAR therapy is depending on the inclusion of lympho-reducing conditioning chemotherapy and the choice of CAR design, both of which are evaluated in ongoing large-scale research efforts. As CAR T-cell therapy requires sophisticated and complex manufacturing and treatment facilities, it is generally only available in a few specialized CAR centers, and is mostly reserved for patients lacking any therapeutic options.

Is allo-HCT still a valid treatment option in the era of novel treatments?

In contrast to novel agents, long-term follow-up from large prospective trials of HCT has almost reached a decade in a few centers. This vast body of experience demonstrates the following:
- Allo-HCT is effective and has curative potential in about half of patients with CLL.
- As allo-HCT has been primarily conducted in high-risk patients, as recommended by internationally accepted guidelines, the negative prognostic impact of high-risk constellations known to confer an adverse prognosis appears to be overcome by this approach. There is currently no prospective data on whether HCT can change the natural biological course of high-risk CLL, but some retrospective data indicates that OS is significantly improved in patients that have a donor versus those lacking a donor.
- However, allo-HCT can only be conducted in selected groups of patients, and comes at the cost of cGvHD and reduction of quality of life, both of which can significantly affect long-term mortality and morbidity.
- While relapse after allo-HCT is generally considered to be difficult to treat, and no standard approach

exists, patients can be successfully rescued and respond to immuno(chemo)therapy.

The advantages and disadvantages of novel substances and HCT are depicted in Table 15.2.

Which patients should be offered allo-HCT in the era of novel agents?

As there are no direct comparisons between HCT and novel agents, and their combinations with each other have not yet been tested within clinical trials, general evidence-based recommendations are very difficult to make. It is therefore essential to understand the limitations of each approach, and carefully weigh their chances and risks on a case-to-case basis. According to the recently published updated recommendations from the EBMT and the European Research Initiative on CLL (ERIC),
- It is feasible to withhold HCT in high-risk patients in first remission, but the lack of curative potential of novel agents in this subgroup must always be considered. This is particularly important in relapsed/refractory high-risk patients, and in patients progressing under novel therapies.
- Allo-HCT should be considered after response to novel therapies, as the success of HCT is highly dependent on the remission state of the time of HCT.
- Individual treatment-histories, patient characteristics, and preferences must always be carefully considered, along with the availability of investigational protocols.

Table 15.2 Overview of advantages and disadvantages of novel substances and allo-HCT.

	Advantages	Disadvantages
BCR signaling inhibitors	• effective • tolerable • prolong PFS • can reduce negative effect of fludarabine-resistance and del17p-	• *so far, short follow-up* • complete responses are rare • mostly only available in clinical trials • very costly • resistance mechanism are emerging • discontinuation observed in about ¼ of patients • dismal outcome after discontinuation • p53 abnormalities remain problematic to manage • numbers in specific subgroups of patients with known high-risk constellations still small • probable lack of chemosensitivity of relapsed disease
Allo-HCT	• long-term follow-up is available • effective • curative potential in ~50% of patients • overcomes negative prognostic impact of high-risk constellations • low early mortality • relapse after allo-HCT can be treated	• only suitable for selected patients • high NRM • cGvHD • reduced quality of life • specialized transplant centers are required

Abbreviations: BCR – B-cell receptor; PFS – progression-free survival; NRM – non-relapse mortality; GvHD – graft-versus-host-disease.

Table 15.3 Who, when, and how of allogeneic HCT for patients with chronic lymphocytic leukemia.

Authors' practice:

A. *PATIENT FACTORS:*

Age:
Reduced intensity allo-HCT is the conditioning of choice for all CLL patients. This approach can be applicable to an increased number of CLL patients and fitness and not age has become the determining factor. We consider this approach suitable for selected patients into their 70s.

Performance Status (PS) and Comorbidity:
Allo-HCT is feasible with low TRM in those with good PS and low co-morbidity scores. We use PS and co-morbidity score as exclusion criteria to lower TRM.
Patients with CLL (<75 years) who have high-risk disease features and who have good PS and low co-morbidity scores are considered allo-HCT eligible at our center.

B. *DISEASE FACTORS:*

Newly diagnosed CLL:

Risk Stratification:
1 Younger patients with progressive disease and del17 or TP53 mutations will undergo tissue typing to identify potential donors. Discussions will be held reviewing the role of RIC allo-HCT *vs.* novel agents in these patients. Currently revised guidelines [6] suggest we should defer allo-HCT in first remission for these patients if novel agents are available and well tolerated.
2 RT
3 Primary refractory CLL – patients who are refractory to front-line chemo-immunotherapy are candidates for allogeneic

Relapsed CLL:
4 Early relapse after chemo-immunotherapy: defined as those relapsing with clinical disease within 2 years after induction or salvage therapy.
5 Failure of, or intolerance of novel agents.
We offer allo-HCT consultation to eligible patients fulfilling the above criteria for short survival with current therapies

C. *DONOR EVALUATION:*

Ideal donor: HLA-MSD or HLA-MUD at all A, B, C, DRB1 loci using high resolution typing.
If an ideal donor has been identified, allo-HCT is offered either on a clinical trial protocol or as standard of care for patients defined here after risks and benefits have been discussed.

Alternative donor: If an ideal HLA-matched donor is not available:
We offer allo-HCT using a HLA-haploidentical or other mismatched donor only on a clinical trial protocol and only for those without an ideal donor

D. *CONDITIONING THERAPY:*
Non-myeloablative regimens are used almost exclusively in CLL because of the age distribution of the disease and the clear evidence of a GvL effect.

E. *POST ALLOTRANSPLANT THERAPY:*
After stopping immune suppressive therapy at 100 days post, patients with no GvHD and adequate PS will be considered for DLI, particularly if mixed donor chimerism or if there are rising levels of MRD.

These recommendations are summarized in Table 15.3. Ideally, biomarkers will be developed to help identify which patients will fail novel agents and which patients are most suitable for HCT.

Table 15.4 highlights points about management of CLL.

Conflict of interest

The authors have sources of conflict of interest to declare that are relevant to this work

Table 15.4 Important points about management of CLL.

1. Standard immunochemotherapy is unsuitable or unsuccessful for patients with TP53 abnormalities and some patients who relapse shortly after initial therapy.
2. These patients are considered "high/highest-risk" and require alternative treatment strategies.
3. Auto-HCT is not an adequate CLL treatment.
4. Allo-HCT offers the only potentially curative approach in the treatment of high-risk CLL patients, but is suitable for only a minority of high-risk patients due to comorbidities and advanced age.
5. Remission status at the time of transplantation and pre-transplant characteristics are predictive of allo-HCT outcome.
6. MRD kinetics aid in the assessment of response and indicate the level of ongoing GvL-mediated immunotherapeutic activity after allo-HCT.
7. Allo-HCT is associated with significant treatment-related mortality and morbidity.
8. Allo-HCT must always be considered in view of other, potentially less toxic therapies.
9. Several new agents demonstrate impressive and durable responses in high-risk patients who might be candidates for transplant, but probably lack curative potential in high-risk CLL patients.
10. Allo-HCT can be withheld in high-risk patients in first remission, but the lack of curative potential of novel agents in this subgroup must always be considered.
11. Allo-HCT should be considered after response to novel therapies.
12. The choice of allo-HCT versus a novel agent is one that must be gauged on a patient by patient basis, and individual treatment-histories, patient characteristics and preferences must always be carefully considered.
13. Until data mature, patients should be treated within clinical trials whenever possible.

Selected reading

1. Hallek M, Fischer K, Fingerle-Rowson G, et al. Addition of rituximab to fludarabine and cyclophosphamide in patients with chronic lymphocytic leukaemia: a randomised, open-label, phase 3 trial. *Lancet*. Oct 2, 2010;**376**(9747):1164–1174.
2. Gribben JG, Riches JC. Immunotherapeutic strategies including transplantation: eradication of disease. *ASH Education Program Book*. Dec 6, 2013;**2013**(1):151–157.
3. Hallek M, Cheson BD, Catovsky D, et al. Guidelines for the diagnosis and treatment of chronic lymphocytic leukemia: a report from the International Workshop on Chronic Lymphocytic Leukemia updating the National Cancer Institute Working Group 1996 guidelines. *Blood*. Jun 15, 2008;**111**(12):5446–5456.
4. Woyach JA, Johnson AJ. Targeted therapies in CLL: mechanisms of resistance and strategies for management. *Blood*. Jul 23, 2015;**126**(4):471–477.
5. Brentjens RJ, Daniyan AF. Chimeric antigen receptor (CAR) T cell therapy for the treatment of B cell malignancies. *J Leukoc Biol*. 2016 Dec;**100**(6):1255–1264.
6. Dreger P, Schetelig J, Andersen N, et al. Managing high-risk chronic lymphocytic leukemia during transition to a new treatment era: stem cell transplantation or novel agents? *Blood*. Dec 18, 2014;**124**(26):3841–3849.
7. Schetelig J, de Wreede LC, van Gelder M, et al. Risk factors for treatment failure after allogeneic transplantation of patients with CLL: a report from the European Society for Blood and Marrow Transplantation *Bone Marrow Transplant*. Jan 23, 2017. doi: 10.1038/bmt.2016.329.

CHAPTER 16

Hodgkin Lymphoma

Anna Sureda and Eva Domingo-Domenech

Clinical Hematology Department, Institut Català d'Oncologia – Hospital Duran i Reynals, Barcelona, Spain

Introduction

Most patients with Hodgkin Lymphoma (HL) achieve sustained remission following first-line chemotherapy (CT) with or without consolidation radiotherapy (RT). However, studies report that 5–10% are refractory to first-line therapy and up to 30% of patients relapse. Recommended second-line treatment, for patients who can tolerate it, is multi-agent salvage CT followed by high-dose chemotherapy and autologous hematopoietic cell transplantation (auto-HCT). Recent literature reports the success rate of auto-HCT as greater than 50%.

Prognosis of patients relapsing after an auto-HCT is poor, showing median survival from relapse of 10.3 months. Salvage options for this population of patients include RT, palliative CT, a second auto-HCT, an allogeneic hematopoietic cell transplant (allo-HCT), monoclonal antibodies, and novel agents. Adapting the treatment to the specific situation of each patient is the primary end-point.

Auto-HCT for Hodgkin Lymphoma: The HD 01 trial

Auto-HCT is the standard of care for those patients with HL in first chemosensitive relapse. The first randomized trial compared auto-HCT with BEAM (BCNU, etoposide, cytarabine, melphalan) to mini-BEAM without any autologous graft support in patients with active HL, in whom conventional therapy had failed. Both 3-year event-free survival (EFS) and progression free survival (PFS) showed significant differences in favor of BEAM plus auto-HCT ($P=0.025$ and $P=0.005$, respectively). No differences in terms of overall survival (OS) were seen.

The second randomized trial (HD01 trial) was published 10 years later; a total of 161 patients were assigned two cycles of DexaBEAM and either two further courses of DexaBEAM or BEAM. There was a significant improvement in 3-year freedom from treatment failure (FFTF) for patients undergoing auto-HCT compared to four cycles of DexaBEAM (55 vs 34%, $P=0.019$). The 3-year FFTF was significantly better for patients treated with BEAM, regardless of whether the first relapse had occurred early (<12 months) (4 vs 12%, $P=0.007$) or late (>12 months) (75 vs 44%, $P=0.02$). Of note, there was no statistically significant difference in OS for any subgroup of patients.

Prognostic factors for long-term outcomes after autologous-HCT

The impact of auto-HCT in the long-term outcome of patients with relapsed/refractory HL is not the same in all subgroups of patients (Table 16.1). Time to relapse (<12 months vs ≥12 months), extranodal disease, advanced stage, and anemia at relapse, B symptoms, and refractory disease were found to be important adverse prognostic factors. The German Hodgkin Lymphoma Study Group (GHSG) was able to construct a retrospective risk factor score from patients that were included in a Phase III prospective clinical trial. The presence of significant anemia at relapse, early or multiple relapses, and stage IV translated into a dismal overall outcome and a 3-year PFS less than 20%. More recently, a positive fluorodeoxyglucose positron emission tomography (FDG-PET) scan at the end of salvage CT and before auto-HCT has also been considered an adverse prognostic factor; in a group of 101 patients with both non-HL and HL (NHL), both FDG-PET after two

Clinical Manual of Blood and Bone Marrow Transplantation, First Edition. Edited by Syed A. Abutalib and Parameswaran Hari.

Table 16.1 Detrimental risk factors before auto-HCT influencing the outcome after the procedure.

Risk Factors	Brice et al., 1997 (n=280)	Josting et al., 2002 (n=422)	Sureda et al., 2005 (n=357)	Moskowitz et al., 2010 (n=241)	Josting et al., 2010 (n=241)	Smith et al., 2011 (n=214)	Hahn et al., 2013 (n=728)
Primary refractory HL/early relapse	XX	XX	XX		XX		
Extranodal disease	XX	XX	XX			XX	XX
B symptoms		XX			XX		
Chemorefractory disease before auto-HCT	XX		XX				XX
Residual disease at auto-HCT			XX				
PET positive status at auto-HCT				XX			
Bulky disease at auto-HCT			XX			XX	
Anemia at Relapse		XX			XX		
Multiple Relapses Before auto-HCT	XX				XX		XX

Abbreviations: HL, Hodgkin Lymphoma; auto-HCT, Autologous hematopoietic cell transplantation; PET, Positron emission tomography.
References: Brice et al. *Bone Marrow Transplant.* 1997;**20**:21–26.
Josting et al. *J Clin Oncol.* 2002;**20**:221–230.
Sureda et al. *Ann Oncol.* 2005;**16**:625–633.
Moskowitz et al. *Br J Haematol.* 2010;**148**:890–897.
Smith et al. *Br J Haematol.* 2011;**153**:358–363.
Hahn et al. *Biol Blood Marrow Transplant.* 2013;**19**:1740–1744.

cycles of CT and clinical risk score were independent prognostic factors for failure-free survival after auto-HCT. Two other studies have added additional information to the prognostic value of FDG-PET; a pretransplant positive PET/gallium scan was able to predict poor outcome after auto-HCT. Finally, in a group of 189 HL patients prospectively included in transplantation protocols, functional imaging status before auto-HCT was the only factor significant for EFS and OS by multivariate analysis and clearly identified poor-risk patients (5-year EFS 31 and 75% for functional imaging-positive and -negative patients, respectively).

> **PRACTICE POINT**
>
> Positive FDG-PET scan at the end of salvage CT and before auto-HCT is considered an adverse prognostic factor.

First-line salvage chemotherapy before auto-HCT

There are no randomized trials to compare the efficacy of CT regimens prior to auto-HCT. However, many single arm phase II trials have reported on the efficacy of a wide range of different regimens (Table 16.2). Overall response rates (ORR) are reported as 70–90% and complete response rates (CRR) as 20–55%. Toxicity for the majority of regimens was mainly hematological, with gastrointestinal toxicity also a common feature of some regimens. Mortality from salvage therapy is low, as expected from the young age of the patients and associated lack of co-morbidities.

> **PRACTICE POINT**
>
> No recommendations can be made as to the most efficacious regimen, the decision should be tailored to individual patient needs (such as avoiding cisplatin in renal impairment or avoiding ifosfamide in patients at high risk of ifosfamide-induced encephalopathy) and using an established regimen which is familiar to the treating center.

Salvage therapy and effect on graft mobilization

In addition to inducing remission, another important attribute of salvage regimens is a lack of toxicity to the hematopoietic cell compartment that would compromise mobilization and harvesting. Little comparative

Table 16.2 Chemotherapy regimens in relapsed classical HL.

Salvage Protocol	ORR (%)	CRR (%)
ICE (ifosfamide, carboplatin, etoposide)	88	26
IVE (ifosfamide, epirubicin, etoposide)	85	37
MINE (mitoxantrone, ifosfamide, vinorelbine, etoposide)	75	34
IVOx (ifosfamide, etoposide, oxaliplatin)	76	32
IGEV (ifosfamide, gemcitabine, vinorelbine)	81	54
GEM-P (gemcitabine, cisplatin, methylprednisolone)	80	24
GDP (gemcitabine, dexamethasone, cisplatin)	70	52
GVD (gemcitabine, vinorelbine, liposomal doxorubicin)	70	19
Mini-BEAM (carmustine, etoposide, cytarabine, melphalan)	84	32
DexaBEAM (dexamethasone, carmustine, etoposide, cytarabine, melphalan)	81	27
ESHAP (etoposide, methylprednisolone, cytarabine, cisplatin)	73	41
ASHAP (doxorubicin, methylprednisolone, cytarabine, cisplatin)	70	34
DHAP (dexamethasone, cytarabine, cisplatin)	89	21
DHAOx (dexamethasone, cytarabine, oxaliplatin)	74	43

ORR, Overall response rate; CRR, Complete remission rate.

data exist on the impact of CT regimens on the success rate of graft collection. A retrospective comparison between collection after mini-BEAM and GDP appears to confirm that differences do probably exist. A collection of $>5 \times 10^6$ CD34$^+$ cells/kg was obtained in 97% of GDP-mobilized patients, but only 57% of mini-BEAM mobilized patients. A similar comparison in both HL and NHL patients between IVE and ICE showed a collection of $>5 \times 10^6$ CD34$^+$ cells/kg was achieved in 72 and 51%, respectively, suggesting superiority for IVE. Previous reports implicate prior exposure to agents that are toxic to stem cells as a risk factor for reduced stem/progenitor cell mobilization and subsequent engraftment.

PRACTICE POINT

Prior to graft collection it is therefore advised that regimens containing alkylating agents, such as melphalan and carmustine, are avoided.

Positive PET-CT and role of second-line salvage for patients eligible for high-dose therapy: The role of brentuximab vedotin

As previously indicated, patients who are PET-positive after first-line salvage CT, as a group, have relatively poor outcomes. Those achieving PET-negative status

following a second line of salvage may have outcomes that are similar to those achieving this status following a single line, at least for those with exclusively nodal disease, although this finding has only been reported in a single study and requires confirmation. Nevertheless, it is recommended that patients should receive an alternative, non-cross reacting chemotherapy regimen in an attempt to achieve PET-negative status prior to auto-HCT. There are no data to support the choice of any particular regimen, though similar considerations apply regarding potential impact on mobilization. Alternatively, these patients may be considered for investigational strategies in the context of clinical trials.

More recently, alternative salvage agents including the anti-CD30 immunoconjugate brentuximab vedotin (BV) and bendamustine have been used as second-line salvage CT. The majority of data using (BV) come from the pivotal phase II study in which patients were only eligible if they had relapsed following auto-HCT. The ORR was 75% with a 34% CRR. Limited experience from small case series of up to 20 transplant-naïve patients has been published more recently. ORR varies from 30 to 58% in "refractory" patients. Two recent studies reported response rates of 53–58% in patients receiving bendamustine. Although most patients had received a prior auto-HCT, response was not influenced by chemosensitivity to previous line of treatment, suggesting this may be a useful second-line salvage option.

Can we improve the results of auto-HCT?

Tandem transplant versus consolidation therapy after auto-HCT

A number of groups have investigated the role of intensive sequential chemotherapy regimens prior to auto-HCT, particularly in the higher risk cohorts, in order to try to improve outcomes. To date any potential benefits have been offset by increased toxicities, with no evidence to suggest any significant overall benefits.

In the H96 trial, with 245 HL patients included, tandem auto-HCT was used in patients with two or more adverse factors (time to relapse <12 months, stage III or IV at relapse, and relapse within previously irradiated sites) and single BEAM-conditioned auto-HCT in the intermediate-risk group (up to one adverse prognostic factor). The 5-year freedom from second failure and OS estimates were 73 and 85%, respectively, for the intermediate-risk group and 46 and 57%, respectively, for the poor-risk group. With this data, tandem auto-HCT cannot currently be recommended outside of clinical trials, although long-term outcome of patients with adverse prognosis disease seems better when treatment includes two cycles of HDT and auto-HCT.

The concept of consolidation therapy after auto-HCT has been very recently verified by the results of the prospective AETHERA Trial. This prospective randomized placebo-controlled trial including 329 patients with high-risk HL candidates for auto-HCT has demonstrated that early consolidation with BV after auto-HCT improved PFS with respect to placebo.

> **PRACTICE POINT**
>
> Consolidation therapy should be part of treatment protocol after auto-HCT in patients with high-risk HL.

Hodgkin Lymphoma relapsing after first auto-HCT: Allogeneic HCT or second auto-HCT?

Patients with HL who relapse after auto-HCT have a very poor long-term outcome; there is little information about prognostic factors in this setting. A retrospective analysis of the Lymphoma Working Party (LWP) of the European Society for Blood and Marrow Transplantation (EBMT) and Gruppo Italiano Trapianto di Midollo Osseo (GITMO) including 511 adult patients with relapsed HL after auto-HCT indicates that after a median follow-up of 49 months, OS of these patients was 32% at 5 years. Independent risk factors for OS were early relapse after auto-HCT, stage IV disease, and bulky disease at the

Table 16.3 Prognostic factors at relapse for patients with Hodgkin Lymphoma relapsing after auto-HCT.

Risk Factor	RR	CI 95%	p Value
Early Relapse (<12 months after auto-HCT)	1.5	1.2–1.9	<0.001
	1.6	1.6–2.1	=0.001
Stage IV disease	1.8	1.1–3.0	=0.044
Bulky disease	3.2	2.3–4.4	<0.001
Bad performance status Age ≥50 years	1.5	1.1–2.3	=0.019

Abbreviations: RR, relative risk; CI, confidence interval; auto-HCT, autologous hematopoietic cell transplantation.

time of relapse, poor performance status, and age 50 years and over (Table 16.3). For patients with no risk factors, OS at 5 years was 62% compared with 37 and 12% for those having one and two or more factors, respectively.

Relapsed disease after auto-HCT represents a clear unmet need. Therapeutic options in this subgroup of patients are very heterogeneous and include salvage CT and/or RT followed or not by a second auto-HCT, palliative care, new drugs, or biological agents. HDC supported by allo-HCT is a suitable approach for patients relapsing after auto-HCT and with early relapsed or refractory HL. A broad spectrum of evidence supports the existence of a graft-versus-Hodgkin lymphoma (GvHL) effect and some studies show a lower rate of relapse after allo-HCT compared with auto-HCT.

> **PRACTICE POINTS**
>
> A second auto-HCT can be eventually considered in patients with late relapses after a first autologous transplantation and with low disease burden. In all other cases, allo-HCT should be considered the standard approach for auto-HCT failures.

Allo-HCT for Hodgkin Lymphoma

Compared to the number of autologous transplants, few patients with HL have undergone an allo-HCT. One of the major obstacles was the unfavorable outcome of allo-HCT in patients with HL reported in all early series. Two large registry-based studies gave disappointing results regarding the role of myeloablative allo-HCT in the high non-relapse mortality (NRM) of the procedure. A total of 100 HL patients allografted from HLA-identical siblings were reported by the International Bone Marrow Transplant Registry (IBMTR). The 3-year-rates for OS, disease-free survival (DFS), and probability of relapse were only 21, 15, and 65%, respectively. Major problems were persistent or recurrent disease or respiratory complications, which accounted for 35–51%

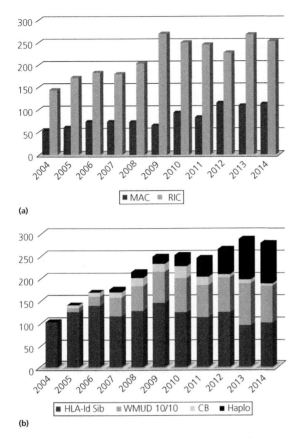

(a)

(b)

Figure 16.1 Allogeneic hematopoietic cell transplants for relapsed/refractory Hodgkin Lymphoma: (a) evolution of allogeneic hematopoietic cell transplantation over time; (a) myeloablative conditioning (MAC) vs reduced-intensity conditioning (RIC) regimens in allogeneic hematopoietic cell transplantation recipients; (b) evolution of HLA-identical sibling allo-HCT, well matched unrelated donors, cord blood transplants (CBT) and HLA-haploidentical transplants (haplo-HCT) over time. The experience of the Lymphoma Working Party (LWP) of the European Society for Blood and Marrow Transplantation (EBMT) (personal communication).

of deaths. A case-matched analysis including 45 allografts and 45 autografts reported to the EBMT did not find significant differences in actuarial probabilities of OS, PFS, and relapse rate (RR) between allo-HCT and auto-HCT (25, 15, and 61% vs 37, 24, and 61%, respectively). NRM at 4 years was significantly higher for allografts than for autografts (48 vs 27%). A potential beneficial effect of allo-HCT was not discernible at this point as results of both studies were hampered by an exceedingly high NRM.

Nonetheless, RR after allo-HCT compared favorably with that after auto-HCT in most instances and gave rise to speculations that there may be a GvHL effect similar to what had been described as the graft-*versus*-leukemia effect in the early 1980s. Reduced-intensity conditioning (RIC) became clinical practice in the mid-1990s. It has certainly been a major factor in the constant rise in the number of patients undergoing allo-HCT for HL in recent years (Figure 16.1).

The EBMT was the first group to retrospectively compare the outcomes after reduced-intensity or myeloablative conditioning in patients with relapsed/refractory HL. NRM was significantly decreased in the RIC/allo-HCT group (23 vs 46% at 1 year). The development of chronic GvHD decreased the incidence of relapse after transplantation, which translated into a better PFS and OS. This analysis indicated that RIC/allo-HCT was able to reduce NRM and improve the long-term outcome of these patients.

Allogeneic transplantation in patients failing after an auto-HCT

Allo-HCT has basically been used in auto-HCT failures. Unfortunately, the information we have in this setting is based on phase II prospective clinical trials that include reduced numbers of patients with short follow-up. In addition, the transplantation procedure is heterogeneous among different studies and comparisons are impossible to perform (Table 16.4). There are no Phase III randomized prospective clinical trials comparing the role of allo-HCT ahead of other therapeutic strategies in this setting. The potential superiority of allo-HCT in front of other "more conventional" treatment strategies has been only demonstrated in donor *vs* no donor analysis. The UK group identified a group of patients who had relapsed following a BEAM autograft who were chemosensitive at relapse and had survived at least 12 months from relapse and who would therefore have been eligible for a reduced-intensity transplant. This was a highly selected group, representing 44% of all relapses that were predicted to have the best survival. These conventionally treated patients were compared to more recently treated ones who received a reduced-intensity allograft. OS from time of diagnosis and time of autograft were significantly improved following allo-HCT, when compared to the historical control group. The estimated current PFS for the allografted patients was 34% at 5 years and 42% if in chemosensitive relapse at the time of trans plant, suggesting the early promising results might translate into a favorable long-term outcome. A recently published study by the Italian Group had similar outcomes and showed an advantage for allo-HCT over chemotherapy alone in patients with poor-risk HL who had relapsed following auto-HCT.

Table 16.4 Review of outcomes of reduced-intensity allo-HCT for relapsed/refractory Hodgkin Lymphoma.

	No. of Patients	Chemosensitivity (%)	PFS (%/years)	OS (%/years)	NRM (%/years)	RR (%/years)
Robinson et al., 2002	52	67	42 (2)	56 (2)	17 (2)	45 (2)
Peggs et al., 2005	49	67	39 (4)	55 (4)	15 (2)	33 (4)
Alvarez et al., 2006	40	50	32 (2)	48 (2)	25 (1)	NA
Todisco et al., 2007	14	57	25 (2)	57 (2)	0	NA
Corradini et al., 2007	32	62	NA	32 (3)	3 (3)	81 (3)
Anderlini et al., 2008	58	52	20 (2)	48 (2)	15 (2)	61 (2)
Devetten et al., 2009	143	44	20 (2)	37 (2)	33 (2)	47 (2)
Robinson et al., 2009	285	59	29 (4)	25 (4)	19 (1)	53 (3)
Sureda et al., 2012	92	67	24 (4)	43 (4)	15 (1)	59 (4)

Abbreviations: PFS, progression free survival; OS, overall survival; NRM, non-relapse mortality; RR, relapse rate.

References: Robinson et al. *Blood.* 2002;**100**:4310–4316.
Peggs et al. *Lancet.* 2005;**365**:1934–1941.
Alvarez et al. *Biol Blood Marrow Transplant.* 2006;**12**:172–183.
Todisco et al. *Eur J Haematol.* 2007;**78**:322–329.
Corradini et al. *Leukemia.* 2007;**21**:2316–2323.
Anderlini et al. *Haematologica.* 2008;**93**:257–264.
Devetten et al. *Biol Blood Marrow Transplant.* 2009;**15**:109–117.
Robinson et al. *Haematologica.* 2009;**94**:230–28.
Sureda et al. *Haematologica.* 2012;**97**:310–317.

PRACTICE POINT

Allo-HCT from a HLA-identical sibling donor or a well matched unrelated donor (MUD) is still considered an adequate therapeutic option for relapses after auto-HCT and chemosensitive disease.

The LWP of the EBMT has also reported the largest retrospective analysis looking at 285 multiply relapsed HL patients; NRM was 12% at 100 days, 20% at 12 months, and to 22% at 3 years; refractory disease was significantly associated with a higher NRM. The 2-year PFS was 29% and it was also significantly worse for patients with chemoresistant disease ($P<0.001$). Development of either acute or chronic GvHD was associated with a lower RR. A total of 40 patients with relapsed/refractory HL undergoing RIC/allo-HCT from an HLA-identical sibling ($N=20$) or a MUD ($N=20$) was reported by Anderlini. The 2-year OS and PFS were 64 and 32%, respectively. There was a trend for the response status prior to allo-HCT to favorably impact PFS ($P=0.07$) and disease progression ($P=0.049$), but not OS. Response rate 3 months after the allo-HCT was 67% in the Spanish experience; 40 HL patients with multiply relapsed disease and adverse prognostic factors were treated with intravenous fludarabine (150 mg/m²) and melphalan (140 mg/m²) with cyclosporine A and methotrexate as GvHD prophylaxis. The 2-year OS and PFS were 48% and 32%, respectively. Refractoriness to chemotherapy was the only adverse prognostic factor for both OS and PFS. The *in vivo* T-cell depletion with alemtuzumab was the basis of the RIC protocol used by

the UK Cooperative Group. NRM was 16% at 2 years and projected 4-year OS and PFS were 56 and 39%, respectively. Finally, the largest phase II trial including 78 patients with multiply relapsed HL and with adverse prognostic factors has been a joint effort of the Spanish Group for Lymphomas and Stem Cell Transplantation (GELTAMO) and the LWP of the EBMT. Median follow-up of the whole series was 4 years. NRM was 8% at 100 days and 15% at 1 year. Relapse was the major cause of failure. Patients that were allografted in CR had a significantly better outcome. PFS was 48% at 1 year and 24% at 4 years and OS 71% at 1 year and 43% at 4 years. Chronic GvHD was associated with a lower relapse incidence and a better PFS.

In the era of new drugs, results of allo-HCT can potentially be improved by using them as a "bridge to transplant." Chen has recently published his experience with 18 patients with multiply relapsed HL undergoing RIC/allo-HCT after being treated with BV as salvage therapy. NRM and acute and chronic GvHD incidence after the allogeneic procedure were not significantly different from that previously described. Although median follow-up was only 12 months, PFS was 100%. A retrospective analysis comparing outcomes after allo-HCT in relapsed/refractory HL patients who received BV and underwent RIC allo-HCT versus those who did not receive BV and still underwent RIC allo-HCT also found that the administration of BV as a bridge to transplant significantly increased the percentage of patients achieving a CR before the procedure, thus improving the comorbidity index of the patients before the procedure, decreasing NRM, RR after the procedure, and improving the overall outcome of the patients. The widespread use of BV in patients with HL

Table 16.5 Review of response rates after donor lymphocyte infusions.

	No. of Patients	RR (%/years)	No. of Patients Receiving DLI	ORR (%)
Alvarez et al., 2006	40	NA	11	54
Anderlini et al., 2008	58	61 (2)	14	43
Peggs et al., 2011	76	33 (4)	24/31	79
Sureda et al., 2012	92	59 (4)	20/40	50

Abbreviations: RR, relapse rate; DLI, donor lymphocyte infusion; ORR, overall response rate; NA, not available.
References: Alvarez et al. *Biol Blood Marrow Transplant.* 2006;**12**(2):172–183.
Anderlini et al. *Haematologica.* 2008;**93**(2):257–264.
Peggs et al. *J Clin Oncol.* 2011;**29**(8):971–978.
Sureda et al. *Haematologica.* 2012;**97**(2):310–317.

relapsing after an auto-HCT will most certainly change the treatment paradigm of this subgroup of patients, either by allowing some patients to avoid the allogeneic procedure or by increasing the pool of potential candidates for allogeneic transplant and thus acting as a "bridge to allo." This consideration is even stronger nowadays with the advent of check point inhibitors.

Moving allo-HCT to earlier phase of the disease

The more recent investigation of a response-adjusted transplantation algorithm identifies a further potential strategy for evaluation of allo-HCT in those deemed to be at high risk of failure of auto-HCT, targeting the intensification to those who have residual FDG-avid disease following salvage therapy. The 3-year PFS of 68% in this high-risk group was encouraging, with 80% current PFS following donor lymphocyte infusion (DLI). Such approaches may require refinement according to delineation of number of lines of salvage, and according to the outcome of prospective studies evaluating consolidation strategies following auto-HCT and it is recommended that they be evaluated within the context of prospective national studies. These results have constituted the basis for a phase II prospective clinical trial (CRUK-PAIReD, EUDRACT-2008–004956–60) already closed for recruitment that is analyzing long-term outcome of relapsed/refractory HL patients who do not achieve a metabolic CR with first-line salvage chemotherapy and undergo an allo-HCT with BEAM protocol as conditioning regimen and the use of Campath 1H as GvHD prophylaxis. Final results of this trial are eagerly awaited by the transplant community.

Do we have any evidence of a GvHL effect?

Despite the theoretical reliance of reduced-intensity transplantation on a GvHL effect, there are relatively few studies that convincingly demonstrate this activity in HL. In the context of RIC transplantation, there is some evidence of a reduction in relapse in association with GvHD.

The most convincing evidence of GvHL activity in HL comes from the use of DLI to treat patients who relapse following allo-HCT (Table 16.5). ORR to DLI have been reported to be between 15 and 60%, with CR seen in around 30% of patients. Many of these patients had received concurrent CT or RT but responses have been seen to DLI alone and some of these have been durable. There appears to be a higher response rate in the UK series and it is not known whether the high incidence of mixed chimerism seen in patients who received alemtuzumab promotes GvHL responses as it does in some animal models. The optimal T-cell dose for GvHL remains unclear, although many groups use an escalating dose schedule to try to reduce the risk of severe GvHD. Unlike follicular lymphoma, there is preliminary evidence that in relapsed HL, GvHL responses are unlikely in the absence of GvHD. However, when DLI is given for mixed chimerism, there appears to be a GvHL effect that is independent of GvHD. Although the DLI responses are impressive in some patients, the majority of patients will not achieve long-term benefit from DLI and further study is needed to optimize this potential effect.

Increasing the pool of donors for HL patients having an allo-HCT: Beyond HLA-MSD and HLA-MUD

In Europe and North America, only around one-third of patients will have an HLA-MSD, so the use of alternative donors is essential to expand the number of patients eligible for the procedure. The advent of molecular techniques has improved the accuracy of tissue typing reports but the associated increase in HLA polymorphism has made finding an exact molecularly matched donor more difficult. However, the continual increase in unrelated donor numbers, the availability of cord blood, and the use of TCD have allowed a rise in the number of alternative donor transplants performed. Although the number of published studies using unrelated donors remains limited at present, the transplant outcomes appear similar to those using sibling donors.

Cord blood transplants in HL

The published experience with cord blood donors in HL is much more limited but may be feasible. A Eurocord–Netcord study showed a 30% PFS at 1 year in patients with relapsed HL. A recently published French study showed that use of a cord blood donor was associated with inferior survival. Longer-term follow-up of these patients will obviously be necessary to determine whether the GvHL activity of the cord blood obviates the need for post-transplant DLI.

HLA-haploidentical transplants in HL

HLA-haploidentical donors have been used in small series indicating that this may also be a useful donor source, although follow-up is too short to determine the long-term impact of this approach. Raiola recently published the results of a group of 26 multiply relapsed HL patients treated with a HLA-haploidentical-HCT, following RIC conditioning with low-dose TBI, as proposed by the Baltimore group. GvHD prophylaxis consisted of high-dose post-transplantation cyclophosphamide, mycophenolate, and a calcineurin inhibitor. The incidence of grade II–IV acute GvHD and of chronic GvHD was 24 and 8%, respectively. With a median follow-up of 24 months, 21 patients were alive and 20 disease free. Cumulative incidences of NRM and relapse were 4 and 31%, respectively, and actuarial 3-year OS and PFS 77 and 63%, respectively. These preliminary results have significantly increased the interest in performing HLA-haploidentical allo-HCT in this setting.

PRACTICE POINT

Allo-HCT from alternative sources (mismatched unrelated donors, cord blood, and haploidentical donors) have been considered a clinical option for those patients with HL relapsing after auto-HCT in the last EBMT indications manuscript.

Relapses after allo-HCT

Disease relapse is the leading cause of treatment failure in patients with HL treated with an allo-HCT, with relapse rate increasing from 45 to 55%. There are no standard treatment options for patients failing an allo-HCT. If the patient does not have active GvHD and has already stopped immunosuppressive therapy, DLI has been extensively used. Although a significant proportion of patients achieve a complete or partial remission with DLI, only a small proportion of them are long-term responders. An exception to the rule is those patients receiving alemtuzumab as part of the GvHD prophylaxis. DLIs are able to convert mixed chimera into full chimeras thus, decreasing the relapse incidence of this specific population of patients. In addition to that, DLIs used to treat relapsed patients are able to achieve long-lasting complete remissions.

BV has also been used in the post-allo-HCT setting as a single drug or in combination with DLI. Gopal has used BV in 25 HL patients with recurrent disease after allo-HCT. Overall and CRR were 50 and 38%, respectively, among 24 evaluable patients. Median time to response was 8.1 weeks, median PFS was 7.8 months, and median OS was not reached. The combination of BV and DLI has been reported by Theurich et al. in four HL patients with disease relapse after an allo-HCT who showed marked clinical and metabolic responses with a median duration of disease control of at least 349 days after treatment initiation, still ongoing in three of them.

More recently, PD-1 inhibitors have demonstrated clinical efficacy even in patients failing BV. Nivolumab has shown efficacy and tolerability in a phase I trial including 23 patients with relapsed/refractory HL with an overall response rate of 83% and a percentage of metabolic complete remissions of 26%. In the same way, pembrolizumab has also shown efficacy and tolerability in a similar group of patients. Both of them are being subject of an extensive clinical development.

Selected reading

1. Schmitz N, Pfistner B, Sextro M, et al. Aggressive conventional chemotherapy compared with high dose chemotherapy with autologous haematopoietic stem cell transplantation for relapsed chemosensitive Hodgkin's disease: a randomised trial. *Lancet* 2002; **359**:2065–2071.
2. Moskowitz CH, Nademanee A, Masszi T, et al. Brentuximab vedotin as consolidation therapy after autologous stem-cell transplantation in patients with Hodgkin's lymphoma at risk of relapse or progression (AETHERA): a randomised, double-blind, placebo-controlled, phase 3 trial. *The Lancet* 2015; **385**:1853–1862.
3. Martínez C, Canals C, Sarina B, et al. Identification of prognostic factors predicting outcome in Hodgkin's lymphoma patients relapsing after autologous stem cell transplantation. *Ann Oncol.* 2013; **24**:2430–2434.
4. Sureda A, Canals C, Arranz R, et al. Allogeneic stem cell transplantation after reduced intensity conditioning in patients with relapsed or refractory Hodgkin's lymphoma. Results of the HDR-ALLO study – a prospective clinical trial by the Grupo Español de Linfomas/Trasplante de Médula Osea (GEL/TAMO) and the Lymphoma Working Party of the

European Group for Blood and Marrow Transplantation. *Haematologica.* 2012; **97**:310–317.

5. Raiola A, Dominietto A, Varaldo R, et al. Unmanipulated haploidentical BMT following non-myeloablative conditioning and postransplantion CY for advanced Hodgkin's lymphoma. *Bone Marrow Transplant* 2014; **49**:190–194.

6. Anderlini P, Saliba R, Acholonu S, Giralt SA, Andersson B, Ueno NT, et al. Fludarabine-melphalan as a preparative regimen for reduced-intensity conditioning allogeneic stem cell transplantation in relapsed and refractory Hodgkin's lymphoma: the updated M.D. Anderson Cancer Center experience. *Haematologica.* 2008 Feb; **93**(2):257–264.

CHAPTER 17

Indolent lymphomas

Narendranath Epperla[1], Hamza Hashmi[2], and Mehdi Hamadani[1]

[1] Division of Hematology and Oncology, Medical College of Wisconsin, Milwaukee, WI, USA

[2] Department of Internal Medicine, Michigan State University, Grand Rapids, MI, USA

Introduction

Indolent lymphomas also referred to as low grade lymphomas present with striking pathobiologies and clinical heterogeneity. The recent advances in the management strategies of indolent lymphomas including combination chemoimmunotherapy, radio-immunoconjugates, and targeted therapies (PI3K inhibitors, BTK inhibitors, lenalidomide, etc.) have led to higher frequency of response in the non-transplant setting. However, due to their indolent nature, these lymphoproliferative disorders remain generally incurable. Although hematopoietic cell transplantation (HCT) is considered a feasible option, its role in indolent lymphomas remains controversial. While high-dose therapy (HDT) and autologous HCT (auto-HCT) has low treatment related mortality (TRM) and morbidity, disease relapse remains a major concern. In addition, long-term toxicities especially the development of secondary myelodysplastic syndrome/acute myeloid leukemia (sMDS/AML) is concerning with this approach. Although myeloablative (MA) allogeneic-HCT (allo-HCT) is a potentially curative modality, it is often associated with prohibitive TRM. Reduced intensity conditioning (RIC) allo-HCT provides an alternative with acceptable TRM while achieving superior response rates.

This chapter provides an overview of contemporary clinical data assessing the role and optimal timing of auto-HCT, along with post-transplant maintenance therapy in indolent B-cell non-Hodgkin lymphomas (NHL) including follicular lymphoma (FL), transformed FL, lymphoplasmacytic lymphoma/Waldenström macroglobulinemia (LPL/WM), mantle cell lymphoma (MCL), marginal zone lymphoma (MZL), and small lymphocytic lymphoma (SLL).

Follicular lymphoma

FL represents 22% of NHL. The median age at diagnosis is generally in the sixth decade and is more common in females. FL is an indolent lymphoma with a disease course characterized by remissions and relapses with conventional chemoimmunotherapies followed by development of resistance and/or transformation to a more aggressive histology. Management strategies range from surveillance, combination chemoimmunotherapy, radio-immunotherapy to HCT (auto-HCT or allo-HCT).

HCT in first remission: Auto-HCT versus allo-HCT

The role of auto-HCT consolidation for FL in first remission has been extensively investigated to improve the depth of response, disease control, and possibly survival. Randomized studies conducted in pre-rituximab and rituximab-era have demonstrated improved progression free survival (PFS) with upfront auto-HCT for FL in first remission, without any overall survival (OS) benefit, and trend toward more sMDS/AML (Table 17.1).

Allo-HCT offers several advantages such as a lymphoma-free graft and the alloreactive donor T-cell mediated graft-versus-lymphoma (GvL) effects. In FL, allo-HCT represents a potentially curative treatment modality. There are no randomized controlled data to support allo-HCT in first remission for chemosensitive FL patients. However, based on limited single institution data there may be role for allo-HCT in a small subset of high-risk FL patients with primary refractory disease, failing to achieve remission despite multiple treatment

Clinical Manual of Blood and Bone Marrow Transplantation, First Edition. Edited by Syed A. Abutalib and Parameswaran Hari.

Table 17.1 Randomized prospective trials addressing the role of autologous transplantation in first remission for FL patients.

Study (Year)	No/Auto	Conditioning Regimen	TRM Auto versus Chemotherapy	EFS/PFS Auto versus Chemotherapy (Years)	OS Auto versus Chemotherapy (Years)	Comments
GLSG (2004)	307/240	CHOP/MCP	<2.5% in both arms	64* vs 33% (5)	Not reported	Significantly more sMDS/AML with auto (3.5* vs 0%; p = 0.02)
GELA (2006)	402/192	CHOP-HDT	Not reported	38 vs 28% (7)	76 vs 71% (7)	Second malignancies similar in both groups; 14 with chemotherapy and 11 with auto-HCT
GITMO (2008)	136/68	Hd Cy Hd Vp16 APO DHAP	N = 3 vs N = 2 at 100 days	61* vs 28% (4)	81 v. 80% (4)	4–year sMDS/AML was higher with HDT (6.6 vs 1.7%)
GOELAMS (2009)	166/86	VCAP Vp16 DHAP	Not reported	64* vs 39% (9)	76 vs 80% (9)	Auto-HCT associated with significantly more second malignancies (n = 12* vs 1; p = 0.01)

Lenz et al. *Blood* 2004;**104**:2667–2674. Sebban et al. *Blood* 2006;**108**:2540–2544. Ladetto et al. *Blood* 2008;**111**:4004–4013. Gyan et al. *Blood* 2009; **113**:995–1001.

GLSG – German low grade lymphoma study group; GELA – Groupe d'Etude des Lymphomes de l'Adulte; GOELAMS - Groupe Ouest-Est des Leucémies et Autres Maladies du Sang; GITMO - Gruppo Italiano Trapianto di Midollo Osseo; TRM – treatment related mortality; HDT – high-dose therapy and autologous HCT arm; C – chemotherapy arm; EFS/PFS – Event/progression free survival; OS – overall survival; sMDS – secondary myelodysplastic syndrome; AML – acute myeloid leukemia

CHOP – cyclophosphamide, doxorobucin, vincristine, prednisone; MCP – melphalan, cyclophosphamide, prednisone; Hd – high-dose; Cy – cytarabine; Vp16 – etoposide; APO- vincristine, adriamycin, and prednisone; DHAP-dexamethasone, cytarabine, cisplatin; VCAP – vincristine, cyclophosphamide, Adriamycin, and prednisolone

attempts. Such high-risk FL patients with primary refractory disease can be considered for an allo-HCT, ideally within the context of a clinical trial.

PRACTICE POINT

Upfront auto-HCT and allo-HCT for FL in first remission is not recommended owing to following considerations:

- Recent advances in the management of FL, including radio-immunotherapy consolidation, rituximab maintenance and/or re-treatment and approval of targeted, highly active oral agents in relapsed setting.
- Risk of secondary malignancies.
- Lack of a clear OS benefit.

HCT for relapsed FL: Auto-HCT versus MA- allo-HCT

Although FL patients generally respond to initial therapy, disease relapse inevitably occurs. The role, optimal timing, and preferred transplant modality (autologous vs allogeneic), in the relapsed setting are some of the questions that lack definitive answers. In the rituximab-era, the lack of randomized data establishing the superiority of auto-HCT over salvage chemoimmunotherapy alone makes it difficult to recommend the routine use of auto-HCT in relapsed FL (Table 17.2). Therefore, the decision to offer an auto-HCT for relapsed FL should be based on careful review of individual patient factors including age, associated comorbidities, risk of secondary cancers, and presence of chemosensitive disease and it should not be offered to heavily pretreated patients with refractory disease.

Registry data from the Center for International Blood & Marrow Transplant Research (CIBMTR) and the European Society for Blood and Marrow Transplantation (EBMT) show a plateau in relapse risk, 2–3 years after allografting, unlike auto-HCT where relapse risk after transplant does not decrease overtime. Despite low relapse rates post allo-HCT (20–25% post allograft compared to 50–55% post auto-HCT at 5 years) there was no difference in OS in both the CIBMTR and EBMT studies, due to high rates of TRM following MA allografts (35–40% compared to 8–15% after auto-HCT) (Table 17.2). Whether younger patients with chemorefractory disease benefit from MA allo-HCT over RIC regimens, is currently not known.

Table 17.2 Retrospective studies with a minimum of 100 patients addressing the role of autologous transplantation in relapsed/refractory FL (2002–2012).

Group (Year)	No. T/Auto	Conditioning Regimen	TRM % (Years)	EFS/PFS % (Years)	OS % (Years)	Comments
FHCRC (2003)	125/ 98	TBI/Cy/VP-16 TBI/Cy Bu-Mel Bu-TT	11% at day 100	29% (5)	53 (5)	Compared to conventional HDT, RIT in transplant conditioning was associated with improved OS % (53 vs 67) and PFS % (29 vs 48)
CIBMTR (2004)	728/ 597 purged 131 unpurged	TBI based	Purged = 14 Unpurged = 8 (5)	Purged = 39 Unpurged = 31 (5)	Purged = 62* Unpurged = 55 (5)	- Chemosensitive disease predicted better outcomes. - OS favored purged autografts
EBMT (2007)	693/378	TBI BEAM BEAC CBV	9 (5)	31 (10)	52 (10)	- CR1 predicted better outcomes. - 9% had second cancers
DFCI/SBH (2007)	121/ 121	Cy/TBI	NR	48 (10)	54 (10)	- 12.4% had sMDS/AML - Greater benefit for FL in CR2
Ottawa (2007)	115/ 115	TBI BEAM CBV	14	56 (5)	72 (5)	- 7% second cancers - Chemosensitive disease had better outcomes - All unpurged autografts
GELF86/94 (2008)	254/96	Cy/Vp16/TBI	NR	RT=67 T=46 R=39 (5)	RT=93 T=63 R=70 (5)	Patients getting rituximab-based salvage at relapse did not benefit from auto-HCT
GITIL (2008)	223/223	Cy/Vp16 cytarabine	~3	74 (5)	55 (5)	Rituximab administration with HDT improved OS and EFS

Gopal et al. *Blood* 2003; 2003; **102**(7): 2351–2357. van Besien et al. *Blood* 2003; **102**(10):3521–3529. Montoto et al. *Leukemia* 2007; **21**(11): 2324–2331. Rohatiner al. *J Clin Oncol* 2007; **25**(18):2554–2559. Sabloff et al. *Biol Blood Marrow Transplant* 2007; **13**(8):956–964. Sebban et al. *J Clin Oncol* 2008; **26**(21):3614–3620. Tarella et al. *J Clin Oncol* 2008; **26**(19): 3166–3175.

* Statistically significant value

CIBMTR = Center for International Blood and Marrow Transplant Research; DFCI = Dana-Farber Cancer Institute; EBMT = European Blood and Marrow Transplant; FHCRC = Fred Hutchinson Cancer Research Center; GITIL = Gruppo Italiano Terapie Innnovative nei linfomi; SBH = St. Bartholomew's Hospital

Cy – cyclophosphamide; Mel – melphalan; Flu – Fludarabine; TBI – total body irradiation; Bu- Busulfan; BEAM – BCNU, etoposide, cytarabine, melphalan; VP-16 – etoposide; TT – thiotepa; CBV – Cytoxan (cyclophosphamide), BCNU (carmustine), and VP-16 (etoposide); BEAC – carmustine (BCNU), etoposide, Ara-C, and cyclophosphamide; TRM – treatment related mortality; PFS – progression free survival; OS – overall survival

---

PRACTICE POINT

Auto-HCT is best reserved for chemosensitive relapsed FL patients after 2–3 lines of prior chemoimmunotherapies (ideally at least one doxorubicin-based line, and a bendamustine based regimen), who are not candidates for allo-HCT due to lack of suitable donor, associated comorbidities, or patient preference.

MA allo-HCT should not be considered as the regimen of choice in patients with FL, especially for those with advanced age and/or with associated medical comorbidities and poor performance status.

HCT for relapsed FL: Auto-HCT versus RIC allo-HCT

RIC regimens were developed to improve applicability of allo-HCT to older, heavily pretreated patients with associated medical comorbidities. These regimens aim at reducing procedure related toxicities and rely more heavily on GvL immunologic effects. A commonly encountered clinical question in relapsed FL (that has progressed through multiple lines of prior therapies) is whether to offer auto- or RIC allo-HCT. Although limited, clinical data has shown that TRM with RIC

Table 17.3 Role of RIC allogeneic transplantation in relapsed FL.

Author/ Year	No	Prior Auto-HCT	Conditioning Regimen	TRM	Chronic GvHD (extensive)	DFS/EFS (median f/u) (%/year)	OS (median f/u) (%/year)	Comments
Rezvani (2008)	62/54	32%	TBI +/- Flu	42%	47%	43% (3 y)	52% (3 y)	- Heavily pretreated group (median of 6 lines of treatment) - Long term survivors had good functional status (KPS – 85%)
Thomson (2010)	82	26%	Flu/Mel/Alem	15%	30% (18%)	76% (3.7 y)	76% (3.7 y)	- Median of 4 lines of prior therapy - Relapse risk was significantly reduced by the use of DLI
Pinana (2010)	37	46%	Flu/Mel	37%	78% (42%)	57% (4.4 y)	54% (4.4 y)	- Majority of the patients had a median of 2–3 prior therapies
Shea (2011)	44/16	0%	Flu/Cy	75%	29% (18%)	81% (4.6 y)	9% (4.6 y)	- Majority of the patients had a median of 2 prior therapies. - All the patients were chemosensitive
Khouri (2012)	47	19%	Flu/Cy/RTX	72%	58% (40%)	78%	21%	- Low frequency of relapse seen after a long f/u is suggestive of probable cure in this patient group - Addition of Y^{90} to the conditioning regimen seems to be effective in chemorefractory patients
	26	0%	Flu/Cy/Y^{90}	8%	39% (24%)	87% [CS] (2.9 y) 80% [CR] (2.9 y)	94% [CS] (2.9 y) 80% [CR] (2.9 y)	

Rezvani et al. *J Clin Oncol* 2008;**26**:211–217. Thomson et al. *J Clin Oncol* 2010;**28**:3695–3700. Pinana et al. *Haematologica* 2010; **95**:1176–1182. Shea et al. *Biol Blood Marrow Transplant* 2011;**17**:1395–1403. Khouri et al. *Blood*. 2012;**119**(26):6373–6378.
Cy – cyclophosphamide; Mel – melphalan; Flu – Fludarabine; TBI – total body irradiation; Alem – Alemtuzumab; Y^{90} – Yttrium 90; RTX – total nodal radiation; TRM – treatment related mortality; PFS – progression free survival; OS – overall survival

allo-HCT is relatively low, with lower risk of disease relapse and no risk of sMDS/AML when compared to auto-HCT (Table 17.3). Based on expert opinion, matched unrelated donor transplants are considered as effective as matched related donor transplants.

PRACTICE POINT

It is appropriate to offer RIC allo-HCT to the following patients with a curative intent:

• Appropriately selected and clinically fit FL patients.

• Available suitable donor.

Auto-HCT can be considered for the following patients with the understanding that cure may not be achievable:

• Medically unfit for RIC allo-HCT.

• No suitable donor available.

HCT for relapsed FL: Chemoimmunotherapy/allo-HCT versus tandem auto/allo-HCT

It is not known whether tandem auto/allo-HCT is superior to effective cytoreduction with chemoimmunotherapy followed by allo-HCT. At the present time, a tandem auto/allo-HCT should be considered investigational.

Post auto-HCT maintenance therapy in FL: Where are we now?

In FL, maintenance immunotherapies (with rituximab) have shown benefit after both frontline and subsequent chemoimmunotherapies. In relapsed FL, EBMT conducted

Table 17.4 Autologous HCT for FL that has undergone histological transformation to large cell lymphoma.

Author (Year)	Number of Patients	Age (Range)	Conditioning Regimen	TRM	PFS	OS	Comments
Friedberg (1999) (26)	21	44 (29–58)	TBI/Cy	NA	46% (5 y)	58% (5 y)	All had minimal disease state. Purged autograft used.
Chen (2001) (30)	25[a]	48 (36–64)	Mel/TBI/VP	28%	36% (5 y)	37% (5 y)	All had chemosensitive disease.
Williams (2001) (29)	50	40 (26–52)	Various regimens	8% (100 days)	30% (5 y)	51% (5 y)	100% had chemosensitive disease. High LDH led to poor outcomes.
Hamadani (2008) (31)	24	56 (47–68)	Bu/Cy BCNU-based	8% (100 days)	40% (3 y)	52% (3 y)	17% had bulky disease and no purged autografts used.
Eide (2011) (32)	30[b]	55 (31–65)	BEAM	NA	32% (5 y)	47% (5 y)	The only prospective trial. All 30 had chemosensistive disease.

Friedberg et al. *Biol Blood Marrow Transplant* 1999;**5**(4):262–268. Williams et al. *J Clin Oncol* 2001;**19**(3):727–735. Chen et al. *Br J Haematol* 2001;**113**(1):202–208. Hamadani et al. *Eur J Haematol* 2008;**81**(6):425–431. Eide et al. *Br J Haematol* 2011;**152**(5):600–610.
TBI – total body irradiation; Cy – cyclophosphamide; Mel – melphalan; VP – etoposide; Bu – busulfan; BCNU – carmustine; TRM – treatment related mortality; PFS – progression free survival; OS – overall survival; LDH – lactate dehydrogenase; BEAM – BCNU, etoposide, cytarabine, melphalan.
[a] Of the 35 patients in the sample, only 25 had true histological transformation to diffuse large B-cell lymphoma.
[b] Of the 47 patients enrolled only 30 underwent autologous HCT.

a randomized prospective trial to assess the efficacy and safety of rituximab, as *in vivo* purging before transplantation and as maintenance treatment immediately after HDT and auto-HCT. At a median follow-up of 8.3 years, rituximab maintenance when compared to observation resulted in superior PFS at 10 years (54 vs 37%), but did not translate into an improvement in OS (73 vs 68%). In addition, maintenance rituximab was associated with a higher (albeit statistically non-significant) rate of late neutropenia.

While rituximab maintenance post auto-HCT appears unlikely to improve survival of FL patients, the role of other novel approaches as maintenance therapies post auto-HCT in FL warrants further investigation. Ongoing post auto-HCT maintenance clinical trials involving FL patients are evaluating the role of immune modulators (NCT01035463; lenalidomide maintenance; phase I/II), and proteasome inhibitors (NCT00992446; bortezomib in combination with vorinostat; phase II) as maintenance options.

Transformed FL: Is there a role for HCT?

Transformation of FL into a more aggressive histology is not uncommon. Studies that investigated the role of auto-HCT in transformed FL are limited due to lack of randomized data and variations in the criteria used to define histological transformation (Table 17.4). Moreover, patients with limited stage at the time of transformation can experience prolonged remissions with chemoimmunotherapy alone and it is unknown whether these patients derive any added benefit from auto-HCT consolidation. Treatment strategies are further complicated by the observation that late relapses do occur with the indolent non-transformed component after auto-HCT in transformed FL. This indicates that while HDT may eradicate the large cell component; the (non-transformed) FL remains incurable. There is limited data available for allo-HCT in transformed FL.

PRACTICE POINT

In patients with FL, maintenance therapies post auto-HCT (including rituximab) should be considered investigational and offered only on a clinical trial.

PRACTICE POINT

Auto-HCT is a reasonable option for transformed patients with minimal disease (non-bulky and chemosensitive).

Mantle cell lymphoma

MCL accounts for approximately 6% of all NHLs, and typically presents with advanced stage and involvement of extra nodal sites. Over the last decade; multi-agent chemoimmunotherapies either alone, or followed by auto-HCT consolidation in first remission have provided higher response rates and improved outcomes of MCL patients (see Chapter 19).

Upfront auto-HCT in MCL: Transplant in first remission

The poor prognosis of relapsed MCL (median survival of ~1–2 years), serves as a rationale for auto-HCT *consolidation* in first remission. Early registry data from EBMT and ABMTR (Autologous Bone Marrow Transplant Registry) supported the role of auto-HCT for MCL in first remission, particularly for patients in CR1. These results were subsequently confirmed by the European MCL Network trial, which randomized MCL patients after first-line induction with CHOP-like regimens to either auto-HCT consolidation or interferon maintenance (Table 17.5). Auto-HCT in this study provided a superior PFS but no survival benefit was seen.

Randomized studies supporting upfront auto-HCT for MCL in rituximab-era are not available. Several uncontrolled prospective studies have, however, reported favorable outcomes with upfront auto-HCT consolidation in MCL, in the chemoimmunotherapy era (Table 17.5). Although the aforementioned prospective studies establish the feasibility and efficacy of upfront auto-HCT in MCL, it is important to acknowledge that while this modality is widely practiced, it is not uniformly accepted by all centers. Mature data from the M.D. Anderson Cancer Center (MDACC) suggest that chemoimmunotherapy with R-Hyper-CVAD (rituximab, fractionated cyclophosphamide, vincristine, doxorubicin, dexamethasone alternating with methotrexate and cytarabine), without an auto-HCT consolidation might be an effective strategy for MCL, with 7-year OS and PFS of 60 and 43%, respectively. These excellent outcomes with R-Hyper-CVAD, however; were not reproduced in a multicenter SWOG (South West Oncology Group) study). The poor outcomes of high-risk MIPI patients, with or without auto-HCT have been reported by several other groups, underscoring the need for evaluating alternative consolidation modalities for such patients (e.g., early use of allogeneic-HCT).

> **PRACTICE POINT**
>
> Upfront auto-HCT consolidation in MCL is a valid option, especially for patients with low- and intermediate-risk MIPI.

Relapsed/refractory MCL: Auto-HCT versus allo-HCT

Auto-HCT might not be an effective strategy for relapsed MCL in general, and chemorefractory patients in particular. However, CIBMTR recently reported 5-year OS of 44% in 159 relapsed, chemosensitive MCL patients undergoing auto-HCT (Table 17.5). Of note, Allo-HCT may still offer some benefit in chemorefractory patients. Hamadani et al reported results of allo-HCT for chemorefractory MCL with MA and RIC regimens with almost similar results (TRM, relapse, PFS, and OS) for the two groups (Table 17.6).

> **PRACTICE POINT**
>
> The authors recommend allo-HCT, with RIC for patients with prior auto-HCT or those who are chemoresistant. In patient with chemosensitive disease, who are not candidates for a potentially curative allogeneic-HCT (due to comorbidities, donor availability, etc.), consolidation with an auto-HCT can be offered, with the understanding that this therapy will not cure the disease.

Waldenström macroglobulinemia

WM is an indolent B-cell lymphoproliferative disorder resulting from the accumulation of clonally related IgM secreting lymphoplasmacytic cells. Symptomatic WM patients can be treated with frontline single agent alkylators (e.g. cyclophosphamide or chlorambucil), nucleoside analogs (e.g., fludarabine) or rituximab), ibrutinib, or combination chemoimmunotherapy. Use of auto-HCT consolidation for WM in first remission should not be considered outside the setting of a clinical trial due to lack of clinical data.

Registry data and several retrospective studies have examined the role of auto-HCT mostly in relapsed/ refractory WM (Table 17.7). The use of purine nucleoside analogs (particularly fludarabine – that can impair stem cell mobilization) should be avoided in potential candidates for auto-HCT in future. Several studies have also looked into allo-HCT for treatment of WM (Table 17.8). However, the good response rates seen with allo-HCT are negated by high TRM (Table 17.8).

> **PRACTICE POINT**
>
> Auto-HCT can be considered in relapsed WM patients with chemosensitive disease, typically after 2–3 lines of prior therapies (preferably consisting of at least one alkylator/ anthracycline-based regimen and a bortezomib-containing regimen).

Table 17.5 Autologous transplantation in mantle cell lymphoma patients in first remission.

Author/Year	N	TRM %	Regimen(s)	Median OS % (Years)	Median PFS % (Years)	Comments
Vandenberghe (2003)	195	-	Chemo+ auto-HCT	50 (5)	33 (5)	Disease status at transplant was the most significant factor affecting survival
Dreyling (2005)	62 / 60	5 / 0	R-CHOP+ auto-HCT / R-CHOP+IFN- α	83 vs 77 (3)	3.3 vs 1.4 (3)	- Performed in pre-R era - No survival benefit
Hermine (2012)	455	4	R-CHOP+ auto-HCT / R-CHOP/RDHAP+ auto-HCT	6.8 vs NR	3.8 vs 7.3	Addition of Ara-C in induction improved OS w/o significant increase in toxicity
Geisler (2008) (2012 update)	160	5	R-Maxi-CHOP+high-dose cytarabine+ auto-HCT	58 (10)	7.4	- Late relapses were seen on long term follow-up - Pre-emptive R used post auto-HCT for molecular relapses
Van't Veer (2009)	87	5	R-CHOP+ high-dose cytarabine+ auto-HCT	66 (4)	36 (4)	BEAM was used for conditioning
Damon (2009)	77	3	R-CHOP+MTX + H-AraC/VP16+ auto-HCT	64 (5)	56 (5)	In vivo purging with R used
Gressin (2010)	113	11	R-VADC+ auto-HCT	62 (3)	4.8	Very low hematologic and extra-hematologic toxicity
Delarue (2012)	60	1.5	R-CHOP/RDHAP+ auto-HCT	75 (5)	64 (5)	11 patients had second malignancies
Touzeau (2014)	396	2.5	High-dose cytarabine based regimen + auto-HCT	83 (3)	67 (3yr)	Age, disease status at time of auto-HCT and use of rituximab were statistically predictive for both PFS and OS
Fenske (2014)	249*	3	Chemo+ auto-HCT [early cohort]	61 (5)	52 (5 yr)	Optimal timing for HCT is early in the disease course
	132**	9	Chemo+ auto-HCT [late cohort]	44 (5)	29 (5)	

Vandenberghe et al. *Br J Haematol*. 2003;**120**:793–800. Dreyling et al. *Blood*. 2005;**105**:2677–2684. Hermine et al. *ASH Annual Meeting Abstracts*. 2012;**120**:151. Geisler et al *Br J Haematol*. 2012;**158**:355–362. van 't Veer et al. *Br J Haematol*. 2009;**144**:524–530. Damon et al. *J Clin Oncol*. 2009;**27**:6101–6108. Gressin et al. *Haematologica*. 2010;**95**:1350–1357. Delarue et al. *Blood*. 2013;**121**:48–53. Touzeau et al. *Ann Hematol*. 2014;**93**:233–242. Fenske et al. *J Clin Oncol*. 2014;**32**:273–281.

* Early cohort-transplantation performed in first PR or CR with no more than two prior lines chemotherapy;
** Late cohort-transplantation performed in the remaining chemosensitive patients.
R-CHOP – Rituxin, cyclophosphamide, doxorobucin, vincristine, prednisone; R-DHAP – Rituxin, dexamethasone, cytarabine, cisplatin; VCAP – vincristine, cyclophosphamide, Adriamycin, and prednisolone, H-AraC – high-dose cytosine arabinoside; MTX-methotraxate; R-VADC – vincristine, doxorubicin, dexamethasone, chlorambucil; VCAP – vincristine, cyclophosphamide, Adriamycin, and prednisolone; IFN-a- interferon alpha; R-Maxi-CHOP – dose-intensified induction immunochemotherapy with rituximab (R) + cyclophosphamide, vincristine, doxorubicin, prednisone; TRM – treatment related mortality; PFS – progression free survival; OS – overall survival

Marginal zone lymphomas

In MZL, the role of auto-HCT is very controversial. There are only few, small retrospective case series for auto-HCT in MZL that show approximately similar PFS to ones reported for FL, with frequent late relapses.

> **PRACTICE POINT**
>
> Salvage auto-HCT can be considered in MZL (with a non-curative intent) in:
> • Patients with chemosensitive disease with multiple relapses.
> • Those who are not candidates for clinical trials (or allo-HCT).

Table 17.6 Allogeneic transplantation in Relapsed/Refractory MCL (minimum of 50 patients).

Author/ Year	n	Conditioning Regimen	TRM	Relapse	cGvHD* [n] (Years)	Median OS % (Years)	Median PFS % (Years)	Comments
Cook (2010)	70	Flu Mel+/- Ale [57] Flu Bu +/- Ale [13]	21%	65%	34% (5)	37% (5)	14% (5)	Age at HCT and <2 prior lines of therapy influenced the OS, whereas <2 prior lines of therapy was the only factor to influence PFS
Hari (2011)	105	RIC/MAC	46%	34%	44% (1)	37% (5)	20% (5)	The incidence of grade 2–4 acute GvHD was 42%
Le Gouill (2012)	70	RIC	32%	NA	12	53% (2)	50% (2)	Disease status at allo-HCT was the only parameter influencing EFS and OS
Hamadani [@] (2013)	128	RIC	43%	32%	36 (1)	30% (3)	25% (3)	Despite a refractory dz state, ~ fourth of MCL patients can attain durable remissions after allo-HCT
	74	MAC	47%	33%	13 (1)	25% (3)	20% (3)	
Fenske (2014)	50	RIC (early)^	25%	15%	-	62% (5)	55% (5)	Either auto-HCT or RIC allo-HCT may be effective in RR dz, albeit the chance for long term remission and survival is lower
	88	RIC (late)^^	17%	38%	-	31% (5)	24% (5)	
Dietrich (2014)	80	RIC	30%	33%	-	46% (2)	NA (2)	Allo-HCT may offer durable survival when performed in pts with a remission duration of >1 y after auto-HCT

Cook et al. *Biol Blood Marrow Transplant* 2010;**16**: 1419–1427. Hari et al. *Ann. Oncol* 2011 (Suppl. **4**) (Abstract 038). Le Gouill et al. *Ann Oncol* 2012;**23**: 2695–2703. Hamadani et al. *Biol Blood Marrow Transplant* 2013;**19**: 625–631. Fenske TS et al. *J Clin Oncol* 2014;**32**: 273–281. Dietrich et al. *Ann Oncol* 2014;**25**: 1053–1058.
* Extensive cGvHD
[@] Restricted to chemoresistant patients
^ Early cohort-transplantation performed in first PR or CR with no more than two prior lines chemotherapy;
^^ Late cohort-transplantation performed in the remaining chemosensitive patients.
Bu – busulfan; Mel – melphalan; Flu – fludarabine; Ale – alemtuzumab; RIC – reduced intensity chemotherapy; MAC – myeloablative;
TRM – treatment related mortality; PFS – progression free survival; OS – overall survival
CIBMTR = Center for International Blood and Marrow Transplant Research; DFCI = Dana-Farber Cancer Institute; EBMT = European Blood and Marrow Transplant; FHCRC = Fred Hutchinson Cancer Research Center

Small lymphocytic lymphomas

There are very limited data for SLL with virtually no large retrospective or prospective studies reported for this histology. Several randomized studies show no benefit of upfront auto-HCT in patients with chronic lymphocytic leukemia/SLL. The approval of several highly active agents for SLL (ibrutinib, idelalisib, obinutuzumab) and many other compounds in pipeline, will likely make HCT an increasingly uncommon therapeutic modality for this lymphoma in coming years (see Chapter 15).

PRACTICE POINT

In patients with SLL auto-HCT is not recommended outside off clinical trial.

Auto-HCT and second malignancies

Is this real?
Yes, there is increased incidence of second malignancies particularly sMDS/AML after auto-HCT. Interestingly majority of the risk factors are non-transplant related (detailed later).

What are the risk factors?
Factors that are associated with an increased risk of second cancers after auto-HCT include:
1 advanced patient age
2 pre-transplant chemotherapy (alkylators, topoisomerase II inhibitors [etoposide] or purine nucleoside analogs [fludarabine])
3 difficult CD34+ cell collection
4 use of total body irradiation (TBI) with transplant conditioning.

Table 17.7 Autologous transplantation for Waldenström macroglobulinemia.

Author/Year	N T/Auto	Conditioning regimen (n)	PFS %	OS %	Comments
Tournilhac (2003)	27/17	Mel or Cy/TBI (13) BEAM (3) Mel (1)	44% (10–34 months)	Not reached (18 months)	TRM was 6%
Anagnostopoulos (2006)	26/10	TBI+/- Other (3) Bu+ Cy+/- Other (2) Other (5)	65% (3 y)	70% (3 y)	- Only 50% of the patients were chemosensitive at the time of auto-HCT - Low NRM [11% at 1 and 5 y]
Dhedin (2007)	54/32	BEAM (13) Mel/TBI or Cy/TBI (16) Other (3)	Median, 32 months	58% (5 y)	- TRM was high (12.5%) - 25% patients were chemoresistant at auto-HCT
Gilleece (2008)	18/9	Mel 200 (3) BEAM (5) Cy/TBI (1)	43% (4 y)	73% (4 y)	TRM at 12 months was 0%
Kyriakou (2010)	158/158	TBI + Other (45) BEAM (46) Other (67)	39.7% (5 y)	68.5% (5 y)	3 or more treatment lines, chemorefractory disease at auto-HCT, male sex and age >50 y were associated with a significantly inferior OS

Tournilhac et al. *Semin Oncol* 2003;**30**:291–296. Anagnostopoulos et al. *Biol Blood Marrow Transplant* 2006;**12**:845–854. Dhedin et al. *Haematologica* 2007;**92**:228. Gilleece et al. *Hematology* 2008;**13**:119–127. Kyriakou et al. *J Clin Oncol* 2010;**28**:2227–2232.
Mel – melphalan; Cy – cyclophosphamide, TBI – total body irradiation; BEAM – BCNU, etoposide, cytarabine, melphalan; TRM – treatment related mortality; PFS – progression free survival; OS – overall survival

Table 17.8 Allogeneic transplantation in Waldenström macroglobulinemia.

Author/ Year	No	Conditioning Regimen	TRM %	cGvHD[*] [n]	PFS/RFS % (median f/u)	OS% (median f/u)	Comments
Tournilhac (2003)	27/10	Cy/TBI (8) Mel/TBI (1) Flu/TBI (1)	40	2	4 relapsed (2–10 months)	60% (20.4 months)	- 9/10 patients had preceding auto-HCT - Response rate was high [80%]
Anagnostop-oulos (2006)	26	TBI/Other (15) Bu/Cy/Other (5) Flu/Other (1) NST (5)	40 (1 y)	3	31 (3 y)	46 (3 y)	- 15 patients had >3 lines of treatment prior to allo-HCT
Dhedin (2007)	11 (MA)	Cy/TBI (9) Other (1)	36	2	54 (5 y)	45	- 36% in the MA and 55% in the RIC group were chemoresistant. - EFS was higher (68% vs 48%) with low TRM with RIC allo-HCT
	11 (RIC)	Flu/TBI (10) Other (1)	27	3	68 (5 y)	NR	
Gillece (2008)	18/9	TBI (2) BEAM (2) Flu/Mel (5)	44 (1 y)	4	44 (4 y)	56 (4 y)	- Disease status at allo-HCT was PR (7) and primary refractory (2)
Kyriakou (2010)	37 (MA)	Cy/TBI(27) Bu/Cy/ Other (10)	33 (3 y)	6	56	62	~67% patients had chemosensitive disease at transplant
	49 (RIC)	Flu/Alk(31) Flu/ TBI (18)	23 (3 yr)	13	49	64	
Garnier (2010)	12 (MA)	Cy/TBI (11) Mel/ TBI (1)	25% (1 yr)	8	58 (5 yr)	67 (5 yr)	- Prior median lines of therapy -3 - 44% of patients had chemorefractory disease at allo-HCT
	13 (RIC)	Flu/TBI (7) Flu/Cy (4) Flu/Mel (2)					

Tournilhac et al. *Semin Oncol* 2003;**30**:291–296. Anagnostopoulos et al. *Biol Blood Marrow Transplant* 2006;**12**:845–854. Dhedin et al. *Haematologica* 2007;**92**:228. Gilleece et al. *Hematology* 2008;**13**:119–127. Kyriakou et al. *J Clin Oncol* 2010;**28**:2227–2232. Garnier et al. *Haematologica* 2010;**95**:950–955.
* Extensive cGvHD
Cy – cyclophosphamide; Mel – melphalan; Flu – Fludarabine; TBI-total body irradiation; Bu – Busulfan; BEAM – BCNU, etoposide, cytarabine, melphalan; Alk – Alkylating agent; RIC – reduced intensity chemotherapy; MA – myeloablative; NST – non-myeloablative hematopoietic cell transplant; TRM – treatment related mortality; PFS – progression free survival; OS – overall survival; RFS – relapse free survival; cGvHD – chronic graft-versus-host disease

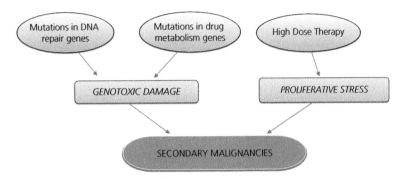

Figure 17.1 Pathophysiology of secondary malignancy in bone marrow transplant patients.

Table 17.9 Recommendations about the current role of autologous transplantation and post auto maintenance therapy in indolent B-cell lymphomas.

	Disease Status	Current Role of Autologous transplantation	Post Auto-HCT Consolidation	Comments
FL	Upfront (after 1st line therapy)	Not recommended	-	-
	Relapsed - Chemorefractory - Chemosensitive	Not recommended Auto-HCT is very appropriate in those who are chemosensitive and not candidates for allo-HCT	- Rituximab improves PFS but not OS and is currently considered investigational. - Immunomodulators (Lenalidomide) and proteasome inhibitors (Bortezomib) are currently being studied in the post auto-HCT setting.	• Immunotransplants • Post-transplant idiotype vaccines • Auto-HCT followed by CD19-direct CART therapy • Tandem auto-allogeneic-HCT
Transformed FL	Chemorefractory Chemosensitive	Not recommended Consider for patients with chemosensitive, non-bulky disease.	-	
WM	Upfront (in 1st remission)	Not recommended	-	Early CD34⁺ cell collection and cryopreservation
	Relapsed - Chemorefractory - Chemosensitive	Not recommended Auto-HCT can be considered after 2–3 lines of prior therapies	-	Bortezomib maintenance
MZL	Upfront (in 1st remission)	Not recommended	-	
	Relapsed	Role is unknown. May consider in chemosensitive patients who are not candidates for allogeneic HCT or clinical trials	-	
SLL		Not recommended*	-	Highly active chemoimmunotherapies show more promising results

What is the pathophysiology?

1 It is hypothesized that second malignancies post auto-HCT are primarily a result of genotoxic damage already incurred by the transplant recipients prior to autografting (Figure 17.1).

2 Data from two randomized clinical trials has revealed increased incidence of secondary malignancies in patients who had received prior therapies. This suggests causative role of HDT in the pathogenesis of secondary malignancy. The hematopoietic reconstitution after auto-HCT exerts a "proliferative stress" on infused progenitor and stem (Figure 17.1).

Strategy to reduce the risk of second malignancies after auto-HCT

1 Limit the exposure to leukemogenic agents before HCT.

2 Use non-TBI based conditioning regimens.

Future efforts directed on improving the role of HCT in indolent lymphomas

Randomized trials clarifying the role and timing of auto-HCT against chemoimmunotherapy for indolent NHL, while urgently needed, are unlikely to be performed in the near future. Cooperative group efforts are needed to incorporate novel potentially curative strategies into modern auto-HCT, rather than solely focusing on therapies merely capable of extending remission duration, without impacting survival. CALGB is evaluating the role of bortezomib maintenance in MCL after auto-HCT (NCT00310037). Maintenance/consolidation with immunomodulatory agents (e.g., lenalidomide; NCT01035463) or newer B-cell monoclonal antibodies (e.g., Ofatumumab, MEDI-551, etc.) warrants investigation in post-transplant setting. Moving forward efforts need to be focused on evaluating novel consolidation or maintenance strategies including "imunotransplant" and post-transplant idiotype vaccination to transform auto-HCT from a remission extending therapy to a more superior curative modality (Table 17.9).

Selected reading

1. Al-Tourah AJ, Gill KK, Chhanabhai M, Hoskins PJ, Klasa RJ, Savage KJ, et al. Population-based analysis of incidence and outcome of transformed non-Hodgkin's lymphoma. *J Clin Oncol* 2008; **26**(32): 5165–5169.

2. Romaguera JE, Fayad LE, Feng L, Hartig K, Weaver P, Rodriguez MA, et al. Ten-year follow-up after intense chemoimmunotherapy with Rituximab-HyperCVAD alternating with Rituximab-high-dose methotrexate/cytarabine (R-MA) and without stem cell transplantation in patients with untreated aggressive mantle cell lymphoma. *Br J Haematol* 2010; **150**(2): 200–208.

3. Bernstein SH, Epner E, Unger JM, Leblanc M, Cebula E, Burack R, et al. A phase II multicenter trial of hyperCVAD MTX/Ara-C and rituximab in patients with previously untreated mantle cell lymphoma; SWOG 0213. *Ann Oncol* 2013; **24**(6): 1587–1593.

4. Brown JR, Gaudet G, Friedberg JW, Neuberg D, Mauch P, Kutok JL, et al. Autologous bone marrow transplantation for marginal zone non-Hodgkin's lymphoma. *Leuk Lymphoma* 2004; **45**(2): 315–320.

5. Li L, Bierman P, Vose J, Loberiza F, Armitage JO, Bociek RG. High-dose therapy/autologous hematopoietic stem cell transplantation in relapsed or refractory marginal zone non-Hodgkin lymphoma. *Clin Lymphoma Myeloma Leuk* 2011; **11**(3): 253–256.

6. Michallet M, Dreger P, Sutton L, Brand R, Richards S, van Os M, et al. Autologous hematopoietic stem cell transplantation in chronic lymphocytic leukemia: results of European intergroup randomized trial comparing autografting versus observation. *Blood* 2011; **117**(5): 1516–1521.

7. Hake CR, Graubert TA, Fenske TS. Does autologous transplantation directly increase the risk of secondary leukemia in lymphoma patients? *Bone Marrow Transplant* 2007; **39**(2): 59–70.

CHAPTER 18

Diffuse large B-cell lymphoma

Syed Abbas Ali[1], Istvan Redei[2], and Syed A. Abutalib[2]

[1] *Sydney Kimmel Comprehensive Cancer Center, Division of Hematologic Malignancies, Johns Hopkins University, Baltimore, MD, USA*

[2] *Department of Hematology and Bone Marrow Transplant, Cancer Treatment Centers of America, Zion, IL, USA*

Introduction

Diffuse large B-cell lymphoma (DLBCL) is the most common aggressive histologic subtype of non-Hodgkin lymphoma (NHL). It is a heterogeneous disease and accounts for approximately 30–40% of cases of NHL in Western countries. Although it can still arise in children, DLBCL's incidence rises with age. Median age at presentation is about 70-years, with a slight male predominance. There are approximately 25,000 new cases every year in the United States, with an estimated 10,000 deaths annually. It can arise *de novo*, or as a transformation of another hematologic malignancy, such as chronic lymphocytic leukemia or follicular lymphoma.

DLBCL is marked by clinical and biological heterogeneity that contributes to the variable patient outcomes seen with standard chemo-immunotherapy. Between 30–40% of patients either have residual disease or relapse after initial therapy. Such patients receive rescue therapy using immunochemotherapy regimens. Transplant eligible patient who have chemotherapy sensitive disease, are candidates for high-dose chemotherapy (HDT) and autologous hematopoietic cell transplantation (HCT).

In this chapter, we discuss the management of patients with relapsed and refractory (R/R) DLBCL, with an emphasis on the role of both autologous- and allogeneic-HCT.

Risk stratification – The Revised International Prognostic Index: Is it still relevant?

Traditionally patients have been stratified according to their risk of treatment failure as determined by widely adopted models first published in 1993, such as the International Prognostic Index (IPI). Other iterations include the revised-IPI (R-IPI), felt to be a better predictor of outcome than the standard IPI treated with rituximab and cyclophosphamide, doxorubicin, vincristine, and prednisone (R-CHOP). More recently, clinically based NCCN-IPI published by Zheng Zhou et al. in 2014 is a more robust prognostic tool relative to IPI model. The 5-year OS ranges from 43 to 84%, and 38 to 96% using the IPI and the NCCN-IPI model, respectively (Tables 18.1 and 18.2).

> **PRACTICE POINTS**
>
> Recent NCCN-IPI provides better risk discrimination among different risk groups in patients with *de novo* (absence of transformation and c-MYC gene rearrangement) DLBCL (Table 18.2).

What is the consensus for auto-HCT in R/R DLBCL?

The standard management of patients with DLBCL who fail first-line therapy comprises salvage chemotherapy followed by high-dose therapy (HDT) and auto-HCT (Table 18.3). This treatment paradigm was established by the PARMA trial (Table 18.4), which demonstrated a significant survival advantage for patients with chemotherapy sensitive disease who were randomized to HDT and an auto-HCT. Since the publication of this study, a number of positive developments have occurred in the treatment of frontline therapy. A major advance has been the incorporation of rituximab into first-line immunochemotherapy leading to a significant improvement in survival. As a consequence, fewer patients

Clinical Manual of Blood and Bone Marrow Transplantation, First Edition. Edited by Syed A. Abutalib and Parameswaran Hari.
© 2017 John Wiley & Sons Ltd. Published 2017 by John Wiley & Sons Ltd.

Table 18.1 Prognostic variables and evulotion of prognostic models in DLBCL.

Prognostic Variables	Evolution of Prognostic Models Over Time $\Longrightarrow$			
	IPI (1993)	aa-IPI (1993)	R-IPI (2007)	NCCN-IPI (2014)
Criteria				
Age				
>40 to <60				1
>60 to ≤ 75	1		1	2
75				3
LDH, normalized				
>1 to ≤ 3	1	1	1	1
>3				2
Ann Arbor stage III-IV	1	1	1	1
Extranodal Disease				
>1 site	1		1	
Any of BM, CNS, GI tract/liver or lung				1
ECOG PS ≥ 2	1	1	1	1
Prognostic Category and Score				
Low	0–1	0	0	0–1
Low-Intermediate	2	1	1–2	2–3
High-Intermediate	3	2		4–5
High	4–5	3	≥3	≥6

IPI = International Prognostic Index, aa-IPI = age-adjusted IPI, R-IPI = Revised-IPI, NCCN-IPI = National Comprehensive Cancer Network IPI, ECOG = Eastern Cooperative Oncology Group, LDH = Lactate dehydrogenase. Adapted from Sehn et al. Blood 2007; Zheng Zhou et al. Blood 2014.

Table 18.2 Comparison between IPI and NCCN-IPI prognostic models.

	IPI				NCCN-IPI			
	Score	N	5-year PFS	5-year OS	Score	N	5-year PFS	5-year OS
Low	0–1	38%	95	90	0–1	19%	91	96
Low-Intermediate	2	26%	66	77	2–3	42%	74	82
High-Intermediate	3	22%	52	62	4–5	31%	51	64
High	4–5	14%	39	54	>6	8%	40	33

IPI = International Prognostic Index, NCCN-IPI = National Comprehensive Cancer Network IPI Adapted from Sehn et al., Blood 2007; Zheng Zhou et al. Blood 2014.

relapse and require salvage therapy and auto-HCT. Some investigators have also suggested than in the era of first-line immunochemotherapy the results of standard salvage therapy may have become less effective. The Collaborative Trial in Relapsed Aggressive Lymphoma (CORAL) study suggested that patients who had received first-line immunochemotherapy and then relapsed within a year had a long-term disease-free survival less than 20% since majority of patients could not get to HDT and auto-HCT rescue (see later). These

Table 18.3 ASBMT Guidelines for hematopoitic cell transplantation in relapsed/refractory DLBCL published in 2011.

Recommended	Not Recommended	Insufficient Evidence/Unable to Comment
Indications validated in 2015		
Auto-HCT if chemosensitive disease	Auto-HCT as first-line therapy is not recommended for any IPI group at this time.	Number of cycles of salvage therapy prior to auto-HCT
Peripheral hematopoietic cell collection preferred	Poorer outcomes with age >60 years, but age is not an absolute contraindication. Creatinine >2.5 mg/dl. Total bilirubin >2.0 mg/dl. NYHA Class III or IV +/- ECOG PS ≥ 3*.	RIC regimens or MAC regimens Routine use of maintenance Rituximab

ASBMT: American Society of Bone Marrow Transplantation; DLBCL: Diffuse large B-cell lymphoma; auto-HCT: autologous hematopoietic stem-cell transplant; NYHA: New York Heart Association; ECOG: Eastern Cooperative Oncology group; PS: PS Oliansky DM, Czuczman M, Fisher RI, et al. The role of cytotoxic therapy with hematopoietic -cell transplantation in the treatment of DLBCL: update of the 2001 evidence-based review. *Biol Blood Marrow Transplant* 2011;**17**:18–19.

important observations highlight the need for improving on currently employed salvage regimens.

> **PRACTICE POINT**
>
> Transplant eligible patients with chemotherapy sensitive disease should proceed to auto-HCT. The treatment of patients who are not candidates for autologous HCT and who fail to respond to second-line chemotherapy therapy, is generally palliative. Age is not a contraindication for autologous HCT, although outcomes in older adults are inferior relative to younger adults.

Should rituximab be part of the first salvage regimen?

Rituximab is a standard component of initial therapy of DLBCL and improves survival rates in this setting. Whether rituximab therapy should be included in the treatment of all patients with R/R DLBCL is controversial. This is primarily because the studies that have demonstrated a benefit from rituximab in this setting have included a few patients who had received rituximab as part of their initial chemotherapy regimen. Some clinicians choose to include rituximab in the treatment of all patients with R/R DLBCL while others reserve the use of rituximab for those patients who relapse more than 6 months after a complete remission (CR) or did not receive rituximab as part of their initial therapy. We favor the latter approach.

In a study conducted by the Dutch-Belgian Hemato-Oncology Cooperative Group (HOVON) group, 239 patients with R/R DLBCL received a salvage regimen consisting of DHAP-VIM-DHAP with or without rituximab followed by auto-HCT. The analysis of the 225 evaluable patients showed that after two courses of chemotherapy, CR/partial response (PR) was obtained in 54% of the patients in the DHAP arm and 75% in the R-DHAP arm (P ≤ 0.01). Post-transplantation PR and CR were obtained in 50 and 73% of the patients, respectively (P = 0.003). A marked difference in favor of the R–DHAP arm was observed at 24 months for failure-free survival (FFS), 50% compared with 24% (P < 0.001), respectively, but not for OS, 52% compared with 59% (P = 0.15), respectively. A Cox regression analysis demonstrated a significant effect of rituximab treatment on FFS and OS when adjusted for time since upfront treatment, age, performance status (PS), and secondary aaIPI (saaIPI). However, <5% of the patients had been exposed to rituximab previously.

In a report of 202 patients with DLBCL relapsing or progressing after treatment with CHOP or CHOP plus rituximab, those treated with a rituximab-containing salvage regimen had a significantly better 2-year survival than those not receiving rituximab (58 vs 24%). The benefit of rituximab was larger among patients who had not received rituximab as part of their initial therapy.

> **PRACTICE POINTS**
>
> We reserve the use of rituximab for patients who relapse more than 6 months after a CR or did not receive rituximab as part of their initial therapy. The role of newer anti-CD20 antibodies in this particular setting is an area of investigation (see later).

Table 18.4 Selected trials – auto-HCT in relapsed or refractory DLBCL.

Author/Year	N	Trial Setting	Regimen	TRM (%)	OS (%, years)	EFS/PFS (%, years)	Comments and Practice Implications
†Philip et al., 1995 (PARMA)	215	Phase III Relapsed	DHAP +/- auto-HCT BEAC +/- IFR + auto-HCT	6%	53 vs 32% at 5-years (p = 0.038)	EFS: 46 vs 12% at 5 y (p = 0.001)	Established auto-HCT as standard of care in pre-rituximab era.
Vose et al., 2001	184	Primary induction failure	Various regimens + HDT/auto-HCT	*7%	37% at 5 y	PFS: 31% at 5 y	ABMTR. Aggressive NHL, ~ 60% DLBCL. No rituximab. Showed primary refractory DLBCL – no CR with induction – can have long-term DFS with HDT auto-HCT.
Kewalramani et al., 2004.	36	Relapsed or refractory	R-ICE + HDT/ auto-HCT	0%	67 vs 56% at 2 y in the auto-HCT cohort	PFS: 54 vs 43% at 2 y (P = 0.25)	Looked at R-ICE vs ICE prior to auto-HCT. Varying conditioning regimens. Historical control – ICE. R-ICE improved CR 53 vs 27%.
Khouri et al., 2005	67	Relapsed	HD-rituximab + salvage	0%	80 vs 53% at 2 y (p = 0.002)	DFS: 67 vs 43% at 2 y (p = 0.004)	Aggressive NHL, 41 with de novo DLBCL. Historical control group at same institution, similar salvage regimens. HD-rituximab with better outcomes with auto-HCT.
Vose et al., 2004	429	First relapse or CR2	CHOP, Adriamycin containing, or other HDT/auto-HCT	-	OS at 3y: CR2 vs Rel1 – 55% vs 38% (p<0.001)	PFS at 3y: CR2 vs Rel1 – 38% vs 28% (p<0.001)	ABMTR. Compared auto-HCT in Rel1 vs CR2. Survival better with HCT in CR2 vs Rel1. Chemotherapy resistance, high initial LDH, relapse in <12months, age ≥40years, use of myeloid growth factors – predictors of worse survival.

Rituximab and radioimmunotherapy (RIT) era
Phase III studies

Author/Year	N	Trial Setting	Regimen	TRM (%)	OS (%, years)	EFS/PFS (%, years)	Comments and Practice Implications
†Gisselbrecht et al., 2010 (CORAL)	396	Phase III	R-ICE vs R-DHAP BEAM/auto-HCT Rituximab vs Observation	-	47 vs 51% at 3 y (p = 0.4)	PFS: 31 vs 42% at 3 y (p = 0.4)	R-ICE and R-DHAP are comparable salvage regimens. Worse outcome if relapse <12mo after diagnosis, prior rituximab, saaIPI 2-3. If relapse >12 months after diagnosis, rituximab exposure does not affect EFS. Standard of care.
Crump et al., 2012 (NCIC CTG-LY.12)	619	Phase III	GDP vs. DHAP Rituximab for CD20+ Auto-HCT	-	39 % vs 39% at 4 y	EFS: 26 vs 26% at 4 y	Included other NHL - 71% of accrued were DLBCL patients. Rituximab added in 2005. GDP is non-inferior, has similar outcomes, but is less toxic. GDP can be delivered outpatient.
Vose et al., 2013 (BMT-CTN 0401) *Rituximab vs RIT*	224	Phase III	R-BEAM vs. Bexxar (B)-BEAM	100 day TRM 4.1% (R-BEAM) vs 4.9% (B-BEAM); P=0.97	2 y OS: 65.6% (R-BEAM) vs 61% (B-BEAM); P = 0.38	2 y PFS 48.6% (R-BEAM) vs 47.9% (B-BEAM); P = 0.94	Addition of RIT was not beneficial relative to conventional conditioning regimen

DHAP – Dexamethasone, high-dose cytarabine, cisplatin; HDT – High-dose therapy. Auto-HCT – Autologous hematopoietic cell transplant; BEAM – BCNU, etoposide, cytarabine, melphalan; BEAC – carmustine, etoposide, cytarabine, cyclophosphamide; IFR – Involved field radiation; ICE – Ifosfamide, carboplatin, etoposide; GDP – Gemcitabine, dexamethasone, cisplatin; ABMTR – Autologous Blood and Marrow Transplant Registry. TRM – Transplant-related mortality. OS – Overall Survival; PFS – Progression-free survival; EFS – Event-free survival; †Landmark trial; *Day 100 mortality rate; Rel1 – first relapse; CR2 – second complete response; NCIC CTG – National Cancer Institute of Canada Clinical Trials Group. RIT – radioimmunotherapy, saaIPI – secondary age-adjusted IPI

Does duration of first remission and exposure to rituximab as part of initial therapy influence subsequent outcome?

In the CORAL trial, 396 patients with DLBCL in first relapse or with primary refractory disease were randomly assigned treatment with rituximab plus ifosfamide, carboplatin, etoposide (R-ICE), or R-DHAP followed by HDT and auto-HCT for responding patients. The initial therapy included rituximab in 62% of patients. When patients were analyzed according to the time of relapse and exposure to rituximab, patients with relapse more than 12 months after initial diagnosis had similar rates of progression-free survival (PFS) whether or not they had received rituximab previously. In contrast, patients relapsing less than 12 months after diagnosis had inferior PFS if they had received prior rituximab.

Is there one best salvage regimen for patients with R/R DLBCL?

Salvage regimens are critical for cytoreduction and establishing chemotherapy sensitivity. Only patients identified with a disease responsive to salvage regimen(s) are eligible for HDT and auto-HCT. Ideal regimens minimize toxicities, maximize response, and do not interfere with hematopoietic cell (HPC) mobilization and collection. Several regimens are available, R-ICE and R-DHAP being the most common in the rituximab era.

The CORAL intergroup trial compared a combination therapy consisting of R-ICE with R-DHAP (Table 18.5). Patients who were DLBCL CD20+ at the time of the first relapse and patients remaining refractory after first-line therapy were randomized between the R-DHAP and R-ICE groups. Responding patients received carmustine, etoposide, cytarabine, and melphalan (BEAM) HDT followed by auto-HCT and were randomized between observation and rituximab maintenance for 1 year. An analysis was conducted on the first 396 randomized patients (R-ICE, n = 202; R-DHAP, n = 194). The median age was 55 years. In 225 patients, a relapse after > 12 months was observed after initial CR. In 166 cases, patients did not achieve initial CR or had early relapses at <12 months. A group of 244 patients (63%) received immunochemotherapy with rituximab as the first-line treatment. At the time of relapse, 226 patients had a saaIPI score of 0–1 and 149 patients had an saaIPI of 2–3. The overall response rate was 63%; 38% of patients achieved CR. There was no difference between the response rates in the R-ICE (63.5; 95% CI, 56–70%) and R-DHAP (62.8; 95 CI, 55–69%) groups. The factors

that affected the response significantly (P < 0.0001) were as follows: R/R at <12 months, with response rates of 46 versus 88%, saaIPI > 1 (52 vs 71%), and prior exposure to rituximab (51 vs 83%). Patients with prior exposure to rituximab had more refractory disease and adverse prognostic factors (Table 18.5).

The NCIC CTG LY.12 compared R-GDP, with R-DHAP in a randomized fashion and demonstrated similar overall response rates (ORR) and outcomes. R-GDP had fewer grade III and IV toxicities and better QoL parameters (Table 18.4).

> **PRACTICE POINTS**
>
> No agent or regimen has demonstrated superiority to another in this setting. Salvage regimens such as GDP, DHAP, ICE with or without rituximab are acceptable options. We prefer to use R-DHAP in patients with germinal center B-cell (GCB) subtype and R-ICE for all other R/R DLBCL patients. R-DHAP is associated with greater toxicity than R-ICE or R-GDP.

Incorporation of Ofatumumab in R/R DLBCL

The initial results of the Orchard Study (OMB110928) were presented at ASH 2014 meeting. In this large international study ofatumumab-DHAP and R-DHAP salvage regimens followed by auto-HCT was compared in R/R DLBCL. In the study 447 patients were randomized to O-DHAP or R-DHAP. Response to salvage regimen was not significantly different between the two study arms. The ORR was 38 with 15% CRs in the O-DHAP cohort and 42 with 22% CRs in the R-DHAP cohort. No differences were found in PFS, EFS, OS, time to recovery of neutrophil and platelet counts, HPC mobilization, time to neutrophil, and platelet recovery post auto-HCT were in the two groups.

> **PRACTICE POINTS**
>
> We prefer to use rituximab (over ofatumumab) based chemotherapy regimens in this particular setting. Obinutuzumab based regimens hold promise and warrants further investigation.

Does cell of origin of *de novo* DLBCL and c-MYC gene rearrangement influence the outcomes with auto-HCT?

Retrospective analysis of CORAL study, Thieblemont et al. evaluated the effect of the cell of origin (COO) on outcomes (Table 18.5). The investigators used the Hans

Table 18.5 Chemosensitive relapsed DLBCL. Data from CORAL study (treatment algorithm: R-ICE vs R-DHAP -> BEAM and auto-HCT ->Rituximab vs Observation).

Question	Answer[1]	Comments
Are R-ICE and R-DHAP comparable salvage regimens	YES	EFS of 26 vs 35% ($P = 0.6$) at 3 years OS 47 vs 51% ($P = 0.5$) at 3 years
Did prior (frontline) rituximab-based regimen effected outcomes differently	YES	Probability of survival was 34 vs 66% with and without rituximab, respectively
Did relapse greater or less than 12 months effected outcomes differently	YES	3 year EFS was 20 vs 45% for relapse > or < 12 months, respectively
Did prior (frontline) rituximab-based regimen effected outcomes differently if relapse was within 12 months of initial therapy	YES	3 year EFS was 21% (<12 months) vs 41% (>12 months)
Did prior (frontline) rituximab-based regimen impact outcomes differently if relapse was > 12 months following initial therapy	NO	No difference in EFS or OS between the 2 subgroups with or without rituximab exposure
Did secondary aaIPI* had any bearing on prognosis	YES	3 year EFS with secondary aaIPI 2–3 was 18 vs 40% for secondary aaIPI 0–1 ($P = 0.0001$)
Did patients with GC-DLBCL responded better to salvage regimen compared to ABC-DLBCL (COO* defined by Hans criteria)	YES	Retrospective analysis of CORAL study showed PFS 70%; OS 74% for GC-DLBCL vs PFS 28%; OS 40% for ABC-DLBCL
Did patients with GC-DLBCL fared better outcomes with R-DHAP compared to R-ICE (COO defined by Hans criteria)	YES	Retrospective analysis of CORAL study showed PFS at 3 years of 100% with R-DHAP and 27% with R-ICE. This needs confirmation by a prospective study
Did patients with ABC-DLBCL fared better outcomes with R-ICE compared R-DHAP (COO defined by Hans criteria)	NO	Retrospective analysis of CORAL study showed equally poor outcomes in ABC-DLBCL (via Hans criteria) with either regimen studied
Incidence of c-myc was greater in GC-DLBCL compared to ABC-DLBCL by Hans criteria	YES	Retrospective analysis showed that c-myc by FISH was positive in 17 patients with GC-DLBCL vs 10 patients with ABC-DLBCL
Incidence of c-myc was greater in GC-DLBCL compared to ABC-DLBCL by GEP analysis	YES	Retrospective analysis showed that c-myc by FISH was more common in GC-DLBCL (n = 3) vs no cases were associated with ABC-DLBCL
R-DHAP showed OS improvement when compared to R-ICE in patients with c-myc (genetically defined) positive relapsed/refractory DLBCL	NO	Retrospective analysis showed that the type of salvage regimen, R-DHAP, or R-ICE, had no impact on survivals, with 4-year PFS rates of 17 vs 19% and 4-year OS rates of 26 vs 31%, respectively
Majority of biological characteristics were similar between diagnosis and relapse in the 45 matched – pair biopsies studied	YES	Retrospective analysis showed this to be true in 87% of the cases
Did maintenance rituximab therapy following HDT/AHCT improved PFS	NO	The 4-year post- autologous transplant EFS rates were 52 and 53% for the 122 patients with rituximab and the 120 patients in the observation group, respectively ($P = 0.7$)

[1] Applicable to patients between the ages 18–65 in CORAL study, *aaIPI: age-adjusted IPI, GC: Germinal center, ABC: Activated B-cell, **COO: cell of origin.

algorithm, a broadly employed surrogate technique that uses immunohistochemistry (IHC) to provide information about GCB and non-GCB subtype using CD10, BCL-6, and MUM-1 expression.

In a multivariate analysis, independent prognostic relevance was found for the interaction between GCB/ non-GCB Hans phenotype and treatment (P = 0.04), prior rituximab exposure (P = 0.0052), secondary aaIPI (P = 0.039), and FoxP1 expression (P = 0.047). Confirmation was obtained by gene-expression profiling (GEP) in a subset of 39 patients. For patients treated with R-DHAP, the 3-year PFS (52 vs 32%) and

OS (61 vs 45%) were higher for the GCB subtype, as compared to non-GCB-DLBCL. However, the 3-year PFS (31 vs 27%) and OS (50 vs 49%) did not differ for GCB and non-GCB-DLBCL treated with R-ICE.

Evaluating a subset of the CORAL study, a univarite analysis. showed that the presence of c-MYC gene rearrangement was the only parameter significantly correlated with both a worse PFS (P = 0.02) and a worse OS (P = 0.04). Of the 161 patients analyzed, 28 (17%) presented with a c-MYC (by FISH not IHC) DLBCL, targeted as either a simple hit (25%) or complex hits (n = 75%), including c-MYC/BCL2, c-MYC/BCL6, and c-MYC/BCL2/BCL6. The outcomes of patients with c-MYC DLBCL were significantly worse than those with without such rearrangement, with the 4-year PFS rate at 18 versus 42% (P = 0.0322), respectively, and the 4-year OS rate at 29 versus 62% (P = 0.0113), respectively. The type of treatment (R-DHAP or R-ICE) had no impact on survival, with the 4-year PFS rate at 17 versus 19%, respectively, and the 4-year OS rate at 26 versus 31%, respectively.

Retrospective analysis showed that GCB-DLBCL had better response overall versus ABC-DLBCL with PFS 70 versus 28%, and OS 74 versus 40%, respectively. ABC-DLBCL by Hans criteria continued to show equally poor outcome with either regimen. Detection of c-MYC by FISH was more commonly observed in the GCB versus the ABC in patients treated on CORAL study (Table 18.5). However, studies by Moskowitz et al. published in Blood in 2005 involving salvage chemotherapy followed by auto-HCT, have not demonstrated IHC determined COO to be predictive of outcome. Although several studies have now confirmed the adverse prognosis associated with the GEP designated ABC subtype, such techniques are not easily or routinely available in the practice setting.

> **PRACTICE POINTS**
>
> These findings underline the heterogeneity of DLBCL; there remains an urgent need to study the effects of new treatments according to the COO and various gene rearrangements. Patients with c-MYC gene rearrangement and R/R DLBCL should be treated on a clinical trial. In such group of patients, we prefer allogeneic-HCT over auto-HCT.

Frontline autologous-HCT: Yes or no?

This strategy has failed to show OS benefit in several randomized clinical trials. A 2008 meta-analysis of 15 randomized clinical trials (RCT) involving more than 3,000 patients, showed better CR rates, similar treatment related mortality (TRM), but no improvement in EFS or OS using auto-HCT consolidation compare to only conventional frontline chemotherapy. However, patients enrolled had both aggressive B- and T-cell NHLs. Two other meta-analyses failed to demonstrate OS benefit of frontline auto-HCT with potential detrimental effect in the low-risk IPI cohort. Among patient with high-intermediate (HI) and high-risk (HR) IPI, auto-HCT consolidation resulted in an EFS of approximately 50% over 3–4 years. LNH-87 trial showed no OS benefit for frontline auto-HCT in aggressive B-cell lymphomas. Interestingly, a subsequent retrospective subset analysis in the HI-IPI and HR-IPI group suggested an improved PFS and OS. However, several previous trials with various designs have failed to demonstrate an OS advantage of this approach in HR-IPI DLBCL. The French GOELAMS 075 study showed a superior 3-year EFS with R-CHOP only over auto-HCT consolidation, 56 versus 36%, respectively, with no impact of IPI risk categories on EFS. The phase III Italian Lymphoma Foundation trial (DLCL04) randomized HR-DLBCL patients between R-CHOP-14 or R-MegaCHOP induction therapy. After finishing induction therapy, patients underwent a second randomization between auto-HCT versus continuation of the original induction regimen. There was a significant 2-year PFS in favor of auto-HCT consolidation compared to the continuation of induction chemotherapy arm, 72 versus 59% (P = 0.008), respectively, but no difference in OS between the two arms.

More recently, the SWOG 9704 trial randomized patient with chemotherapy sensitive, HI-IPI, and HR-IPI disease, between conventional induction therapy only and auto-HCT consolidation. The 2 years PFS was superior (69 vs 55%, P= 0.005) in the auto-HCT arm. There was no significant OS difference (74 vs 71%, P = 0.30) between the two arms. Interestingly, a subset analysis in the HR-IPI cohort demonstrated a significant 2-year OS (84 vs 64%) benefit of the auto-HCT. However, only half of the patients received rituximab as part of the therapy and only limited numbers of patients had HR-IPI disease.

> **PRACTICE POINTS**
>
> Although some studies suggest a PFS benefit of frontline auto-HCT in the HR- IPI group; we do not advocate frontline auto-HCT in patients with de novo (absence of transformation and c-MYC gene rearrangement) DLBCL.

What is the ideal conditioning regimen for auto-HCT?

Numerous regimens have been tried and tested in an attempt to optimize outcomes. These include chemotherapy alone, chemotherapy in combination with total body irradiation (TBI) such as Bu/Mel/TBI, and recently attempts at radioimmunotherapy (RIT) in combination with chemotherapy (Table 18.4; BMT-CTN 0401 RCT).

High dose BEAM regimen continues to be our favorite; this regimen has low morbidity, and mortality (3–5%). BEAM and CBV (cyclophosphamide, carmustine and VP-16) are the most commonly used regimens according to a CIBMTR report published in 2014. Others conditioning regimens include Bu/Cy (busulfan and cyclophosphamide) and Bu/Cy/VP-16 (busulfan, cyclophosphamide and etoposide). Large studies comparing the latter to BEAM have failed to show improvements in outcome.

A further attempt to develop a more effective therapeutic strategy for R/R DLBCL patients consists of the combination of radioimmunotherapy (RIT) with standard chemotherapy regimens. In a promising phase II data with 90Y-ibritumomab tiuxetan combined with BEAM (Z-BEAM) was superior to a historical control in the salvage of patients with high saaIPI scores. To further increase the therapeutic potential of RIT, a dose escalation study for Z-BEAM and auto-HCT has been performed. The delivered RIT dose could safely reach 70 mCi, twice the standard dose, in 44 patients. Careful dosimetry was required to avoid toxicity rather than weight-based dose escalation. A follow-up small positive phase III randomized study with 43 patients reported by in 2012 compared Z-BEAM to BEAM alone as conditioning for aggressive B-cell NHLs. There was significant improvement with OS of 91 versus 62% at 2 years after Z-BEAM and BEAM treatments, respectively (P = 0.05). However, a larger randomized phase III multicenter trial (BMT-CTN 0401) with 244 patients reported by Vose et al. published in the JCO, compared 131Iodine-tositumomab+BEAM with R-BEAM, and showed no difference in 2-year PFS (48 vs 49%), with slightly higher mucositis in the RIT arm.

> **PRACTICE POINT**
>
> BEAM remains the most common conditioning regimen. There are no strong data to support the superiority of any alternative regimen. Regimen related toxicity, Karnofsky performance score (KPS), and comorbidities are all important considerations in selecting a regimen. The use of RIT outside of a clinical trial is not supported by current evidence. Proponents of RIT believe that escalation of RIT dose might favor this strategy; however, this concept remains to be investigated in RCT.

Rituximab as post-transplant maintenance therapy: Yes or no?

Relapse remains the leading cause of death after auto-HCT. The focus should be on preventing relapses. Post-auto-HCT rituximab maintenance has been evaluated to tackle minimal residual disease (MRD) and prevent relapses.

A large randomized multicenter trial with The Groupe d 'Etude des Lymphomes de l'Adulte (formerly GELA, now the LYSA group) reported the results of a cohort of 476 patients with newly diagnosed "high-risk" DLBCL. Patients were randomized to two different induction regimens, and 330 of these patients proceeded to auto-HCT with a subsequent second randomization to maintenance rituximab, or observation. There was no significant difference in EFS between the two arms after a median follow-up of 4 years. Another study by the Canadian Transplant Group randomized patients with R/R aggressive B-cell and T-cell lymphomas to one of two induction regimens. This was followed by auto-HCT and a second randomization after transplant. Patients with CD20+ NHL were randomized to rituximab maintenance *versus* observation.No significant differences were seen in the primary endpoint of 2-year EFS between the maintenance versus observation arms (64 vs 51%, respectively, P = 0.11).

Patients in the CORAL study were first randomized for salvage regimen, and then subsequent to auto-HCT were randomized again to either an observation, or rituximab maintenance (Table 18.5). At a median follow-up of 44 months, when compared with observation, rituximab maintenance resulted in similar rates of EFS (52 vs 53%, P = 0.7), PFS (52 vs 56%), and OS (61 vs 65%) at 4 years There was a significantly higher rate of infection-related adverse events in the maintenance arm. However, subset analysis demonstrated a significantly higher PFS in female patients as compared to male patients on the maintenance arm versus the observation arm. This was attributed to faster clearance of rituximab in males, leading to a shorter duration of exposure and leads one to think that maybe higher dose of rituximab in the male patients could have resulted in favorable outcomes.

> **PRACTICE POINTS**
>
> Maintenance rituximab does not improve clinical outcomes after auto-HCT and is associated with increased long-term toxicities. Pharmacokinetic-based prospective trials designed to exploit the full therapeutic potential of rituximab in post-transplant setting are warranted.

Post-auto-HCT maintenance therapy: Novel approaches are underway

Several agents are being studied in the post-auto-HCT setting (Table 18.6).

Table 18.6 Molecular targets and corresponding agents for treatment of DLBCL.

Drug	Molecular Target	N	Phase of Study	ORR%
Nivolumab	Anti-PD-1 mAb	-	I	-
Pembrolizumab	Anti-PD-1 mAb	-	I	-
Pidilizumab	Anti-PD-1 mAb	35	I/II	51
Ipilimumab	Anti-CTLA-4 mAb	-	I	-
Everolimus	mTOR inhibitor	47	II	30
Temsirolimus	mTOR inhibitor	32	II	28
Lenalidomide	Immunomodulatory drug	134	II	27
Ibrutinib	BTK inhibitor	60	II	22
Idelalisib	PI3K inhibitor	9	I	0
BAY 80–6946	PI3K inhibitor	17	II	12
IPI-145	PI3K inhibitor	10	I	0
BKM-120	PI3K inhibitor	-	I	-
ABT-199	BCL-2 inhibitor	9	I	33
E7438	EZH2 inhibitor	-	I	-
Fostamitinib	SYK inhibitor	23	I	22
MK-2206	AKT inhibitor	-	I	-
OTX015	BET inhibitor	7	I	14
CPI-0610	BET inhibitor	-	I	-
Bortezomib	Proteosome inhibitor	28	I	0
Carfilzomb	Proteosome inhibitor	-	I	-
Enzastaurin	PKC-β inhibitor	55	II	22
Sotrastaurin	PKC-β inhibitor	-	I	-
Obinatuzomab	Anti-CD20 monoclonal Ab	25	II	29
Ofatumomab	Anti-CD20 monoclonal Ab	81	II	11
Dacetuzumab	Anti-CD40 monoclonal Ab	50	I	12
Brentuximab	Anti-CD30 Ab/drug conjugate	19	II	47
Inotuzumab	Anti-CD22 Ab/drug conjugate	25	I	15
CAR Tcells	Anti-CD19 T-cell therapy	9	I	86%

ORR = Overall response rate (%); PD-1 – Programmed Death receptor; CTLA4 – cytotoxic T-lymphocyte associated protein 4; mTOR – mammalian target of rapamycin; BTK – Bruton's tyrosine kinase; PI3k – phosphoinositid-3-kinase; BCL – B-cell CLL/lymhpoma-2; EZH2 – enhancer of zeste homolog -2; SYK – spleen tyrosine kinase; AKT – protien kinase B; BET – bromodomain and extra-terminal motif; PKC – protein kinase C; CAR – chimeric antigen receptor

Promising new developments involve the use of immune checkpoint inhibitors. Pidilizumab (CT-011) is a humanized mAb that binds to programmed death-1 (PD-1) receptor. This leads to mitigation of the apoptotic processes of effector memory T- and NK-cells. A Phase II study was conducted in patients with DLBCL and other NHLs undergoing auto-HCT enrolled 72 chemosensitive patients who after auto-HCT received three doses of Pidilizumab every 6 weeks. Compared with historical controls at 18-months post auto-HCT, Pidilizumab demonstrated improved PFS and OS. Phase III trials are planned.

Chimeric Antigen Receptor (CAR) T-cells targeting CD19, a normal and malignant B-cell specific antigen. CARs are murine derived ("chimeric") fusion proteins incorporating antigen-recognition domains and T-cell activation domains. Genetically modified T-cells expressing anti-CD19 CARs recognize and kill CD19⁺ target cells. In 2015, a phase I trial where they treated 15 patients with advanced B-cell malignancies, nine of whom had DLBCL, and observed eight CRs. These included four of seven evaluable DLBCL patients who had chemorefractory disease. CAR T-cell therapy has shown striking responses in several studies with B-cell malignancies and multiple trials are currently enrolling.

PRACTICE POINTS

Many agents and strategies are being evaluated in the post auto-HCT setting to prevent relapse.

Outcomes of auto-HCT in patients who failed the first salvage regimen

The CORAL study showed that salvage therapies for DLBCL are not always effective and that only half of the patients will proceed to desired auto-HCT. The exact therapeutic strategy is even less clear in patients who require second salvage regimen. Van Den Neste et al. (BMT Journal 2016) reported outcomes of 203 patients who could not proceed to scheduled auto-HCT (due to lack of response to R-DHAP or R-ICE) in the CORAL study. In the intent-to-treat analysis, ORR to second salvage regimen was 39%, with CR or CR unconfirmed in 27%, and PR in 12%. Among the 203 patients, 64 (31.5%) were eventually transplanted (auto-HCT= 56, allo-HCT = 8). Median OS of the entire population was 4.4 months. The OS was significantly improved in patients with lower tertiary IPI, patients responding to third-line treatment and patients transplanted with a 1-year OS of 41.6% compared with 16.3% for patient who were not transplanted (P < 0.0001). In multivariate analysis, IPI at relapse ("second relapse") (hazard ratio (HR) 2.409) and transplantation (HR 0.375) independently predicted OS.

PRACTICE POINTS

Autologous HCT is still a viable option in patients who achieve CR to second salvage regimen. Alternatively, allogeneic HCT can be considered in appropriately selected individuals. When available, enrollment in a clinical trial is encouraged

---

Allogeneic-HCT for DLBCL: Eligibility and timing

Allogeneic HCT may be considered in patients with mobilization failure or relapse following an autologous HCT (Figure 18.1). Allo-HCT is a curative therapy and provides tumor-free hematopoietic graft as well as a possible graft *versus* lymphoma effect (Figure 18.2). approximately, 19% of patients who relapse after auto-HCT undergo allo-HCT. In addition, non-relapse mortality (NRM) is significant after allo-HCT in patients who have failed auto-HCT. In order to effectively employ allo-HCT in relapsed DLBCL, it might be reasonable consider allo-HCT over auto-HCT highly selected group of, for instance, patients with early first relapse (<6 months) and/or high saaIPI after first-line rituximab-containing chemotherapy. This could potentially make allo-HCT the preferred second-line approach in some cases. Proving such hypothesis in favor of allo-HCT over auto-HCT would require a prospective RCT. To date, neither has such a trial been completed, nor is one likely to be undertaken. As a result, there is no consensus on how best to identify such "high risk" group of patients who are deem to fail auto-HCT (Figure 18.1).

PRACTICE POINTS

Adequate disease control is essential prior to allo-HCT, but it is often difficult to achieve in patients who have relapsed or progressed after auto-HCT. Selected "high-risk" patients might be better served with allo-HCT as opposed to auto-HCT, at first relapse.

What are the results of allo-HCT in DLBCL?

Two retrospective analyses were published evaluating the results of allo-HCT in patients with DLBCL who failed auto-HCT. The analysis of the EBMT database included 101 patients; conditioning regimens were non-myeloablative (NMA) in 64 patients. The 3-year PFS and OS were 41 and 53%, respectively. Patient with long remissions after auto-HCT and those with chemotherapy sensitive disease before allo-HCT had the best outcomes. Analysis of 165 patients whose data were reported to the Gruppo Italiano Trapianto di Midollo Osseo (GITMO) registry; 70% of the patients received NMA conditioning regimens. The 1-, 3-, and 5-year OS were 55, 42, and 39%, respectively. The NRM was 28%. Interestingly, the 3-year OS was 27% in chemotherapy refractory patients.

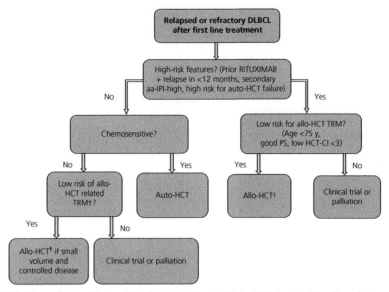

†RIC if >60 years of age; aa-IPI – age-adjusted International Prognostic Index; HCT – hematopoietic cell transplant; TRM – treatment-related mortality; PS – performance status; HCT-CI – Hematopoietic Cell Transplant Comorbidity Index.

Figure 18.1 Approach to relapsed and refractory DLBCL.

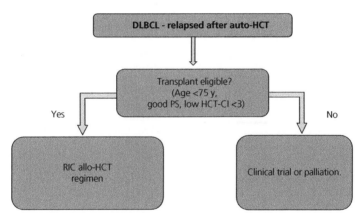

Allo-HCT – allogeneic hematopoietic cell transplant; TRM – treatment-related mortality; PS – performance status; HCT-CI – Hematopoietic Cell Transplant Comorbidity Index; RIC – reduced intensity conditioning regimen

Figure 18.2 Potential schema for allo-HCT in patients who relapse after auto-HCT and have controlled disease.

PRACTICE POINTS

Two retrospective registry studies that include relatively large number of patients indicate a role for allo-HCT in patient with DLBCL relapsing after auto-HCT. These data are also suggestive of a possible GvL effect because both PFS and OS curves seem to form a plateau in a heavily pretreated population of patients. Enrollment into clinical trials is also a reasonable option; however, in this particular setting there is no new or "novel" agent or combination therapy with curative potential.

GvL effect: Does it apply in DLBCL?

There are well-documented GvL effects for certain lymphoma subtypes such as follicular and mantle cell lymphoma. Although the evidence is less extensive, there are data suggesting such an effect in DLBCL as well. These include regression of lymphoma (1) after withdrawal of immunosuppression, (2) following donor lymphocyte infusion (DLI), and (3) lower relapse rates after allo-HCT compared to auto-HCT especially in patients who develop GvHD. Bishop et al. reported

Table 18.7 Who, when, and how of HCT (auto and allo) for *de novo* DLBCL.

Authors' practice:

A. PATIENT FACTORS:
Auto-HCT: Suitable* patients at first relapse with chemosensitive disease are considered for auto-HCT. Age is not a contraindication for auto-HCT, although outcomes in older adults are inferior relative to younger adults.
Allo-HCT: Suitable* patients who are <75 years of age with low comorbidity scores are considered for RIC allo-HCT.

B. DISEASE FACTORS:
High risk for auto-HCT failure: Relapse or progression <12 months after CR1, refractory disease with rituximab based frontline chemotherapy, high saa-IPI of 2–3, less than CR at the time of transplant
High risk for allo-HCT failure: Less than CR at the time of allo-HCT.

C. FIRST SALAVGE REGIMEN:
We prefer to use DHAP in patients with germinal center B-cell (GCB) subtype and ICE for all other R/R DLBCL patients. We incorporate rituximab with these regimens except in a patient who face very early (<6 months) relapse after frontline rituximab-based chemotherapy. Well-designed clinical trial is a reasonable option.

D. CONDITIONING REGIMEN FOR AUTO-HCT:
In majority of our patient we use BEAM regimen (see text).

E. CANDIDACY FOR ALLO-HCT-DISEASE FACTORS:
Allogeneic-HCT may be considered in patients with CD34+ cell mobilization failure or relapse following an auto-HCT

F. INTENSITY OF CONDITIONING REGIMEN FOR ALLO-HCT:
RIC is the preferred after failed auto-HCT. Well-designed clinical trial is a reasonable option

---

* Recipient suitability refers to issues that relate to the general health or medical fitness of the recipient to undergo hematopoietic cell transplant

18 R/R DLBCL patients who underwent allo-HCT following a reduced intensity conditioning (RIC) regimen. Eleven of the 15 patients who were not in CR on day +100 after transplant or developed relapse were initially treated by withdrawal of immunosuppression or DLI alone, whereas four patients received DLI with prior chemotherapy. Clinical responses, even to withdrawal of immunosuppression alone were seen in 9 of the 15 patients. Five responders developed GvHD. Six of the nine responders were alive in remission after a median follow-up of 68 months. Similar results were seen in 5 of 12 patients following DLI in another study.

PRACTICE POINTS

Clinical evidence suggests that GvL effect is operative to some extent in DLBCL and an attempt should be made to harness it in patients who relapse after allo-HCT.

Conditioning regimen for allogeneic HCT: What is the correct intensity?

Several, mostly retrospective, studies indicate an increased NRM and decreased relapse incidence after the use of myeloablative conditioning (MAC) regimens. Allo-HCT with MAC regimen seems to have no clear OS advantage over RIC but it should be considered in highly selected groups of patients (over RIC), that is, young and fit patients, with high-risk disease (not in CR) and without prior history of auto-HCT. For patients with prior history of auto-HCT, RIC is preferred over MAC. Nonmyeloablative might be considered in selected older adults who are deemed unfit for RIC undergoing HLA-matched transplant. option.

PRACTICE POINTS

Current data and guidelines are not definitive enough to provide a preferred conditioning intensity (MAC vs RIC) for HLA-matched transplants. RIC is the preferred in adult undergoing allo-HCT after failed auto-HCT.

Selected reading

1. Philip T, Guglielmi C, Hagenbeek A, et al. Autologous bone marrow transplantation as compared with salvage chemotherapy in relapses of chemotherapy sensitive non-Hodgkin's lymphoma. *N Engl J Med* 1995;**333**(23):1540–1545.
2. Stiff PJ, Unger JM, Cook JR et al. Autologous transplantation as consolidation for aggressive non-Hodgkin's lymphoma. *N Engl J Med*. 2013 Oct 31;**369**(18):1681–1690.
3. Gisselbrecht C, Glass B, Mounier N, et al. Salvage regimens with autologous transplantation for relapsed large B-cell lymphoma in the rituximab era. *J Clin Oncol* 2010;**28**(27):4184–4190.
4. Hamadani M, Saber W, Ahn KW, Carreras J, Cairo MS, Fenske TS *et al.* Impact of pretransplantation conditioning regimens on outcomes of allogeneic transplantation for chemotherapy-unresponsive diffuse large B cell lymphoma and grade III follicular lymphoma. *Biol Blood Marrow Transplant* 2013;**19**:746–753.
5. van Kampen RJ, Canals C, Schouten HC, Nagler A, Thomson KJ, Vernant JP *et al.* Allogeneic stem-cell transplantation as salvage therapy for patients with diffuse large B-cell non-Hodgkin's lymphoma relapsing after an autologous stem-cell transplantation: an analysis of the European Group for Blood and Marrow Transplantation Registry. *J Clin Oncol: Official Journal of the American Society of Clinical Oncology* 2011 Apr 1;**29**(10):1342–1348.
6. Gisselbrecht C. Futility of relapsed diffuse large B cell lymphoma transplantation? *Biol Blood Marrow Transplant* 2014;**20**:1667–1669.
7. Vose JM, Carter S, Burns LJ, Ayala E, Press OW, Moskowitz CH, et al. Phase III randomized study of rituximab/carmustine, etoposide, cytarabine, and melphalan (BEAM) compared

with iodine-131 tositumomab/BEAM with autologous hematopoietic cell transplantation for relapsed diffuse large B cell lymphoma: results from the BMT-CTN 0401 trial. *J Clin Oncol: Official Journal of the American Society of Clinical Oncology.* 2013;**31**(13):1662–1668.

8. Jacobsen ED, Sharman JP, Oki Y, Advani RH, Winter JN, Bello CM et al. Brentuximab vedotin demonstrates objective responses in a phase 2 study of relapsed/refractory DLBCL with variable CD30 expression. *Blood.* 2015 Feb 26;**125**(9):1394–402.

9. Brudno JN, Somerville RP, Shi V, Rose JJ, Halverson DC, Fowler DH et al. Allogeneic T cells that express an anti-CD19 chimeric antigen receptor induce remissions of B-cell malignancies that progress after allogeneic hematopoietic stem-cell transplantation without causing graft-versus-host disease. *J Clin Oncol: Official Journal of the American Society of Clinical Oncology* 2016 Apr 1;**34**(10):1112–1121.

10. Majhail NS, Farnia SH, Giralt SA, LeMaistre CF et al. Indications for Autologous and Allogeneic Hematopoietic Cell Transplantation: Guidelines from the American Society for Blood and Marrow Transplantation. *Biol Blood Marrow Transplant.* 2015 Nov;**21**(11):1863–1869. doi: 10.1016/j.bbmt.2015.07.032. Epub 2015 Aug 7.

11. Zheng Zhou Z, Sehn K, Rademaker A, et al. An enhanced International Prognostic Index (NCCN-IPI) for patients with diffuse large B cell lymphoma treated in the rituximab era. *Blood* 2014 Feb 6;**123**(6):837–842.

12. Thieblemont C, Briere J, Mounier N, et al. The germinal center/activated B-cell subclassification has a prognostic impact for response to salvage therapy in relapsed/refractory diffuse large B-cell lymphoma: a bio-CORAL study. *J Clin Oncol* 2011;**29**(31):4079–4087.

13. Crump M, Kuruvilla J, Couban S, MacDonald DA, Kukreti V, Kouroukis CT *et al.* Randomized comparison of gemcitabine, dexamethasone, and cisplatin vs. dexamethasone, cytarabine, and cisplatin chemotherapy before autologous stem-cell transplantation for relapsed and refractory aggressive lymphomas: NCIC-CTG LY.12. *J Clin Oncol* 2014; **32**:3490–3496.

14. Glass B, Hasenkamp J, Wulf G, Dreger P, Pfreundschuh M, Gramatzki M *et al.* Rituximab after lymphoma-directed conditioning and allogeneic stem-cell transplantation for relapsed and refractory aggressive non-Hodgkin lymphoma (DSHNHL R3): an open-label, randomised, phase 2 trial. *Lancet Oncol* 2014;**15**:757–766.

15. Bacher U, Klyuchnikov E, Le-Rademacher J, Carreras J, Armand P, Bishop MR, et al. Conditioning regimens for allotransplants for diffuse large B-cell lymphoma: myeloablative or reduced intensity? *Blood.* 2012;**120**(20):4256–4262.

CHAPTER 19

Mantle cell lymphoma

Narendranath Epperla and Timothy S. Fenske

Division of Hematology and Oncology, Medical College of Wisconsin, Milwaukee, WI, USA

Introduction

Mantle cell lymphoma (MCL) is a distinct subtype of B-cell non-Hodgkin lymphoma (NHL) characterized by cyclin D1 overexpression resulting from the t(11;14)(q13;32) translocation. MCL is more common in Caucasians compared to African Americans with a median age of over 65 years and male predominance (3:1). MCL is a heterogeneous disease with biologic and morphological variants that define a spectrum of disease, with "indolent" MCL on one end of the spectrum and the aggressive blastoid variant MCL on the other end.

Despite the advent of newer "targeted" agents such as bortezomib, lenalidomide, and ibrutinib, MCL remains a challenging clinical problem with most patients experiencing repeated relapses and ultimately succumbing to the disease. As a result, hematopoietic cell transplantation (HCT) is an important tool and continues to be commonly used in the management of MCL. Currently, there is a lack of consensus regarding optimal frontline therapy, indications for high dose therapy (HDT) and autologous HCT (auto-HCT), and maintenance therapy following auto-HCT. In this chapter, we discuss the current state of the art in the management of MCL, with an emphasis on the continued important role of autologous HCT, even in this era of multiple new and novel agents.

Risk stratification

The MCL International Prognostic Index (or "MIPI score") uses age, performance status, lactate dehydrogenase (LDH), and leukocyte count to classify MCL into three prognostic groups: low, intermediate, and high risk with corresponding 5-year overall survival (OS) rates of 83, 63, and 34%, respectively. Proliferation index (as measured by Ki-67 staining), gene expression profile signature, complex karyotype, and minimal residual disease (MRD) after frontline therapy also provide prognostic information, however in routine clinical practice, there is lack of consensus in how to best use these tools to select treatment for an individual patient.

PRACTICE POINT

A MCL-specific risk-stratification index, the MIPI score, has been validated to predict outcomes following frontline therapy, including auto-HCT. However, there is insufficient data at this time to recommend risk-adapted therapy based on the MIPI score.

Front line therapy in MCL

There is no standard frontline therapy for MCL. In general, more aggressive approaches are utilized in "younger, fit" patients (often including upfront HCT), to achieve prolonged first remissions. On the other hand, more conservative non-transplant approaches are favored for older and/or less fit patients, to minimize toxicity. Achievement of complete response (CR) prior to HCT is associated with longer progression-free survival (PFS). With intensive treatment approaches, a median PFS of >5 years can be expected in younger "fit" patients who achieve CR and then undergo auto-HCT in first CR. However, the chance for a longer first remission comes with a cost, and all treatment choices must be weighed against potential toxicities. For determining appropriate frontline therapy, patients can be stratified into "younger/fit" patients, "elderly/unfit" patients

Clinical Manual of Blood and Bone Marrow Transplantation, First Edition. Edited by Syed A. Abutalib and Parameswaran Hari.
© 2017 John Wiley & Sons Ltd. Published 2017 by John Wiley & Sons Ltd.

(those felt to be able to withstand standard chemo-therapy but not HDT) and "frail" patients (those unlikely to even withstand standard chemotherapy).

Younger, fit patients

For patients <60–65 years of age, with a good functional status and no significant comorbidities, it is reasonable to aim for a long (>5 year) first remission. When that is the goal, more intensive induction chemotherapy, potentially followed by consolidation with auto-HCT should be considered.

Is the addition of rituximab and/or cytarabine to frontline therapy beneficial?

The German Low Grade Lymphoma Study Group (GLSG) demonstrated improved overall response rate (ORR) with the addition of rituximab to CHOP (cyclo-phosphamide, doxorubicin, vincristine, and predni-sone), which was the frontline therapy in that study. In a more recent randomized phase III trial conducted by Hermine et al., R-CHOP was compared with R-CHOP alternating with R-DHAP (rituximab, dexamethasone, high dose Ara-C and cisplatin) prior to auto-HCT. An OS benefit was seen in the R-CHOP/R-DHAP arm. There have now been several phase III and phase II studies suggesting improved outcomes with the incorporation of rituximab and high dose Ara-C prior to auto-HCT (Table 19.1).

Is intensification of induction therapy beneficial?

Another dose-intensified approach, R-HyperCVAD (rituximab, hyper-fractionated cyclophosphamide, vin-cristine, doxorubicin, and dexamethasone) alternating with R-MTX/AraC (rituximab, high dose methotrexate/cytarabine) also achieved a favorable ORR and PFS, in a single-center phase II study (Table 19.1). However, the treatment dropout rate was high at 29%, particularly from toxicity related to R-MTX/AraC part of the reg-imen. In addition, in retrospect, 50% of patients in this study had low MIPI scores. Two subsequent multicenter studies, using the same regimen, confirmed high rates of ORR and CR, but with very high treatment dropout rates of 63 and 39%, respectively (Table 19.1). In addition, the treatment related mortality (TRM) with this regimen is approximately 8%, which is significantly higher than the rate of TRM with auto-HCT currently. However, to date there have been no prospective com-parative studies comparing R-HyperCVAD (without auto-HCT) to an auto-HCT based approach.

Recently, a U.S. SWOG/Intergroup study was designed as a randomized phase II comparison of R-HyperCVAD-MTX/AraC induction followed by consoli-dation with auto-HCT versus R-bendamustine followed by auto-HCT, for patients <65 years with untreated MCL. Unfortunately, this study was closed early into accrual due to an unacceptably high incidence of failed peripheral blood stem cell collection in the R-HyperCVAD-MTX/AraC arm.

PRACTICE POINT

For younger fit patients, induction therapy with a rituximab/chemotherapy combination that includes high-dose cytarabine is recommended. The authors recommend R-CHOP alternating with R-DHAP, the Nordic MCL-2 regimen, or R-DHAP x 4 cycles, followed by auto-HCT as the most effective available regimens to accomplish this while maintaining a relatively low toxicity profile.

Elderly or "unfit" patients (unfit to receive auto-HCT)

Treatment strategies for older (over 60–65 years of age) fit patients and young patients ineligible for transplanta-tion (due to comorbid conditions) are similar. In a study conducted by the EBMT, outcomes with auto-HCT for patients ≥65 years were compared with patients <65 years age. The two groups were found to have sim-ilar rates of OS, PFS, and TRM. This suggests that age should not be used as the sole factor to determine auto-HCT eligibility. Instead, age, performance status, and comorbidity profile all need to be considered in deter-mining transplant eligibility.

However, despite the ability to offer HCT to older patients, the fact remains that many patients over age 60–65 will not be good candidates for HCT due to comorbidities. The overall treatment strategy for such patients typically involves the use of an effective induction regimen with a tolerable side effect profile, followed by maintenance therapy, with the hopes of prolonging the remission duration.

Multiple combination therapies have been studied (Table 19.2); however, the recommended induction reg-imen for elderly patients is chemoimmunotherapy, typ-ically R-CHOP or R-Bendamustine (BR). BR has been shown to be non-inferior with better tolerability when compared to R-CHOP. However, in a large randomized trial, R-CHOP followed by maintenance rituximab led to excellent PFS. Recently the results of the StiL trial were presented at ASCO 2016 wherein, at a median follow-up of 4.5 years, 2 years of rituximab maintenance after BR did not demonstrate PFS or OS benefit. The other

Table 19.1 Studies investigating the role of first-line dose-intensified chemotherapy in MCL.

Author/Year	Study Design	N	Regimen(s)	TRM	OS (Years)	PFS (Years)	Comments
			Auto-HCT based regimens				
Dreyling (2005)	Randomized Phase III	62	R-CHOP+IFN-α	0%	77	1.4	- Performed in pre-R era
		60	R-CHOP+ auto-HCT	5%	vs 83% (3 y)	vs 3.3 (3 y)	- No survival benefit
Hermine (2016)	Randomized Phase III	455	R-CHOP+ auto-HCT / RCHOP/RDHAP+ auto-HCT	4%	6.8 vs NR	3.8 vs 7.3	Addition of AraC in induction improved OS w/o significant increase in toxicity
Le Gouill (2016)	Prospective phase III	299	R-DHAP+ auto-HCT	-	82.6% (3 y)	73.7% (3 y)	Patients who did not reach at least a PR after 4 courses of R-DHAP could receive 4 additional courses of R-CHOP
Geisler (2008) (NORDIC MCL-2)	Phase II	160	R-Maxi-CHOP+ high dose cytarabine+ auto-HCT	5%	58% (10 y)	7.4	- Late relapses were seen on long-term follow up - Pre-emptive R used post auto-HCT for molecular relapses
Van't Veer (2009)	Phase II	87	R-CHOP+ high dose cytarabine+ auto-HCT	5%	66% (4 y)	36% (4 y)	BEAM was used for conditioning. The ORR was 70% but the remissions are not durable
Damon (2009)	Phase II	77	R-CHOP+MTX + H-AraC/VP16+ auto-HCT	3%	64% (5 y)	56% (5 y)	In vivo purging with R used
Delarue (2012)	Phase II	60	RCHOP/RDHAP+ auto-HCT	1.5%	75% (5 y)	64% (5 y)	11 patients had second malignancies
Touzeau (2014)	Phase II	396	High dose cytarabine based regimen+ auto-HCT	2.5%	79.5% (3 y)	63.5% (3 y)	For patients transplanted upfront age, disease status at auto-HCT and use of R were predictive for both OS and PFS
Chen (2015)		18	R-HyperCVAD+ auto-HCT		88% (2 y)	82% (2 y)	Study closed early due to excessive failed stem cell mobilization in R-HyperCVAD arm
		35	BR+ auto-HCT		87% (2 y)	81% (2 y)	
			Non-auto-HCT based regimens				
Romaguera (2010)	Phase II Single center	97	R-HyperCVAD	8%	NR	4.6	Treatment dropout rate 29%
Merli (2012)	Phase II multicenter	60	R-HyperCVAD	6.5%	NR	NR	Treatment dropout rate 63%
Bernstein (2013)	Phase II multicenter	49	R-HyperCVAD	2%	6.8	4.8	Treatment dropout rate 39%

Dreyling et al. *Blood.* 2005;**105**:2677–2684. Hermine et al. *Lancet.* 2016;**388**:565–575. Le Gouill et al. ASH Annual Meeting Abstracts 2016. Geisler et al. *Br J Haematol.* 2012;**158**:355–362. van't Veer et al. *Br J Haematol.* 2009;**144**: 524–530. Damon et al. *J Clin Oncol.* 2009;**27**: 6101–6108. Delarue et al. *Blood.* 2013;**121**:48–53. Touzeau et al. *Ann Hematol.* 2014;**93**: 233–242. Chen et al. *Br J Haematol.* 2016 Dec 19 [Epub ahead of print]. Romaguera et al. *Br J Haematol.* 2010;**150**:200–208. Merli et al. *Br J Haematol.* 2012;**156**:346–353. Bernstein et al. *Ann Oncol.* 2013;**24**:1587–1593.

TRM – treatment related mortality; OS – overall survival; PFS – progression-free survival; ORR – overall response rate; R-CHOP – Rituximab, cyclophosphamide, doxorubicin, vincristine, prednisone; IFN-α – Interferon alpha; DHAP – Dexamethasone, high dose cytarabine, cisplatin; HyperCVAD – Cyclophosphamide, vincristine, doxorubicin, dexamethasone; BR – Bendamustine, rituximab

Table 19.2 Frontline chemotherapy options for transplant-ineligible patients.

Author/Year	Study Design	N	Regimen(s)	Conventional chemoimmunotherapy			Comments
				ORR %	mOS (Years)	mPFS (Months)	
Lenz (2005)	Randomized Phase III	112	CHOP	75	76% (2 y)	14	Toxicity was acceptable, with no major differences between the two therapeutic groups
			R-CHOP	94	76% (2 y)	21	
Herold (2007)	Randomized Phase III	90	MCP	63	52% (4 y)	18	Patients receiving R-MCP had more grade 3 or 4 leukopenia compared with patients treated with MCP, but this did not translate into an increased rate of infections
			R-MCP	71	56% (4 y)	20	
Kluin-Nelemans (2012)	Randomized Phase III	560	induction: FCR vs R-CHOP	78 vs 86	47 vs 62% (4 y)	26 vs 28	The influence of maintenance therapy with rituximab on the duration of remission was detected in patients who received R-CHOP but not in those who received R-FC
		316	Maintenance: IFN-α vs R	-	67 vs 79% (4 y)	-	
Rummel (2013)	Randomized Phase III	94 (MCL subset)	R-CHOP	91	NR	21	BR has comparable OS but prolonged PFS with fewer toxic effects
			BR	93	NR	35	
Robak (2015)	Randomized Phase III	244	R-CHOP	89	56.3 mo	14.4 mo	VR-CAP was associated with improved OS vs R-CHOP but had increased hematologic toxicity
		243	VR-CAP	92	NR	24.7 mo	
Combination with newer agents							
Visco 2013	Phase II	20	R-BAC	82	100% (2 y)	2 y 95%	R-BAC is well tolerated in elderly patients and is effective in MCL
Ruan 2014	Phase II	36	R-CHOP + Bevacizumab	82	82% (3 y)	18	The addition of bevacizumab to the standard R-CHOP regimen did not improve efficacy beyond that observed from previous studies using R-CHOP alone

Lenz et al. *J Clin Oncol.* 2005;**23**:1984–1992. Herold et al. *J Clin Oncol.* 2007;**25**:1986–1992. Kluin-Nelemans et al. *N Engl J Med.* 2012;**367**:520–531. Rummel et al. *Lancet.* 2013;**381**:1203–1210. Robak et al. *N Engl J Med.* 2015;**372**:944–953. Visco et al. *J Clin Oncol.* 2013;**31**:1442–1449. Ruan et al. *Clin Lymphoma Myeloma Leuk.* 2014;**14**:107–113.

ORR – overall response rate; mOS – median overall survival; mPFS – median progression-free survival; R-CHOP – Rituximab, cyclophosphamide, doxorubicin, vincristine, prednisone; MCP – Mitoxantrone, chlorambucil, prednisone; FCR – Fludarabine, cyclophosphamide, prednisone; IFN-α – Interferon alpha; BR- Bendamustine, rituximab; VR-CAP – Bortezomib, rituximab, cyclophosphamide, adriamycin, prednisone; R-BAC – Rituximab, Bendamustine, cytarabine.

regimen that may be considered in this patient population is VR-CAP regimen (in which bortezomib is substituted for vincristine in R-CHOP) that demonstrated improved outcomes (including overall survival) compared to R-CHOP but at the expense of increased hematological toxicity.

PRACTICE POINT

Age, performance status, and comorbidity profile, along with chemosensitivity should all be considered in determining if a patient is a candidate for auto-HCT. For elderly patients (or those unfit to undergo auto-HCT) we encourage clinical trial enrollment. Off protocol we recommend induction with BR, or R-CHOP or VR-CAP. Maintenance rituximab has been shown to improve survival following R-CHOP; it is unclear at this time whether maintenance rituximab improves outcomes after BR or VR-CAP.

Frail patients

Relatively limited options are available for very elderly or frail patients with MCL. Observation is a reasonable option for patients with asymptomatic disease and low disease burden, with treatment deferred until the development of symptoms. If treatment is required, oral chlorambucil as a single agent, chlorambucil in combination with rituximab, or rituximab with low dose bendamustine, are all potential therapeutic options. Newer agents such as bortezomib, lenalidomide, and ibrutinib are not approved as first-line therapy but could be considered as soon as a first-line therapy is deemed ineffective or not well tolerated.

Consolidation/maintenance treatment after frontline therapy

After frontline therapy for MCL, consolidation, or maintenance therapy should be considered, based on the patient's transplant eligibility status.

For transplant eligible patients (young "fit" patients)

The European Mantle Cell Lymphoma (EMCL) Network carried out a randomized prospective trial to evaluate the role of auto-HCT consolidation following frontline therapy for MCL. In that study, patients who responded to frontline (CHOP-like) therapy were then randomized to either undergo consolidation with HDT (total body irradiation (TBI)+cyclophosphamide) and auto-HCT versus maintenance therapy with interferon-α. The auto-HCT arm had a longer median PFS (39 vs 17 months) compared with maintenance therapy with interferon-α. However, while a trend was seen (p=0.18) no survival benefit was proven with auto-HCT. This is

likely due to the crossover design of the study (since patients not assigned to upfront auto-HCT were able to undergo auto-HCT at relapse), and also potentially because the auto-HCT conditioning regimen used was TBI-based, which is associated with higher TRM than chemotherapy conditioning regimens. In a CIBMTR study evaluating timing of transplant in chemosensitive MCL patients, there was a survival benefit noted to those who underwent auto-HCT early in the disease course compared to those transplanted later. Table 19.3 summarizes the results of studies reporting outcomes of upfront auto-HCT consolidation in MCL.

PRACTICE POINT

Given the collective available data on outcomes with auto-HCT consolidation and relatively low TRM of <5% using non-TBI-based preparative regimens, and until similar or superior data is available with newer non-transplant strategies, the authors feel that younger fit patients are best served with consolidative auto-HCT in first remission. This approach leads to excellent outcomes especially in patients achieving CR prior to transplant, with a median PFS in the 5–10 years range.

For transplant-ineligible patients (elderly patients)

In elderly patients not eligible for auto-HCT, the European MCL Network conducted a randomized phase III trial comparing induction with R-CHOP versus R-FC (rituximab, fludarabine, and cyclophosphamide), with a second randomization comparing maintenance rituximab versus interferon-α. Patients who received maintenance rituximab after R-CHOP therapy had significantly better 4 year OS compared to interferon-α, with a median PFS of 75 months compared to 27 months (Table 19.4). The Eastern Cooperative Oncology Group (ECOG) conducted a phase II study (E1405) in previously untreated MCL patients in which patients were treated with rituximab, bortezomib and modified hyper-CVAD (VcR-CVAD) chemotherapy followed by maintenance rituximab. The ORR and CR with induction therapy were 95 and 68%, respectively. At a median follow up of 3 years, PFS and OS were 72 and 88%, respectively (Table 19.4).

It is not known whether offering maintenance rituximab following bendamustine+rituximab (BR) induction therapy improves outcomes over BR alone. One randomized trial presented at the 2016 ASCO meeting showed no benefit for maintenance rituximab after BR induction. An ongoing intergroup trial (ECOG 1411) is investigating the role of rituximab maintenance either

Table 19.3 Studies evaluating consolidation of first remission with auto-HCT in MCL.

Author/Year	Study Design	N	Regimen(s)	TRM	OS (Years)	PFS (Years)	Comments
Dreyling (2005)	Randomized Phase III	62	CHOP+ auto-HCT	5%	83	3.3	- Performed in pre-R era
		60	CHOP+ IFN-α	0%	vs 77% (3 y)	vs 1.4 (3 y)	- No survival benefit (in part due to crossover design)
Hermine (2016)	Randomized Phase III	455	R-CHOP+ auto-HCT RCHOP/RDHAP+ auto-HCT	4%	6.8 vs NR (median OS)	3.8 vs 7.3 (median PFS)	Addition of AraC improved OS w/o increase in toxicity
Vandenberghe (2003)	Registry study	195	Chemo+auto-HCT	-	50% (5 y)	33% (5 y)	Disease status at transplant was the most significant factor affecting survival
Geisler (2012- update) (NORDIC MCL-2)	Phase II	160	R-Maxi-CHOP+ high dose cytarabine+auto-HCT	5%	58% (10 y)	7.4	- Late relapses were seen on long-term follow up - Pre-emptive R used post auto-HCT for molecular relapses
Van't Veer (2009)	Phase II	87	R-CHOP+ H-AraC + auto-HCT	5%	66% (4 y)	36% (4 y)	BEAM was used for conditioning. The ORR was 70% but the remissions are not durable
Damon (2009)	Phase II	77	R-CHOP+ MTX+high dose cytarabine/ VP16+ auto-HCT	3%	64% (5 y)	56% (5 y)	In vivo purging with R used
Delarue (2012)	Phase II	60	RCHOP/RDHAP+ auto-HCT	1.5%	75% (5 y)	64% (5 y)	11 patients had second malignancies
Touzeau (2014)	Phase II	396	High dose cytarabine based regimen+auto-HCT	2.5%	83% (3 y)	67% (3y)	For patients transplanted upfront age, disease status at auto-HCT and use of R were predictive for both OS and PFS
Fenske (2014)	Registry study	249*	Chemo+auto-HCT (early cohort)	3%	61% (5 y)	52% (5 y)	Optimal timing for auto-HCT is early in the disease course. Outcomes best if transplanted in CR

Dreyling et al. *Blood.* 2005;**105**:2677–2684. Hermine et al. *Lancet.* 2016;**388**:565–575. Vandenberghe et al. *Br J Haematol.* 2003;**120**:793–800. Geisler et al. *Br J Haematol.* 2012;**158**: 355–362. van 't Veer et al. *Br J Haematol.* 2009;**144**:524–530. Damon et al. *J Clin Oncol.* 2009;**27**:6101–6108. Delarue et al. *Blood.* 2013;**121**:48–53. Touzeau et al. *Ann Hematol.* 2014;**93**:233–242. Fenske et al. *J Clin Oncol.* 2014;**32**:273–281.

* Early cohort-transplantation performed in first PR or CR with no more than two prior lines of chemotherapy

TRM – treatment related mortality; mOS – median overall survival; mPFS – median progression-free survival; ORR – overall response rate; R-CHOP – Rituximab, cyclophosphamide, doxorubicin, vincristine, prednisone; IFN-α – Interferon alpha; DHAP – Dexamethasone, high dose cytarabine, cisplatin; BR – Bendamustine, rituximab

Table 19.4 Prospective studies evaluating the role of maintenance therapies after frontline non-transplant therapies in MCL patients.

Author/Year	Study Design	N	Induction Regimen	Maintenance Regimen	OS (Years)	PFS (Years)	Comments
Kluin-Nelemans et al. (2012)	Randomized Phase III	485	R-CHOP vs. R-FC	INF-α Rituximab (1 dose q 2mo, until disease progression)	63% vs 87% (4)	(Median) 27 mo vs 75 mo	- OS benefit with maintenance R in R-CHOP induction arm - No benefit of maintenance R in FC induction arm
Kenkre (2011)	Phase II	22	Modified R-HyperCVAD	Rituximab (4 weekly doses, every 6 mo for 2 years)	70 mo (5)	37 mo (5)	Feasibility of R maintenance in MCL was established
Dunleavy (2012)	Randomized Phase II	43	Bortezomib + DA-EPOCH-R	Bortezomib Observation	80% (4)	50% (4)	No benefits of Bortezomib maintenance seen
Chang (2014)	Phase II	44	VcR-CVAD	Rituximab (4 weekly doses, every 6 mo for 2 years)	88% (3)	73% (3)	
Rummel (2016)	Randomized Phase II	120	BR	Observation (n=61) Rituximab (one dose every 2 mo for 2 years) (n=59)	Median NR vs 69.6 (4.5)	Median 54.7 vs NR (4.5)	At a median follow-up of 4.5 years, there was no benefit demonstrated for R maintenance after BR i

Kluin-Nelemans et al. *N Engl J Med.* 2012;**367**:520–531. Kenkre et al. *Leuk Lymphoma.* 2011;**52**:1675–1680. Dunleavy et al. *Blood ASH Annual Meeting Abstracts* 2012;**120**: 3672. Chang et al. *Blood.*2014;**123**:1665–1673. Rummel et al. ASCO Meeting Abstracts 2016.

OS – Overall survival; PFS – Progression-free survival; CHOP – Cyclophosphamide, doxorubicin, vincristine, prednisone; IFN-α – Interferon alpha; R – Rituximab; FC- Fludarabine, cyclophosphamide; HyperCVAD- Cyclophosphamide, vincristine, doxorubicin, dexamethasone; DA-EPOCH-R – Dose adjusted etoposide, prednisone, vincristine, cyclophosphamide, doxorubicin, rituximab; VcR-CVAD – Rituximab, bortezomib, cyclophosphamide, vincristine, doxorubicin, dexamethasone; BR – Bendamustine, rituximab.

alone or in combination with lenalidomide after BR (± bortezomib) induction in MCL (NCT01415752). The optimal duration of rituximab maintenance in MCL is also not clearly defined. The European MCL Network study continued maintenance rituximab until disease progression. Whether maintenance rituximab continued until disease progression is superior to maintenance over a defined period of time (e.g., 2–3 years), and whether such extended rituximab dosing leads to toxicities (such as clinically significant hypogammaglobulinemia) warrants further investigation.

PRACTICE POINT

For patients who are not candidates for auto-HCT, maintenance rituximab is reasonable following R-CHOP-like induction. One randomized trial (only presented in abstract form so far) found no benefit for rituximab maintenance after BR, although based on the benefit seen after RCHOP, and due to the more favorable toxicity profile of BR versus RCHOP, it has become common practice to treat transplant-ineligible MCL patients with BR followed by maintenance rituximab.

Is maintenance therapy a suitable alternative for auto-HCT in transplant eligible patients?

To date, there are no randomized studies comparing auto-HCT versus maintenance therapy after induction with rituximab and H-AraC based regimens. In the ECOG 1405 study, 75 patients received VcR-CVAD induction followed by maintenance rituximab or auto-HCT. Importantly, the decision to pursue auto-HCT was at the discretion of the treating physician and was not a randomization. In addition, the study was not powered to detect a difference in these two consolidation approaches. With these important caveats in mind, there was no significant difference between the maintenance rituximab (n = 44) and auto-HCT (n = 22) groups in terms of PFS, OS, or toxicities (Table 19.4). However, in order to confirm these findings, a much larger randomized clinical trial would be required.

PRACTICE POINT

At this time, there is no data to suggest superiority or non-inferiority of maintenance strategies over auto-HCT consolidation in younger patients. As a result, for transplant-eligible patients, outside of a clinical trial we do not currently recommend maintenance rituximab as substitute for consolidation with auto-HCT.

What is the role of radioimmunotherapy consolidation in MCL?

Radioimmunotherapy (RIT) entails delivery of a radio-isotope chemically linked to a monoclonal antibody, to a lymphoma in a targeted fashion. Currently there is only one anti-CD20 radioimmunotherapy agent (^{90}Y-ibritumomab tiuxetan) approved and available in the U.S. for B-cell NHL. Since MCL is generally radiosensitive and expresses CD20, there is a good rationale for using anti-CD20 RIT in MCL. ECOG 1499 was a phase 2 study in which RIT consolidation was given after four cycles of chemoimmunotherapy (R-CHOP). In this study of 22 patients, RIT improved responses achieved after four cycles of R-CHOP, leading to an ORR of 82% (and CR rate of 50%) at completion of therapy. No unexpected toxicities were observed.

PRACTICE POINT

RIT consolidation after R-CHOP induction in MCL is feasible. However, due to lack of randomized data comparing RIT consolidation versus observation, maintenance rituximab and/or auto-HCT, we recommend that RIT consolidation only be offered within the context of a clinical trial.

Conditioning regimen for auto-HCT in MCL – Does it matter?

The most commonly used preparative regimens for auto-HCT are BEAM, BEAC, CBV, and regimens incorporating TBI. Over the last decade, the use of TBI-based regimens has declined due to increased toxicities associated with TBI. In a recent comparison of patients treated on the Nordic MCL2, HOVON 45, and European MCL Younger trials, there was a trend toward improved PFS for patients who received TBI and transplanted in first partial remission. However, variable doses of H-Ara-C given in these studies may also account for the difference noted.

In a recent study by the CIBMTR, patients with chemo-sensitive MCL who underwent a first HCT were analyzed. For the auto-HCT patients, nearly 80% received non-TBI conditioning, reflecting recent practice patterns. For patients transplanted in CR1 (with one line of therapy), CR1 (with two lines of therapy), or PR1, the 5-year PFS was 70, 56, and 30%, respectively. Patients failing to achieve CR with one or two lines of therapy may therefore benefit from an approach other than a standard BEAM auto-HCT. In non-CR patients prior to auto-HCT, the role of RIT (90Y-ibritumomab-tiuxetan) added to BEAM/BEAC was evaluated by the Nordic MCL3 study. Improved outcomes were not seen with the addition of 90Y-ibritumomab-tiuxetan.

PRACTICE POINTS

- For patients in first CR, we recommend a non-TBI-based conditioning regimen such as BEAM, BEAC, or CBV.

- Patients who are not in CR prior to upfront transplant represent a group of patients unlikely to achieve long-term remission with a standard non-TBI auto-HCT. For such patients, it is reasonable to consider a second line of therapy in hopes of achieving CR prior to auto-HCT.

- If a CR still is not achieved despite two lines of therapy, it is unclear what the optimal treatment strategy is. Auto-HCT is still a reasonable option, with the understanding that a remission >2–3 years is unlikely. In this setting various other options should be considered including a TBI-based auto-HCT, a RIC allo-HCT, or investigational maintenance/consolidation approaches.

Post–auto-HCT maintenance therapy in MCL – are we there yet?

In MCL, prevention of relapse or progression after auto-HCT is an important goal, since the outcome for those who relapse after auto-HCT is poor. Historically the median survival of patients relapsing after auto-HCT is in the range of 19–23 months. Maintenance rituximab after induction chemoimmunotherapies has been shown to improve OS in older patients with MCL. This has led to the investigation of this concept post auto-HCT. Several retrospective studies using maintenance rituximab after auto-HCT (Table 19.5), have suggested an improvement in PFS associated with maintenance rituximab after auto-HCT. In the recently presented LyMA trial at ASH 2016, the 4 year PFS (p=0.0005) and OS (p=0.0413) were significantly improved with 3 years of maintenance rituximab, compared to observation (Table 19.5). This will likely establish maintenance rituximab after auto-HCT for MCL as a new standard of care.

Several novel agents are being currently being studied in the post auto-HCT setting, such as lenalidomide and ibrutinib. A randomized phase III study is ongoing in Italy to evaluate the role of lenalidomide maintenance after upfront auto-HCT consolidation in MCL (NCT02354313). There is also a European randomized prospective study (the "TRIANGLE" study) looking at the impact of adding ibrutinib to induction and maintenance therapy for first-line treatment of MCL.

PRACTICE POINT

Maintenance rituximab has shown to have a survival benefit after auto-HCT in MCL. Hence the authors feel that maintenance rituximab should be incorporated into the treatment paradigm post auto-HCT.

Relapsed/refractory MCL – what are the options?

Treatment of patients with relapsed/refractory MCL depends on several factors including HCT eligibility, disease status (chemosensitivity, disease burden, CNS involvement), and donor availability.

Relapsed/refractory patients eligible for transplant

This group can be divided into three categories based on their previous treatment history:

1 *Chemosensitive patients who have not undergone auto-HCT previously* – options include either auto-HCT or allo-HCT. Allo-HCT offers the potential of long-term remission/cure, albeit with a significantly higher risk of TRM in the first 1–2 years. Auto-HCT, while carrying a lower TRM, does not appear to be curative whether administered in the frontline or relapsed/refractory setting, since most patients eventually do relapse. Auto-HCT later in the disease course can achieve remissions lasting 2–4 years while allo-HCT shows a trend toward lower relapse albeit with a high risk of TRM. Certain factors can be used to predict relapsed/refractory MCL patients more likely to have an extended remission with auto-HCT. A lack of B symptoms at diagnosis, a MIPI score <4, and a "remission quotient" >5 were found to predict for a better outcome with auto-HCT. The remission quotient is calculated as (months since diagnosis)/(total lines of therapy), and is essentially a measure of whether the patient has generally had short remissions with prior therapy. The decision regarding allo-HCT versus auto-HCT in this patient group should be based on perceived risk/aggressiveness of the lymphoma, patient age, comorbidity profile, and donor availability.

2 *Patients who have undergone auto-HCT previously* – allo-HCT is the only option with a significant chance and track record for long-term remission in this setting. In such patients allo-HCT may still offer the potential for cure, although the chance is lower than if allo-HCT is applied earlier in the disease course. Two studies have studied this scenario, one from the EBMT and one from the CIBMTR. In both studies, approximately 40% of patients who underwent an allo-HCT after a

Table 19.5 Studies using maintenance rituximab after auto-HCT in MCL.

Author/Year	Study Design	n	Maintenance	PFS/EFS (%) (Years)	OS (%) (Years)	Comments
Le Gouill (2016)	Prospective phase III	240 R=120 Obs=120	Rituximab 375 mg/m² IV (every 2 months for 3 y)	82.2 * vs 64.6 (O) (4 y)	88.7 * vs 81.4 (O) (4 y)	All patients received 4 courses of R-DHAP followed by auto-HCT. Conditioning regimen was R-BEAM (R=500 mg/m²).
Lim (2008)	Retrospective	8	Rituximab 375 mg/m² (q 3 mo for 2 y starting day+100)	57	67	Delayed immunoglobulin reconstitution was seen in all patients and persisted beyond the rituximab maintenance period.
Graf (2014)	Retrospective	157 R=50 Obs=107	Rituximab 375 mg/m² (variable dosing schedule but median doses=8)	HR of 0.33 favoring R maintenance	HR of 0.40 favoring R maintenance	In the landmark analysis at D 100 after auto-HCT 3y PFS&OS were statistically better in the MR compared to the no MR group.
Dietrich (2014)	Retrospective	72 R=22 Obs=50	Rituximab 375 mg/m² (every 3 months for 2 y)	90 * vs 65 (O)	90 * vs 84 (O)	Patients in both the arms were well matched. The median observation time was 56 months.

Le Gouill et al. ASH Annual Meeting Abstracts 2016. Lim et al. *Br J Haematol.* 2008; **142**(3):482–484. Graf et al ASH Annual Meeting Abstracts 2014. Dietrich et al. *Leukemia* 2014; **28**:708–709.

CS – chemosensitive, PFS – progression-free survival, EFS – event free survival, OS – overall survival, MR – maintenance rituximab, HR – hazard ratio, R- Rituximab arm, O – Observation arm, EFS – event free survival, ORR – overall response rate, CR – complete remission, R-DHAP – Rituximab, Dexamethasone, Cytarabine, and Cisplatin, R-BEAM – Rituximab, Carmustine, Etoposide, Cytarabine, and Melphalan.

failed auto-HCT enjoyed long-term survival. In particular, in patients who had a remission of >1 year following auto-HCT, who then relapse and undergo allo-HCT, a 50% long-term survival can be expected, with a clear plateau in the survival curve.

3 *Patients with chemoresistant disease* – Allo-HCT may still offer some benefit. A recent study from the CIBMTR reported results of allo-HCT for chemorefractory MCL with myeloablative and RIC regimens. The results were similar regardless of conditioning intensity, with 25–30% OS and 20–25% PFS seen at 3 years post-transplant.

PRACTICE POINTS

- For patients who relapse following auto-HCT, we recommend allo-HCT with reduced-intensity conditioning for those who are allo-HCT candidates.

- For patients who are chemoresistant (without a large disease burden or actively progressing disease), allo-HCT offers a modest chance (20–25%) for long-term remission.

- For those with chemosensitive disease and no prior history of auto-HCT, either auto-HCT or allo-HCT, can be considered depending on perceived aggressiveness of the lymphoma, donor availability, patient comorbidity profile, performance status, and chemosensitivity.

Relapsed/refractory patients ineligible for transplant

Patients with relapsed/refractory disease who are not candidates for transplantation should be considered for clinical trials. If a clinical trial option is not available, several non-protocol options can be considered as well. In selecting therapies, one needs to consider prior therapies given, the duration of remission with prior regimens, underlying comorbidities of the patient, and possible side effects of the various agents being considered. If the duration of remission was several years with the first line of therapy, the same regimen can be considered again, given there are no dose-limiting or cumulative toxicities. Alternatively, any regimen listed in Table 19.2 or novel agents (see Table 19.6) can be considered.

Conundrums in MCL

Is a risk-adapted approach feasible?

1 *High risk patients*: Several tools (such as MIPI score, proliferation index, blastoid histology, post-treatment PET scan, or MRD analysis) could theoretically be used to target patients at high risk of relapse. Such patients could then undergo a risk-adapted (i.e., more intensified) treatment approach. As an example, those patients with high MIPI score or "blastoid variant"

could be treated with allo-HCT as opposed to auto-HCT in first remission. While on the surface this approach may seem logical, early application of allo-HCT may also expose many patients to unnecessary risk. One small prospective study has shown that early incorporation of allo-HCT for MCL is feasible. However, a large CIBMTR registry study comparing allo-HCT versus auto-HCT early in the disease course failed to show improved long-term survival with early allo-HCT. It is important to note that these studies were not stratified based on prognostic factors. A prospective trial looking at allo-HCT specifically in "high risk" MCL patients to date has not been completed. Other interventions such as early incorporation of novel agents, maintenance therapies or "pre-emptive" therapies (based on MRD analysis during remission) may eventually be shown to improve outcomes such that allo-HCT may be safely reserved for relapsed patients. Alternatively, ongoing research may eventually identify a very select high risk group of MCL patients in whom the risk of allo-HCT early in the disease course may be justified.

2 *Low risk patients*: Currently there is no data to indicate that therapy de-escalation (e.g., omission of auto-HCT) can be implemented without compromising outcomes. An ongoing study in Europe (MCL Younger II, the "TRIANGLE" study) is evaluating this question. A U.S. Intergroup trial, expected to activate in mid 2017, will compare up-front versus deferred auto-HCT in low risk patients, defined as those who achieve MRD-negativity with first-line induction therapy.

PRACTICE POINT

Due to insufficient data, we feel that it is not possible to define a risk-adapted approach for MCL patients at this time, outside of a clinical trial. We do recommend enrollment of high-risk patients in clinical trials to evaluate novel approaches such as early allo-HCT, and enrollment of low-risk patients in clinical trials to evaluate whether auto-HCT can be deferred.

Novel agents – what are the challenges faced?

Currently three novel agents are FDA approved in the U.S. for relapsed and refractory MCL – bortezomib, lenalidomide, and ibrutinib. In addition, many agents are currently under evaluation in MCL, including bcl2 inhibitors, histone deacetylase inhibitors, newer proteasome inhibitors, cell cycle inhibitors, novel immunomodulatory therapies, new monoclonal antibodies, and antibody/drug conjugates (Table 19.6). With a plethora of new agents and approaches emerging in MCL, new questions arise relative to the optimal sequencing of therapy.

1 *Can therapy with novel agents preclude the need for auto-HCT consolidation?* Although tempting to adopt a

Table 19.6 Novel agents in the treatment of relapsed/refractory MCL (minimum of 20 patients).

Author/Year	Study Design	N	Regimen(s)	ORR %	CR %	Median PFS/EFS/TTP (Months)	Median DOR (Months)	Median OS (Months)
			Proteasome inhibitors					
Goy (2009)	Phase II	141	Single agent Bortezomib	33	8	6.7	9.2	23.5%
Kouroukis (2011)	Phase II	25	Bortezomib + Gemcitabine	60	11	11.4	-	NA
			Immunomodulatory drugs (Imids)					
Harel (2010)	Retrospective	58	Thalidomide +/- Bortezomib +/- Rituximab	50	21	NR (1 y TTF 29%)	-	NR (1 y OS 62%)
Ruan (2010)	Phase II	22	Metronomic regimen RT-PEPC	73	32	10	-	NR (2 y OS 45%)
Wang (2012)	Phase II	44	Lenalidomide + Rituximab	57	36	11.1	18.9	24.3
Zaja (2012)	Phase II	33	Lenalidomide + Dexamethasone	52	24	12	18	20
Goy (2013)	Phase II	134	Lenalidomide	28	8	4.0	16.6	19
Zinzani (2013)	Phase II	57	Lenalidomide	35	12	8.8	16.3	NR
			mTOR inhibitors					
Witzig (2005)	Phase II	34	Temsirolimus	38	3	6.5	6.9	12
Ansell (2008)	Phase II	27	Temsirolimus	41	4	6.0	6	14
Hess (2009)	Randomized Phase III	54	Temsirolimus 175 mg per 75 mg	22	2	4.8	7.1 (n=5)	12.8
		54	Temsirolimus 175 mg per 25 mg	6	0	3.4	3.6 (n=6)	10
		53	Investigator's choice	2	2	1.9	NA (n=0)	9.7

(Continued)

Table 19.6 (Continued)

Author/Year	Study Design	N	Regimen(s)	ORR %	CR %	Median PFS/EFS/TTP (Months)	Median DOR (Months)	Median OS (Months)
Ansell (2011)	Phase II	69	Temsirolimus+Rituximab	59	19	9.7	10.6	29.5
Renner (2012)	Phase II	35	Everolimus	20	6	5.5	17	NA
BCR signaling								
Wang (2013)	Phase II	111	Ibrutinib (BTK inhibitor)	68	21	13.9	17.5	NR (1.5 y OS 58%)
Wang (2016)	Phase II	50	Ibrutinib+Rituximab	88	44	NR	NR	NR
Radioimmunotherapy								
Wang (2009)	Phase II	32	90Y-ibritumumab tiuxetan	31	16	6.0	28	21

Goy et al. *Ann Oncol* 2009;**20**:520–525. Kouroukis et al. *Leuk Lymphoma* 2011;**52**:394–399. Harel et al. *Blood* (ASH Annual Meeting Abstracts) 2010;**116**:1794. Ruan et al. *Cancer.* 2010;**116**:2655–2664. Wang et al. *Lancet Oncol.* 2012;**13**:716–723. Zaja et al. *Haematologica.* 2012;**97**:416–422. Goy et al. *J Clin Oncol.* 2013;**31**:3688–3695. Zinzani et al. *Ann Oncol.* 2013;**24**:2892–2897. Witzig et al. *J Clin Oncol.* 2005;**23**:5347–5356. Ansell et al. *Cancer.* 2008;**113**:508–514. Hess et al. *J Clin Oncol.* 2009;**27**:3822–3829. Ansell et al. *Lancet Oncol.* 2011;**12**:361–368. Renner et al. *Haematologica.* 2012;**97**:1085–1091. Wang et al. *N Engl J Med.* 2013;**369**:507–516. Wang et al. *J Clin Oncol.* 2009;**27**:5213–5218.

ORR – Overall response rate, CR – Complete response, PFS – progression-free survival, EFS – event free survival, TTF – Time to failure, DOR – duration of response, OS – overall survival, TTP – Time to progression, BTK – Bruton tyosine kinase, EFS – Event free survival.

potentially less toxic therapy, outside of a clinical trial, we feel it would be premature to abandon the use of consolidative auto-HCT given its track record of being able to produce long remissions. We do encourage continued enrollment of patients on clinical trials that hopefully will eventually help define subgroups of MCL patients who may, using non-transplant approaches, be able to achieve outcomes similar to that seen with upfront auto-HCT.

2 *Can new/novel agents be incorporated prior to auto-HCT to help improve response?* For patients who are not auto-HCT candidates, early incorporation of bortezomib into induction therapy appears to improve outcomes, as discussed before. Whether early incorporation of bortezomib or other newer agents will improve outcomes for patients destined to undergo auto-HCT in first remission is not yet known but is a focus of some ongoing clinical trials.

3 *Can new/novel agents be incorporated following auto-HCT to extend the duration of first remission?* Only the LYSA study, comparing maintenance rituximab to observation after auto-HCT, has addressed this question so far (see discussion previously). Newer agents such as ibrutinib are being evaluated as maintenance therapy following auto-HCT as well. However, such studies are in very early stages and data are not yet available. It may ultimately be most cost-effective to use MRD analysis to identify patients most likely to benefit from this approach. Such issues will hopefully be addressed in clinical trials that are currently ongoing or soon to open.

Minimal residual disease analysis – is it ready for prime time?

In the Nordic MCL-2 trial, after completion of auto-HCT, an MRD monitoring strategy was employed using PCR (polymerase chain reaction). For those who became MRD-positive ("molecular relapse"), pre-emptive treatment with rituximab was given (as four weekly infusions). Of the 26 patients who experienced molecular relapse (without overt clinical relapse), pre-emptive rituximab led to molecular remission in 92%. Importantly, for those who achieved molecular remission after pre-emptive rituximab, the clinical relapse-free survival after rituximab was 3.7 years, which is considerably longer than that expected following molecular relapse. Though this strategy appears feasible and promising, this approach warrants further investigation before it can be widely recommended, particularly now with data showing survival benefit when rituximab maintenance is applied to all patients (without MRD monitoring) post auto-HCT.

> **PRACTICE POINT**
>
> Techniques to monitor MRD after auto-HCT are now available in routine clinical practice. This approach allows for the application of pre-emptive therapy which may prevent or delay clinical relapse. Whether this approach will improve long-term survival, and which pre-emptive treatment is most effective, remains unknown at this time.

Conclusions

MCL is a relatively uncommon form of NHL that ranges from an indolent form on one end of the spectrum to a highly aggressive (blastoid) variant on the other end. Given this clinical heterogeneity and variable patient factors (age, frailty, comorbidity), a single treatment for MCL cannot be recommended. Despite the availability of multiple treatment options for frontline and relapsed MCL, the clinical decision making is still a challenge due to the relative paucity of published prospective randomized trials. We present an algorithm (Figure 19.1a and 19.1b) to summarize our recommended treatment approach.

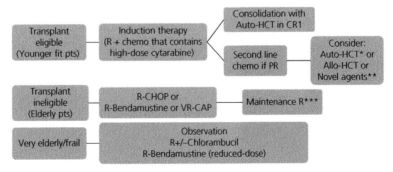

Figure 19.1 (a) Treatment options for newly diagnosed MCL.
*For patients going to auto-HCT in PR, TBI conditioning may offer benefit
**Novel agents as listed in Table 19.6
***Unclear that maintenance rituximab offers benefit after VR-CAP or R-Bendamustine

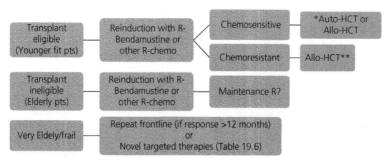

Figure 19.1 (b) Treatment options for relapsed MCL.
*Consolidation with allo-HCT if previously received auto-HCT otherwise auto-HCT is also an option.
**Allo-HCT not recommended if high disease bulk and/or rapidly progressing disease.

Several new/novel agents have shown improved response rates in recent studies and are currently being tested on a larger scale. Whole genome sequencing studies have helped identify recurrently mutated genes and pathways that contribute to lymphomagenesis in cooperation with the t(11;14) translocation. In addition, MRD monitoring (with potential application of pre-emptive or risk-adapted therapies) and new immuno-therapies such as chimeric antigen receptor (CAR) T-cell therapy (employing HDT as a lymphodepleting platform for CAR T-cell therapy) and programmed death-1 (PD-1) and programmed death ligand 1 (PDL1) inhibitors appear promising and have generated a great deal of enthusiasm and hope of transforming auto-HCT from a "remission extending" therapy to a potentially curative modality.

Selected reading

1. Hoster E, Dreyling M, Klapper W, et al. A new prognostic index (MIPI) for patients with advanced-stage mantle cell lymphoma. *Blood.* 2008;**111**: 558–565.

2. Hermine O, Hoster E, Walewski J, et al. Addition of high-dose cytarabine to immunochemotherapy before autologous stem-cell transplantation in patients aged 65 years or younger with mantle cell lymphoma (MCL Younger): a randomized, open-label, phase 3 trial of the European Mantle Cell Lymphoma Network. *Lancet.* 2016;**388**: 565–575.

3. Dreyling M, Lenz G, Hoster E, et al. Early consolidation by myeloablative radiochemotherapy followed by autologous stem cell transplantation in first remission significantly prolongs progression-free survival in mantle-cell lymphoma: results of a prospective randomized trial of the European MCL Network. *Blood.* 2005;**105**: 2677–2684.

4. Fenske TS, Zhang MJ, Carreras J, et al. Autologous or reduced-intensity conditioning allogeneic hematopoietic cell transplantation for chemotherapy-sensitive mantle-cell lymphoma: analysis of transplantation timing and modality. *J Clin Oncol.* 2014;**32**: 273–281.

5. Le Gouill SL, Thieblemont C, Oberic L, et al. Rituximab Maintenance after autologous stem cell transplantation prolongs survival in younger patients with Mantle cell lymphoma: Final results of Randomized phase 3 LyMa trial of the Lysa/Goelams group. *ASH Annual Meeting Abstracts.* 2016.

CHAPTER 20

T-cell lymphoma

Adrienne A. Phillips and Koen van Besien

Division of Hematology and Oncology, Department of Medicine, Weill Cornell Medical College, New York, NY, USA

Introduction

Peripheral T-cell Lymphomas (PTCLs) are uncommon malignancies, accounting for 10–15% of all non-Hodgkin lymphomas (NHL). Geographic variation has been well documented and may reflect exposure to specific pathogenic viruses, such as Epstein–Barr Virus (EBV) and Human T-cell leukemia virus-1 (HTLV-1) in Asian countries. The World Health Organization (WHO) classifies over 20 subtypes of PTCL, each with unique characteristics. Because of the rarity and heterogeneity of these diseases, until recently, large clinical trials have not been conducted and optimal therapy is not well defined. Most subtypes are treated with similar combination chemotherapy regimens as used for "aggressive" B-cell NHLs (e.g., diffuse large B-cell lymphoma (DLBCL), but with poorer outcomes. New treatment combinations and novel agents have recently been explored and several new PTCL therapies are now available but the treatment results remain suboptimal. There is some uncontrolled prospective and retrospective data to suggest autologous hematopoietic cell transplantation (auto-HCT) in first remission (CR1) may have clinical benefit in PTCL (with exception of ALK-positive anaplastic large-cell lymphoma (ALK⁺ ALCL) and the role for allogeneic hematopoietic cell transplantation (allo-HCT) is evolving.

Interest in PTCL is driven by:

1 Advances in our understanding of molecular alterations of PTCL and improved diagnostic ability to distinguish subtypes
2 Poor outcomes when PTCL is treated with regimens used for "aggressive" B-cell NHL
3 Better international collaborations to conduct large clinical trials.

What are the subtypes of PTCL and what are their geographic distributions?

PTCLs are a subset of NHL that arise from lymphocytes at the post-thymic stage ("mature") of maturation which display T-cell or natural killer (NK)-cell immunophenotypes. In the broadest sense, any mature T-cell NHL is considered a PTCL with the exception of lymphoblastic lymphoma (i.e. the lymphoma counterpart of T-cell acute lymphoblastic leukemia). Advances in our understanding of T-cell biology and molecular alterations of T-cell NHL over the past decade have led to a refinement of the WHO classification system. The 2008 WHO classification of T-cell neoplasms was designed to integrate the morphologic, immunophenotypic, genetic, and clinical characteristics of these diseases. T-cell neoplasms can be characterized as conditions with primarily cutaneous, extranodal, nodal, or leukemic presentations and currently, comprise over 20 biologically and clinically distinct entities (Table 20.1). Importantly, the term "peripheral" in "peripheral T-cell lymphoma" does not refer to the site of involvement but rather to the immunophenotype of tumors derived from post-thymic, or mature, T-cells. Cutaneous T-cell lymphoma (CTCL)/mycosis fungoides (MF) is generally considered indolent in its early stages with variety of distinct therapy(ies) when compared to other mature T-NHLs therefore will not be discussed in this chapter.

Worldwide, PTCLs represent approximately 10–15% of all NHLs. Ethnic and geographic variations account for differences in prevalence however, with rates ranging from 24% in Asia to 4% in North America. The incidence in the United States between 1992 and 2005 has increased 7.9% annually. The reason behind the geographic variation is not entirely clear but may be related

Clinical Manual of Blood and Bone Marrow Transplantation, First Edition. Edited by Syed A. Abutalib and Parameswaran Hari.

Table 20.1 Mature T- and NK-cell neoplasms: The WHO Classification.

WHO Classification 2008	
Leukemic	T-PLL
	T-LGL
	Chronic LPDs of NK-cells
	Aggressive NK-cell leukemia
	ATLL (HTLV-1+)
	Systemic EBV+ T-cell LPDs of childhood
Nodal	AITL
	ALCL, ALK+
	ALCL, ALK−
	PTCL-NOS
Extranodal	Extranodal NK-/T-cell lymphoma, nasal type
	Enteropathy-associated T-cell lymphoma
	Hepatosplenic T-cell lymphoma
	Subcutaneous panniculitis-like T-cell lymphoma
Cutaneous	Mycosis fungoides
	Sézary syndrome
	Primary cutaneous CD30+ T-cell LPD
	-Primary cutaneous aggressive epidermotropic CD8+ TCL[c]
	-Primary cutaneous small/medium CD4+ TCL[c]
	Primary cutaneous γδ TCL

T-PLL – T-cell prolymphocytic leukemia; T-LGLL – T-cell large granular lymphocytic leukemia; T-LGL – T-cell large granular lymphocytic leukemia; ATLL – Adult T-cell leukemia/lymphoma; HTLV-1 – human T-lymphotropic virus, type I; LPD – lymphoproliferative disorder; PTCL-U – peripheral T-cell lymphoma, unspecified; PTCL-NOS- peripheral T-cell lymphoma, not otherwise specified; ALCL – anaplastic large-cell lymphoma; ALK – anaplastic lymphoma kinase
[c] A provisional entity

to exposure or genetic susceptibility to pathogenic agents in Asian countries, notably HTLV-1 infection and adult T-cell leukemia/lymphoma (ATLL) and EBV infection and NK-/T-cell lymphoma (NKTCL). An international collaborative study also suggests geographic variation for other PTCL subtypes (Table 20.2). Overall, the most common PTCL subtypes identified were PTCL, not otherwise specified (PTCL-NOS 25.9%), angioimmunoblastic T-cell lymphoma (AITL 18.5%), NKTCL (10.4%), and ATLL (9.6%). With few exceptions, the course of most PTCL subtypes is aggressive and the clinical outcome is poor.

What is the standard evaluation for a patient suspected to have PTCL?

The diagnostic workup of PTCL is similar to that performed for other types of lymphomas however patients with PTCLs and B-NHLs frequently have different clinical characteristics (Table 20.3). An essential part of the initial workup is a complete physical examination with attention to nodal areas. Patients are also assessed for the presence of B symptoms. Similar to aggressive B-NHLs (e.g., DLBCL), the Ann Arbor system is used to stage PTCL. The value of utilizing positron emission tomography (PET) scans in patients with PTCL, however, has been questioned. Recent studies suggest PET scans might be as useful in these patients as in those with aggressive B-NHLs however the maximum standardized uptake value (SUV_{MAX}) in patients with PTCLs is somewhat lower than in DLBCL, and that the SUV_{MAX}

Table 20.2 Major PTCL subtypes by geographic region in the International T-cell lymphoma project.

PTCL subtype	Overall (%)	North America (%)	Europe (%)	Asia (%)	5 y PFS (%)	5 y OS (%)
PTCL-NOS	25.9	34.4	34.3	22.4	20	32
AITL	18.5	16.0	28.7	17.9	18	32
ALCL, ALK+	6.6	16.0	6.4	3.2	60	70
ALCL, ALK−	5.5	7.8	9.4	2.6	36	49
NKTCL	10.4	5.1	4.3	22.4	29	42
ATLL	9.6	2.0	1.0	25	12	14
Enteropathy-type TCL	4.7	5.8	9.1	1.9	4	20
Hepatosplenic TCL	1.4	3.0	2.3	0.2	0	7
SCPTCL	0.9	1.3	0.5	1.3	24	64

PTCL-NOS – peripheral T-cell lymphoma, not otherwise specified, AITL – angioimmunoblastic T-cell lymphoma, ALCL – anaplastic large-cell lymphoma, ALK – anaplastic kinase, NKTCL – natural killer T-cell lymphoma, ATLL – adult T-cell leukemia/lymphoma, TCL – T-cell lymphoma, SCPTCL – subcutaneous panniculitis-like T-cell lymphoma

Table 20.3 Characteristics of PTCLs and B-NHLs.

	PTCLs (%)	B-NHLs (%)
Stage III/IV disease	78	58
B symptoms	57	40
Bone marrow involvement	31	17
Skin lesions	21	4

in extranodal PTCLs might be lower than in those presenting primarily in nodal sites.

One challenge in diagnosing PTCL is that some patients will present with extranodal involvement with a high degree of necrosis such that a biopsy specimen is too small for thorough examination. In fact, the diagnostic agreement rate among expert hematopathologists is only 75%. Diagnostic information can be derived from sufficient formalin-fixed, paraffin-embedded tissue from which histology and immunohistochemistry is carried out. Fresh tissue is required for flow cytometry and cytogenetic studies. Although approximately 90% of PTCLs demonstrate cytogenetic abnormalities, none is specific for any PTCL subtype except for the translocation of the anaplastic lymphoma kinase (ALK) gene on chromosome 2p23. There are several recognized translocations and inversions involving ALK, most commonly t(2;5) encoding a nuclear phosphoprotein (NPM)/ ALK fusion protein in 70–75% of cases of ALK-positive anaplastic large-cell lymphoma (ALK$^+$ ALCL), which has a distinctly better clinical outcome than ALK-negative ALCL (ALK$^-$ ALCL). Clonal T-cell receptor (TCR) gene rearrangements are usually, but not always detected and immunoglobulin (Ig) genes are usually germline.

Is there a standard upfront regimen for T-NHLs (excluding CTCL/MF)?

The optimal therapeutic strategy for most PTCL subtypes is unknown. A low overall incidence and prevalence of PTCLs combined with disease heterogeneity has made it challenging to conduct randomized or multi-institutional trials. Regimens used for aggressive B-cell NHL are frequently used. With the exception of ALK$^+$ ALCL, which has an excellent outcome with anthracycline-based combination chemotherapy, other PTCLs have poor outcomes. The tendency for poor survival in PTCL suggests that the same regimens may not be equally efficacious in patients with aggressive B- and T-cell NHL. New combinations of therapy, dose intensified therapies, and novel agents are necessary.

Patients with PTCL were treated until the rituximab era with the same approach as B-cell NHL. *Outside of a clinical trial*, cyclophosphamide, doxorubicin, vincristine and prednisone (*CHOP*) or CHOP-like chemotherapy regimens (e.g., *EPOCH*- etoposide, prednisone, vincristine, cyclophosphamide, doxorubicin or *hyperCVAD*- hyperfractionated cyclophosphamide, vincristine, doxorubicin, and decadron alternating with high-dose methotrexate and cytarabine) *are considered reasonable options*. The large Intergroup trial, which established that CHOP was equally efficacious and less toxic than other chemotherapy combinations (ProMACE-CytaBOM, MACOP, mBACOD) in aggressive NHL however was performed in an era when routine immunophenotyping to distinguish B- and T-cell lineage was not performed. Unfortunately, with the notable exception of ALK$^+$ ALCL, outcomes with CHOP in PTCL have been poor. Despite these suboptimal results, few studies have compared CHOP to other regimens in the initial treatment of PTCL. The German High-Grade Non-Hodgkin's Lymphoma Group (DSHNHL) evaluated the outcome of 289 patients with ALK$^+$ ALCL, ALK$^-$ ALCL, PTCL-unclassified (PTCL-U now PTCL-NOS), and AITL treated on their protocols. Treatment consisted of 6–8 cycles of CHOP or etoposide plus CHOP (CHOEP). Three-year event free survival (EFS) and overall survival (OS) was 75.8 and 89.8% (ALK$^+$ ALCL), 50.0 and 67.5% (AITL), 45.7 and 62.1% (ALK$^-$ ALCL), and 41.1 and 53.9% (PTCL-NOS), respectively. For younger patients, the addition of etoposide improved response rates. The difference in EFS for younger patients and ALK$^+$ ALCL treated with CHOP or CHOEP was impressive (3-year EFS for CHOEP patients was 91.2 vs 57.1% for patients treated with CHOP, P=0.12), and a statistically not significant difference was seen in the remaining patients when ALK$^+$ ALCL was excluded (3-year EFS for CHOEP patients 60.7 vs 48.3% for patients treated with CHOP, P=0.57). Although this difference was not statistically significant, the authors concluded that CHOP plus etoposide should be administered to younger patients with T-cell lymphoma as first-line therapy.

> **PRACTICE POINT**
>
> Our preferred regimen for the upfront treatment of younger patients with ALK-negative PTCL outside of a clinical trial is dose adjusted-EPOCH.

What agents are available for relapsed or refractory disease?

Unfortunately, most patients with PTCL will either not achieve remission or will relapse. There is a paucity of data regarding the treatment of such patient and the general approach has been to administer further treatment with the hope of attaining a response and offering auto-HCT or allo-HCT given the potential for long-term DFS. Traditional regimens for patients who are transplant candidates include regimens such as ICE (ifosfamide, carboplatin, etoposide), DHAP (dexamethasone, high-dose cytarabine, and cisplatin), ESHAP (etoposide, methyl-prednisolone, cytarabine, and cisplatin), single-agent gemcitabine, GDP (gemcitabine, cisplatin, and dexamethasone), or gemcitabine and oxaliplatin. With these regimens, response rates for patients with PTCL are approximately 40–50% however the published experience is limited to case reports and phase II trials with a heterogeneous patient population.

Four novel agents are now approved for single-agent treatment of relapsed or refractory PTCL specifically-brentuximab, pralatrexate, romidepsin, and belinostat and are summarized in Table 20.4.

Data for HCT (auto and allo) in PTCL

The poor results with conventional chemotherapy have led to the exploration of high-dose chemotherapy supported auto-HCT or allo-HCT in PTCL however to date, this has not been investigated in a randomized trial. A number of uncontrolled prospective and retrospective studies suggest that upfront high-dose chemotherapy with auto-HCT as consolidation in patients who attained complete remission (not PR; see later) following first-line therapy may result in superior disease control and improved OS. The use of allo-HCT has typically been limited to patients with relapsed PTCL however prospective studies are ongoing. Table 20.5 highlights prospective studies of HCT (auto and allo) in PTCL. Notably, many studies exclude the more favorable ALK+ ALCL subtype and unfortunately, a significant proportion of patients do not proceed to transplant due to progressive disease, an important selection bias.

Role of frontline auto-HCT

In the largest prospective study by the Nordic Lymphoma Group (NLG) reported by d'Amore et. al., 160 patients with PTCL (excluding ALK+ ALCL) underwent induction with biweekly CHOEP followed by auto-HCT in patients with chemotherapy-sensitive disease. The median age was 57 years, the post-induction therapy CR rate was 51.2% and partial response (PR) rate was 30.6%. 26% of patients experienced treatment failure and did not proceed to transplant. Following conditioning with BEAM or BEAC, the TRM was 4% and at 5 years, median OS and PFS was 51 and 44%, respectively. The majority of relapses (18%) were seen within the first 2

years post-transplant and only 7% experienced relapse more than 2 years post-transplant. Reimer, et. al. conducted the second largest prospective study of upfront auto-HCT for patients with PTCL. Of 83 patients enrolled, the median age was 46.5 years and induction therapy consisted of CHOP. 34% of patients did not undergo transplantation because of progressive disease or death. For those transplanted, the conditioning regimen was high-dose cyclophosphamide and total body irradiation (TBI) and there were no reported mobilization failures. TRM was 3.6% and at 3 years, OS and PFS were 48 and 36%, respectively. Other smaller studies are listed. Taking into account the acceptable toxicity of auto-HCT and the poor prognosis of most patients with PTCL, most experts recommend autologous consolidation for patients with PTCL in CR1 – exceptions to this recommendation are patients with stage I-II disease at diagnosis or those with ALK+ ALCL.

PRACTICE POINT

We recommend auto-HCT for patients with PTCL in CR1 – exceptions to this recommendation are patients with stage I-II disease at diagnosis or those with ALK+ ALCL.

Role of frontline allo-HCT

The role of allogeneic transplantation has also been preliminarily investigated and ongoing clinical trials are testing its role in the upfront setting. Corradini et. al. recently updated their clinical trial of chemo-immuno-therapy in patients with PTCL followed by either auto-HCT or allo-HCT. Twenty-three patients had allo-HCT of which 13 were from a matched related donor (MRD) and 10 from a HLA-matched unrelated donor (MUD). One patient died from early toxicity and 22 patients were evaluable for graft-versus-host disease (GvHD). Chronic GvHD (cGvHD) occurred in 52% and survival outcomes of patients who had received allo-HCT were similar to those who had auto-HCT (4-year OS of 69% versus 92%) and the authors were not able provide a conclusive statement on superiority of either approach. In a single institution, prospective study, Loirat reported 49 newly diagnosed PTCL patients who underwent upfront allo-HCT following induction with CHOP. Twenty-nine patients (60%) proceeded to transplant: 45% from a MRD, 28% from a MUD, 11% from an unmatched-related donor, and 17% from a cord-blood donor. 28% had cGvHD and 1- and 2-year OS were 76 and 72.5%, respectively, with a TRM of 8.2%. The obvious limitations of allogeneic transplant including donor availability, high early, and severe chronic

Table 20.4 Selected studies of approved single-agent therapies for relapsed or refractory in PTCL.

Study	Agent	Mechanism of Action	Patient Number (n)	Indication	ORR (%)	Duration of Response (months)	Median PFS (months)	Notable Toxicities
Pro (2012)	Brentuximab	anti-CD30 drug conjugate (MMAE)	58	ALCL	86	12.6	13.3	Peripheral sensory neuropathy, nausea, fatigue, pyrexia
Piekarz (2011) Coiffier (2012 and 2014)	Romidepsin	HDAC inhibitor	45 130	PTCL and CTCL PTCL	38 25	8.9 28	NR 4	Nausea, fatigue, thrombocytopenia, and anemia
O'Connor (2015)	Belinostat	pan-HDAC inhibitor	120	PTCL	26	8.3	NR	Thrombocytopenia, neutropenia, anemia
O'Connor (2011)	Pralatrexate	Anti-folate	109	PTCL	29	10.1	3.5	Thrombocytopenia, neutropenia, mucositis, and anemia

ORR – overall response rate; PFS – progression free survival; MMAE – monomethylauristatin; HDAC – histone deacetylase; NR – not reported

Table 20.5 Prospective trials for upfront HCT (auto or allo) in PTCL (excluding CTCL/MF).

Author	N total N allo	Trial Setting	Conditioning	cGvHD allo-HCT	TRM	OS	PFS	Comments and Practice Implications
d'Amore (2012)	160/-	Prospective study of upfront auto-HCT in PTCL (excluding ALK+ ALCL)	BEAM/BEAC	-	4%	5 y OS 51%	5 y PFS 44%	Largest prospective study of auto-HCT in PTCL; induction regimen biweekly CHOEP if ≤60 y; 26% did not undergo transplantation.
Reimer (2009)	83/-	Prospective study of upfront auto-HCT in PTCL	CyTBI	-	3.6%	3 y OS 48%	3 y PFS 36%	34% did not undergo transplantation for progressive disease/death.
Corradini (2006)	62/-	Two prospective phase II studies of upfront auto-HCT in PTCL	BEAM Mito+MEL	-	4.8%	12 y OS 34%	12 y PFS 30%	74% completed entire treatment program. 12 y OS and PFS for ALK+ ALCL was 62 and 54% (significantly better). CR prior to auto-HCT was associated with significant clinical benefit.
Rodriguez (2007)	26/-	Prospective phase II study of upfront auto-HCT in PTCL	BEAM	-	0%	3 y OS 73%	3 y PFS 53%	Induction regimen with MegaCHOP×3 then gallium scan, if negative one additional cycle followed by auto-HCT. If positive, IFE×2.
Mercadal (2008)	41/-	Prospective phase II study of intensive chemotherapy and auto-HCT for upfront PTCL	BEAM/BEAC	-	0%	4 y OS 39%	4 y PFS 30%	Age≤65, excluded ALK+ ALCL. Induction regimen CHOP/ESHAP. Trend for shorter survival for AITL. No clear benefit for auto-HCT.
Corradini (2014)	64/23	Phase II study of chemo-immunotherapy in newly diagnosed PTCL <60 y with allo-HCT pending donor availability	Thiotepa, FLU, Cy (n=23) BEAM (n=14)	52% -	13% NR	4 y OS 49% At 32 m all but 1 pt alive	4 y PFS 44% NR	30% did not undergo transplantation for progressive disease/death; induction therapy included AL; first prospective study of upfront allo-HCT in PTCL; no difference in outcomes between auto-HCT and allo-HCT.
Loirat (2015)	49/29	Upfront allo-HCT in PTCL, single center	FLU/BU	28%	8.2%	2 y OS 55%	2 y PFS 51%	80% had HLA-matched donor but only 60% proceeded to transplant.

BEAM – carmustine, etoposide, cytarabine, melphalan; BEAC – carmustine, etoposide, cytarabine, cyclophosphamide; cGvHD – chronic graft-versus-host disease; TRM – treatment related mortality; OS – overall survival; PFS – progression free survival; AL – alemtuzumab; Cy – cyclophosphamide; TBI – total body irradiation; Mito – mitoxantrone; MEL – melphalan FLU – fludarabine; BU– busulfan

Table 20.6 Select trials for allo-HCT in relapsed or refractory PTCL.

Author	N total N allo	Trial Setting	Conditioning	cGvHD allo-HCT (%)	TRM (%)	OS	PFS	Comments and Practice Implications
Corradini (2004)	17/17	Pilot study of RIC followed by allo-HCT	Thiotepa, FLU, Cy	50	6	3 y OS 81%	3 y PFS 64%	DLI induced response in 2 patients progressing after allo-HCT; median age 41
Dodero (2012)	52/52	Retrospective study of RIC and allo-HCT	Thiotepa-based RIC regimens +/– TBI	27	12	5y OS 5 0%	5 y PFS 40%	Largest retrospective series; several patients failed auto-HCT; median age 47
Le Gouill (2008)	77/77	Retrospective study of allo-HCT for aggressive T-cell lymphomas	Varied– 74% MA, 26% RIC	NR	34	5 y OS 57%	5 y EFS 53%	Trend for better TRM when time from diagnosis to allo-HCT was <12 m; median age 36
Voss (2013)	14/8	Retrospective study of allo-HCT for HSTCL	NR	NR	25	Median OS 59 mos	Median PFS 13.3 mos	Non-CHOP induction followed by early HCT may improve survival for HSTCL subtype of PTCL
Kyriakou (2009)	45/45	Retrospective study of allo-HCT for AITL	Varied– 55.5% MA, 44.4% RIC	56	25	3 y OS 64%	3 y PFS 66%	Allo-HCT is a valid therapeutic option for AITL

RIC – reduced intensity conditioning; FLU – fludarabine; Cy – cyclophosphamide; DLI – donor lymphocyte infusion; TBI – total body irradiation; MA – myeloablative; TRM – treatment related morality

BEAM – carmustine, etoposide, cytarabine, melphalan; BEAC – carmustine, etoposide, cytarabine, cyclophosphamide; cGvHD – chronic graft-versus-host disease; TRM – treatment related mortality;

OS – overall survival; PFS – progression free survival; AL – alemtuzumab; Cy – cyclophosphamide; Mito – mitoxantrone; MEL – melphalan; BU – busulfan;

morbidity are steadily improving because of advances in donor selection, conditioning, GvHD prophylaxis, and supportive care. Upfront allo-HCT is feasible with a low TRM and continues to be investigated.

PRACTICE POINT

We recommend allogeneic transplantation for patients who have responsive disease but fail to obtain initial CR and for those with recurrent disease.

With regard to salvage therapy, auto-HCT appears to be less effective for relapsed or refractory disease except for possibly patients with ALK⁺ ALCL. allo-HCT has been studied in small prospective cohorts and few retrospective series suggesting the existence of a graft versus lymphoma effect. Table 20.6 highlights select studies. The largest retrospective study of allo-HCT for PTCL was reported by Le Gouill et al. Conditioning regimens varied in this study and included both myeloablative (MA) and reduced intensity conditioning (RIC) and 5-year OS was 57% and TRM was 34%. There was a trend for improved TRM with a shorter time from diagnosis to allo-HCT. Corradini et al. reported a small prospective

pilot study using RIC followed by allo-HCT for relapsed or refractory PTCL and 3-year OS was 81% and TRM was just 6% suggesting using RIC results in a lower TRM. Small retrospective studies suggest hepatosplenic T-cell lymphoma and AITL may have particular benefit from frontline allo-HCT.

PRACTICE POINTS

In patients with PTCL, enrollment on a clinical trial is preferred as there is no standard therapy and prognosis for all subtypes except ALK⁺ ALCL is poor.

For patients with relapsed disease who are potential transplant candidates, options include traditional combination salvage regimens which are preferred over single agents because of their higher ORR that can serve as a bridge to transplant. For patients who are not transplant candidates, sequential single-agent therapy is preferred to minimize toxicity. An important exception is to use brentuximab rather than other agents in patients with CD30⁺ ALCL.

Auto-HCT is recommended for all subtypes of PTCL in CR1 with the exception of ALK⁺ ALCL and early stage disease. Allo-HCT may be a promising option for select patients who fail to achieve CR1 or who have relapsed disease as early studies suggest a graft-versus T-cell *lymphoma effect.*

Table 20.7 Who, when, and how of HCT for PTCL.

Authors' practice:

A. PATIENT FACTORS:
Age: Age is a poor predictor of transplant tolerance and we do not have specific age cut-offs for either autologous or allogeneic transplant.
Performance Status (PS) and Co morbidity: Outcomes are heavily influenced by performance status, comorbidity score, and frailty. Patients who are frail with a very poor performance status or many comorbidities are considered ineligible for allo-HCT.

B. DISEASE FACTORS:
Autologous transplant is recommended for all subtypes of newly diagnosed PTCL in CR1 with the exception of ALK⁺ ALCL and patients with early stage disease.
Allogeneic transplant is recommended for all subtypes of PTCL who fail to achieve CR1 or who relapse after initial therapy.

C. DONOR EVALUATION:
Ideal donor: An HLA- matched sibling or an unrelated donor matched at A, B, C, DRB1 loci using high resolution typing is preferred. Recent evidence indicates that matching or permissive mismatching for HLA-DP is important as well.
Alternative donor: If an ideal matched donor is not available, excellent outcomes have been reported with HLA mismatched donor transplant. Options include HLA haplo-transplant, cord-blood transplant, or haplo-cord transplant in context of clinical trial.

D. CONDITIONING THERAPY:
We use the BEAM regimen for both frontline autologous and frontline allogeneic transplant conditioning (see text). The optimal conditioning regimen or type of GvHD prophylaxis remain a matter of debate. There is increasing evidence that over time, the toxicity and mortality associated with chronic GvHD outweighs its effect on relapse rates. We therefore recommend stringent GvHD prophylaxis and incorporate ATG and/or alemtuzumab in our conditioning regimens. For those who fail autologous transplant or who have contraindications for high-dose BCNU, we use fludarabine, and melphalan conditioning with ATG or alemtuzumab.

E. POST ALLOTRANSPLANT THERAPY:
There are no published studies of maintenance therapy after HCT in PTCL. Case reports of brentuximab vedotin, denileukin diftitox, and romidepsin in few PTCL subtypes have been reported. Decision is made on case by case basis

Selected reading

1. Vose J, Armitage J, Weisenburger D. International peripheral T-cell and natural killer/T-cell lymphoma study: pathology findings and clinical outcomes. *Journal of Clinical Oncology: Official Journal of the American Society of Clinical Oncology.* 2008;26(25):4124–4130.

2. Schmitz N, Trumper L, Ziepert M, Nickelsen M, Ho AD, Metzner B, et al. Treatment and prognosis of mature T-cell and NK-cell lymphoma: an analysis of patients with T-cell lymphoma treated in studies of the German High-Grade Non-Hodgkin Lymphoma Study Group. *Blood.* 2010;116(18): 3418–3425.

3. d'Amore F, Relander T, Lauritzsen GF, Jantunen E, Hagberg H, Anderson H, et al. Up-front autologous stem-cell transplantation in peripheral T-cell lymphoma: NLG-T-01. *Journal of Clinical Oncology: Official Journal of the American Society of Clinical Oncology.* 2012;30(25):3093–309.

4. Reimer P, Rudiger T, Geissinger E, Weissinger F, Nerl C, Schmitz N, et al. Autologous stem-cell transplantation as first-line therapy in peripheral T-cell lymphomas: results of a prospective multicenter study. *Journal of Clinical Oncology: Official Journal of the American Society of Clinical Oncology.* 2009;27(1):106–013.

5. Corradini P, Vitolo U, Rambaldi A, Miceli R, Patriarca F, Gallamini A, et al. Intensified chemo-immunotherapy with or without stem cell transplantation in newly diagnosed patients with peripheral T-cell lymphoma. *Leukemia.* 2014;28(9):1885–1891.

6. Loirat M, Chevallier P, Leux C, Moreau A, Bossard C, Guillaume T, et al. Upfront allogeneic stem-cell transplantation for patients with nonlocalized untreated peripheral T-cell lymphoma: an intention-to-treat analysis from a single center. *Annals of Oncology: Official Journal of the European Society for Medical Oncology/ESMO.* 2015;26(2):386–392.

7. Le Gouill S, Milpied N, Buzyn A, De Latour RP, Vernant JP, Mohty M, et al. Graft-versus-lymphoma effect for aggressive T-cell lymphomas in adults: a study by the Societe Francaise de Greffe de Moelle et de Therapie Cellulaire. *Journal of Clinical Oncology: Official Journal of the American Society of Clinical Oncology.* 2008;26(14):2264–2271.

8. Corradini P, Dodero A, Zallio F, Caracciolo D, Casini M, Bregni M, et al. Graft-versus-lymphoma effect in relapsed peripheral T-cell non-Hodgkin's lymphomas after reduced-intensity conditioning followed by allogeneic transplantation of hematopoietic cells. *Journal of Clinical Oncology: Official Journal of the American Society of Clinical Oncology.* 2004;22(11): 2172–2176.

9. Coiffier B, Pro B, Prince HM, Foss F, Sokol L, Greenwood M, et al. Romidepsin for the treatment of relapsed/refractory peripheral T-cell lymphoma: pivotal study update demonstrates durable responses. *Journal of Hematology & Oncology.* 2014;7:11.

10. O'Connor OA, Pro B, Pinter-Brown L, Bartlett N, Popplewell L, Coiffier B, et al. Pralatrexate in patients with relapsed or refractory peripheral T-cell lymphoma: results from the pivotal PROPEL study. *Journal of Clinical Oncology: Official Journal of the American Society of Clinical Oncology.* 2011;29(9):1182–1189.

11. Corradini P, Tarella C, Zallio F, Dodero A, Zanni M, Valagussa P, et al. Long-term follow-up of patients with peripheral T-cell lymphomas treated up-front with high-dose chemotherapy followed by autologous stem cell transplantation. *Leukemia.* 2006;20(9):1533–1538.

12. Rodriguez J, Conde E, Gutierrez A, Arranz R, Leon A, Marin J, et al. Frontline autologous stem cell transplantation in high-risk peripheral T-cell lymphoma: a prospective study from The Gel-Tamo Study Group. *European Journal of Haematology.* 2007;79(1):32–38.

13. Dodero A, Spina F, Narni F, Patriarca F, Cavattoni I, Benedetti F, et al. Allogeneic transplantation following a reduced-intensity conditioning regimen in relapsed/refractory peripheral T-cell lymphomas: long-term remissions and response to donor lymphocyte infusions support the role of a graft-versus-lymphoma effect. *Leukemia.* 2012;26(3):520–526.

14. Voss MH, Lunning MA, Maragulia JC, Papadopoulos EB, Goldberg J, Zelenetz AD, et al. Intensive induction chemotherapy followed by early high-dose therapy and hematopoietic stem cell transplantation results in improved outcome for patients with hepatosplenic T-cell lymphoma: a single institution experience. *Clinical Lymphoma, Myeloma & Leukemia.* 2013;13(1):8–14.

15. Kyriakou C, Canals C, Finke J, Kobbe G, Harousseau JL, Kolb HJ, et al. Allogeneic stem cell transplantation is able to induce long-term remissions in angioimmunoblastic T-cell lymphoma: a retrospective study from the lymphoma working party of the European group for blood and marrow transplantation. *Journal of Clinical Oncology: Official Journal of the American Society of Clinical Oncology.* 2009;27(24): 3951–3958.

CHAPTER 21

Primary CNS lymphoma

Henry C. Fung, Philip Pancari, and Patricia Kropf

Fox Chase Cancer Center, Temple Health, Philadelphia, PA, USA

Introduction

Primary central nervous system lymphoma (PCNSL) is an uncommon subtype of extra-nodal lymphomas arising in and confined to the brain, eyes, spinal cord, and leptomeninges. This chapter will specifically focus on B-cell PCNSL. Over the past few decades, PCNSL has evolved from a uniformly fatal disease to a potentially curable disease, largely due to the incorporation of high-dose methotrexate (HDMTX) based induction regimens. Remarkably, approximately 20% of patients with PCNSL can achieved durable remission with this strategy. Combining whole-brain radiation therapy (WBRT) with HDMTX improves disease control and perhaps survivals; however, the utility of this approach is limited by long-term neurological toxicity especially if WBRT is given at conventional doses (not low-dose WBRT). Recent studies utilizing chemo-immunotherapy induction followed by non-myeloablative consolidation therapy have resulted in significant improvement in outcomes. The optimal consolidation however remains to be determined. High-dose chemotherapy (HDT) followed by autologous hematopoietic cell transplant (auto-HCT) is emerging as an effective consolidation treatments for patients with PCNSL. Here, we will review the management of PCNSL specifically addressing the role of auto-HCT in the treatment of PCNSL.

Epidemiology, pathology, and clinical presentation

The estimated incidence of PCNSL is 7 per million per year. It accounts for approximately 5% of all primary brain tumors. Most commonly, PCNSL presents as diffuse and multifocal supratentorial brain masses. After routine lymphoma staging, up to 10% patients initially thought to have PCNSL were found to have occult systemic lymphoma. Therefore, body CT scan and or PET-CT and bone marrow biopsy need to be part of initial staging. In addition, a detailed ophthalmologic examination including slit lamp examination, CSF analysis, and serum lactate dehydrogenase level, HIV, and hepatitis serology should be performed during the initial work-up.

MRI scan is the preferred radiological study for initial diagnostic work-up. The tumor usually appears as single or multiple lesions on nonenhanced T1-weighted images, hyperintense tumor, and edema on T2 or FLAIR images and densely enhancing masses after administration of gadolinium. Stereotactic biopsy is the diagnostic procedure of choice. The majority of PCNSL are diffuse large B-cell lymphomas, germinal center subtype. Primary T-cell lymphomas and low-grade lymphoma account for less than 10 % of PCNSL.

Auto-HCT in the setting of recurrent or refractory PCNSL: Does it work?

Soussain et al. reported 20 patients with recurrent or refractory PCNSL receiving a high-dose chemotherapy combination of Thiotepa, Busulfan, and cyclophosphamide (TBC) followed by auto-HCT. The estimated 3-year event-free survival was 53%. In a subsequent prospective study from the same group, out of 43 patients with progressive disease or recurrent disease, 27 (63%) patients proceeded to transplant, including 12 with progressive disease. For all transplanted patients, the 1-year OS was 78%, with a median survival of 59 months. The median survival for patients who responded to salvage chemotherapy was 64 months

Clinical Manual of Blood and Bone Marrow Transplantation, First Edition. Edited by Syed A. Abutalib and Parameswaran Hari.

versus 9 months for those who were transplanted with progressive disease.

In a retrospective study from seven French centers that included 79 patients with a median follow-up of 56 months, the estimated 5-year overall survival for patients with chemosensitive versus chemo-refractory disease were 62 and 36.2%, respectively. However, only 2 of the 18 patients with chemo-refractory disease were alive in CR at the last follow-up at 45 and 56 months.

It is reasonable to consider auto-HCT for selected patients with chemosensitive relapsed or refractory PCNSL. On the other hand, these data may not apply to patients who failed modern chemo-immunotherapy and intensive chemotherapy consolidation as this may represent a subgroup of patients with more refractory disease. The role of auto-HCT for patients with chemo-refractory relapsed PCNSL is very limited if any.

PRACTICE POINT

Patients with chemosensitive relapsed or refractory PCNSL could be considered for auto-HCT. The outcomes are inferior in chemotherapy refractory patients and those with progressive disease.

Auto-HCT as front line treatment: Is there a straightforward answer?

Investigators from Memorial Sloan Kettering Cancer Center (MSKCC) conducted a phase II prospective study utilized an induction regimen with HDMTX and cytarabine, followed by consolidation with BEAM (carmustine (BCNU), etoposide, cytarabine, and melphalan). By an intent-to-treat (ITT) analysis, 3-year EFS was 25%. The poor outcomes from this study were likely due to suboptimal response to induction with an overall response rate of 57% and perhaps a "less effective" transplant-conditioning regimen (BEAM) utilizing drugs that have limited CNS penetration.

This strategy was then modified using an enhanced chemo-immunotherapy induction regimen that consisted of the combination of rituximab, HDMTX, procarbazine, and vincristine (R-MPV), and utilized TBC as a conditioning regimen that has better CNS penetration. Following 5–7 cycles of R-MPV, the response rate was 97% which compared favorably to their previous trial using HDMTX/cytarabine. After a median follow-up of 45 months, the median PFS has not been reached and there were no events after 2 years, and the estimated 5-year PFS and OS were 79% (95% CI, 58–90) and 81% (95% CI,63–91) respectively. The median follow-up for survivors was 45 months (range: 7–86).

Kasenda et al. treated 43 immunocompetent patients with newly diagnosed PCNSL according to two different high-dose methotrexate-based protocols followed by high-dose carmustine/thiotepa (BCNU/TT) and auto-HCT (±whole-brain irradiation). Median OS was 104 months. Two- and 5-year OS were 81 and 70%, respectively. In a large retrospective multicenter study that included data on 105 immuno-competent patients from 12 German centers; with a median follow-up of 47 months, median PFS and OS were 85 and 121 months respectively with estimated 5-year survival of 79%. Other phase II studies as summarized in Table 21.1 also suggest that auto-HCT as consolidation without WBRT is an effective treatment for patients with PCNSL and may contribute to the overall improvement of outcomes.

Given this data, despite the absence of a phase III randomized study; induction with chemo-immunotherapy followed by consolidation with auto-HCT can be considered an excellent treatment approach for transplant eligible patients.

PRACTICE POINT

HDMTX induction followed by auto-HCT consolidation is an effective treatment for patients with PCNSL in the frontline setting.

Comparison between types of consolidation: Non-myeloablative chemotherapy versus auto-HCT

Parallel to a transplant consolidation approach, investigators from CALGB adopted the UCSF approach utilizing high-dose etoposide and cytarabine (EC) without hematopoietic cell support. Forty-two patients with newly diagnosed PCNSL received MT-R (methotrexate, temozolomide, and rituximab) induction followed by consolidation with EC. Sixty-six percent of patients achieved CR with induction. With a median follow-up of 4.9 years, the 2-year PFS was 57 and 77% for patients who completed consolidation.

Despite the limitations on possible bias from patient selection, the results from MSKCC, CALGB and registry studies clearly demonstrate that the outcomes of patients with PCNSL have improved significantly and WBRT is no longer indicated in the context of front line consolidation. It also highlighted the importance of the modern chemo-immunotherapy as remission induction (rituximab and combined chemotherapy) followed by consolidation with either EC or auto-HCT. On the other hand, the best approach for treatment of PCNSL remains to be determined. An ongoing intergroup study

Table 21.1 Summary of published data on autologous hematopoietic cell transplantation for patients with Primary CNS Lymphoma.

Author (Year)	No. Patients	Induction Regimen	ORR to Induction (%)	WBR	Median FU (months)	PFS	Outcomes
Abrey (2003)	28	MTX cytarabine	57	No	28	ITT 3-y: 25%	ITT 3-y 60%
Colombat (2006)	25	MBVP Ifo/cytarabine	84	Yes	34	ITT 3-y 58%	ITT 3-y 64%
Illerhaus (2006)	30	MTX cytarabine/TT	80	Yes	63	NA	ITT 3-y 69%
Montemurro (2007)	23	MTX	61	Post-AHCT WRR to < CR	15	ITT 3-y 48%	ITT 2-y 48%
Illerhaus (2008)	13	MTX cytarabine TT		No	72		5-y OS 77%
Yoon (2011)	11	MTX cytarabine		No	10		2-y OS 89%
Schorb (2012)	105	MTX/cytarabine/TT (77%)	Multicenter Retro-studies	34	47		5-y OS 79%
Kasenda (2012)	43	MTX/cytarabine/TT	NA	70%	120		5-y OS 70%
Omuro (2015)	32	R-MVP	97%	No	45	ITT 3-y 79%	ITT 3-y 81%

Abbreviations: Auto-HCT, autologous hematopoietic cell transplantation; cytarabine, cytarabine; BCNU, carmustine; BEAM, carmustine, etoposide, melphalan, and cytarabine; BU, busulfan; Cy, cyclophosphamide; VP-16, etoposide; FU, follow-up; Ifo, ifosfamide; MBVP, methotrexate, carmustine, VP-16

Regimens	References
BEAM (BCNU, etoposide, cytarabine, melphalan)	Abrey (2003)
BCNU/TT (BCNU, thiotepa)	Kasenda (2012)
BuTTCTX (BCNU, thiotepa, cyclophosphamide	Omuro (2015)

comparing EC consolidation with auto-HCT will provide invaluable data to determine the best post-induction treatment strategy for patients with PCNSL.

> **PRACTICE POINT**
>
> Due to the rarity of the disease, the optimal consolidation strategy for patients with PCNSL remains to be determined. At least two clinical trials are underway. The first, NCT01511562 (CALGB 51101), randomizes patients to non-myeloablative consolidation (EC) or carmustine, thiotepa, and auto-HCT. The second, NCT01011920, randomizes patients to methotrexate-based combinations after which complete responders are again randomized to either WBRT or myeloablative chemotherapy with auto-HCT.

Eligibility criteria for auto-HCT

All patients with PCNSL should be potential candidates for auto-HCT and they should be assessed by a transplant specialist soon after diagnosis. The eligibility criteria for transplant for PCNSL is similar to the criteria used for any auto-HCT with emphasis on comorbidity, performance status, and chemosensitivity.

> **PRACTICE POINT**
>
> Age by itself should not be a contraindication for auto-HCT.

Is HIV associated Primary CNS lymphoma a contraindication for auto-HCT?

Patients with HIV associated Hodgkin and non-Hodgkin lymphoma have similar transplant outcomes when compared with non-HIV patients. Several HIV positive PCNSL patients have been transplanted and this in itself should not be a contraindication.

> **PRACTICE POINT**
>
> HIV sero-positivity by itself should not be a contraindication for auto-HCT.

What is the best induction regimen before auto-HCT?

HDMTX with leucovorin rescue is the single most effective treatment for PCNSL. Dose of methotrexate used ranged from 1–8 g/m^2. Retrospective analysis from MSKCC and others have demonstrated that addition of intrathecal methotrexate did not affect the outcome on patients treated with HDMTX at a target dose of 3–3.5 g/m^2 including in patients with lymphomatous meningitis at diagnosis. There is also evidence to suggest that greater than four cycles of methotrexate-based therapy may be necessary to achieve remission before consolidation using non–cross-resistant agents in consolidative therapy.

In a randomized phase II study (IELSG no. 20), Ferreri and colleagues evaluated four courses of MTX 3.5 g/m^2, alone or combined with cytarabine (4 doses of 2 g/m^2). The addition of cytarabine resulted in improved response rates (CR: 46 vs 18%; $P = 0.006$) and survival rates (3-year OS: 46 vs 32%; $P = 0.07$) compared with HDMTX. However, as discussed earlier; four cycles of HDMTX may not be the optimal schedule. On the other hand, despite the lack of phase III data, some investigators considered MTX-cytarabine combination as the current standard of care for induction.

Although rituximab improves outcomes in patients with almost every subtype of CD20$^+$ B-cell lymphoma; patients with PCNSL was considered a possible outliner because less than 1% of systemic rituximab penetrates the leptomeningeal compartment. Nevertheless, several studies demonstrate that intravenous rituximab may induce responses of contrast-enhancing lesions of CNS lymphoma, suggesting selective activity in the setting of a disrupted blood-brain barrier and supporting the rationale for incorporating of rituximab into PCNSL induction regimens. Although we do not have a phase III

study to determine the true impact of outcomes on adding Rituxan to the PCNSL regimens, we recommend all patients with CD20$^+$ PCNSL to receive rituximab. Multiple studies have used a higher dose of rituximab of 500 mg/m^2 instead of the regular dose of 375 mg/m^2; we do not have a strong opinion on this practice and it is doubtful that we can ever show any differences between the two dosing regimens.

In summary, monotherapy HDMTX (8 g/m^2) and HDMTX (2.5–3.5 gm/m^2) based combination chemotherapy yielded similar efficacy, but the former requires more frequent dose reductions because of impaired creatinine clearance. Monotherapy with lesser dose such as MTX 3.5 g/m^2 has demonstrated variable results as described previously though the less favorable outcomes could be the results of giving inadequate number of cycles of therapy. Thus, we advocate the MSKCC induction regimen, that is, R-MPV for 6–8 cycles, which is well tolerated, easily manageable, associated with very high response rates and without the need forintrathecal prophylaxis (see below). R-MPV consists of rituximab 500 mg/m^2 IV on day 1; methotrexate 3.5 mg/m^2 IV (over 2 hours) on Day 2 and vincristine 1.4 mg/m^2 (capped at 2.8 mg) and procarbazine 100 mg/m^2 per day on days 2–8 during odd cycles.

> **PRACTICE POINT**
>
> In the absence of randomized prospective data, we favor the use of the chemo-immunotherapy that contains HDMTX in range of 3–3.5 gm/m^2, rituximab +/− vincristine and procarbazine for 6–8 cycles without intra-thecal chemotherapy.

Is achievement of complete remission necessary before proceeding to consolidation with auto-HCT?

In general, patients who are transplanted while in CR as defined by MRI with gadolinium, tend to have better outcomes. The role of PET-CT in PCNSL remains to be determined. On the other hand, for patients with PCNSL who achieve a PR with HDMTX containing induction chemotherapy, the role of transplant is still unclear. In a recent MSKCC report, 7 of 26 transplanted patients were in PR, and 4 converted to CR after transplant; subgroup survivals were not reported though the 5-year PFS of 81% was noted to be remarkable.

> **PRACTICE POINT**
>
> Auto-HCT in patients achieving PR after appropriate chemo-immunotherapy is a reasonable approach.

Conditioning regimen: Is there a standard?

As shown in Table 21.1, various conditioning regimens have been used and it is unlikely that we will have a phase III randomized study to identify the best regimen. BEAM is not favored because of the poor outcomes in the original MSKCC trial though as discussed above, this could be due to suboptimal disease control before transplant. In a phase II study from GOELAMS, the combination of BEAM and WBRT results in 3-year PFS and OS of 58 and 64%, respectively. In our opinion, BEAM is as an option specifically in circumstances when thiotepa is not available. Thiotepa/Busulfan +/− cyclophosphamide or thiotep/BCNU based conditioning regimen, however, is associated with better CNS penetration and excellent results have been reported both for patients with relapsed and refractory disease and when used in front line setting.

> **PRACTICE POINT**
>
> No standard conditioning regimen currently exists and thiotepa based regimen is preferable based on phase II data.

What is the role of WBRT?

WBRT was the treatment of choice before the advent of modern chemotherapy. The response rates of WBRT alone (36–40 Gy) was up to 90% though median survival was limited to approximately 1 year and many patients experienced progression of lymphoma within the irradiated field. In the SG-1 trial; a large phase III randomized study that included 551 patients; after front line HDMTX, patients were randomized between observation and WBRT. Although WBRT resulted in modest improvement in PFS after methotrexate-based induction, this did not translate into improved overall survival partly because of the severe neurotoxicity caused by WBRT. Post-WBRT neurotoxicity presents as dementia, ataxia, and urinary incontinence and the risk is particularly high in patients who receive combined modality therapy. Due to the unacceptable neurotoxicity, there is no role for WBRT in preparation of patients for auto-HCT with intent to cure. We reserve WBRT for frail patients who are not candidates for systemic chemotherapy and selected patients who relapse after transplant or as palliative care in patients with refractory disease.

> **PRACTICE POINT**
>
> With an intent to achieve long-term durable remission and possible cure, in our opinion there is no role for high-dose (conventional) WBRT as consolidation therapy.

What is the role of intrathecal chemotherapy?

We do not recommend upfront intrathecal chemotherapy when MTX above 3.5 gm/m² every 2 weeks is given as induction.

Conclusion

PCNSL is a potential curative disease when treated with induction chemo-immunotherapy based on HDMTX and rituximab and consolidation with auto-HCT. See Table 21.2 for an overview of the authors' practice.

Table 21.2 Who, when, and how of auto-HCT for PCNSL.

Authors' practice:

A. PATIENT FACTORS:

Age:
Auto-HCT is the transplant option for patients with PCNSL. All patients with PCNSL are potential candidate for auto-HCT, patients should not be excluded from transplant solely based on age. Similar to all other patients with lymphoma/myeloma, we consider this approach suitable for selected patients up to their mid-70s.

Performance Status (PS) and Comorbidity:
Auto-HCT is feasible with low TRM in those with good PS and low comorbidity scores. We use PS and comorbidity score as exclusion criteria to lower TRM.
Patients with PCNSL (age <75 years) who have chemo-responsive disease and who have good PS with low comorbidity scores are considered for auto-HCT at our center.

Table 21.2 (Continued)

B. DISEASE FACTORS:

Newly diagnosed PCNSL:

1 All patients who have achieved CR are potential candidate for consolidation with auto-HCT.

2 All patients with chemo-responsive disease after treatment with chemo-immunotherapy and achieve a PR are potential candidate for consolidation with auto-HCT.

3 Patients with refractory or progressive disease are not eligible for auto-HCT

Relapsed PCNSL:

1 All patients who have achieved CR2 or PR2 after salvage chemotherapy are potential candidate for consolidation with auto-HCT.

2 Patients with progressive disease are not eligible for auto-HCT

C. INDUCTION REGIMEN

For patients with newly diagnosed PCNSL, we treated them with 6–8 cycles of HDMTX (3.5 g/m^2), procarbazine and vincristine (R-MPV) with rituximab.

D. CONDITIONING THERAPY:

There is no standard conditioning regimen. We favor the use of thiotepa, busulfan, and cyclophosphamide (TBC; MSKCC regimen) or consider BEAM regimen when thiotepa is not available.

E. ADDITIONAL THERAPY POST AUTO-TRANSPLANT:

Not recommended

Selected reading

1. Kasenda B, Schorb E, Fritsch K, Finke J and Illerhaus G. Prognosis after high-dose chemotherapy followed by autologous stem-cell transplantation as first-line treatment in primary CNS lymphoma – a long-term follow-up study. *Ann Oncol* 2015;**26**(3):608–611.

2. Ferreri AJ, Reni M, Foppoli M, et al. High-dose cytarabine plus high-dose methotrexate versus high-dose methotrexate alone in patients with primary CNS lymphoma: A randomized phase II trial. *Lancet* 2009;**374**:1512–1520.

3. Abrey LE, Moskowitz CH, Mason WP et al. Intensive methotrexate and cytarabine followed by high-dose chemotherapy with autologous stem-cell rescue in patients with newly diagnosed primary CNS lymphoma: an intent-to-treat analysis. *J Clin Oncol* 2003;**21**:4151–4156.

4. Colombat P, Lemevel A, Bertrand P et al. High-dose chemotherapy with autologous stem cell transplantation as first-line therapy for primary CNS lymphoma in patients younger than 60 years: a multicenter phase II study of the GOELAMS group. *Bone Marrow Transplant.* 2006 Sep;**38**(6):417–420.

5. Illerhaus G, Marks R, Ihorst G et al. High-dose chemotherapy with autologous stem-cell transplantation and hyperfractionated radiotherapy as first-line treatment of primary CNS lymphoma. *J Clin Oncol.* 2006 Aug 20;**24**(24):3865–3870.

6. Montemurro M, Kiefer T, Schüler F. Primary central nervous system lymphoma treated with high-dose methotrexate, high-dose busulfan/thiotepa, autologous stem-cell transplantation and response-adapted whole-brain radiotherapy: results of the multicenter Ostdeutsche Studiengruppe Hämato-Onkologie OSHO-53 phase II study. *Ann Oncol* 2006;**18**(4):665–671.

7. Illerhaus G, Müller F, Feuerhake F et al. High-dose chemotherapy and autologous stem-cell transplantation without consolidating radiotherapy as first-line treatment for primary lymphoma of the central nervous system. *Haematologica January* 2008;**93**:147–148.

8. Yoon DH, Lee DH, Choi DR et al. Feasibility of BU, CY and etoposide (BUCYE), and auto-SCT in patients with newly diagnosed primary CNS lymphoma: a single-center experience. *Bone Marrow Transplantation* 2011;**46**:105–109; doi:10.1038/bmt.2010.71.

9. Schorb E, Kasenda B, Atta J, et al. Prognosis of patients with primary central nervous system lymphoma after high-dose chemotherapy followed by autologous stem cell transplantation. *Haematologica.* 2013;**98**(5):765–770. doi: 10.3324/haematol.2012.076075.

10. Kasenda B, Schorb E, Fritsch K, et al. Prognosis after high-dose chemotherapy followed by autologous stem-cell transplantation as first-line treatment in primary CNS lymphoma – a long-term follow-up study. *Ann Oncol.* 2012 Oct;**23**(10):2670–2675.

11. Omuro, A, Correa, DD, DeAngelis, LM, et al. R-MPV followed by high-dose chemotherapy with TBC and autologous stem-cell transplant for newly diagnosed primary CNS lymphoma. *Blood.* 2015;**125**(9):1403–1410.

CHAPTER 22

Autologous hematopoietic transplant in multiple myeloma

Nisha S. Joseph, Ajay K. Nooka, and Sagar Lonial

Department of Hematology and Medical Oncology, Emory University School of Medicine, Atlanta, GA, USA

Introduction

The use of high-dose therapy (HDT) and autologous bone marrow transplantation in the treatment of multiple myeloma (MM) was first initiated in the late 1980s and early 1990s. Initially, transplantation was introduced as a means for treating refractory and relapsed myeloma, but given significant success in these end-stage patients, further investigation into its utility in the larger myeloma population followed. This led to several large randomized clinical trials demonstrating the benefit of HDT and bone marrow transplantation, ultimately autologous hematopoietic cell transplantation (auto-HCT), as part of the initial treatment for transplant-eligible patients. The success was measured not only in improved duration of remission, but also in terms of improved overall survival. The benefit noted with HDT was also associated with a higher complete remission (CR) rate, as well as improved depth of response when compared with standard therapy, resulting in HDT becoming the standard of care. As the era of novel agents has progressed and their use in induction regimens has increased, many have called into question the ongoing benefit of HDT in view of the high CR rates achieved with modern induction regimens alone. However, to date, trials continue to demonstrate a benefit of auto-HCT in terms of duration of remission as well as overall survival (OS). In this chapter, we will review some of the data that surrounds the use of auto-HCT as it relates to myeloma patients, with particular focus on issues such as age, induction, conditioning, and future directions in cellular therapy for myeloma.

What is the role of induction therapy prior to auto-HCT?

Backbone of VD: Prior to the advent of novel therapies, HDT/auto-HCT was considered the standard of care for younger MM patients. The ability to attain CR or at least very good partial response (VGPR) translated to better overall outcomes. One method in which to improve upon the CR+VGPR rate in transplanted patients was to better the induction regimens. Novel agents are now routinely used as part of the induction regimen prior to transplantation and this has led to significant improvements in the depth of response achieved before auto-HCT, and ultimately OS. In an era when the utility of HDT was limited to the ability to achieve CR following relatively ineffective induction therapy (namely steroid and alkylator-based regimens), it was clear that the survival benefit associated with transplant was in part correlated with a higher CR rate post-transplant. Now in the era of modern induction, using agents such as bortezomib, thalidomide, and lenalidomide, it is no longer uncommon for patients to achieve a CR following four cycles of induction alone.

Traditionally, prior to routine use of novel therapies, the standard induction regimen consisted of high-dose dexamethasone alone or in combination with vincristine and adriamycin (VAD). A randomized trial conducted by the IFM showed that bortezomib and dexamethasone (VD) when compared to VAD had significantly improved CR+VGPR rates both before and after HDT and auto-HCT (6 and 16% with VD vs 1 and 9% with VAD), which established VD as the new standard induction regimen.

Clinical Manual of Blood and Bone Marrow Transplantation, First Edition. Edited by Syed A. Abutalib and Parameswaran Hari.

Addition of third agent with a backbone of VD: Is that a standard?

The next step was the evaluation of three-drug combination regimens utilizing VD with the addition of a novel agent in comparison to VAD and VAD-like regimens.

Several phase 3 trials have showed improved VGPR rates from using three-drug combinations with a VD backbone and the addition of a third agent such as thalidomide or lenalidomide. In a trial from the Italian Myeloma Group, a randomization between VTD or TD demonstrated significant benefit favoring the three-drug induction, nearly doubling the VGPR or better rate associated with an improvement in post-transplant progression free survival (PFS).

The French group, in a prospective phase 3 trial comparing VTD to VCD, were the first to demonstrate that an IMiD (thalidomide) as a partner to VD resulted in superior responses post induction, compared to cyclophosphamide as a partner.

These positive results lead to three-drug combinations including VD to be the current standard of care prior to auto-HCT (Table 22.1).

However, it should be noted that all regimens have not yet to date been compared directly to each other, so there is not a specific regimen that has been established as standard of care.

Is auto-HCT reasonable after excellent responses from three-drug combination?

Despite encouraging response with induction alone, early transplant remains an important adjunct to treatment in transplant-eligible patients. There have been two trials presented or published by Palumbo and colleagues that utilized Rd (lenalidomide and dexamethasone) induction followed by a randomization between transplant or alternative consolidation using melphalan or cyclophosphamide +Rd. In the most mature of these trials, despite a similar CR rate between the transplant and non-transplant arm, the PFS and OS favored the group that had an early transplant. So, despite encouraging results after induction, these studies repeatedly demonstrate that among patients who receive more modern induction, there continues to be benefit for HDT consolidation even after achieving a major response with modern drug induction.

In the same vein, the E4A03 trial assessed survival and duration of remission in a non-randomized fashion, evaluating patients who went on to transplant versus those who elected not to proceed to transplant. What was found was a significant improvement in OS and PFS favoring those who underwent early transplant despite the fact that the pre-transplant CR rate was higher among those who opted not to continue on to transplant.

Similarly, an Italian trial directly compared Rd followed by HDT and AHCT versus consolidative cyclophosphamide and Rd in 256 untreated transplant eligible patients. Additionally, patients underwent a second randomization to lenalidomide versus lenalidomide and prednisone maintenance. The median PFS for cohort that underwent transplant was 43.3 months versus 28 months, and the 4-year overall survival was 86% versus 71%, showing a 58% risk reduction favoring the transplant arm.

More recently, the French reported their results from the IFM/DFCI trial that compared 3 drug induction (RVD) followed by early versus delayed transplant. The initial results suggest early transplant offered deeper responses and higher minimal residual disease (MRD) negative rates and resulted in PFS benefit (4 yr PFS: 47% vs 35%, hazard ratio 0.69).

On the same note, EMN02/H095 MM trial randomized newly diagnosed myeloma patients to receive auto-HCT versus VMP consolidation among 1192 newly diagnosed myeloma patients who had undergone VCD induction therapy. In a second randomization, patients received either VRD consolidation followed by lenalidomide maintenance or lenalidomide maintenance alone. Again, upfront AHCT was associated with superior PFS and this benefit was retained across all patients.

PRACTICE POINTS

Optimal choice of induction remains unclear, however the use of a three-drug induction is now a standard for transplant-eligible patients. The advantage of a three-drug induction is a higher overall response rate and VGPR rate before transplant, in addition to the fact that fewer patients require salvage therapy for failure to achieve at least a PR. If a patient achieves a PR or better, there is insufficient data supporting switching to a second induction regimen simply because patients have failed to achieve CR or VGPR prior to transplant. Finally, based upon new phase III data supporting VTD and phase II data with the IMID/PI combination (RVD, KRD) is superior to the PI/Cyclophosphamide (VCD, KCD) or IMID/Cyclophosphamide (CTD, CRD) combination.

What about patients who achieve sCR or are MRD negative after RVD/triple therapy-should they undergo frontline auto-HCT? The goal of front line auto-HCT is to deepen the response that is achieved post-induction therapy. If a patient achieves sCR or a much deeper response such as MRD negativity after triplet induction

Table 22.1 Induction regimens.

Author, year	Regimen	N	Median f/u (m)	Best response (%) after induction			Best response (%) after transplant 1			Best response (%) post-transplant			PFS
				≥PR	≥VGPR	CR/nCR	≥PR	≥VGPR	CR/nCR	≥PR	≥VGPR	CR/nCR	
Harousseau 2010	VD	223	31.2	79	38	15	80	54	35		68#	40#	36 m
	VAD	218		63	15	6	77	37	18		47#	23#	29.7 m
Rajkumar 2010	Rd	222	35.8	70	26	4							65% (2y)
	RD	223		81	33	5							63% (2y)
Rosinol 2012	TD	127	35.2	62	29	14			24				28.2 m
	VTD	130		85	60	35			46				56.2 m
Cavo 2010	TD	238	30.4	79	28	11	84	58	31	89#	74#	54#	56% (3y)
	VTD	236		93	62	31	93	79	52	96#	89#	71#	68% (3y)
Moreau 2011	VD	99	32	81	36	22	86	58	29				30 m
	vTD	100		88	49	31	89	74	61				26 m
Sonneveld 2012	PAD	413	41	78	42	11	88	62	31	90$	76$	49$	35 m
	VAD	414		54	14	5	75	36	15	83$	56$	34$	28 m
Moreau 2016	VTD	170		92.3	66.3	13							
	VCD	170		83.4	56.2	8.9							
Reeder 2009	VCD	33		96	71	46	100	74	70				
Richardson 2010	RVD	66	21	100	67	39							75% (1.5y)
Jakubowiak 2012	CRD	53	13	98	81	62							92% (2y)
Sonneveld 2015	CTD	91	23	90	68	25	96	76	33	96*	89*	58*	72% (3y)
Zimmerman 2015	CRD	62	9.7	98	78	24	100	97	69	100*	100*	100*	100% (1y)

Vd: bortezomib and dexamethasone, Rd: lenalidomide and dexamethasone, RD: lenalidomide and high-dose-dexamethasone, TD: thalidomide and dexamethasone, VTD: bortezomib, thalidomide, and dexamethasone, vTD: low dose bortezomib, thalidomide, and dexamethasone, PAD: bortezomib, adriamycin, and dexamethasone, VAD: vincristine, adriamycin, and dexamethasone, VCD: bortezomib, cyclophosphamide, and dexamethasone, CTD: carfilzomib, thalidomide, and dexamethasone, RVD: lenalidomide, bortezomib, and dexamethasone, CRD: carfilzomib, lenalidomide, and dexamethasone, f/u: follow up, PFS: progression free survival, PR: partial response, VGPR: very good partial response, CR: complete response, nCR: near complete response, m: months, y: years, * received consolidation, # received auto-HCT2, $ received maintenance.

therapy with RVD, the authors certainly favor consolidating the response with an auto-HCT. Based on the IFM phase 2 trial that has evaluated triplet RVD induction therapy followed by auto-HCT and lenalidomide maintenance, the 3-year PFS among the patients that achieved MRD negativity was 100% signifying the importance of achieving a deeper response. The usage of a combination induction approach followed by consolidation with front line auto-HCT delivers high quality deeper molecular responses and lengthier PFS supporting our initial treatment approach.

Similar results were reported from the IFM/DFCI trial, where early transplant conferred higher MRD negative rates, which translated to PFS benefit.

What is the role of chemotherapy induced mobilization?

Cyclophosphamide or chemotherapy based mobilization is useful when patients have received extensive number of cycles of induction prior to referral to a transplant center. Cyclophosphamide based mobilization also has the advantage of potentially shortening the number of days of collection due to a more rapid mobilization effect. However, the use of chemomobilization does carry with it the risk of complications during the period of aplasia such as bleeding or infections, though these events occur rarely. In general, the use of growth factor mobilization or growth factors + plerixafor have significantly reduced the need for chemomobilization. Patients who have received more than six cycles of lenalidomide based induction may be considered for chemotherapy based mobilization. However, the collection failure rate for patients who receive RVD based induction for four cycles followed by growth factor mobilization is very low suggesting that the use of chemotherapy is not needed for most patients who are referred early in their induction course for HPC collection.

Choice of conditioning

The standard approach for conditioning before auto-HCT in myeloma has traditionally been melphalan (Mel) 200 mg/m^2. In a randomized trial from the IFM, patients were randomized to receive either Mel 140 mg/m^2 + total body irradiation (TBI) or standard melphalan 200 mg/m^2. This was done based on the knowledge that plasma cell disorders appear to be exquisitely sensitive to radiation-based therapy, and was an attempt to enhance the efficacy of the transplant process. The significance of this trial was the realization that though PFS and OS were similar, the associated toxicity was much higher in the group that received TBI. As such, the conclusion from that study was that Mel 200 mg/m^2 was to remain the standard of care.

Is there anything better than Mel 200 mg/m^2?: There have been many trials suggesting the benefit of alternative conditioning regimens to improve upon this step of the HDT procedure that either include or do not include melphalan as part of the regimen. Additional agents studied in combination with melphalan include bortezomib, bendamustine, or intravenous busulfan.

A retrospective analysis compared outcomes for HDT treating either with Mel 200 mg/m^2 or busulfan/cyclophosphamide/etoposide (Bu/Cy/VP-16). Findings revealed no difference between the arms, but again raised concern for higher rates of toxicity for the polychemotherapy arm. A more recent analysis evaluated the benefit related to combining busulfan with melphalan (Bu/Mel) compared against Mel 200 mg/m^2 in a retrospective cohort of patients. In this trial, there was a higher incidence of toxicity associated with the use of busulfan (particularly VOD) but there was also a suggestion of improved PFS compared with Mel 200 mg/m^2. There was no difference in OS between the groups, leaving the final analysis to be that additional study is clearly needed before concluding adding additional chemotherapy to the Mel 200 mg/m^2 regimen is beneficial. Several trials compared various conditioning regimens to Mel 200 mg/m^2, as summarized in Table 22.2, but did not prove to be efficacious than Mel 200 mg/m^2.

The addition of bortezomib appears to add benefit

Along the same lines, two groups have worked on combining the proteasome inhibitor (PI) bortezomib with Mel 200 mg/m^2 as part of a conditioning strategy for transplant. In a phase 1 trial, Lonial et al. demonstrated that bortezomib could be safely combined with Mel 200 mg/m^2, and that when sequence of administration was considered (before Mel or after), the optimal sequence was a single dose after administration of Mel in order to optimize the potential synergy between the alkylating agent and the bortezomib. This was proven using marrow samples collected on each patient in the trial before and after transplant to assess for differences in plasma cell apoptosis. A parallel trial was conducted by the IFM evaluating the combination of bortezomib with melphalan, two doses before and after melphalan, and demonstrated that there was also a positive interaction when both agents are combined. Both trials suggested a higher post-transplant CR rate when bortezomib was added to the conditioning, and that additional trials are needed to further explore this approach.

Table 22.2 Studies with conditioning regimens for auto-HCT.

Author, year	N	Conditioning Regimen	Median f/u	Best response (%) after transplant			PFS (m)	OS (m)	Complications
				≥PR	≥VGPR	CR/nCR			
Moreau 2002	140	Mel 140 +TBI	20	89	55	29	21	43	↑ incidence of transfusion requirements, mucositis, TRM (3.6%), VOD (<1%)
	142	Mel 200		94	43	35	20.5	NR	Quicker engraftment, TRM (0%)
Fenk 2005	26	Idarabucin+ Cy+ Mel 200	51	85	50		20	46	↑ incidence of transfusion requirements, mucositis, TRM (20%)
	30	Mel 100 x 2		93	33		16	66	TRM (0%)
Vela-Ojeda 2007	28	BCNU+VP-16+ Mel 140 (PO)	34.2				25	36	TRM 14%, no significant differences in engraftment parameters or toxicity
	26	Mel 200 (IV)					38	86	TRM 11.5%
Lahuerta 2010	225	Busulfan + Mel 140	72	90		51	41	79	↑ incidence of TRM (8.4%), VOD (8%)
	542	Mel 200	47	92		53	31	71	TRM 3.5%, VOD (0.4%)
Benson 2007	62	BuCyVP-16		77		24	26.7	31.2	TRM (3.2%), no significant differences in engraftment parameters
	48	Mel 200		74		23	25	NR	TRM (0%)
Palumbo 2010	149	Mel 200 x 2	44.6	78.5	36.9	14.8	31.4	NR	TRM (3.1%), ↑ incidence of transfusion, antibiotic requirements, mucositis
	149	Mel 100 x 2		71.8	21.5	8.1	26.2	60	Similar rate of TRM (2.9%)
Lonial 2010	19	BTZ→Mel200		79	47	11		NR	↑ incidence of diarrhea, nausea, mucositis
	20	Mel200→BTZ		95	55	30		60	↑ incidence of febrile neutropenia
Sharma 2012	12	Mel 200+AA+ ATO	36	85	60	20	19.5	NR	no significant differences in engraftment parameters or toxicity
	9	Mel 200+AA+ ATO+ BTZ 1 mg/m²		90	60	10	17.2	NR	
	6	Mel 200+AA+ ATO+ BTZ 1.5 mg/m²		95	65	10	20.5	NR	

Mel: Melphalan, TBI: Total Body Irradiation, Cy: Cytoxan, BTZ: Bortezomib, AA: ascorbic acid, ATO: arsenic trioxide. PO: per os, IV: intravenous, f/u: follow up, m: months, NR: not reported, PR: partial response, VGPR: very good partial response, CR: complete response, nCR: near complete response, PFS: progression free survival, OS: overall survival, ↑: increase TRM: transplant-related mortality, VOD: veno-occlusive disease,

Consolidation therapy

Success with use of novel agents has been demonstrated in consolidation and maintenance regimens as well. As the goal of effective consolidation therapy is to enhance the responsiveness of disease while minimizing toxicity, use of novel agents in consolidation therapy has proven effective in several phase II/III trials. However, to date, these therapies have not been approved for use in the post-auto-HCT setting and thus need to be tailored on an individual patient basis.

Tandem auto-HCT as consolidation

Prior to the introduction of novel agents, tandem auto-HCT was found to be beneficial in patients who had insufficient responses to the initial transplant. This therapeutic option was initially reserved for patients who did not achieve at least VGPR after their first transplant. Now with novel therapy, tandem auto-HCT is reserved for specific patient groups. An analysis of several phase 3 studies looked at 606 patients following single (254 patients) or double (352 patients) auto-HCT with prior bortezomib induction and divided them into groups based on specific high-risk prognosticators, namely International Staging System (ISS) stage 3, high-risk cytogenetics, and failure to achieve CR post-induction. The conclusion was that in patients with more than two poor prognosticators, there was improved PFS and OS with tandem auto-HCT.

A randomized phase 3 study conducted by Palumbo et al. compared tandem auto-HCT versus consolidation therapy with six cycles of lenalidomide, melphalan, and prednisone following induction with Rd. An improved PFS was seen in the tandem auto-HCT arm demonstrating the continued important role auto-HCT plays in the treatment of myeloma.

The EMN02/H095 MM trial incorporated the question of upfront-single versus double auto-HCT in their phase 3 trial. In this trial, 3 year PFS was 73.6 versus 62.2%; p = 0.05 favoring the double auto-HCT. Patients with high risk cytogenetics seemed to benefit the most (3 year PFS: 64.9 vs 41.4%; p = 0.046). Shorter follow up and suboptimal induction regimen in this trial warrants that no formal conclusions can be drawn, particularly when the same question from the phase III staMINA trial from

the BMT CTN did not confer any additional benefit to double auto-HCT compared to a single auto-HCT followed by maintenance.

Combination of novel agents in consolidation after auto-HCT

There are many studies to date that demonstrated better depth of response with novel therapy-based consolidation regimens. A significant randomized phase 3 trial conducted by the International Myeloma Group compared VTD versus TD as both induction and maintenance regimens before and after auto-HCT, and found superior CR rates (62 vs 45%) and longer 3-year PFS (68 vs 56%) in the VTD group. The EMN02/H095 MM trial in their second randomization addressed the role of RVD consolidation for two cycles followed by maintenance. PFS was prolonged in patients randomized to VRD, but limited to patients with standard risk cytogenetics However, consolidation therapy with RVD in the phase III staMINA trial from the BMT CTN did not confer benefit compared to a single auto-HCT followed by maintenance.

Choice of maintenance therapy

Unlike with consolidation therapy, maintenance therapy is given on a long-term basis with the goal of prolonging response with minimal toxicities. The first agent studied for use as maintenance therapy following auto-HCT was Thalidomide. Six randomized control studies demonstrated improved PFS, improved response rate and half of the studies showed improved OS. However, drawbacks to thalidomide as long-term maintenance therapy include toxicities such as peripheral neuropathy as well as observed resistance in patients with high-risk cytogenetics. In a meta-analysis of six randomized control studies involving 2786 patients, Kagoya et al. found that though patients treated with thalidomide had increased PFS and mildly improved OS, there were was also increased risk of venous thrombosis and peripheral neuropathy compared with controls.

The current best option for maintenance therapy is lenalidomide. There are three large studies that have looked at the efficacy of lenalidomide post-transplant. In a randomized placebo-controlled study done for the IFM,

614 patients aged less than 65 years were randomized to either a placebo group or to receive daily lenalidomide as maintenance following either single or tandem transplantation. Patients on lenalidomide maintenance therapy had an improved PFS of 46 months versus 24 months in the placebo group with similar rates of grade III and IV peripheral neuropathy among both groups. Another similar randomized study conducted by the CALGB assigned 460 patients one hundred days post-auto-HCT to either a placebo or lenalidomide arm until disease progression. Findings at a median follow up of 65 months included an improved OS (NR vs 76 months, p = 0.001)) as well as prolonged time to progression (TTP) (53 months in lenalidomide group vs 26 months in the placebo group). Adversely, there was found to be an increased risk of grade 3 and 4 hematologic AEs and grade 3 non-hematologic AEs, as well as increased risk of secondary primary malignancies (11 vs 4%). However, the side effects were considered manageable with less than 30% of patients needing to discontinue therapy due to inability to tolerate. The third major study was conducted by the GIMEMA group, in which patients underwent two randomizations. The first was to either receive six cycles of lenalidomide, melphalan and prednisone after induction, or to tandem transplant. Patients were then again randomized to lenalidomide maintenance versus placebo. Again, PFS was improved on lenalidomide maintenance (41.9 vs 21.6 months) though no significant improvement was seen in 3-year OS.

Bortezomib has also been studied as maintenance therapy, notably in two phase 3 studies. Sonneveld et al. conducted a study first randomizing patients to either receive induction with bortezomib-doxorubicin-dexamethasone or vincristine-doxorubicin-dexamethasone, and then randomized patients post-transplant to receive maintenance therapy with either thalidomide versus Intravenous (now preferred route of administration is subcutaneous) bortezomib, respectively. Maintenance was continued for 2 years post-auto-HCT. PFS and OS were statistically improved in the bortezomib arm with a median follow up of 74 months. In addition, toxicities were noted to be manageable though 35% of patients in that arm did discontinue or require dose reduction.

In another large randomized phase 3 study conducted by the Spanish Myeloma Group, in patients again with differing induction regimens, maintenance was compared between bortezomib-thalidomide (VT) versus interferon versus thalidomide alone. Though no difference in OS was found, there was significant increase in PFS in the VT arm.

Associated toxicities and effect on quality of life (QoL) is an important consideration as well when deciding on maintenance therapy. Only a few studies to date have specifically analyzed this effect. One such study assessed QoL with Td following auto-HCT, and found that patients reported worse QoL citing decreased cognitive functioning, difficulty with breathing, constipation, dry mouth, and balance issues. More study in this area is needed with currently employed maintenance therapies. Selected maintenance studies are summarized in Table 22.3.

PRACTICE POINTS

Nearly all studies have shown a benefit for maintenance therapy in terms of PFS, and the CALGB has shown a benefit for OS that continues to hold up with longer follow up. The duration of PFS for low dose maintenance appears to be longer than the salvage duration of PFS for Len/dex suggesting a longer benefit for maintenance. The use of bortezomib maintenance appears to offer benefits for the t(4;14) patients, and for high-risk patients, the use of RVD maintenance appears to offer benefit in PFS and OS.

Age as a factor for auto-HCT: What is the upper limit?

Initial evaluation for transplantation involves determination of eligibility and ability to tolerate HDT and auto-HCT. It is important to note that eligibility cannot focus on age alone. The use of HDT and auto-HCT has been generally considered for patients who are young and fit, and as such, there have been artificial age considerations for suitability for HDT and auto-HCT. In Europe, 65 years old is generally accepted as the cut off for transplant eligibility. In the US, there has been a shift toward incorporating performance status (PS) and assessment of comorbidities more so than age alone when considering the use of HDT and auto-HCT. In fact, Medicare will cover autologous transplant for a myeloma patient up to age 78 pending overall health. Given the growing elderly population in the US and Europe, the fact that this cohort is underrepresented and understudied in major clinical trials is even more concerning. Charleston et al have worked to develop a frailty score, and method of estimating risk of death from comorbid disease in longitudinal studies. This could be of use moving forward with attempts to better study tolerability of myeloma therapies and auto-HCT. It is important to take into account overall health, as well as further define and study appropriate dose-reductions needed in the geriatric population.

There are a number of different series of patient that have been reported above age 65 by US investigators that demonstrate the benefit for HDT in older patient. One such study is a recently published analysis from the

Table 22.3 Studies with different maintenance regimens after auto-HCT.

Author, year	N	Maintenance regimen	Median f/u (m)	Best response (%) on maintenance			PFS (m)	OS (m)	SPM (%)
				≥PR (%)	≥VGPR(%)	≥CR (%)			
Barlogie 2006	323	Thalidomide	42			62	56% (5y)	65%	NR
	323	Observation				43	44% (5y)	65%	NR
Attal 2006	200	Observation	39	92	55		38% (3y)	77% (4y)	NR
	196	Pamidronate		94	57		39% (3y)	74% (4y)	NR
	201	Thalidomide and pamidronate		97	67		51% (3y)	87% (4y)	NR
Lokhorst 2010	268	Alpha-interferon	52	79	54	23	25	60	NR
	268	Thalidomide		88	66	31	34	73	NR
Spencer 2009	129	Prednisolone	36		44		23% (3y)	75% (3y)	NR
	114	Thalidomide and prednisolone			65		42% (3y)	86% (3y)	NR
Maiolino 2012	52	Dexamethasone	27		48		19	70% (2y)	NR
	56	Thalidomide and dexamethasone			50		36	85% (2y)	NR
McCarthy 2012	231	Lenalidomide	65				53	NR	11
	229	Observation					26	76	4
Attal 2012	307	Lenalidomide	67	99	84	29	46	82	9.7
	307	Observation		99	76	27	24	81	5.9
Palumbo 2014	126	Lenalidomide	51.2	86.2	62.1	34.5	41.9	88% (3y)	4.3
	125	Observation		82.6	52.2	28.7	21.6	79.2% (3y)	4.3
Sonneveld 2012	413	Bortezomib	41	90	76	49	35	61% (5y)	NR
	414	Thalidomide		83	56	34	28	55% (5y)	NR
Rosinol 2012	89	Bortezomib and thalidomide	34.9			70	PFS benefit for VT arm (p<0.0009)	OS not different	NR
	87	Thalidomide				66			NR
	90	Alpha-interferon				68			NR
Nooka 2014	45	Lenalidomide, bortezomib, and dexamethasone (RVD)	26	100	96	51	32	93% (3y)	NR

f/u: follow up, m: months, y: years, VT: bortezomib and thalidomide, NR: not reported, PR: partial response, VGPR: very good partial response, CR: complete response, nCR: near complete response, PFS: progression free survival, SPM: second primary malignancy.

CIBMTR that suggests that the benefit for HDT is the same in patients older than 65 as it is for younger patients. Hailemichael et al reviewed outcomes for patients with MM who were older than age 65 and older than age 70, and demonstrated that in suitable patients with good PS, outcomes for these well-chosen patients was superior to that of similarly matched SEER patients. This suggests that while not all elderly patients may be suitable candidates, age alone is not sufficient to exclude patients at the outset. In an older paper from Badros and colleagues at the University of Arkansas, it is also clear that in order to reduce the toxicity of older patients with myeloma, lower doses of melphalan should be used. In this case, they identified that for patients older than 70, Mel 140 mg/m^2 should be the dose used for transplant, similar to what is recommended for patients with severe renal dysfunction. Trials evaluating transplant outcomes by age groups are summarized in Table 22.4.

PRACTICE POINTS

Data series from many groups have now shown that the benefit of HDT is not limited to patients younger than age 65. Benefit is clear for well selected older patients up to age 78. Reduced dose melphalan (Mel 140 mg/m^2) represents a standard for patients older than 70, and mitigates potential toxicity for these patients while preserving benefit.

Allogeneic HCT

For newly diagnosed myeloma, the benefit for early allogeneic transplant continues to evolve (see Chapter 23 by Hari). Though randomized clinical trials have failed to demonstrate benefit for standard or high-risk patients to date, there does continue to be interest in pursuing this course for younger patients. The role of allogeneic hematopoietic cell transplant (allo-HCT) as salvage therapy for relapsed or refractory myeloma remains unclear. The limitations on the benefit for allogeneic transplant are related in part to significant improvements in outcomes for patients with relapsed MM through the availability of new drugs. This is coupled with increased treatment related mortality associated with the older age of the average MM patient, limiting the overall efficacy and safety of the allogeneic transplant approach. When evaluated by genetics at relapse, patients with standard risk myeloma can have a very long median OS (5–7 years) while those with poor risk genetics likely have a disease biology that is too proliferative to allow for impactful graft versus tumor effect to take hold. Though a small proportion of patients may derive long-term benefit, the mortality and morbidity in form of acute/chronic graft-versus-host disease associated with allo-HCT

strongly outweighs the benefits as viewed by multiple published series to date. The probability of benefit from an allo-HCT in a patient with aggressive relapse or among patients with high-risk myeloma also remains unproven. Among high-risk patients who achieve a good quality response with salvage therapy, allo-HCT may be considered, although with high risks of transplant-related mortality, preferably in the setting of a clinical trial and employing newer agents like bortezomib for graft modulation post-transplant.

PRACTICE POINTS

The use of allogeneic transplant for myeloma has demonstrated a clear graft vs tumor effect, however the price for the benefit remains quite high. Randomized clinical trials have failed to demonstrate a benefit for allo- versus tandem auto-HCT even among high-risk myeloma patients. Currently the use of allogeneic transplant is limited to younger patients with suitable donors, in the context of well-designed clinical trials.

Cellular therapy

Beyond the use of allogeneic transplant, other cellular based treatments are currently in development for myeloma as well. These include the use of methods to augment or give targeted cellular infusions, the use of CAR T-cells, as well as dendritic cell based vaccines.

NK-cells

Natural Killer (NK)-cells are members of the innate immune system that play a key role in defense against viruses and tumors. Though their role is myeloma is not fully understood, they have been shown to play a key role in myeloma cell neutralization predominantly through two receptors: the natural cytotoxicity receptor (NCR) and NK receptor member D of the lectin-like receptor family (NKG2D). Due to depression of NK activity in advanced myeloma, enhancement of NK efficacy could potentially improve anti-myeloma activity and has led to ongoing trials exploring the utility of NK-cell-based therapy in myeloma. The use of NK based cellular infusions has been pioneered in the context of HLA-haploidentical transplantation, and in the myeloma world, there are groups evaluating the use of NK-cell infusions as part of a therapeutic treatment for patients also receiving bortezomib-based salvage therapy (ClinicalTrial.gov # NCT01313897).

Additional work is being done evaluating the use of antibodies directed at KIR (Killer cell immunoglobulin-like receptor) on NK-cells with the idea of trying to induce anti-tumor activity among endogenous NK-cells.

Table 22.4 Studies with auto-HCT in older patients with MM.

Author, year	N	Age groups (y)	Response (%) prior to transplant			Melphalan dosing§			PFS (m)	p-value	OS	p-value	NRM
			≥PR (%)	≥VGPR (%)	≥CR (%)	<140	140–180	≥180					
Sharma 2014	5818	18–59	90	42	12	2%	6%	86%	42% (3y)	NS	78 (3y)	<0.001	3% (2y)
	4666	60–69	91	44	14	3%	12%	80%	38% (3y)		75 (3y)		2% (2y)
	946	≥70	90	41	14	5%	37%	51%	33% (3y)		72 (3y)		0% (2y)
Auner 2015	1729	<40	73								61.5 (5y)*		
	8696	40–49	84.8								62.8 (5y)		
	21,791	50–59	85.4								59.9 (5y)		
	12,989	60–64	86.7								58.8 (5y)		
	7131	65–69	85								53.2 (5y)		
	1339	≥70	82.5								49.7 (5y)		
Qazilbash 2007	26	≥70				0%	4%	96%	39% (3y)		65 (3y)		
Hailemichael 2012	734	<65									88 m		
	114	65–69									62 m		
	45	70–74									56 m		
	8	≥75									42 m		
Bashir 2012	84	≥70	82	20		0%	10%	90%	27% (5y)		67 (5y)		

* 5y survival, 2006–2010, § expressed as mg/m², f/u: follow up, m: months, y: years, PR: partial response, VGPR: very good partial response, CR: complete response, PFS: progression free survival, OS: overall survival, NRM: non-relapse mortality.

Table 22.5 Who, when, and how of auto-HCT for MM. Authors' practice.

A. PATIENT FACTORS	**Age of patient:** • Age is becoming a lesser important determinant of auto-HCT eligibility, mainly due to the proven benefit of auto-HCT among elderly and decreased TRM among this age group. • We consider this approach safe and suitable for most patients up to age 78. **Performance Status and Comorbidities:** • Using Charleston's frailty score, a method of estimating risk of death from comorbid disease will help to assess tolerability of auto-HCT among geriatric population. • We recommend that overall health should be taken into consideration while assessing auto-HCT eligibility.
B. DISEASE FACTORS:	**Newly diagnosed myeloma:** • For standard risk myeloma patients, though the benefit of auto-HCT is proven, the timing of auto-HCT is unclear. In the absence of any contraindications, we favor early auto-HCT, following the initial induction therapy. • For, high-risk myeloma patients with del 1p, del 17p, t(4;14), t(14:16), t(14;20) or plasma cell leukemia, we favor an early auto-HCT followed by intense maintenance therapy. • Use of allogeneic transplant is limited to younger high-risk patients with suitable donors, only in the context of well-designed clinical trials. **Salvage transplant for myeloma:** • Though data limited, salvage auto-HCT benefits certain patients that are chemo sensitive. • Younger, fit patients that have previously derived prolonged benefit from an auto-HCT, or those that could not receive an upfront auto-HCT may be considered for salvage auto-HCT at relapse. • Early relapses after an auto-HCT may not benefit from a salvage auto-HCT (lesser benefit among patients that received <2 year PFS benefit with no maintenance and <3 year PFS benefit while on maintenance after auto-HCT) **Tandem transplants for myeloma:** • While routine use of tandem transplants is discouraged, there may be a role for tandem transplants among patients that have achieved <PR post auto-HCT
C. DONOR EVALUATION:	**Disease related assessments:** • Comprehensive disease evaluation with serum and urine paraprotein evaluations, imaging, and bone marrow biopsy are required prior to transplant. **Patient related assessments:** • Other patient related assessments at a minimum should include evaluating cardiac and pulmonary functions, infectious disease markers prior to proceeding with autologous transplant.
D. CONDITIONING THERAPY:	**Younger transplant-eligible patients:** • Melphalan 200 mg/m² is the recommended conditioning regimen **For selected patients:** • For patients ≥70 years old, patients with creatinine clearance ≤40 ml/min, a dose reduction of 1/3rd dose to 140 mg/m² is recommended.
E. POST AUTO-HCT THERAPY:	**High-risk patients:** • The use of bortezomib maintenance offers benefit for the t(4;14) patients, and the use of RVD maintenance appears to benefit all high-risk patients. **Standard risk patients:** • Almost all studies evaluating the benefit of maintenance have shown a benefit in terms of PFS, CALGB study evaluating lenalidomide maintenance has shown a benefit for OS. • Increased risk of secondary primary malignancies observed with lenalidomide maintenance should be discussed with patients.

Auto-HCT: autologous hematopoietic cell transplant, PS: performance status, PR: partial response, PFS: progression free survival, OS; overall survival, RVD: lenalidomide, bortezomib, and dexamethasone

In myeloma patients, tumor cells upregulate the expression of ligands to the inhibitory NK-cell KIR receptor. Therefore, interfering with the KIR-ligand interaction and subsequent inhibitory signaling pathways can lead to enhanced NK-cell cytotoxicity against myeloma cells. Benson et al. conducted a study assessing the efficacy of IPH2101, a human IgG4 mAb against KIR2DL-1, KIR2DL-2, and KIR-2DL3 in conjunction with lenalidomide. Lenalidomide specifically has been shown to enhance NK-cell proliferation and activity against malignant cells. Preclinical data suggests that the use of an antibody that blocks KIR-ligand interaction combined with lenalidomide is able to induce significant response in murine models, though early clinical trials have to date failed to demonstrate significant anti-tumor activity as yet.

CAR T-cells

The more recent excitement over the use of chimeric antigen receptor on T-cells (CAR T-cells) based technology has also been investigated in the context of myeloma. T-cells target malignant cells through various signaling pathways, one of which being the binding of the T-cell receptor (TCR) with the Major Histocompatibility Complex (MHC) on the tumor cell. The tumor cell's means of evading detection is via mutations in the MHC. However, CAR T-cells have been genetically modified to have a different extracellular antigen binding site known as scFv, a single chain antibody, which allows T-cells to identify malignant cells without the use of the MHC. To date, most studies have been done showing success with targeting CD-19 positive B-cell malignancies similar to what has been so successful for ALL, though the data for myeloma remains very limited. Additional MM surface antigens that are being studied include CS1, BCMA (B-cell maturation antigen), CD38, CD56, and CD74. A downside to some of these targets is high expression in non-myeloma cells. Approaches using CS1 and BCMA may offer additional clinical benefits as their expression on myeloma cells is significantly higher than what is seen with these other surface proteins, rendering them potentially a better overall target with less cytotoxicity when utilizing this approach in the setting of myeloma.

Dendritic cell vaccines

Finally, the use of cellular therapy through dendritic cell vaccines is yet another method for cellular therapy that is currently being tested in relapsed and smoldering myeloma. Tumor immunotherapy is a promising area in myeloma research and thus vaccines aimed at developing myeloma-specific immunity have become a major area of focus. Currently there are several groups that are working on either whole cell, or antigen specific dendritic cell vaccines as a method by which innate immunity can be enhanced for an anti-tumor effect. Currently, these approaches are in phase I and combination studies to date with only minimal clinical response to yet be demonstrated.

Conclusion

Summary of our recommendations are included in Table 22.5. Additional methods to enhance the benefit associated with autologous transplant include more attention on the induction, consolidation, and maintenance phases to try and achieve low levels or MRD, which will be associated with a higher rate of "cured" patients. The use of allogeneic transplant remains an experimental approach for most patients, and should be conducted in the context of well-designed clinical trials. Finally, the use of cellular therapies represents an important step forward in the future, whether they are related to cellular based treatments (NK-cell based) or CAR T-cell based, or dendritic vaccines, they represent the next frontier of potential ways to enhance innate immunity in the hopes of long-term disease control.

Selected reading

1. Moreau, P., Hulin, C., Macro, M., et al., VTD is superior to VCD prior to intensive therapy in multiple myeloma: results of the prospective IFM2013-04 trial. *Blood*, 2016. **127**(21):p. 2569–2574.
2. Gay, F., Oliva, S., Petrucci, M.T., et al., Chemotherapy plus lenalidomide versus autologous transplantation, followed by lenalidomide plus prednisone versus lenalidomide maintenance, in patients with multiple myeloma: a randomised, multicentre, phase 3 trial. *Lancet Oncol*, 2015. **16**(16):p. 1617–1629.
3. Attal, M., Lauwers-Cances, V., Hulin, C. et al., Autologous transplantation for multiple myeloma in the era of new drugs: A phase III study of the Intergroupe Francophone Du Myeloma (IFM/DFCI 2009 Trial). *Blood*, 2015. **126**(23):p. 391.
4. Cavo, M., Beksac, M., Dimopoulos, M.A., et al., Intensification Therapy with bortezomib-melphalan-prednisone versus autologous stem cell transplantation for newly diagnosed multiple myeloma: An Intergroup, Multicenter, Phase III study of the European Myeloma Network (EMN02/HO95 MM Trial). *Blood*, 2016. **128**(22): p. 673.
5. Roussel, M., Lauwers-Cances, V., Robillard, N., et al., Frontline transplantation program with lenalidomide, bortezomib, and dexamethasone combination as induction and consolidation followed by lenalidomide maintenance in patients with multiple myeloma: A phase II study by the Intergroupe Francophone du Myélome. *Journal of Clinical Oncology*, 2014. **32**(25): p. 2712–2717.
6. Moreau, P., Facon, T., Attal, M., et al., Comparison of 200 mg/m(2) melphalan and 8 Gy total body irradiation plus 140 mg/m(2) melphalan as conditioning regimens for peripheral blood stem cell transplantation in patients with newly diagnosed multiple myeloma: final analysis of the Intergroupe Francophone du Myeloma 9502 randomized trial. *Blood*, 2002. **99**(3): p. 731–735.
7. Moreau, P., Attal, M. and Facon, T., Frontline therapy of multiple myeloma. *Blood*, 2015. **125**(20): p. 3076–3084.
8. Cavo, M., Salwender, H., Rosinol, L., Moreau, P., Petrucci, M.T., Blau, I.W., et al, Double vs single autologous stem cell transplantation after bortezomib-based induction regimens for multiple myeloma; an integrated analysis of patient-level data from Phase European III Studies. *ASH Annual Meeting Abstracts*, 2013: p. 767.
9. Palumbo, A., Cavallo, F., Gay, F., et al., Autologous transplantation and maintenance therapy in multiple myeloma. *N Engl J Med*, 2014. **371**(10): p. 895–905.
10. Sonneveld, P., Beksac, M., van der Holt, B., et al., Consolidation followed by maintenance therapy versus maintenance alone in newly diagnosed, transplant eligible patients with multiple myeloma (MM): A randomized

phase 3 study of the European Myeloma Network (EMN02/HO95 MM Trial). *Blood*, 2016. **128**(22): p. 242.

11. Attal, M., Lauwers-Cances, V., Marit, G., et al., Lenalidomide maintenance after stem-cell transplantation for multiple myeloma. *N Engl J Med*, 2012. **366**(19): p. 1782–1791.

12. McCarthy, P.L., Owzar, K., Hofmeister, C.C., et al., Lenalidomide after stem-cell transplantation for multiple myeloma. *N Engl J Med*, 2012. **366**(19): p. 1770–1781.

13. Benson, D.M., Jr., Hofmeister, C.C., Padmanabhan, S., et al., A phase 1 trial of the anti-KIR antibody IPH2101 in patients with relapsed/refractory multiple myeloma. *Blood*, 2012. **120**(22): p. 4324–4333.

14. Ayed, A.O., Chang, L.J. and Moreb, J.S. Immunotherapy for multiple myeloma: Current status and future directions. *Crit Rev Oncol Hematol*, 2015. **96**(3): p. 399–412.

15. Sharma, M., Khan, H., THrall, P.F., et al., A randomized phase 2 trial of a preparative regimen of bortezomib, high-dose melphalan, arsenic trioxide, and ascorbic acid. *Cancer*, 2012. **118**(9): p. 2507–2515.

16. Bashir, Q., Shah, N., Parmar, S., et al., Feasibility of autologous hematopoietic stem cell transplant in patients aged >/=70 years with multiple myeloma. *Leuk Lymphoma*, 2012. **53**(1): p. 118–122.

CHAPTER 23

Allogeneic hematopoietic transplant in multiple myeloma

Parameswaran Hari and Binod Dhakal

Medical College of Wisconsin, Milwaukee, WI, USA

Introduction

Due to our inability to cure MM with current therapies, including autologous transplant (auto-HCT), there has been a sustained interest in allo-HCT since this technique uses a myeloma free donor cell graft and allows a donor driven, immune mediated graft-versus-MM effect. Based on reporting to the Center for International Blood and Marrow Transplant Research (CIBMTR), fewer than 200 patients per year in the US undergo an allo-HCT for MM.

Interest in allo-HCT for MM is driven by:

1 The use of a myeloma free donor cell graft.
2 Evidence of donor driven, immune mediated graft-versus-MM effect.
3 The inability to cure myeloma with autologous transplant and non-transplant therapies.

Allogeneic transplant in MM: How did we get here?

Allo-HCT preceded by classic myeloablative conditioning as practiced in the 1990s was associated with unacceptable treatment related mortality (TRM) of 40–60%. The allo-HCT arm of the US Intergroup S9321 study was terminated after an early TRM of 53% was observed. Notably allo-HCT survivors in this study demonstrated a plateau survival after year 2 with no late relapse events indicating a likely cure.

Non-myeloablative and reduced intensity conditioning (NST/RIC) approaches in the 2000s a major practice change. Such lower intensity conditioning led to:

1 Reduction in the use of myeloablative conditioning and lower TRM.
2 Expanded allo-HCT eligibility with older patients considered for transplant.

3 increasing numbers of allo-HCT performed after auto-HCT in a tandem auto-allo-HCT fashion (including several clinical trials).

However, retrospective data comparisons suggest that the decline in TRM was negated by an increase in relapse risk in later years. Several phase II studies reported a strategy of an initial auto-HCT followed (usually 3–6 months later) by lower intensity allo-HCT using NST/RIC. The rationale was to uncouple myeloablation (achieved by the auto-HCT) from the immune mediated graft-versus-MM benefits of the allo-HCT approach. Excellent short term (24 month) outcomes could be achieved with TRM ranging from 11% (for related donor grafts) to 26% (for unrelated donor grafts). Randomized studies were performed testing this tandem auto-followed by allo-HCT strategy against tandem auto-HCT.

What are the randomized data regarding the role of upfront allo-HCT in MM?

Modern randomized trials (summarized in Table 23.1) have evaluated tandem auto-allo-HCT approach versus tandem auto-HCT in the upfront transplant setting in newly diagnosed patients after induction. The results have been discordant with two published studies indicating a survival benefit for the allogeneic approach while the largest study showed no benefit in progression free or overall survival. Studies restricting eligibility to higher-risk patients (variably defined) and comparing the approaches have also been reported with discordant results. Knop et al. indicate a PFS benefit for the allo-HCT arm and a survival benefit for those with 17p deletion. However, two other studies did not indicate survival benefit.

Clinical Manual of Blood and Bone Marrow Transplantation, First Edition. Edited by Syed A. Abutalib and Parameswaran Hari.
© 2017 John Wiley & Sons Ltd. Published 2017 by John Wiley & Sons Ltd.

Table 23.1 Allogeneic hematopoietic cell transplantation in multiple myeloma with reduced intensity/non-myeloablative conditioning-upfront setting.

Reference	N total / N allo	Trial Setting	Conditioning	cGvHD allo-HCT (%)	TRM (%)	OS	PFS	Conclusion
Bruno et al., 2007	245/58	Post-induction biological assignment based on sibling match donor	MEL ASCT followed by TBI 2 Gy vs MEL doses 100–200 mg/m²	32	10	Median 80 vs 54 months (p = 0.01)	Median 35 vs 29 months (p = 0.02)	Clear benefit for allotransplant in intention to treat donor versus no-donor analysis.
Garban et al., 2006/IFM 9903–04	284/65	Parallel prospective studies limited to high-risk disease	MEL 200 ASCT followed by FLU-BU + ATG allotransplant vs MEL 200 ASCT	42	11	Median 34 vs 48 months (p = 0.07)	Median 19 vs 22 months (p = 0.58)	30% did not complete allotransplant. No benefit to allotransplant in this study.
Rosinol et al., 2008	110/25	Limited to patients not in CR after a first ASCT	FLU-MEL allotransplant vs ASCT	66	16	Median NR vs 58 months (p = 0.9)	Median 20 vs 26 months (p = 0.4)	Higher CR rate after allotransplant but no survival benefit.
Knop et al., 2008	199/126	Limited to patients with 13q- by FISH, unrelated donor grafts in 60%	MEL 200 ASCT followed by FLU-MEL vs MEL 200 ASCT	N/R	12	Median NR @ 49 months	Median 34.5 vs 22 months (p = 0.005)	Largest trial in high-risk patients and with unrelated donors. De117p subgroup with OS benefit.
Garton et al., 2013/EBMT-NMAM	357/108	Post-induction biological assignment based on sibling match donor	MEL 200 ASCT followed by FLU–TBI 2 Gy vs MEL 200 ASCT	54	13	8-y OS 49% vs 39 % (p = 0.03)	8-y PFS 22% vs 12% (p = 0.02)	Allotransplant with lower risk of relapse and improved PFS. Benefit for higher-risk del 13 subset.
Krishnan et al., 2011/BMT CTN 0102	710/226	Post-induction biologic assignment based on matched sibling donor	MEL 200 ASCT followed by TBI 2 Gy allotransplant vs MEL 200 ASCT	54	11	3-y OS 77% vs 80%	3-y PFS 43% vs 46%	No benefit to allotransplant in this study.
Lokhorst et al., 2012/HOVON 54	Not strictly a randomized study – donor vs no-donor analysis of HOVON 50		MEL 200 ASCT followed by TBI 2 Gy allo-HCT	64	16	6-y OS 55% in both groups	6-y PFS 28% (donor group) vs 22% (no-donor group)	No benefit to having a related donor but allotransplant was by center preference. Relapse lower for those with donors.

MEL – Melphalan, Flu – Fludarabine, BU-Busulfan, Gy – Gray, TBI – Total body irradiation, ATG – Anti-thymocyte globulin, N/R – not reported

Meta analyses of the published allo-HCT versus auto-HCT studies suggest:

1 CR rates are higher for allo-HCT.
2 Consistent survival benefit cannot be demonstrated.
3 Allo-HCT provides superior anti-relapse potential compared with auto-HCT.
4 TRM rates are higher after allo-HCT.

In addition, the long term (8-year follow up) results of the EBMT-NMAM study have indicated that patients who relapsed/progressed following allo-HCT had a longer OS than those who relapsed after tandem auto-HCT. The graft-versus-MM effect is thought to have played a major role in this phenomenon.

In the absence of a clear-cut survival advantage across studies and with recent improvements in induction and maintenance therapy, enthusiasm for allo-HCT in MM waned. Given results from European studies, investigators are pursuing allo-HCT based approaches in younger patients with high-risk MM where the benefits of novel therapy are modest. In order to improve the risk benefit ratio of allo-HCT, it is instructive to analyze the reasons for the disparate results obtained in randomized studies.

Why is there discrepancy between randomized study results?

The discordant outcomes are likely due to variations in:
1 conditioning regimens employed (TBI 2 Gy vs fluodarabine – Busulfan/Melphalan)
2 patient selection
3 MM risk profile definition (modern definitions of risk not used)
4 length of follow up (shorter for the negative BMT CTN study)
5 use of agents such as ATG (antithymocyte globulin) in conditioning that could have reduced the potential for graft-versus-MM effect.

Graft-versus-MM effect: Does it exist?

Several lines of evidence have been presented for a graft-versus-MM effect:
1 Myeloma (idiotype) specific CD4 T-cell response could be transferred from an immunized marrow donor to patients in early studies.
2 DLI (donor lymphocyte infusions) in patients with residual or progressive MM after allo-HCT can lead to responses. Although the durability of responses after DLI is modest, the occurrence of GvHD (acute or chronic) after DLI seems to be the most powerful predictor of a response.
3 The prospective BMT CTN 0102 study and a retrospective CIBMTR study also found that the occurrence of chronic GvHD after allo-HCT correlated with freedom from progressive MM.
4 *In vitro* or *in vivo* T-cell depletion has been associated with higher relapse rates and the need for DLI after allo-HCT in MM.

Selection of patients for allo-HCT – Defining risk

The term "ultra-high risk" MM is used to characterize patients who by baseline risk stratification have an estimated median survival of 24 months or less. This subgroup includes those presenting with International Stage (ISS) stage 3 disease and with specific genetic abnormalities such as deletion 17p, immunoglobulin-heavy chain gene translocations t(4;14) or t(14;16) and chromosome 1q21 amplification (>3 copies). A sub-analysis of the HOVON-65-GMMG-HD4 study identified a high-risk subgroup (comprising approximately 18% of patients) characterized by the presence of del(17p13)/t(4;14)/1q21 (>3 copies) and a high ISS score of II or III. Median PFS for this group was only 18.7 months. The outcomes for these patients remain poor despite the best available alternative therapies. Those relapsing early (within 12–18 months from transplant) after auto-HCT represent a group with an expected survival of <12 months from relapse. Such patients with poor prognosis may be considered for allo-HCT despite the risk of higher TRM and GvHD.

Deciding on allo-HCT for the high-risk MM patient in practice

High-risk MM patients may acquire new clonal abnormalities and present with aggressive rapidly growing relapses and sometimes secondary plasma cell leukemia. An aggressive approach to therapy including allo-HCT with the intent to produce a deep CR and prevent further relapse is warranted in these patients. In the absence of an effective established standard of care, these patients should be enrolled in allo-HCT clinical trials whenever possible.

Does allo-HCT benefit high-risk patients or after relapse?

Knop et al. presented the results of a study restricted to MM patients with del13q by FISH. After initial auto-HCT, patients received either allo-HCT from HLA matched related or unrelated donors following fludarabine and melphalan conditioning versus another melphalan based auto-HCT. At 49 months of follow up, PFS was superior for the allo-HCT group and in the highest risk subgroup with additional del17p abnormality, OS and PFS were superior for the allo-HCT cohort. In an update of the European Group for Blood and Marrow Transplantation (EBMT-NMAM) study, at a median follow up of 96 months, 21% of patients with the higher-risk del 13 abnormality receiving tandem auto-allo-HCT were progression free versus 5% in the tandem AHCT group.

Patriarca et al. reported a donor versus no-donor analysis of consecutive patients who had relapses after auto-HCT and then were considered for allo-HCT with RIC. At 2 years, TRM was high at 22% in the donor group, while PFS was 42% for the donor group versus 18% in the no-donor group (p < 0.001). Karyotype and chemosensitivity to salvage were associated with survival.

> **PRACTICE POINT**
>
> In patients with ultra-high-risk MM, allo-HCT should be one of the considerations ideally in the setting of a clinical trial.
>
> The authors offer allo-HCT either on a clinical trial or as standard of care to younger eligible patients with well-defined high-risk features (Table 23.2). This philosophy is based on the proven benefit of allo-HCT in multiple randomized trials as the best anti-relapse strategy and also with the expectation that with careful patient selection TRM can be reduced significantly. The benefits of a prolonged PFS after allo-HCT in patients with high-risk disease while exciting, may still be enhanced by maintenance strategies (see later). The risks associated with the procedure in terms of TRM and GvHD have to be acknowledged.

Table 23.2 Who, when, and how of allogeneic HCT for MM.

Authors' practice

A. PATIENT FACTORS:

Age:
Approximately 15% of patients with MM are <55 years old. Allo-HCT is an option in these patients:

Performance Status (PS) and Comorbidity:
Allo-HCT is feasible with low TRM in those with good PS and low comorbidity scores. We use PS and comorbidity score as exclusion criteria to lower TRM.
Younger patients with MM (<55 years) with good PS and low comorbidity scores should be considered allo-HCT eligible.

B. DISEASE FACTORS:

Newly diagnosed MM:
Myeloma Risk Stratification:
Karyotyping, plasma cell enriched FISH based and/or Gene Expression Profiling (GEP) based risk stratification in allo-HCT eligible patients at diagnosis.
If any of the following are discovered – we proceed to donor search:
1 Ultra-high-risk MM – defined by R-ISS stage 3 or a high plasma cell proliferation index AND the presence of any or a combination of the following specific genetic changes: del(17p), chromosome 1 q gains, t(14:20), t(14:16) OR a high-risk gene expression profile.
2 Primary Plasma Cell Leukemia
3 Primary Refractory MM: patients who are refractory to or progressing on combination therapy involving both full doses of Lenalidomide and a proteasome inhibitor (bortezomib/carfilzomib) after four cycles

Relapsed MM:
4 Early relapse after AHCT: defined as those relapsing with clinical disease (NOT biochemical progression) within 18 months after induction and AHCT. These patients are considered if they achieve a VGPR or better disease status with salvage therapy.
We offer allo-HCT consultation to eligible patients fulfilling the above criteria for short survival with current therapies and AHCT.

C. DONOR EVALUATION:
Ideal donor: Matched Sibling or an unrelated donor matched at all A, B, C, DRB1 loci using high resolution typing.
If an ideal donor has been identified, allo-HCT is offered either on a clinical trial protocol or as standard of care for patients defined previously after risks and benefits have been discussed.

Alternative donor: If an ideal matched donor is not available:
We offer allo-HCT using a haploidentical or other mismatched donor only on a clinical trial protocol and only for those without an ideal donor.

D. CONDITIONING THERAPY:
We offer fludarabine and melphalan based reduced intensity regimens. Non-myeloablative regimens with low dose TBI are not used. For patients receiving allo-HCT as their first ever transplant (e.g., primary plasma cell leukemia), myeloablative regimens have been used.

E. POST-ALLOTRANSPLANT THERAPY:
At day 100, patients with no GvHD and adequate PS, we initiate maintenance therapy either on a clinical trial or as standard of care with lenalidomide or bortezomib with intent to continue such therapy for 3 years.

Timing of allo-HCT: Upfront or at early relapse or late relapse?

As a curative intent procedure and as an adjunct/alternative to an auto-HCT, allo-HCT has the best long term outcomes and highest curative potential when it is part of a planned upfront strategy in newly diagnosed patients. Since deferring allo-HCT to relapse helps avoid the potential early TRM, there is interest in offering it to patients relapsing after auto-HCT.

A CIBMTR analysis and several single center studies have suggested that for the multiply relapsed patient in the salvage setting, allo-HCT does not offer significant advantages in survival or a prospect of cure. In the CIBMTR study, 152 patients, all of whom received a NST/RIC allo-HCT after relapse following a prior ASCT (50% relapsing within 24 months) were analyzed. Even with a relatively acceptable TRM of 13% in the first year, the 3 year PFS and OS were 6 and 20%, respectively. From data presented by Patriarca et al., it appears that the benefit is highest when allo-HCT is used earlier in the disease course and when used as a strategy for consolidation of a remission induced by salvage therapy.

> **PRACTICE POINT**
>
> In relapsed MM, it is the author's policy to offer allo-HCT to patients who are in therapy sensitive early relapse and after they achieve a deep remission such as VGPR or CR. Allo-HCT in multiply relapsed patients and in those with uncontrolled MM is likely futile.

Plasma cell leukemia and allo-HCT

Primary PCL is an aggressive neoplasm and patients generally present at a younger age and with worse performance status at diagnosis compared to MM patients. Also, PCL patients have a higher incidence of extra medullary involvement with extensive bone disease. Genetic abnormalities such as the t(4;14), del(1p21), and *MYC* gene rearrangements have been associated with poor outcomes.

In a comparison from the EBMT, patients with PCL receiving auto-HCT (compared to MM patients) were more likely to suffer TRM and achieve a CR but OS was inferior to the MM patients since responses were not sustained. A CIBMTR study of 97 primary PCL patients reported a 3 year PFS and OS at 3 years of 34 and 64%, respectively, while 50 allo-HCT recipients (16 with NST/RIC regimens) demonstrated a PFS of 18% and OS of 56% in the NST/RIC cohort with a significant relapse rate of 39%. Although inconclusive, these data suggest that in PCL (as in MM), the benefits of lower relapse rates following allo-HCT are often offset by the high TRM.

> **PRACTICE POINT**
>
> In young persons with PCL, given the extremely high-risk of relapse after an auto-HCT, the option of allo-HCT should be explored and its risks and benefits should be discussed.

Planned post-transplant maintenance or cell therapy after allo-HCT

Current post allo-HCT maintenance strategies involve two major approaches:
1 Lenalidomide based:
   a In addition to its anti-myeloma activity lenalidomide also up regulates NK-cells and NK T-cells. Lenalidomide maintenance after allotransplant is attractive since the GvM effect could be augmented by lenalidomide induced stimulation of the alloreactive lymphocytes and NK-cells.
   b In a phase I/II study, within the first week of lenalidomide treatment, peripheral CD4 and CD8 T-cells increased with improved NK-cell derived anti-myeloma activity and was followed by a delayed increase in the regulatory T-cells. Objective responses to salvage treatment with lenalidomide were noted in 83% of patients (including 29% CR) relapsing after an allotransplant. On lenalidomide therapy, 31% developed or exacerbated an acute GvHD episode that was significantly associated with an improved anti-myeloma response.
   c However, the feasibility of lenalidomide maintenance after allotransplant is controversial. The HOVON 76 trial which assessed maintenance lenalidomide starting 1–6 months after allotransplant reported a 37% acute GvHD rate (at a median of 18 days on lenalidomide) leading to premature discontinuation of therapy. A similar US phase II study reported the use of post-allotransplant lenalidomide maintenance starting at a median of 96 days post-transplant in 30 high-risk patients. The cumulative incidence of PCM progression from start of maintenance was 37% with a low TRM of 11%. Acute GvHD was noted in 37% while PFS and OS at 18 months from initiation of lenalidomide was 63 and 78%, respectively, suggesting a benefit and manageable GvHD risk in this high-risk subgroup.
2 Proteasome inhibitors (PI) based:
   a PI are known to suppress GvHD without significantly mitigating the GvM effect. Therefore, bortezomib has been explored for post-allotransplant

maintenance. Kroger et al. investigated the use of bortezomib, for at least two cycles and a median of 8 months following a RIC allotransplant. In patients with measurable disease, CR was seen in 30%, PR in 50%, and a minor response was seen in 20% of patients. There was no major increase in GvHD.

b A national US trial led by the BMT CTN is currently exploring this further for high-risk PCM patients either in the upfront setting or after an early relapse following AHCT. This trial incorporates a proteasome inhibitor (bortezomib) in the conditioning regimen (fludarabine+melphalan+bortezomib) and also the second-generation oral proteasome inhibitor (ixazomib) in planned post-allotransplant maintenance.

Minimal residual disease (MRD) evaluation in allo-HCT

Deeper levels of remission (described as minimal residual disease negativity) after therapy in MM correlate with superior PFS. In studies of patients in CR following auto or allo-HCT, those who were negative for plasma cell clone-specific markers, or negative for aberrant plasma cells by multi parameter flow cytometry were more likely to be relapse-free at 5 years. Similarly, re-appearance of MRD markers often heralds overt relapse. Compared with auto-HCT recipients, allo-HCT recipients were more likely to be in complete remissions and also molecular CR (MCR). Current data support the concept that while an MRD negative state is associated with longer relapse-free survival and reduced relapse rates, the presence of MRD does not uniformly equate with impending relapse. Also, a level of remission that equates to a cure has not been defined. Consensus criteria for MRD monitoring need to be validated in the allo-HCT setting and MRD driven post-transplant interventions are an area of research.

Relapse after allo-HCT in MM

Treatment options for relapsed MM after allo-HCT include DLI alone or in combination with salvage chemotherapy. Novel agents and combinations involving novel agents have been used successfully. A higher-risk of GvHD has been reported in those treated with LEN but special precautions other than close monitoring are not needed.

Emerging immunotherapy approaches

Immunotherapy, excluding the proven graft-versus-myeloma effect from alloreactive T-cells administered in conventional stem cell allografts, is an attractive option

yet remains in its early development. Recent efforts to generate activated chimeric antigen receptor T lymphocytes (CAR T-cells), a technology with proven efficacy in B-cell malignancies expressing CD19, is just being explored in MM to other potential targets such as BCMA (B-cell maturation antigen). Cellular therapy is perhaps the most under-utilized but may be the most potent modality for disease control in MM. Similarly, the platform of allogeneic hematopoietic cell transplant, may present further opportunities for newer immunotherapy approaches like monoclonal antibodies, immune check point blockade, and CAR T-cell therapy.

SUMMARY

1 Allo-HCT is a consideration for high-risk MM patients who are unlikely to benefit from standard approaches.
2 Reduced Intensity Conditioning regimens for allo-HCT have lowered TRM in recent years.
3 Conditioning regimen intensity of moderate anti-MM potential (such as fludarabine – melphalan) are preferred over non-myeloablative regimens (such as 2 Gy TBI).
4 Planned post-transplant therapy is an area of interest and active research.
5 Lenalidomide based maintenance is associated with increased risk of GvHD.
6 The benefits of allo-HCT with/without further maintenance for high-risk are being assessed in the US in the BMT CTN 1302 clinical trial designed for this subgroup of patients.
7 Treatment options for relapse after allo-HCT include DLI alone or in combination with salvage chemotherapy.
8 Alternative donor approaches (haplo identical/cord grafts) should only be pursued in clinical trials.

Selected reading

1. Bruno B, Rotta M, Patriarca F, Mordini N, Allione B, Carnevale-Schianca F, et al. A comparison of allografting with autografting for newly diagnosed myeloma. *N Engl J Med* 2007; **356**: 1110–1120.
2. Garton G, Iacobelli S, Bjorkstrand B, Hegenbart U, Gruber A, Greinix H, et al. Autologous/reduced-intensity allogeneic stem cell transplantation vs autologous transplantation in multiple myeloma: long-term results of the EBMT-NMAM2000 study. *Blood* 2013; **121**: 5055–5063.
3. Knop S, Liebisch P, Hebart H, et al. Allogeneic stem cell transplant versus tandem high-dose melphalan for front-line treatment of deletion 13q14 myeloma – an interim analysis of the German DSMM V trial. *ASH Annual Meeting Abstracts* 2009; **114**: 51.
4. Patriarca F, Einsele H, Spina F, Bruno B, Isola M, Nozzoli C, et al. Allogeneic stem cell transplantation in multiple myeloma relapsed after autograft: a multicenter retrospective study based on donor availability. *Biol Blood Marrow Transplant* 2012; **18**: 617–626.

5. Kroger N, Zabelina T, Ayuk F, et al. Bortezomib after dose-reduced allogeneic stem cell transplantation for multiple myeloma to enhance or maintain remission status. *Exp Hematol* 2006; **34**: 770–775.

6. Garban F, Attal M, Michallet M, et al. Prospective comparison of autologous stem cell transplantation followed by dose-reduced allograft (IFM99-03 trial) with tandem autologous stem cell transplantation (IFM99-04 trial) in high-risk de novo multiple myeloma. *Blood* 2006; **107**: 3474–3480.

7. Rosinol L, Perez-Simon JA, Sureda A, et al. A prospective PETHEMA study of tandem autologous transplantation versus autograft followed by reduced-intensity conditioning allogeneic transplantation in newly diagnosed multiple myeloma. *Blood* 2008; **112**: 3591–3593.

8. Krishnan A, Pasquini MC, Logan B, Stadtmauer EA, Vesole DH, Alyea E, et al. Autologous haemopoietic stem-cell transplantation followed by allogeneic or autologous haemopoietic stem-cell transplantation in patients with multiple myeloma (BMT CTN 0102): a phase 3 biological assignment trial. *Lancet Oncol* 2011; **12**: 1195–1203.

9. Lokhorst HM, van der Holt B, Cornelissen JJ, et al. Donor versus no-donor comparison of newly diagnosed myeloma patients included in the HOVON-50 multiple myeloma study. *Blood* 2012; **119**: 6219, 25.

10. Tricot G, Vesole DH, Jagannath S, Hilton J, Munshi N, Barlogie B. Graft-versus-myeloma effect: proof of principle. *Blood* 1996; **87**: 1196–1198.

11. Alsina M, Becker PS, Zhong X, Adams A, Hari P, Rowley S, et al. Lenalidomide maintenance for high-risk multiple myeloma after allogeneic hematopoietic cell transplantation. *Biol Blood Marrow Transplant* 2014; **20**: 1183–1189.

CHAPTER 24

Light-chain amyloidosis

Amara S. Hussain and Anita D'Souza

Medical College of Wisconsin, Milwaukee, WI, USA

Introduction

Light-chain (AL) amyloidosis, also known as primary systemic amyloidosis, is a plasma cell dyscrasia with multiple paraneoplastic manifestations. Similar to multiple myeloma (MM), there is a clonal proliferation of plasma cells. However, unlike MM, the overall clonal plasma cell burden is usually low in AL amyloidosis. However, these plasma cells secrete immunoglobulin light chains that have an unfortunate predilection to misfold. These resultant misfolded, insoluble fibrils deposit in various organs such as the heart, kidney, liver, and nerves among others, causing organ dysfunction. This disease tends to have a progressive course due to uncontrolled tissue damage from extracellular amyloid deposition and can be rapidly fatal without treatment. Treatment is directed at eliminating the underlying plasma cell clone and in turn the source of the amyloidogenic light chain, by use of chemotherapy. In this chapter, we will review the evidence and utility of autologous hematopoietic cell transplantation (auto-HCT) in AL amyloidosis in the context of other treatment options.

History and current data of transplantation for AL amyloidosis

Since the late 1980s, high dose melphalan with auto-HCT has been identified as a successful therapeutic option in MM. The first report of use of auto-HCT in AL amyloidosis was in 1993 with the use of busulfan and melphalan followed by infusion of CD34+ cells from bone marrow and peripheral blood. While the patient died of complications, she nonetheless had full engraftment. Subsequently, a report from the Netherlands demonstrated a successful syngeneic allogeneic transplant using cyclophosphamide with total body irradiation followed by bone marrow transplantation. The patient had a hematologic and clinical response. The first report of a successful auto-HCT using high dose melphalan was reported by Moreau, et al. in 1996 and immediately thereafter followed by a report of five patients treated with high dose melphalan at Boston University with success. With an increase in the experience of transplant in AL amyloidosis, it became apparent that there was a much higher morbidity and mortality seen among patients with AL amyloidosis compared to patients with MM. A transplant-related mortality (TRM) of as high as 43% was reported in this early transplant period. Additionally, a retrospective study from the Mayo Clinic suggested that patients who met transplant eligibility had good outcomes with non-transplant therapies thus showing the possibility of a selection bias in single center non-randomized studies.

In the early 2000s, larger transplant series from the Boston University, Mayo Clinic, and a multicenter CIBMTR study each showed decreasing TRM of under 20% with refinements in the selection of patients to undergo transplant, along with hematologic responses in 30–40% and organ responses ranging 44–58%.

The much-anticipated randomized phase III clinical trial comparing high dose melphalan and auto-HCT compared to standard melphalan/dexamethasone chemotherapy was published in 2007, and failed to show a survival benefit for transplant compared to chemotherapy. This study, although a commendable effort for a large multicenter trial in a rare disease, was criticized for the high mortality (24%) in the transplant arm, 13 of 50 transplant-randomized patients not getting planned transplants and the lowering of melphalan conditioning

Clinical Manual of Blood and Bone Marrow Transplantation, First Edition. Edited by Syed A. Abutalib and Parameswaran Hari.
© 2017 John Wiley & Sons Ltd. Published 2017 by John Wiley & Sons Ltd.

Table 24.1 Who, when, and how of auto-HCT for AL amyloidosis.

A. PATIENT FACTORS:
Karnofsky performance score of <80% has been associated with lower progression-free and overall survival in AL.

B. ELIGIBILITY FACTORS FOR AUTO-HCT:
1 Cardiac biomarkers: NT-proBNP <5000, TnT <0.06
2 Fewer than three organs involved with AL
3 Non-severe autonomic neuropathy
4 Non-advanced cardiac involvement (NYHA ≤ 2, left ventricular ejection fraction ≥40%)

C. CONDITIONING THERAPY:
High dose melphalan therapy has remained the standard of choice. Dose reductions in melphalan have been associated with lower PFS and increased relapse rate in the current era of novel triplet therapy.

D. POST-TRANSPLANT THERAPY:
Consolidation with bortezomib/dexamethasone at 3 months post-transplant if patients have obtained less than complete hematologic response.

---

chemotherapy in a third of the transplanted patients. What was clear again was that careful selection of patients was necessary for good outcomes.

The identification of the NT-proBNP and troponin T as biomarkers of severity of amyloid involvement led to a simple staging system in 2004; and further refined in 2012 resulting in identification of AL patients that have early mortality of as high as 40% regardless of therapy. It was clear that similar factors that help define the degree of cardiac AL involvement are also critical in post-transplant AL outcomes. Table 24.1 shows factors associated with a high risk of post-transplant mortality and poor survival in AL amyloidosis.

We recently conducted a large CIBMTR analysis of all auto-transplants conducted in North America between 1995 and 2012. In this largest transplant series to date, which included over 1500 patients, we saw decreasing rates of early mortality post-transplant in more recent years (down to 5% in 2007–2012 vs 20% in 1995–2000) and improvement in 5-year OS from 55% in 1995–2000 to 77% in 2007–2012. Further, this study showed that centers performing at least four AL transplants each year had better success in lowering early post-transplant mortality thus emphasizing the need for center experience in this rare disease.

Do patients need induction chemotherapy prior to auto-HCT?

Most patients with AL amyloidosis have low plasma cell burden, and there is no data to date showing a benefit of induction chemotherapy prior to auto-transplant. Prospective studies using melphalan and prednisone induction prior to chemotherapy showed a detriment from this approach, owing to organ progression leading to transplant ineligibility as a result. However, bortezomib therapy is being studied in the setting of a clinical trial, and retrospective data of use of bortezomib and dexamethasone with/out cyclophosphamide appears to have good outcomes, allowing for some transplant ineligible patients being converted to transplant eligible. Again, one has to consider the possibility of selection bias with retrospective data and induction therapy should be used with caution so that there is no further deterioration of organ function.

PRACTICE POINTS

In patients who are eligible for transplantation, we recommend upfront auto-transplant. In patients who are ineligible, we consider bortezomib and dexamethasone with/out cyclophosphamide, and re-evaluate transplant eligibility for 3–6 cycles of chemotherapy.

Mobilization and collection of CD34+ cells

A dose of CD34+ cells $\geq 5 \times 10^6$ cells/kg is targeted. Chemomobilization has been associated with increased complications, and therefore essentially abandoned. Granulocyte-Colony Stimulating Factor (G-CSF) has been reported to cause weight gain, pulmonary edema, capillary leak, splenic rupture, and even death. Indeed, marked fluid retention during mobilization leading to an increase in weight by two percent forecasts a higher mortality rate. Patients have to be monitored closely (sometimes inpatient) during mobilization process. Recently, success has been seen with the use of plerixafor in combination with G-CSF resulting in fewer days of exposure to G-CSF leading to lesser weight gain and no mobilization failures. Patients with autonomic neuropathy and cardiac involvement can develop hypocalcemia and citrate toxicity from the use of citrate as an anticoagulant during apheresis; this risk is reduced by the use of heparin as anticoagulant during apheresis.

PRACTICE POINT

We use citrate as an anticoagulant during apheresis with careful monitoring for symptoms of hypocalcemia.

Conditioning chemotherapy

High dose melphalan remains the standard of care. A risk-adapted approach was proposed based on creatinine clearance, number of organs involved with amyloidosis and presence of cardiac involvement with adjustment of melphalan dose between 100–200 mg/m². It is noteworthy to point out that lowering the dose of melphalan < 140 mg/m² is associated with lower hematologic response as well as higher rate of hematologic relapse.

Supportive care: Important aspects in candidates for auto-HCT

In addition to refinements in selecting patients, improvement in supportive treatment during the peri-transplant period has led to improved TRM in AL amyloidosis. Patients with AL amyloidosis are at an increased risk of becoming volume overloaded. Diuresis ought to be undertaken judiciously, as even mild intravascular depletion, can precipitate gastrointestinal upset, including nausea and vomiting, or worse, induce cardio-renal syndrome. As a result, diuresis and albumin infusions may be necessary to achieve euvolemia. Post-transplantation complications that may be unique and more amplified in AL patients include gastrointestinal bleeding, cardiac arrhythmias, and unresponsive hypotension in selected patients with AL amyloidosis. Patients can develop severe gastrointestinal bleeding from mucositis related to chemotherapy. Patients with orthostatic hypotension may need midodrine and fludrocortisone. However, fludrocortisone can cause resultant fluid retention. Table 24.2 describes various examples of supportive care that may be needed during the peri-transplant period highlighting the need for a multi-disciplinary team approach.

Post-transplant consolidation

Post-transplant consolidation has been used in a risk-adapted chemotherapy approach. In this approach, patients with persistent clonal disease following transplant receive further therapy with novel agents (thalidomide/dexamethasone, bortezomib/dexamethasone). This has been associated with low TRM, and high overall hematologic and organ response rates. Using the CIBMTR cohort, we analyzed day 100 responses to transplant based on the 2012 hematologic response criteria. We found that patients with VGPR or better had excellent outcomes, while those with less than VGPR had uniformly poor progression-free and overall survival.

> **PRACTICE POINT**
>
> We consider post-transplant bortezomib-based consolidation based on sub-optimal day-100 hematologic response (<VGPR).

Response to treatment

Hematologic response is measured using the 2012 criteria proposed by Palladini, et al. and summarized in Table 24.3. Noteworthy is the absence of bone marrow plasma cell clearance in response criteria (unlike with MM) as well as the importance of absolute reduction in the free light-chain excess (rather than the M-protein). Hematologic response correlates with organ response and OS. Organ responses are described for cardiac, renal, and hepatic amyloidosis in Figure 24.1A–C. There is a suggestion that patients without a complete response after transplant may benefit from the use of consolidative chemotherapy with thalidomide or bortezomib with deepening of hematologic response.

> **PRACTICE POINTS**
>
> We follow monoclonal protein studies in blood and urine (serum protein electrophoresis with immunofixation, free light chains), bone marrow biopsy, and organ amyloid measures such as cardiac (NT-proBNP, Troponin T), renal (creatinine, urine protein/creatinine ratio), hepatic (alkaline phosphatase) at day 100 post-transplant, and every 3 months thereafter in the first year. Following that, depending on response patients may continue to be seen at 3-monthly intervals or slightly less frequently. In patients with cardiac amyloidosis, we perform cardiac imaging with 2D echocardiogram with strain imaging or cardiac magnetic resonance at day 100 post-transplant and 1 year post-transplant.

Role of allogeneic transplant in AL amyloidosis

There are individual case reports and small series suggesting a role for allogeneic transplant in AL amyloidosis. The largest data is reported from the European Group for Blood and Marrow Transplantation (EBMT) registry and describes 15 patients with allogeneic and four patients with syngeneic allogeneic transplant. The TRM was high at 40%, with seven long-term survivors at a median follow up of 19 months.

> **PRACTICE POINT**
>
> At this point, allo-HCT is not a modality that can be recommended in most AL patients.

Table 24.2 Supportive care during peri-transplant period.

	Helpful	Caution
Fluid retention and weight gain	Loop diuretics, Spironolactone Periodic thoracentesis may be needed	Fludrocortisone/salt tablets for hypotension
Heart failure	Diuretics Salt and fluid restriction	Calcium channel blockers Digoxin (can bind to amyloid fibrils leading to digoxin toxicity) Beta blockers may cause decompensation Afterload reduction (ACE-I, ARBs) poorly tolerated
Cardiac arrhythmias (atrial fibrillation, ventricular arrhythmias, Sudden Cardiac Death)	Amiodarone AV nodal ablation and pacemaker AICD in select patients may be considered	Rate lowering calcium channel blockers, beta blockers, digoxin
Orthostatic hypotension	Waist-high elastic stockings Midodrine Salt tablets, Fludrocortisone (can worsen fluid retention) Continuous noradrenalin infusion (for refractory hypotension)	
Neuropathic pain	Gabapentin Pregabalin Duloxetine Amitriptyline Nortriptyline Topical agents (lidocaine, TCA, ketamine)	
Nephrotic syndrome	Diuretics Low dose ACE-I (if patient is not hypotensive)	
Renal failure	Dialysis Patients may need pre-transplant midodrine (particularly in those with autonomic neuropathy)	
Gastroparesis causing nausea and vomiting	Anti-emetics, metoclopramide	
Intestinal pseudo-obstruction	Neostigmine	
Diarrhea	Fiber supplements, Bile salt binding agents Loperamide Octreotide (in refractory cases)	
Malnutrition	Dietician consultation early Parenteral nutrition may be needed in those with severe steatorrhea	
Anti-coagulation	May be needed in patients with cardiomyopathy, atrial fibrillation	Check factor X levels Higher risk of GI bleeding

Role of solid organ transplant in AL amyloidosis

The United Network for Organ Sharing data in both renal and cardiac transplant suggest poor outcomes in amyloidosis, however, there may be a role for organ transplant in AL amyloidosis. The danger is for recurrence of the amyloid process in the transplanted organ, in the setting of an incurable underlying clonal disease. In select patients with amyloid cardiomyopathy, cardiac transplantation may be of benefit either following chemotherapy or with an adjuvant auto-HCT post-cardiac transplant. This has been reported with varying success in the form of case reports and few case series

Table 24.3 Active agents in AL amyloidosis. (Combinations of novel agents preferred over single agent therapy in frontline setting.)

Drug	Trial Phase	Mechanism of Action	Major Findings	Adverse Side Effects	Other
Melphalan-Dexamethasone	-	Alkylating Agent	Standard of care in those ineligible for stem cell transplantation	Cytopenias	* Well-tolerated in the elderly and those with baseline neuropathy * No effect on CD34+ cell collection
Thalidomide	II	IMID	Rapid response compared to MEL-DEX	Fluid retention and cardiac issues including progression of congestive heart failure, increase of biomarkers, and arrhythmias	Stem Cell Sparing Common Regimen: cyclophosphamide-thalidomide-dexamethasone; large issue with toxicity, hence caution with those with advanced cardiac involvement
Bortezomib	I/II	Proteasome Inhibitor	Rapid Hematologic Response	Neuropathy	* Administer via SQ to ↓ toxicity * Administer via IV if concern for poor gut absorption * Common Regimen: Bortezomib-Cyclophosphamide-Dexamethsone (BoCyD)
Lenalidomide	II	IMID	Benefit seen as salvage therapy (failed at least two lines), with use of dexamethasone	Cytopenia Rashes Fatigue GI toxicity	
Pomalidomide	II	IMID	Second-line	Neutropenia, Fatigue	
Ixazomib	III	Oral proteasome Inhibitor	Studies currently underway		
Doxycycline	II	In vivo disruption of amyloid accumulation	Studies currently underway		
NEOD001	III	monoclonal against AL fibrils	Studies currently underway		
CPHPC + Anti-SAP antibody	I	Small molecule that clears SAP from circulation combine with anti-SAP antibody	Studies currently underway		

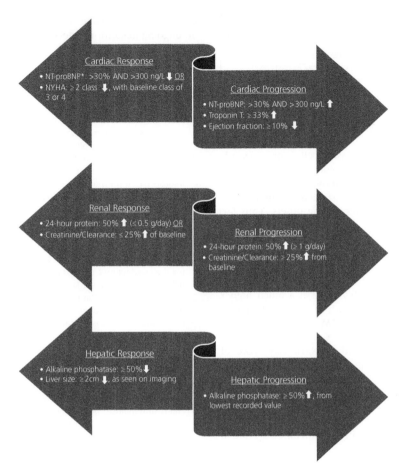

Figure 24.1 Organ responses for renal and hepatic amyloidosis.

from around the world. Successful renal transplant has also been reported before or after auto-transplant from high-volume specialized amyloid centers such as the National Amyloid Center in the UK, Mayo Clinic, and Boston University in a small series.

Non-transplant chemotherapy options

Melphalan and dexamethasone is the only chemotherapy that has shown to be beneficial based on a randomized phase 3 clinical trial thus far, which showed superiority of this regimen over auto-transplant. In the last 15 years, as novel agents revolutionized treatment of MM, it was natural that these agents would next be tried in AL amyloidosis. The most exciting of these drugs is bortezomib, which has been shown to cause prompt (and deep) hematologic responses with organ improvement resulting in patients becoming transplant eligible in some instances.

There is no randomized clinical trial comparing bortezomib with melphalan but a multicenter, international study (NCI 1277016) comparing melphalan and dexamethasone versus bortezomib, melphalan, and dexamethasone is underway.

There has been no improvement in the initial mortality of as high as 40% within the first year of diagnosis of AL amyloidosis, particularly among those with advanced cardiac amyloidosis. This thus highlights the need for adjunctive treatments that help in fibril breakdown or clearance. Doxycycline has been of interest as an anti-fibril agent and is currently undergoing prospective testing. The monoclonal antibody, NEOD001, which targets a cryptic epitope on amyloid fibrils, is another exciting drug is currently in phase 3 testing. The hope is that fibril-directed therapies can help hasten organ responses while chemotherapy helps control the underlying amyloidogenic malignant clone.

PRACTICE POINT

Anti-fibril therapies are entering the phase of clinical testing. The role of these drugs will be key in hastening organ responses and lowering early mortality seen in AL.

Current status and future directions

AL amyloidosis is a clonal plasma cell disorder associated with multi-systemic involvement from AL deposition. The resultant disease morbidity and mortality stems from the deposition of misfolded, insoluble fibrils in the heart, kidneys, nerves among others. Thus far, treatments have focused on chemotherapeutics that target the underlying plasma cell clone, the source of the amyloidogenic light chains. Auto-HCT is one such modality that is associated with deep hematologic responses, organ responses as well as long-term survival. Unfortunately, patients with AL are at a much higher risk of complications and death after transplantation when compared to those with MM. Thus, patient selection is of utmost importance. Current features that permit transplantation include a Karnofsky score of >80%, not extensive cardiac involvement (including NT-proBNP < 5000 ng/L, troponin T < 0.06 ng/mL, NYHA < 2, and LVEF ≥40%), and no more than three organs with amyloid. In addition, extensive supportive care during various phases of auto-transplant – before, during, and after transplantation – outcomes, decline in early TRM and OS have improved considerably. There is an ongoing need for the development of amyloid fibril-directed therapy.

Selected reading

1. Moreau P, Milpied N, de Faucal P, et al. High-dose melphalan and autologous bone marrow transplantation for systemic AL amyloidosis with cardiac involvement. *Blood* 1996;**87**:3063–3064,
2. Palladini G, Dispenzieri A, Gertz MA, et al. New criteria for response to treatment in immunoglobulin light chain amyloidosis based on free light chain measurement and cardiac biomarkers: impact on survival outcomes. *J Clin Oncol* 2012;**30**:4541–4549.
3. Jaccard A, Moreau P, Leblond V, et al. High-dose melphalan versus melphalan plus dexamethasone for AL amyloidosis. *New England Journal of Medicine* 2007;**357**(11):1083–1093.
4. Comenzo R, Reece D, Palladini G, et al. Consensus guidelines for the conduct and reporting 1of clinical trials in systemic light-chain amyloidosis. *Leukemia* 2012;**26**(11):2317–2325.
5. Dispenzieri A, Kyle Ram Lacy M, et al. Superior survival in primary systemic amyloidosis patients undergoing peripheral blood stem cell transplantation: a case-control study. *Blood* 2004;**103**(10):3960–3963.
6. Kumar S, Gertz M, Lacy M, et al. Recent improvements in survival in primary systemic amyloidosis and the importance of an early mortality risk score. *Mayo Clinic Proceedings* 2011;**86**(1):12–18.
7. D'Souza A, Dispenzieri A, Wirk B, et al. Improved outcomes after autologous hematopoietic cell transplantation for light chain amyloidosis: A Center for International Blood and Marrow Transplant Research Study. *Journal of Clinical Oncology* 2015;**33**(32):3741–3749.

CHAPTER 25

Autoimmune disorders

Adam Bryant[1] and Harold Atkins[2,3,4]

[1] Bone Marrow Transplant Fellow, Memorial Sloan Kettering Cancer Center, New York, NY, USA

[2] Blood and Marrow Transplant Program, The Ottawa Hospital, Ottawa, Ontario, Canada

[3] Cancer Therapeutics Program, The Ottawa Hospital Research Institute, Ottawa, Ontario, Canada

[4] Division of Hematology, University of Ottawa, Ottawa, Ontario, Canada

Introduction

Autoimmune diseases (AIDs) are common with a worldwide prevalence estimated at 5%. AIDs can affect any organ and while heterogeneous in manifestations and severity, all AIDs degrade quality of life. Immuno-suppressive therapies, including steroids, cytotoxic agents, and biologic therapies are often effective in controlling disease but also attenuate protective immune responses. Rarely, patients are refractory to these agents and develop severe, life-threatening, or even fatal AID-related complications.

Autologous hematopoietic cell transplant (HCT) has been used to treat patients with severe and refractory AID for the last 20 years. The basis for its role includes:

1 AID remissions in patients with coincident AID undergoing HCT for a hematologic malignancy,

2 Success in remitting AID in experimental animal models using HCT, and

3 Cohort studies and clinical trials using autologous HCT to treat patients with neurologic, rheumatologic, gastrointestinal, endocrine, and hematologic AID.

Strategies employing HCT in AID

A variety of strategies have been employed to mitigate or eradicate autoimmunity. These include:

1 Autologous umbilical cord blood or bone marrow infusions.

    Marrow can stimulate organ repair in animal models but there has been little or no effectiveness shown in early phase trials for patients with autoimmune diseases.

2 High-dose cytotoxic therapy without hematopoietic cell support.

Increased immune suppression is presumed to correlate with more effective and prolonged control of autoreactivity. High-dose cyclophosphamide induces responses for patients with aplastic anemia, MS, systemic lupus erythematosus, and other AIDs, with about 20% of patients demonstrating 5 year event-free survival.

3 High-dose chemotherapy followed by autologous hematopoietic cell rescue.

Following autologous hematopoietic cell graft collection, a conditioning regimen is administered to suppress or ablate the immune system. Conditioning regimens employ chemotherapy of varying intensity and immune depleting antibodies. Autologous HCT reduces the duration of cytopenias and contributes to the reconstitution of the immune system. Given that immune responses can be transferred through a hematopoietic cell graft, most investigators employ methods, either cyclophosphamide (CY) for mobilization or *ex-vivo* selection to deplete the graft of immune cells. There have not been systematic head-to-head comparisons of the different approaches.

Eradication of autoimmunity has been demonstrated by clinical improvement, ability to withdraw from all immune suppression, and where measurable, disappearance of auto-antibodies. Evidence supports the reconstitution of a tolerant, functional immune system following transplantation.

4 High-dose chemotherapy followed by allogeneic hematopoietic cell transplantation.

Allogeneic HCT has been used in the context of pediatric autoimmune cytopenias, showing benefit despite substantial overall toxicity. The small number of adult patients undergoing allogeneic HCT for AID (Table 25.1) limits any meaningful conclusions. Allogeneic HCT is rarely used for patients with AID

Clinical Manual of Blood and Bone Marrow Transplantation, First Edition. Edited by Syed A. Abutalib and Parameswaran Hari.

because of its substantial treatment related mortality and the limited data regarding disease control. Allogeneic HCT is generally discouraged in consensus statements and guidelines.

Transplant activity, indications, and outcomes

An overview of the number of HCT and the disease indication reported to the Center for International Blood and Marrow Transplant Research (CIBMTR) and the European Society for Blood and Marrow Transplantation (EBMT) is summarized in Table 25.1. The predominant indications for HCT have evolved over time, in part, due to the introduction of alternative therapies (i.e., biologic agents

for rheumatoid arthritis). Currently, the most common indications are MS, Systemic Sclerosis (SSc), Crohn's Disease (CD), and autoimmune cytopenias.

1 MS

MS begins with episodic autoimmune attack of oligodendrocytes in the central nervous system causing transient disabilities interspersed with periods of remissions (relapsing-remitting MS; RRMS). As central nervous system damage progresses to include axonal transection, there is an accumulation of permanent disabilities (secondary progressive MS; SPMS). Currently available conventional immunomodulatory therapies, used to reduce the risk of relapse in RRMS include; glatiramer-acetate, β-interferon, natalizumab, fingolimod, teriflunomide, dimethyl fumarate, daclizumab, and alemtuzumab. They are ineffective in

Table 25.1 Indications for HCT in North America, South America, and Europe 1996–2011. This table was adapted from data presented in reports from the Center for International Blood and Marrow Transplant Research (CIBMTR) data dating from 1996–2009, representing more than 400 centers in North and South America, and the European Group for Blood and Marrow Transplantation (EBMT) dating from 1996–2011, representing more than 500 centers from across Europe and Great Britain.

	Allogeneic		Autologous		Total	
	n	%	n	%	n	%
Neurologic Disease	4	1	698	99	702	43
Multiple sclerosis	3	0	662	100	665	41
Other neurologic disease including myasthenia gravis	1	3	36	97	37	2
Rheumatologic and Vasculitic Disease	12	2	710	98	722	44
Systemic sclerosis	0	0	363	100	363	22
Systemic lupus erythematosus	2	2	122	98	124	8
Rheumatoid arthritis	2	2	86	98	88	5
Juvenile chronic arthritis	3	4	71	96	74	5
Polymyositis/dermatomyositis	0	0	16	100	16	1
Other rheumatologic and vasculitic diseases	5	9	52	91	57	3
Autoimmune Hematologic Disease	34	43	45	57	79	5
Immune thrombocytopenia	4	13	28	88	32	2
Autoimmune hemolytic anemia	5	36	9	64	14	1
Evan's syndrome	12	71	5	29	17	1
Other hematologic disease including pure red cell aplasia	13	81	3	19	16	1
Inflammatory Bowel Disease	7	11	58	89	65	4
Crohn's disease	1	2	56	98	57	3
Ulcerative colitis	3	75	1	25	4	0
Other inflammatory bowel disease	3	75	1	25	4	0
Type 1 Diabetes	0	0	32	100	32	2
Others	8	26	23	74	31	2
TOTALS	*65*	*4*	*1566*	*96*	*1631*	

preventing or alleviating the course of patients with SPMS. Mitoxantrone has been used to temporarily slow progression in SPMS.

The indications for autologous HCT are based on clinical trial experience and registry data. The goal is to identify patients who are at risk of rapid and severe disease progression early (≤5 years) after diagnosis. Optimally, these patients demonstrate:

- An aggressive disease course denoted by multiple relapses and/or the onset of permanent disability within a few years after diagnosis,
- Clinical and imaging (MRI) evidence of CNS inflammation,
- Non-response to other immunomodulatory therapies.

Specific criteria, adapted from prominent clinical trials, are presented in Table 25.2.

The benefits reported for patients with RRMS and SPMS that have undergone autologous HCT include:

- Reduction in the occurrence of further clinical relapses,
- Reduction in the development of new lesions on MRI scanning,
- Delay or prevention of further disability,
- Improvement of disability.

Disease specific outcomes and TRM of selected trials are presented in Table 25.3.

2 Systemic sclerosis

Systemic sclerosis (SSc) is an autoimmune condition with lymphocyte-mediated diffuse endothelial damage and cytokine-mediated connective tissue fibrosis. Patients with limited SSc typically only have sclerosis of the hands, face, and neck. Some may develop a syndrome of calcinosis, Raynaud phenomenon, esophageal dysmotility, sclerodactyly, and teleangiectasia. Diffuse cutaneous systemic sclerosis manifests with more extensive skin sclerosis with involvement of the lungs, gastrointestinal tract, kidneys, and cardiovascular system. The mainstay of treatment, prolonged administration of CY, has shown only modest benefits. With few effective treatments, patients with active diffuse SSc have 5-year survival rates of 50–80%. Data from registries, cohort studies and a randomized clinical trial show a benefit for HCT over conventional doses of CY for selected patients with diffuse SSc. There is a dramatic long-term survival benefit for patients treated with HCT over those receiving monthly intravenous CY despite a higher regimen-related mortality during the first year following HCT. Additionally, HCT recipients experience improvement of skin and pulmonary sclerosis. Suggested patient selection criteria are summarized in Table 25.2 while disease specific outcomes and TRM of selected trials are presented in Table 25.3.

3 Autoimmune cytopenias other than aplastic anemia

Most patients with autoimmune cytopenias are successfully managed with a combination of supportive transfusions, immunomodulatory (intravenous immunoglobulin) or immunosuppressive agents (corticosteroids, azathioprine, cyclosporine, monoclonal antibodies), and adjunctive therapies (splenectomy, thrombopoietin agonists). Chronic immune suppression may be required for patients with persistent cytopenias. The estimated mortality rate is 10–30% in pediatric patients with autoimmune hemolytic anemia (AIHA), Evans syndrome (ED) and thrombotic thrombocytopenic purpura (TTP). A significant proportion of patients achieved sustained and clinically relevant responses following either autologous or allogeneic HCT despite having long-standing disease that had failed multiple treatments. The selection of candidates should weigh the effectiveness of alternate approaches against the potential effectiveness and inherent risks of allogeneic or autologous HCT.

4 Crohn's disease (CD)

CD is an inflammatory bowel disease characterized by transmural inflammation of the digestive tract. The pathogenesis is thought to involve both genetic and environmental components. It typically runs a chronic course with intermittent relapses and remissions. Symptoms arise when any portion of the gastrointestinal tract is affected. Sustained inflammation may lead to fibrostenosis of the bowel. There may be extra-intestinal involvement affecting joints, eyes, liver, and the skin. Conventional therapies include corticosteroids, immune suppressants (methotrexate, thiopurines), and biologic agents (tumor necrosis factor inhibitors, anti-interleukins). Surgical interventions play a role for patients with localized but severe bowel wall inflammation or for those with fistulae or abscesses.

The role of autologous HCT in the management of patients with severe refractory disease is uncertain (Table 25.2). While cohort studies suggest benefit for anti-TNF refractory recipients of HCT, a randomized clinical trial did not demonstrate sustained disease response after 1 year of follow-up. (Table 25.3). Many patients will need to restart medical therapy with biologic agents but they are less likely to need steroids for disease control after HCT.

5 Other AIDs

HCT has been employed for other less common AIDs (Table 25.1). HCT could be considered when:

- Patients are experiencing severe disability, morbidity, or life-threatening AID-related complications,
- The patient is refractory to conventional immunotherapies,
- The patient does not have permanent, severe AID-related visceral organ damage, and
- The patient does not have relative or absolute contraindications to HCT.

Table 25.2 Suggested selection criteria for HCT for patients with autoimmune disease adapted from guidelines and clinical trials.

	Suggested Selection Criteria	Suggested Contraindications
All Autoimmune Disease	• Disease refractory to conventional therapy • Disease of sufficient severity to affect quality of life, morbidity, or mortality • Patient of suitable age group and health status to tolerate and benefit from HCT	• Severe cardiac dysfunction with LVEF <40%, Uncontrolled ventricular arrhythmia or Pericardial effusion > 1 cm • Severe renal dysfunction with CrCl < 30 ml/min per m² • Severe respiratory disease with DLCO < 40% • Uncontrolled infection • Pregnancy

Multiple Sclerosis	**RRMS patients**
	• 18–45 years
	• Expanded Disability Status Score (EDSS) between 3.0 and 6.0
	• <5 years from initiation of first therapy
	• Highly active RRMS, defined as
	  ○ ≥1 severe relapses (ΔEDSS ≥1 and Fatigue Severity Scale (FSS) of ≥2 in motor, cerebellar or brain stem deficit (or documented changes in neurological examination consistent with this level of disability) and/or incomplete recovery from clinically significant relapses
	and
	  ○ ≥1 gadolinium-positive (Gd+) lesion of diameter ≥ 3 mm or accumulation of ≥ 0.3 T2 lesions/month in two consecutive MRI 6–12 months apart.
	• Failure of between one and three lines of best available medical therapy
	SPMS patients considered for auto-HCT if
	• Evidence of active inflammation
	  ○ clinical relapses
	  ○ gadolinium enhancing lesions
	  ○ new T2 MRI lesions on two subsequent scans
	• Sustained and clinically relevant increase in disability over the last year
		• ≥ 45 years (low probability to fit inclusion criteria, fast shift to SPMS)
		• advanced impairment of mobility (EDSS ≥6.5)

Systemic Scleroderma	• 18–65 years
	• Diffuse cutaneous SSc according to American Rheumatism Association criteria
	• Disease duration < 4 years
	• Minimum modified Rodnan skin score (mRSS) ≥15
	• Visceral involvement
	  ○ renal: proteinuria >0.3 g/24 h
	  ○ cardiac: conduction disturbance, left axis deviation, rhythm disturbance, pericarditis
	  ○ pulmonary: DLCO ≤70% or FVC ≤70% and evidence of interstitial lung disease
		Severe visceral involvement indicated by:
		• renal: CrCl < 40 ml/min per m²
		• cardiac: LVEF < 50%
		• pulmonary: mean PaP > 50 mm Hg

Crohn's Disease	• 18–65 years • Confirmed diagnosis of CD • Endoscopic and pathologic evidence of severe active bowel inflammation • Refractory to at least three immunosuppressive agents • Impaired quality of life related to CD (Karnofsky, EuroQOL-5D, IBDQ)	• Pregnancy • Severe comorbidity • Short bowel-related diarrhea • Significant malnutrition (BMI ≤18, serum albumin < 20 g/L) • Previous poor compliance • High infectious risk

Table 25.3 Disease specific outcomes and treatment related mortality in select trials of autologous HCT in AID.

Trial	n	Outcomes		TRM
		Multiple Sclerosis		
Atkins et al.	24	Relapses (in 179 patient-year follow-up) Progression-free survival (with median follow-up of 6.7 yrs) Improvement in EDSS	0 70% 40% at 7.5 yrs	4%
Nash et al.	24	3-year relapse-free survival 3-year event-free survival (no death, clinical or MRI MS event),	86% 78%	0%
Burt et al.	151	4-year relapse-free survival 4-year progression-free survival	80% 87%	0%
Mancardi et al.	21 • 9 HCT • 12 MiTX	Autologous HCT vs Mitoxantrone (MiTX) • Reduction in new T2 lesions - risk ratio: • Reduction in annualized relapse rate - risk ratio: • Reduction in disease progression Not statistically significant	0.21 (95% CI 0.10–0.48, p < 0.001) 0.36 (95% CI 0.15–0.88, p = 0.026) 57 vs 48% (p = 0.5)	0%
		Systemic Sclerosis		
ASSIST	19 • 10 HCT • 9 CTX	Autologous HCT vs monthly Cyclophosphamide (CTX) • mRSS score improvement at 1 year - odds ratio: Disease progression	110 (95% CI 14 to inf, p < 0.001) 0 vs 89% (p < 0.001)	0%
ASTIS	156 • 79 HCT • 77 CTX	Auto-HCT vs pulsed Cy • 2-year event-free survival - odds ratio: • 4-year event-free survival - odds ratio:	0.35 (CI 0.16–0.74) 0.34 (CI 0.16–0.74)	10 v 0%
		Crohn's Disease		
Burt et al.	24	1-year retreatment-free survival 2-year retreatment-free survival 5-year retreatment-free survival 5-year steroid-free remission	91% 63% 19% 80%	0%
Hawkey et al.	23 HCT 22 Standard	1-year sustained disease remission	8.7% vs 4.5% (p = 0.6)	4%

Autologous hematopoietic cell mobilization and collection

No systematic reviews or studies have compared mobilization chemotherapy for patients with AID but the majority receive intravenous CY at a dose between 1.5 and 4 g/m². The following principles guide the mobilization and collection of an autologous hematopoietic cell graft from patients with an AID:

1 Consideration should be given to reducing or discontinuing immune suppression prior to mobilization however this may be not be feasible if the AID is active.
2 Cytokine mobilization has been associated with flares of the underlying AID. Consideration should be given to concurrent administration of steroids to prevent this.
3 Intravenous CY:
  a Enhances hematopoietic CD34+ cell mobilization,

  b Can prevent AID flares sometimes seen with G-CSF alone and obviate the need for additional steroids, and
  c Can reduce the number of reactive immune cells in the graft.
4 Mesna and judicious hyperhydration may be used to prevent hemorrhagic cystitis associated with CY administration.
5 Mobilized hematopoietic CD34+ cells are favored for their ease of collection and rapid engraftment.
6 A minimum of 2×10^6/kg CD34+ cells is suggested to optimize engraftment.
7 The role of *ex-vivo* immune cell depletion of the graft, through immunomagnetic CD34+ selection, is controversial with no high-quality evidence to support or refute its use. However, the selection process is expensive, time consuming, and may necessitate higher CD34+ harvest thresholds.

Table 25.4 Potential complications that may occur during mobilization and collection of patients with selected AIDs.

Indication	Caution
Multiple Sclerosis	Neurologic deterioration due to disease reactivation; consider prevention or treatment with by concomitant corticosteroids. Bladder dysfunction leading to cyclophosphamide induced hemorrhagic cystitis. Consider bladder catheterization but this may increase the risk of bacterial urinary tract infection.
Systemic Scleroderma	Potentially fatal cardiac complications.
Systemic Lupus Erythematosus	Potentially fatal cardiac complications.
Crohn's disease	Neutropenia and life-threatening sepsis has been reported. Consider prophylactic antibiotics and close monitoring in an inpatient setting.
Immune Thrombocytopenia, Evan's Syndrome	Profound thrombocytopenia and fatal bleeding has been reported. Lowest effective chemotherapy dose or GCSF alone could be considered, followed by close in- or out-patient monitoring.
Juvenile Idiopathic Arthritis	Life-threatening macrophage activation syndrome has been reported.

Table 25.5 Conditioning regimens commonly used for selected AIDs.

Disease	Regimen	Dosing	Days
Multiple Sclerosis	BEAM-ATG • Carmustine (BCNU) • Etoposide • Cytosine arabinoside (Ara-c) • Melphalan • Rabbit anti-thymocyte globulin	300 mg/m^2 $200 \text{ mg/m}^2/\text{d}$ $200 \text{ mg/m}^2/\text{d}$ 140 mg/m^2 3.75 mg/kg/d	−6 −5 to −2 −5 to −2 −1 +1 to +2
Systemic Sclerosis	Cy-ATG • Cyclophosphamide • Rabbit anti-thymocyte globulin	50 mg/kg/d 2.5 mg/kg/d	−5 to −2 −4 to −2
Crohn's Disease	Cy-ATG • Cyclophosphamide • Rabbit anti-thymocyte globulin	50 mg/kg/d 2.5 mg/kg/d	−5 to −2 −4 to −2

8 There is no reported experience using the mobilizing agent plerixafor in patients with active AID.

Considerations that are specific to individual AIDs are outlined in Table 25.4.

Conditioning regimens for autologous HCT

Conditioning regimens were derived from regimens used for aplastic anemia and hematologic malignancies because of the wealth of experience and knowledge existing with regards to regimen-related toxicities and supportive care requirements. Ablation of lymphocytes is augmented with the inclusion of anti-thymocyte preparations (ATG) or other antibodies that target and destroy immune cells. Systematic studies of different conditioning regimens have not been performed. It is difficult to draw strong conclusions by comparing studies because of differences in disease and patient characteristics. There is a suggestion, looking across all the reported studies, that increasing the intensity of the conditioning regimen results in improved disease control but at the cost of higher rates and severity of toxicity and TRM. Investigators have, by enlarge, adopted intermediate intensity regimens such as BEAM-ATG (BCNU, etoposide, cytarabine, melphalan with ATG) that balance adequate disease control with acceptable TRM. Lower intensity regimens, such as CY with ATG, have better toxicity profiles with acceptable efficacy which may be appropriate for subpopulations at high risk of toxicity, such as patients with scleroderma. With the availability of intravenous busulfan, serum drug level monitoring, and effective supportive care, higher intensity regimens using busulfan, CY, and anti-thymocyte globulin may result in more effective disease control with acceptable toxicity profiles. A summary of the most commonly used AID-specific conditioning regimens is outlined in Table 25.5.

Table 25.6 Supportive care and prophylaxis for patients with AID undergoing autologous HCT.

Prior to auto-HCT

- Appropriate patient selection, with exclusion of patients with severe comorbidities or conditions that may increase the risk of short and long-term complications,
- Comprehensive testing prior to HCT to assess for active infection or treatment-limiting organ dysfunction,
- Consult fertility specialists prior to treatment to mitigate the risk of HCT-induced infertility as appropriate.

During and after the HCT hospitalization

- Supportive blood and platelet transfusions administered as per local protocols, using irradiated blood products.
  - Use CMV-negative leukodepleted blood products for CMV-negative recipients
- Antimicrobial prophylaxis including:
  - Broad spectrum antibacterial prophylaxis during neutropenia,
  - Antifungal prophylaxis against mucocutaneous candidiasis,
  - Pneumocystis jirovecii (PJP) prophylaxis for 6 to 12 months after HCT,
  - Toxoplasma prophylaxis if anti-toxoplasma antibody-positive (as per PJP prophylaxis)
  - Herpes virus prophylaxis for 6–12 months after HCT,
- Treatment of fever and proven infection should follow center-specific policies and protocols.
  - Consider engraftment syndrome if fever coincides with neutrophil recovery.
- Close viral surveillance and pre-emptive therapy of patients receiving ATG or selected autologous grafts including:
  - CMV PCR or antigenemia screening regularly for the first 100 days following HCT,
  - EBV PCR screening regularly for the first 100 days following HCT,
  - Anti-CMV therapy (ganciclovir, valganciclovir, or foscarnet) for patients with CMV viremia or antigenemia,
  - Intravenous immune-globulin in selected cases where benefits outweigh risks and costs of administration.

After the HCT hospitalization and for long-term follow-up

- Regular follow-up with a transplant specialist for at least the first 100 post-transplant days or longer.
- Counsel the patient and monitor for secondary autoimmune phenomenon.
- Annual combined follow-up with a transplant specialist and referring AID physician to monitor for disease activity and late complications.

Early and late complications of HCT and supportive care during HCT

Patients with AID may experience complications that are not typical for those undergoing autologous HCT for lymphomas or multiple myeloma. Immunocompromised due to immunosuppressive treatments prior to HCT, additional immunosuppression associated with the conditioning regimen augment the risk of opportunistic infections before immune reconstitution can occur, 6–12 months after autologous HCT. Infectious and other complications that are more frequent in HCT recipients with AID include:

1 Increased rates of herpes-family viral reactivation. EBV-mediated post-transplant lymphoproliferative disorder (PTLD) and CMV viremia, infections typically associated with allogeneic HCT, have been observed following autologous HCT. Shingles is common and acyclovir prophylaxis is recommended.

2 An engraftment syndrome with non-infectious fevers, lassitude, and rash with or without eosinophilia and pulmonary symptoms.

3 Fever and infection induced pseudo-relapses with worsening of clinical symptoms have been observed. This can be mistaken as a clinical relapse for patients with MS but is generally transient and resolves once the underlying fever or infection resolves.

4 An increased risk of UTI related to urinary bladder catheterization (inserted to reduce the risk of hemorrhagic cystitis from high-dose CY) for patients with reduced mobility from their AID.

5 A secondary autoimmune disease that differs from the original indication may occur within the first 5 years after HCT in about 10% of patients. Thyroid disease or autoimmune cytopenias are the most common manifestations.

The risks of early and late HCT-related complications can be minimized by appropriate patient selection, prophylactic and pre-emptive strategies, and good supportive care. Important risk-reducing measures are summarized in Table 25.6.

Summary key points

1 Autologous HCT is a viable treatment for select patients with severe AID, particularly SSc and MS, that are refractory to conventional treatment,

2 The indication for autologous HCT is unique for each AID and patient selection must be made on a case-by-case basis in association with an AID specialist,

3 Attentive care during and careful monitoring after autologous HCT is required to reduce the chance of a poor outcome attributable to the unique complications of patients with AID,

4 As experience with auto-HCT accumulates further clarification of the role, timing, and optimal patient selection for autologous HCT in AID is anticipated.

5 Allogeneic HCT for AID is generally discouraged owing to its high rate of TRM and lack of supportive data.

Selected reading

The following articles provide concise and comprehensive information about the role of HCT for patients with AID:

1 High Dose Chemotherapy without stem cell support

1. DeZern AE, Petri M, Drachman DB, et al. High-dose cyclophosphamide without stem cell rescue in 207 patients with aplastic anemia and other autoimmune diseases. *Medicine (Baltimore)*. Mar 2011;**90**(2):89–98.

2 Updated EBMT guidelines for auto-HCT in AID.

2. Snowden JA, Saccardi R, Allez M, et al. Haematopoietic SCT in severe autoimmune diseases: updated guidelines of the European Group for Blood and Marrow Transplantation. *Bone Marrow Transplantation*. Jun 2012;**47**(6):770–790

3 Summary report of HCT for AID in North and South America.

3. Pasquini MC, Voltarelli J, Atkins HL, et al. Transplantation for autoimmune diseases in north and South America: a report of the Center for International Blood and Marrow Transplant Research. *Biology of Blood & Marrow Transplantation*. Oct 2012;**18**(10):1471–1478

4 HCT in Systemic Sclerosis.

4. van Laar JM, Farge D, Sont JK, et al. Autologous hematopoietic stem cell transplantation vs intravenous pulse cyclophosphamide in diffuse cutaneous systemic sclerosis: a randomized clinical trial. *JAMA*. Jun 2014;**311**(24):2490–2498.

5. Burt RK, Shah SJ, Dill K, et al. Autologous non-myeloablative haemopoietic stem-cell transplantation compared with pulse cyclophosphamide once per month for systemic sclerosis (ASSIST): an open-label, randomised phase 2 trial. *Lancet*. Aug 2011;**378**(9790): 498–506.

5 HCT in Autoimmune Cytopenias

6. Passweg JR, Rabusin M. Hematopoetic stem cell transplantation for immune thrombocytopenia and other refractory autoimmune cytopenias. *Autoimmunity*. Dec 2008;**41**(8):660–665.

6 HCT in Crohns Disease

7. Burt RK, Craig RM, Milanetti F, et al. Autologous non-myeloablative hematopoietic stem cell transplantation in patients with severe anti-TNF refractory Crohn disease: long-term follow-up. *Blood*. Dec 2010;**116**(26): 6123–6132.

8. Hawkey CJ, Allez M, Clark MM, et al. Autologous hematopoetic stem cell transplantation for refractory Crohn disease: A randomized clinical trial. *JAMA*. Dec 2015;**314**(23):2524–2534.

7 HCT in MS

9. Atkins HL, Bowman M, Allan D, et al. Immunoablation and autologous haemopoietic stem-cell transplantation for aggressive multiple sclerosis: a multicentre single-group phase 2 trial. *Lancet*. Aug 2016;**388**(10044): 576–585.

10. Nash RA, Hutton GJ, Racke MK, et al. High-dose immunosuppressive therapy and autologous hematopoietic cell transplantation for relapsing-remitting multiple sclerosis (HALT-MS): a 3-year interim report. *JAMA Neurol*. Feb 2015;**72**(2):159–169.

11. Burt RK, Balabanov R, Han X, et al. Association of non-myeloablative hematopoietic stem cell transplantation with neurological disability in patients with relapsing-remitting multiple sclerosis. *JAMA*. Jan 2015;**313**(3): 275–284.

12. Mancardi GL, Sormani MP, Gualandi F, et al. Autologous hematopoietic stem cell transplantation in multiple sclerosis: a phase II trial. *Neurology*. Mar 2015;**84**(10):981–988.

CHAPTER 26

Testicular cancer

Moshe C. Ornstein[1], Navneet S. Majhail[2,3], and Timothy Gilligan[1]

[1] Cleveland Clinic Taussig Cancer Institute, Cleveland, OH, USA

[2] Cleveland Clinic Lerner College of Medicine, Cleveland Clinic, Cleveland, OH, USA

[3] Blood & Marrow Transplant Program, Cleveland Clinic, Cleveland, OH, USA

Introduction

Germ cell tumors (GCT) are the most common malignancy among men between 15 and 35 years of age and their incidence has been increasing over the past century. As a result of their extreme sensitivity to cisplatin-based chemotherapy, they are highly curable even in the metastatic setting. However, certain groups of GCT patients continue to have a poorer prognosis, including those with primary mediastinal nonseminoma, those who present with metastatic disease to organs other than the lungs or with very high serum tumor markers, and those who progress or relapse after first-line chemotherapy for metastatic disease. Since the mid-1980s, high-dose chemotherapy (HDCT) with autologous hematopoietic cell transplant (AHCT) rescue has provided a therapeutic option for patients needing second- or third-line chemotherapy, although it has never been shown in a randomized controlled trail to result in longer survival.

Prognostic factors

GCTs are broadly characterized as seminomas and non-seminomas (NSGCT). The International Germ Cell Cancer Collaborative Group (IGCCCG) further categorizes GCTs into poor-risk, intermediate-risk, and good-risk disease which, for NSGCTs, have cure rates of about 90, 80, and 50%, respectively. For seminomas, the cure rates are roughly 85 and 70% in the good- and intermediate-risk categories. There are no poor-risk seminomas. The IGCCCG prognostic score is based on a variety of features including location of primary tumor, metastatic sites, and serum tumor marker levels at the time that chemotherapy is initiated (LDH, AFP, and hCG). However, the IGCCCG risk stratification is the risk score given to patients at the time they begin first-line chemotherapy rather than to patients with relapsed or refractory disease.

Factors that predict outcomes in the relapsed refractory setting have been investigated by numerous groups. Small studies and retrospective reviews identified multiple poor-prognostic factors for patients undergoing HDCT in the relapsed setting including primary mediastinal-NSGCT, hCG > 1,000 IU/1, IGCCCG poor-risk group (stage IIIC) at time of first-line chemotherapy, HDCT as third-line or later therapy, and more than three metastatic sites. There are inherent limitations in these data from small studies and retrospective reviews from specialized centers. Therefore, the International Prognostic Factor Study Group (IPFSG) reviewed a cohort of 1,594 patients treated in 38 sites worldwide who progressed after standard cisplatin-based chemotherapy to develop a prognostic score for patients with relapsed/refractory GCTs. In multivariate analyses, 10 prognostic factors were identified including primary tumor site, prior response, AFP and hCG values prior to salvage therapy, and progression-free interval. These factors comprise a complex scoring system that risk-stratifies patients into five groups to predict PFS at 2 and 3 years (Table 26.1). Such prognostic scoring systems are important to help clinicians and patients balance the risks and benefits of HDCT versus conventional-dose chemotherapy (CDCT) in the initial salvage setting.

PRACTICE POINT

Prognostic scores are available for metastatic GCT in the treatment-naïve and refractory/relapsed settings and should be used to help guide therapy decisions.

Clinical Manual of Blood and Bone Marrow Transplantation, First Edition. Edited by Syed A. Abutalib and Parameswaran Hari.
© 2017 John Wiley & Sons Ltd. Published 2017 by John Wiley & Sons Ltd.

Table 26.1 International Prognostic Factor Study Group (IPFSG) score for cisplatin-refractory or relapsed metastatic GCT (adapted with modifications from Feldman *et al.* Urol Oncol. 2015 Mar 30 and Lorch *et al.* *J Clin Oncol.* 2010 **28**(33):4906–4911).

Prognostic Factors	Points per Prognostic Factor					Total Points per Row
	−1	**0**	**1**	**2**	**3**	
Primary tumor site		Testis	RP		Mediastinal nonseminoma	____
Response to first-line chemotherapy		CR/PRm−	PRm+/SD	PD		____
Duration of progression-free interval (month)		>3	≤3			____
AFP prior to salvage chemotherapy		Normal	≤1,000 ng/ml	>1,000 ng/ml		____
HCG prior to salvage chemotherapy		≤1,000 IU/1	>1,000 IU/1			____
Presence of liver, brain, or bone metastases		Absent	Present			____
Initial risk score						____ (sum of rows 1–6)
Reclassify initial risk score		0	1 or 2	3 or 4	≥5	____
Histology	Pure seminoma	NSGCT or MGCT				____
Final score:						____ (sum of row 8–9)
IPFSG risk group by final score and predicted OS	**−1 = Very low**	**0 = Low**	**1 = Intermediate**	**2 = High**	**3 = Very high**	
2-y PFS	75%	51%	40%	26%	6%	
3-y OS	77%	66%	58%	27%	6%	

AFP: alpha fetoprotein; CR: complete remission; HCG: human chorionic gonadotropin; MGCT: Mixed germ cell tumor; NSGCT: Non-seminomatous germ cell tumor; PD: progressive disease; PR(+): partial remission with positive biomarkers; PR(−): partial remission with negative biomarkers; RP: retroperitoneum; SD: stable disease

AHCT for GCT: What are the outcomes and which patient should be considered?

In the front-line setting, patients with good-risk disease should not be considered for HDCT and should instead be treated with standard CDCT with bleomycin, etoposide, and cisplatin (BEP). For patients with intermediate-risk and poor-risk disease, multiple single-arm Phase II trials demonstrated high response rate and survival using HDCT/AHCT compared to historical controls treated with CDCT. These initial data were encouraging and provided evidentiary support for conducting randomized controlled trials to assess the use of HDCT/AHCT in the front-line setting for these high-risk patients. However, three Phase III trials failed to demonstrate a disease-free or overall survival benefit to HDCT/AHCT compared to CDCT. As such, patients with intermediate- or poor-risk disease should be treated with standard-dose cisplatin-based chemotherapy in the front-line setting and HDCT/AHCT should be considered only for patients with relapsed or refractory disease.

Things are more complicated with regard to relapsed and refractory disease. There remains debate as to whether HDCT/AHCT should be used as initial salvage therapy (i.e., after failure of first-line therapy) or if it should be reserved for progressive and refractory disease after conventional-dose salvage chemotherapy or if it should be reserved for clinical trials. There is no doubt that many people can be cured with HDCT/AHCT; the question is whether the results are superior to CDCT. The only prospective randomized trial comparing initial salvage HDCT/AHCT and CDCT did not demonstrate a statistically or clinically significant difference in event-free or overall survival between the two groups. It is worth noting that this study had several limitations. The most important were that only a single cycle of high-dose chemotherapy was administered, whereas more favorable results have been reported when two cycles are given. Furthermore, the HDCT was preceded by three cycles of CDCT with the result that a large proportion of patients randomized to high-dose chemotherapy never in-fact received it due to toxicity or progression during the cycles of CDCT.

So why does widespread use of HDCT/AHCT for relapsed GCTs continue?

Numerous case series and uncontrolled studies have reported outcomes that are superior to historical controls. For instance, a matched-pair study reported an absolute improvement in overall 2-year survival of 10% with HDCT/AHCT.

HDCT/AHCT as initial salvage is associated with reduced toxicity and improved efficacy when compared with HDCT/AHCT use in the subsequent salvage setting, arguing for its use as initial salvage therapy. Conversely, studies using initial salvage therapy with conventional-dose ifosfomide and cisplatin in addition to paclitaxel (TIP), vinblastine (VeIP), or etoposide (VIP) have reported sustained complete response (CR) rates of approximately 60–70% and would spare many of these patients from the toxicities associated with HDCT/AHCT in the initial salvage setting. Large retrospective and non-randomized prospective data indicate that HDCT/AHCT as initial salvage is associated with improved progression-free and overall survival compared to standard-dose salvage regimens. An international collaborative cooperative group randomized prospective study (Randomized Phase III Trial of Initial Salvage Chemotherapy for Patients with Germ Cell Tumors – TIGER) is ongoing to answer this important question.

Until the results of TIGER trial are available, one approach to the decision of HDCT/AHCT versus CDCT is based on patient's risk of sustained CR. Patients with risk factors that predict good response to chemotherapy, including gonadal or retroperitoneal primary site and prior CR lasting greater than six months, may be considered for CDCT as initial salvage therapy. Since these patients can have CR rate as high as 70%, CDCT will spare them the toxicity associated with HDCT/AHCT. Conversely, patients with poor risk factors (mediastinal primary site, incomplete response to front-line therapy, or CR lasting less than six months) should be offered HDCT/AHCT as initial salvage therapy as it has lower toxicity and mortality compared with its use as second and third-line salvage therapy. An additional factor to consider is access to high-volume centers, where the best results with HDCT/AHCT have been reported. Patients treated at centers without experience using HDCT/AHCT for GCTs may be better off receiving CDCT given the greater complexity and risk of HDCT/AHCT.

Over the past few decades, with increasing HDCT/AHCT experience and enhanced supportive care measures, patient outcomes have improved. treatment-related mortality (TRM) is currently in the low single-digits and sustained remission rates are reported to be in the 40–63% range depending on patient risk factors and timing of treatment (Table 26.2). A critical component to this success is the use of experienced and multidisciplinary transplant teams that work in close collaboration with their colleagues from urologic oncology. Hence, patients who may be candidates for HDCT/AHCT should be referred to cancer centers with appropriate experience and resources.

Table 26.2 Selected prospective clinical trials for HDCT/AHCT as salvage therapy for GCT.

Author	Phase	Total Patients	Trial Setting	Regimen*	TRM (p value)	OS** (p value)	EFS** (p value)	Comments and Practice Implications
Pico et al. (2005)	III	263	First relapse following CR or PR after cisplatin-based therapy	Arm A: PEI or VeIP × 4 Arm B: PEI or VeIP followed by HDCT CECy × 1	3 vs 7% (NR)	53 vs 53% (1.0)	35 vs 42% (0.16)	*Trial results:* One cycle HDCT not better than CDCT. Largest randomized trial in this patient population but with minimal practice implications given significant limitations including: • Study did not address benefit of sequential HDCT. • Many patients in Arm B did not receive HDCT. • Patients refractory to first-line platinum therapy were excluded.
Lorch et al. (2007)	III	211	Relapsed/refractory after at least 1 cycle cisplatin-based chemo	Arm A: VIP × 1 followed by HDCT CE × 3 Arm B: VIP × 3 followed by HDCT CECy × 1	4 vs 16%	48 vs 46% (0.19)	47 vs 45% (0.44)	Study stopped early given high toxicity rates in arm B. *Practice implication:* a less intensive triple sequential transplant is more effective and less toxic than single cycle HDCT with 3 drugs.
Einhorn et al. (2007)	Case series	135	First relapse following prior cisplatin-based therapy (n=135) Relapse following two (n=45) or more (n=4) prior cisplatin-based regimens	HDCT CE × 2	N.A.	66% at 5 years	70% vs 45%	This is a single-institution consecutive case series of patients treated 1996–2004 rather than a clinical trial. 20% of patients had relapsed pure seminoma Doses of CE were higher than some series (Carboplatin 700mg/m²/day for days −5, −4, −3 and etoposide 750mg/m²/day for days −5, −4, −3) There were three acute drug-related deaths and three patients later developed acute leukemia.
Motzer et al. (1996)	I/II	58	Incomplete response following first-line cisplatin-based therapy or incomplete response or relapse after cisplatin-based salvage	HDCT CECy × 2	12%	31% (2 y)	21% (2 y)	Study was predominantly in pts with poor-prognostic factors to CDCT. Study conducted in 1990s so despite good survival outcomes, TRM is very high. Compare with later trials.
Rick et al. (2001)	II	80	Relapse/refractory following first-line cisplatin therapy	TIP × 3 (with or without an additional TI × 1) followed by HDCT CETh × 1	1%	30%	25%	*Practice point:* The addition of a third agent did not change outcome but resulted in increased toxicity suggesting that a third agent in HDCT is not warranted.
Feldman et al. (2010)	II	107	Recurrence after at least one cycle of cisplatin therapy as well as either extragonadal primary or incomplete response to prior salvage	TI × 2 followed by HDCT CE × 3	2%	52% (5 y)	47% (5 y)	*Practice implication:* Study demonstrated impressive survival rates of ~50% with low TRM in patients who based on poor risk factors would be unlikely to have a good response to CDCT.

* All HDCT were followed by AHCT rescue

** OS and EFS are at 3 yr mark unless otherwise indicated.

CDCT: conventional dose chemotherapy; CE: carboplatin, etoposide; CECy: carboplatin, etoposide, cyclophosphamide; CETh: carboplatin, etoposide, thiotepa; CR: complete response; HDCT: high-dose chemotherapy; PEI: cisplatin, etoposide, ifosfomide; PR: partial response; TI: paclitaxel,ifosfomide; TIP: paclitaxel, ifosfomide, cisplatin; VeIP: vinblastine, ifosfomide, cisplatin; TRM: treatment-related mortality; VelP: vinblastine, ifosfomide, cisplatin;

Dr. L. Einhorn at Indiana University (see recommended reading 1 and next the section on the number of cycles).

> **PRACTICE POINT**
>
> Front-line therapy for all GCT risk groups should be cisplatin-based CDCT. HDCT/AHCT should be reserved for the refractory/relapsed setting. The use and timing of HDCT/AHCT in the relapsed/refractory setting should be determined on an individual basis depending on patient's prognostic factors and the availability of physicians with experience and expertise in treating relapsed GCTs.

> **PRACTICE POINT**
>
> Tandem HDCT/AHCT in relapsed/refractory GCT are most widely studied. There are no persuasive data to justify the addition of a third chemotherapeutic agent in the preparative regimen.

HDCT/AHCT: How is it done?

The first step in the HDCT/AHCT is mobilizing hematopoietic progenitor cells so that they can be collected via leukopheresis. Methods for mobilization, collection, and cryopreservation of peripheral hematopoietic cells are discussed in previous chapters. If hematopoietic cell mobilization and collection cannot begin within 2 weeks, it is generally prudent to give the patient one or two cycles of CDCT to keep the cancer under control while waiting to begin HDCT/AST. CDCT will mobilize hematopoietic cell circulation and can be used for that purpose. However, if mobilization and collection of hematopoietic cells can be initiated within two weeks, and the patient has chemosensitive disease (without marrow involvement), then CDCT is not generally indicated and mobilization can be accomplished with administration of colony stimulating factors.

Two early studies of relapsed or refractory GCT patients treated with HDCT/AHCT established carboplatin and etoposide as the backbone chemotherapy for this treatment approach. The typical myeloablative preparative regimen includes carboplatin $700\,mg/m^2$ and etoposide $750\,mg/m^2$ daily on days 4, 3, and 2. On day 1 (day prior to transplant) no chemotherapy is given. Day 0 is the day of infusion of autologous CD34+ cells. The addition of a third chemotherapeutic agent is associated with increased toxicity and no significant improvement in outcomes compared with two agents.

Following administration of HDCT and subsequent infusion of AHCT there is a 3–12-week recovery time period prior to the subsequent HDCT/AHCT. During this time, restaging CT scans of the chest, abdomen, and pelvis are done to demonstrate a minimum of stable disease prior to proceeding with the second transplant. If imaging does not declare progressive disease, then the standard of care is to move forward with similar myeloablative HDCT (same preparatory regimen) followed by second autologous transplant. The concept of tandem (i.e., more than one) transplants for GCTs was established as a standard by

Efficacy and Toxicity: How can we maximize efficacy while limiting the toxicity?

Numerous strategies have been attempted to improve efficacy in patients undergoing HDCT/AHCT. Studies with higher doses of carboplatin and etoposide demonstrated improved durable remission rates. However, most of these patients were treated in the initial salvage setting and patients with poor-prognostic factors such as primary mediastinal-NSGCT and late relapse were excluded. Studies investigating the addition of a third agent have not demonstrated sufficient improvement in outcomes to justify the added toxicity and are thus not recommended. Likewise, the previously mentioned retrospective study of almost 1,600 patients conducted by the IPFSG demonstrated improved outcomes in patients who received two or more cycles (i.e., sequential) compared to those who received only one cycle HDCT. There are insufficient data to determine a difference in outcome between two and three HDCT cycles, so the use of more than two cycles is best reserved for clinical trials.

Toxicity rates of HDCT/AHCT vary depending on the timing and regimen of HDCT/AHCT. In studies of HDCT/AHCT as first-line salvage therapy, the most common grade three or greater toxicities were gastrointestinal, hepatobiliary, and pulmonary, occurring in approximately 42, 24, and 15% of patients, respectively. These rates are higher than those in patients receiving CDCT. Rates of febrile neutropenia in HDCT/AHCT vary widely across clinic trials and range from approximately 40–70%.

The use of HDCT/AHCT earlier in salvage therapy is associated with less toxicity than when it is used in later in the disease course. Additionally, the combination of autologous peripheral blood grafts with G-CSF

Table 26.3 Author's practice: Who, when, and how of AHCT for GCT.

A. PATIENT FACTORS:
Age: Majority of patients diagnosed with GCT; those eligible for HDCT/AHCT usually will be between 15 and 40 years of age.
Performance Status (PS) and Comorbidity: Fewer comorbidities and a good performance status (ECOG 0–1; Karnofsky >70%) are critical for patients undergoing HDCT/AHCT to reduce TRM. Patients with significant cardiac, pulmonary, renal, or hepatic toxicity will be excluded per institutional protocols.
B. DISEASE FACTORS:
Newly diagnosed GCT: We do not recommend HDCT/AHCT as front-line therapy for patients with any risk GCT. Patients should be treated with standard of care cisplatin-based chemotherapy.
Relapsed/Refractory: HDCT/AHCT can cure 40–63% of patients with relapsed/refractory GCT but should not be used as first-line therapy. Patient's risk factors should guide the use of HDCT/AHCT vs chemotherapy only as initial salvage therapy. Patients with favorable risk factors at relapse may be considered for salvage chemotherapy alone while those with poor risk factors (see text) should be offered HDCT/AHCT as initial salvage therapy.
C. HDCT REGIMEN (same for second transplant as well): There are a variety of options for the HDCT regimen prior to AHCT. Our recommendations reflect a well-established standard for tandem transplants using etoposide 750 mg/m² IV daily for three doses and carboplatin 700 mg/m² IV daily for three doses. Both drugs are given daily from day 4 to day 2 following by a day of rest on D-1 with autologous graft infusion occurring on D-0. Addition of third chemotherapeutic agent to preparative regimen has no clinical benefit
D. Interval between the two transplant: Tandem HDCT/AHCT are better than one but it's unclear if three are better than two. The second cycle of high-dose chemotherapy should be administered as soon as the patient has recovered normal platelet and granulocyte counts after the first cycle. Given that a randomized controlled trial comparing standard-dose salvage chemotherapy to a single course of HDCT found no difference in outcome (53% survival in each arm), there is little rationale for proceeding with only a single cycle of HDCT.
E. POST HDCT/AHCT THERAPY: Patients should have daily CBC counts following HDCT/AHCT until ANC >500 uL and platelet count >20,000 uL then weekly for the first 6 weeks following transplant. While inpatient, chemistry profiles, and coagulation studies should be collected as clinically indicated. Long-term follow-up including basic blood-work, tumor biomarkers, and imaging should follow published guidelines.

AHCT: autologous hematopoietic cell transplant; CDCT: conventional-dose chemotherapy; CR: complete response; GCT: germ cell tumor; HDCT: high-dose chemotherapy; IR: incomplete response; RP: retroperitoneal

administration to promote engraftment, improved infectious disease and supportive care protocols, and increased experience with HDCT/AHCT have improved efficacy while minimizing toxicity. As a result of these factors, TRM rates have decreased from over 20% in the initial HDCT studies to reported TRM rates of approximately 2–3% in present day studies.

PRACTICE POINTS

Although there is evidence that higher doses of carboplatin and etoposide with autologous hematopoietic stem cell rescue can improve outcomes in men with relapsed germ cell tumors, this has not been demonstrated in randomized controlled trials. Data exist to support the use of two cycles of HDCT/AHCT ("tandem transplant") rather than one cycle. It is unknown whether administering more than two cycles improves outcomes (see Table 26.3).

Selected reading

1. Pico JL, Rosti G, Kramar A, *et al.* A randomised trial of high-dose chemotherapy in the salvage treatment of patients failing first-line platinum chemotherapy for advanced germ cell tumours. *Ann Oncol* **16**:1152–1159, 2005.
2. Lorch A, Kollmannsberger C, Hartmann JT, *et al.* Single versus sequential high-dose chemotherapy in patients with relapsed or refractory germ cell tumors: a prospective randomized multicenter trial of the German Testicular Cancer Study Group. *J Clin Oncol* **25**:2778–2784, 2007.
3. Einhorn LH, Williams SD, Chamness A, *et al.* High-dose chemotherapy and stem-cell rescue for metastatic germ-cell tumors. *N Engl J Med* **357**:340–348, 2007.
4. Motzer RJ. High-dose carboplatin, etoposide, and cyclophosphamide for patients with refractory germ cell tumors: treatment results and prognostic factors for survival and toxicity. *Journal of Clinical Oncology* **14**: 1098–1105, 1996.
5. Rick O, Bokemeyer C, Beyer J, *et al.* Salvage treatment with paclitaxel, ifosfamide, and cisplatin plus high-dose carboplatin,

etoposide, and thiotepa followed by autologous stem-cell rescue in patients with relapsed or refractory germ cell cancer. *Journal of Clinical Oncology* **19**:81–88, 2001.

6. Feldman DR, Sheinfeld J, Bajorin DF, *et al.* TI-CE high-dose chemotherapy for patients with previously treated germ cell tumors: results and prognostic factor analysis. *J Clin Oncol* **28**:1706–1713, 2010.

7. Einhorn LH, Williams SD, Chamness A, *et al.* High-dose chemotherapy and stem-cell rescue for metastatic germ-cell tumors. *N Engl J Med* **357**:3403–3408, 2007.

8. Lorch A, Beyer J. High-dose chemotherapy as salvage treatment in germ-cell cancer: when, in whom and how. World J Urol, 2016.

9. Lorch A, Bascoul-Mollevi C, Kramar A, et al. Conventional-dose versus high-dose chemotherapy as first salvage treatment in male patients with metastatic germ cell tumors: evidence from a large international database. *J Clin Oncol* **29**:2178–2184, 2011.

10. International Prognostic Factors Study G, Lorch A, Beyer J, et al. Prognostic factors in patients with metastatic germ cell tumors who experienced treatment failure with cisplatin-based first-line chemotherapy. *J Clin Oncol* **28**: 4906–4911, 2010.

CHAPTER 27

Sickle cell disease

Sonali Chaudhury[1] and Shalini Shenoy[2]

[1] Division of Pediatric Hematology/Oncology/Stem Cell Transplantation, Ann & Robert H. Lurie Children's Hospital of Chicago, Northwestern University Feinberg School of Medicine, Chicago, IL, USA

[2] Division of Pediatric Hematology/Oncology/Stem Cell Transplantation, Washington University School of Medicine, St. Louis Children's Hospital, St. Louis, MO, USA

Introduction

The importance of tracking the natural history of sickle cell disease (SCD)

- SCD is the most common inherited disorder of hemoglobin in the United States.
  - Over 100,000 children and adults live with the disease in the US and millions more across the world.
- The severity of SCD varies between individuals and between different locations of geographic origin.
  - The most severe manifestations are found in patients with hemoglobin (Hb) SS and Sβ[0] thalassemia and progress with age.
  - Morbidity, poor quality of life (QoL), and early mortality are related to sickle related vasculopathy that targets vital organs such as the central nervous system (CNS) (silent and overt strokes), eyes (proliferative retinopathy), lungs (acute chest syndrome and pulmonary hypertension), kidneys, bone, and joints (avascular necrosis), and painful vaso-occlusive episodes (VOE).
- Interventions such as penicillin prophylaxis, red cell transfusions, erythrocytapheresis, iron chelation, and hydroxyurea have revolutionized treatment and increased survival especially in children. Despite this, complications set in with age. Median age at death in 2005 was 42 and 38 years for females and males with SCD, respectively. Cardiopulmonary and renal complications primarily contributed to mortality.

- Additional measures of well-being also deteriorate with age resulting in a gradual decline in IQ, performance status, and QoL measures. Increased health care utilization, narcotic dependence, and lowered education and job retention capabilities add to dealing with disease burden.
- In addition to supportive care, it is important to consider and discuss with patients and families the pros and cons of curative therapies such as allogeneic hematopoietic cell transplant (allo-HCT) and in the future, potentially gene therapy options as available.

> **PRACTICE POINT**
>
> SCD now rarely results in mortality in the first two decades of life in developed countries due to improved supportive care strategies. However, despite adequate supportive care the vasculopathy progresses during subsequent decades, to organ damage often resulting in morbidity and premature mortality.

The changing indications for allo-HCT in SCD

Approximately 500 transplants have been reported to the Center for International Blood and Marrow Transplant Research (CIBMTR) from US centers. Of these, 75% are from human leukocyte antigen (HLA)-matched sibling donors (MSD). Most SCD transplants are performed following "severe" disease manifestations. Recommended indications for allo-HCT are summarized in Table 27.1.

Clinical Manual of Blood and Bone Marrow Transplantation, First Edition. Edited by Syed A. Abutalib and Parameswaran Hari.
© 2017 John Wiley & Sons Ltd. Published 2017 by John Wiley & Sons Ltd.

Table 27.1 Indications for transplantation in sickle cell disease.

HLA-Matched Sibling Donor	HLA-Matched Unrelated Donor or Haploidentical Donor
Consider early transplant: With onset of symptoms	Stroke
Stroke – overt or silent	Elevated TCD velocity unresponsive to transfusions
Elevated TCD velocity	Recurrent ACS despite supportive care
Recurrent acute chest syndrome	Recurrent severe VOE despite supportive care
Recurrent VOE requiring medications	Red cell alloimmunization + indication for chronic red cell transfusion therapy
Indication for chronic red cell transfusion therapy	Pulmonary hypertension
Pulmonary hypertension	Sickle nephropathy
Recurrent priapism	
Sickle nephropathy	
Bone and joint involvement	
Sickle retinopathy	
TRV >2.5 m/s	
Sickle related liver injury or iron overload	

TCD – Transcranial Doppler, TRV – tricuspid regurgitation velocity, VOE – venocclusive episode

Traditional indications for allo-HCT

- Overt stroke or elevated transcranial Doppler velocities (TCD) > 200 cm/s by the non-imaging technique or >185 cm/s by the imaging technique especially when unresponsive to chronic transfusion therapy (high risk for stroke)
- Recurrent severe acute chest syndrome (ACS) – especially with episodes of respiratory failure
- Chronic ongoing or acute intermittent debilitating VOE interfering with lifestyle, activity, and requiring prolonged narcotics/hospitalization.

Additional indications that signal severity of SCD but can add to allo-HCT toxicities

- Nephropathy
- Retinopathy
- Red cell alloimmunization
- Early pulmonary hypertension
- Recurrent priapism
- Avascular necrosis, osteonecrosis

Relative contraindications to allo-HCT in SCD-will increase allo-HCT related morbidity/mortality

- Biopsy-proven bridging hepatic fibrosis or cirrhosis
- Severe pulmonary hypertension
- Poor performance status (such as severe sequelae from stroke)

> **PRACTICE POINTS**
>
> **1** From a disease perspective, severity and progression of organ damage dictate consideration of allo-HCT. Since outcomes are very good, HLA-MSD transplants should be discussed with all patients who have a major hemoglobinopathy, if applicable. The caveat, however, is an associated GvHD or mortality risk, albeit small, and donor availability. Alternate donor transplants have higher risks of toxicity, GvHD, rejection, and mortality. Consideration of HCT should be based on disease severity, weighing the pros and cons carefully with the patient and their family.
> **2** Transplant outcomes also vary based on age of the patient, graft source, preparative regimen, GvHD incidence and prophylaxis, and compliance. All these factors should be considered when discussing expected/desired outcomes following allo-HCT.

Donor availability for allo-HCT

- Only 14% of SCD patients will have HLA -MSD available for allo-HCT in SCD.
- Donors with sickle trait are eligible to donate. Engrafted hematopoietic cells from sickle trait positive donors are able to stem SCD complications post-HCT.
- Only 19% of patients will find HLA-matched unrelated donors (HLA-matched at 8/8 major HLA loci – A, B, C, and DRB1) (MUD donors) in the voluntary donor registries. This low number is due in

part to fewer minority donors in the registry and efforts are underway to expand these numbers.

- However, 76% of African Americans will find a one-antigen HLA-mismatched registry donor. HLA-mismatched unrelated donor (mMUD) transplants, however, can be expected to have even higher toxicity than HLA-MUD transplants.
- Both HLA-MUD and HLA-mMUD transplants should be considered only in clinical trial settings at an experienced center.
- Fully HLA-matched (HLA-matched at six major loci A, B and DRB1) umbilical cord blood (UCB) is only available in 2–6% of patients; though a HLA-matched (6/6) UCB product could have some advantage over graft from marrow, outcomes are further subject to optimum cell dose requirements (ideally >5.0×10^7/kg total nucleated cells [TNC]) and intensity of preparative regimen.
- UCB HLA-matched at 5/6 HLA loci are more prevalent; 58% for children (<20 years) and 24% for adults based on cell dose adequacy for malignant disorders (2.5×10^7/kg TNC). Due to increased risks of graft rejection in non-malignant disorders (due to immune competency of the patient) higher doses of cells in the graft are desired, that is, ideally >5.0×10^7/kg TNC.
- More recently, HLA-haplo-identical (HI) hematopoietic cell transplant (HCT) methodology has advanced to allow consideration of HI-HCT options for SCD in trial settings. Options include traditional myeloablative or reduced intensity non-ablative regimens with CD34$^+$ selected infusions with measured T-cell replete marrow or peripheral blood cells with post-transplant cyclophosphamide to prevent alloreactive T-cell expansion, and αβ+T and B-cell (CD19) depleted products. Toxicity and engraftment remain obstacles that have prompted the development of clinical trials researching the best way to overcome these.

PRACTICE POINT

Allo-HCT from HLA-MSD is established with good outcomes and enables an informed transplant discussion. Of note, GvHD and mortality risks associated with HLA-MSD also increase with age. Alternate donor transplants should be undertaken only in patients with severe disease and in a clinical trial setting. Studies seek to improve outcomes and overcome risks of mortality, GvHD, infections, graft rejection, and acute and/or late organ toxicities.

Transplant trials in SCD – Preparative regimens

History – The first transplant for SCD was reported in 1984 – and was performed from a HLA-MSD for acute myeloid leukemia. The recipient was cured of both disorders which triggered interest in treating SCD with

transplantation. Table 27.2 (parts A and B) summarizes published HCT efforts for SCD.

- Myeloablative transplants for SCD have been performed in approximately 800 patients to date, primarily in Belgium, France, United States, United Kingdom, and Italy. Of over 500 transplants reported to the CIBMTR for SCD, 75% were from HLA-MSD (preferred donor).
- The majority of transplants performed to date with HLA-MSD marrow (BMT) or cord (UCBT) have utilized myeloablative regimens, the commonest being busulfan and cyclophosphamide. The addition of hydroxyurea and rabbit antithymocyte globulin (rATG) to the preparative regimen resulted in a significant decrease in graft rejection rates.
- Myeloablative conditioning followed by HLA-matched (6/6) unrelated donor (URD) UCBT had lower than desired DFS (50%).
- "Reduced toxicity" myeloablative regimens combining busulfan or treosulfan with fludarabine/alemtuzumab/thiotepa in HLA-MSD HCT had comparable efficacy and reduced exposure to combination chemotherapy.
- Lowering the intensity of the preparative regimen is well tolerated but had variable success in small reports. Graft rejection rates increased with lowered intensity. Recently, immunoablation with an alemtuzumab, fludarabine and melphalan in a reduced intensity conditioning (RIC) trial yielded comparable results to myeloablative transplants for hemoglobinopathy in a large series of HLA-MSD HCT in children.
- Donor cell (graft) tolerance induction following very low intensity conditioning was used by investigators at the NIH focusing on adults with severe sickle cell disease who had a HLA-MSD. Alemtuzumab was used with low dose radiation followed by infusion of granulocyte- colony stimulating factor (G-CSF) mobilized peripheral blood cells. Recipients continued sirolimus based immunosuppression post-HCT to stimulate donor T regulatory cell activity and maintain mixed donor-recipient chimerism. Immunosuppression was continued for extended periods of time if donor T-cell engraftment was <50%. About half of the patients continue on long-term immunosuppression to maintain engraftment of >50% donor T-cells.
- RIC regimens were unable to support engraftment when unrelated UCB was used as a graft source. Intensification of RIC regimens have shown better engraftment kinetics in recent pilot studies of URD UCBT.
- A HLA-MUD bone marrow transplant trial (the SCURT trial from the Bone Marrow Transplant Clinical Trials Network) in children using a RIC regimen has recently completed accrual. Engraftment rates were similar to HLA-MSD but GvHD rates following transplant from unrelated donors were higher, leading to lower survival than HLA-MSD HCT. Alternate approaches to tackle GvHD are necessary for HLA-MUD grafts.

Table 27.2 (A) Outcomes of myeloablative HLA-matched sibling donor transplants for hemoglobinopathy*.

Author (Journal)	Graft Source (Numbers)	Conditioning Regimen	Graft Rejection (%)	Acute/Chronic GvHD (%)	OS (%)	EFS (%)
Vermylen C et al. (BMT 1998)	BM (48) UCB (2)	Bu/Cy ± rATG ±TLI	10	40/20	93	82
Bernaudin F et al. (Blood 2007)	BM/PBHC (75) UCB (12)	Bu/Cy ± rATG	22 (pre-ATG) 3 (post-ATG)	20/11	93	86 (before 2000) 95 (after 2000)
Panepinto J et al. (BJH 2007)	BM/PBHC 63 UCB 4	Bu/CY (6 others)	13	10/22	97	85
Walters MC et al. (BBMT 2001)	BM (59)	Bu/Cy +/-rATG +/-Alemtuzumab	9	12/14	93	85
*Locatelli F et al. (Blood 2013)	BM (389) UCB (97)	Bu+/-Cy+/-Flu+/-TT +/-ATG/ALG	6 9	21/11 10/7	97 95	85 83
Lucarelli G et al. (BMT 2014)	BM (40)	Bu/Cy/rATG+/-Flu	None	50/5 (severe)	91	91
Dedeken L et al. (BJH 2014)	BM (39) UCB (3) BM+UCB (7) PBHC (1)	Bu/Cy/±rATG ± HU	4 (None after HU+ ATG)	22/20	94	85 (97 with HU)

* Patient overlap present between reports

Outcomes include thalassemia and sickle cell disease

Table 27.2 (B) Outcomes of RIC or myeloablative reduced toxicity conditioning (RTC) regimens with HLA-MSD transplant for hemoglobinopathies.

Author (Journal)	Graft Source (Numbers)	Conditioning Regimen	Graft Rejection (%)	Acute/Chronic GvHD (%)	OS (%)	EFS (%)
*King A et al. (Am J H 2015)	BM (46) BM+UCB (5) UCB (1)	Flu/Mel/ Alemtuzumab	2	23/13	94	92
Hseih M et al. (JAMA 2014)	PBHC (30) (young adults)	Alemtuzumab, TBI+Sirolimus	13	0	97	87
Bhatia M et al. (BMT 2014)	BM (15) UCB (3)	Bu/Flu/Alemtuzumab	None	17/11	100	100
Horan et al. (BBMT 2015)	BM (11) BM+UCB (2) UCB (1)	Dose de-escalation Bu/Flu/CY/equineATG	None	14/14	100	100
Krishnamurti et al. (BBMT 2008)	BM (7)	Bu/Flu/equine ATG/TLI	None	12/12	100	85

* Patient overlap present between reports

Outcomes include thalassemia and sickle cell disease

BM – Bone marrow, PBHC – peripheral blood hematopoietic cells, UCB – umbilical cord blood, TLI – Total lymphoid irradiation; rATG – (rabbit) antithymocyte globulin, ALG – antilymphocyte globulin, Bu – Busulfan, Flu – fludarabine, Cy – cyclophosphamide, HU – hydroxyurea, Me – melphalan, TT – thiotepa

- HI-HCT if successful, has the potential to benefit the most number of patients due to the ease of donor availability. A full intensity regimen utilizing chemotherapy and lymphoid irradiation, followed by CD34$^+$ selected cells (adopted from Italian thalassemia experience) is being tested but short and long-term outcomes need to be tracked. Reduced intensity approaches (using combinations of hydroxyurea, thymoglobulin or alemtuzumab, fludarabine, cyclophosphamide) utilizing unmanipulated BM or peripheral blood hematopoietic cells (PBHC) are based on the premise that high dose cyclophosphamide immediately post-transplant is able to prevent expansion of allo-reactive mismatched donor T-cells to offset GvHD. Initial attempts at such transplants were well tolerated without mortality but had high rates of graft rejection (43%). Strategies to intensify preparative regimens in this setting to allow better engraftment are under investigation.

- The majority of transplants for SCD have been performed in children with HLA-MSD except for the NIH trial (SCURT – BMT CTN 0601). Adult transplant attempts from alternate donors have been otherwise limited by toxicity likely due to pre-existing disease related organ damage (kidneys, lungs, heart). Recent additional efforts are underway to investigate HCT for SCD in adolescents and young adults. The STRIDE trial is a reduced toxicity myeloablative transplant trial for adults accepting related and HLA-matched unrelated grafts. Similarly, a reduced intensity HI-HCT trial with post-HCT cyclophosphamide is in development for pediatric and adult patients with SCD.

PRACTICE POINT

Myeloablative regimens have yielded good outcomes following HLA-MSD bone marrow transplants. RICs that are immunoablative are more recent, have shorter follow up, but are promising for comparable results with myeloablative regimens with HLA-MSD. CBT have an increased risk of graft rejection with RIC and the best outcomes to date (with MSD UCB) utilize myeloablation. Tolerability and regimen related toxicity, such as organ dysfunction and sterility, is expected to be lower with RIC regimens but have to be tracked long-term.

Outcomes of HCT for SCD

- The bulk of the data for HCT outcomes is from MSD (responsible for >75% of HCT reported to registries).
- HLA-MSD BMT results in overall survival (OS) of 94–100% with DFS between 85–92%.
- HLA-MSD (6/6) UCBT results are similar with OS >95% and EFS between 80–90% – of note, with myeloablative conditioning.
- Transplant-related mortality (TRM) is low in HLA-MSD BMT but not absent. HLA-MSD HCT can be expected to have a mortality of up to 5–6%.

- RIC transplants are able to achieve similar survival rates with potentially lowered toxicity but long-term follow up is necessary to prove their safety and efficacy.
- Very low intensity transplants can render patients disease free often with continued immune suppression to maintain grafts. Such transplants have targeted older patients in their second or third decade to avoid more intense conditioning agents in order to minimize TRM.
- Unrelated donor transplants are experimental. Unrelated UCBT has yielded 50% DFS. The DFS with bone marrow following RIC is expected to be in the 70–75% range. Thus, unrelated UCBT has had the poorest outcomes to date. However, unrelated UCBT with modified RIC regimens, or with UCB products expanded in vitro have had early results that are more promising. However, unrelated UCBT with modified RIC regimens, or with UCB products expanded *in vitro* have had early results that are more promising. GvHD incidence of 50–60% with URD, needs to be tackled.
- HI-HCT are the most recent addition to armamentarium. The approach is undergoing modifications to improve outcomes and offset graft rejection. The goal is to successfully maintain stable donor engraftment (current results with 43% rejection rate) that can sustain donor derived erythropoiesis.
- Transplants in older patients with alternate donors are just gaining momentum (HI-HCT, the STRIDE trial). These will evaluate whether disease related sequelae can be stemmed or reversed by transplant and extend duration and QoL following HCT in adults.

PRACTICE POINT

HLA-MSD transplants should be discussed in the presence of such a donor in all patients with SCD given the excellent outcomes especially in the young patients. The balance between the low risk of mortality and the ongoing disease related damage with age should be addressed. HLA-MSD HCT is definitely in the best interest of patients with ongoing disease manifestations, poor QoL, or with the necessity for chronic red cell transfusion therapy. Unrelated and haploidentical donor transplants are experimental and should be performed as part of clinical trials that address and track rejection and GvHD risks carefully. The goal of such trials would be to achieve HCT outcomes comparable to HLA-MSD HCT. In addition to graft source, age, disease status, compliance, regimen intensity, and immunologic status of the recipient will influence HCT outcomes.

Toxicities and supportive care – Not to be forgotten after HCT

SCD related risks/precautions

- Toxicities can be divided into those that are SCD related and those that are HCT related. Transplant care for SCD patients has several special characteristics.
- HCT toxicities are primarily organ dysfunction or failure, infections, and GvHD.

- The iron deposition and sickle vasculopathy are risk factors for hepatic sinusoidal obstruction syndrome (SOS) and can be exacerbated during transplant by hepatotoxic medications (busulfan, azoles) or the inflammatory cytokines of engraftment. Medications with efficacy against hepatic SOS such as defibrotide should be available for use as needed. Though there has been concern raised about the use of Granulocyte Colony Stimulating Factor (GCSF) post allo-HCT in an inflammatory setting, transplant trials (e.g., the SCURT trial) have used the drug to hasten recovery of white cells and no major toxicities have been reported.
- Pulmonary toxicity of infectious or GvHD origin can be exacerbated by compromised lung volumes (SCD with recurrent ACS) or by pulmonary hypertension and should be monitored carefully and treated promptly.
- SCD patients have a low threshold for seizures and CNS toxicity such as posterior reversible leukoencephalopathy syndrome (PRES) are common depending on the type of transplant and risk factors such as hypertension, steroids and calcineurin inhibitors. The incidence reported ranges between 5 and 34%. This is likely due to cerebral vasculopathy and CNS vulnerability during the changes of HCT. Seizure prophylaxis is mandatory for all SCD patients undergoing transplant until patients are off immunosuppression. Levetiracetam is preferred for seizure prophylaxis. It is commenced at the time of commencing conditioning therapy and continued until calcineurin inhibitors used for GvHD prophylaxis or treatment are discontinued.
- Hypertension is a pre-empting event or an early sign of impending PRES. Of note, SCD patients have blood pressures that are lower than established norms for age. Patients are pre-disposed to hypertension during HCT due to shifts in fluid balance, disease induced renal dysfunction, and medications such as calcineurin inhibitors or steroids. Hypertension control should be strictly followed and inciting factors avoided if possible.
- Electrolyte imbalance due to renal tubular dysfunction can be expected to worsen with age and SCD related renal damage requiring close follow up and supplementation as needed. Nephrotoxic agents should be avoided if possible.
- Predisposition to ischemic or hemorrhagic stroke – the acute inflammatory changes post-transplant have been known to predispose to acute CNS events and radiographic changes early post-HCT. This risk improves with time and donor engraftment renders stability to the CNS long-term presumably by halting progression in cerebral vasculopathy.
- Bleeding risks are higher in the presence of vasculopathy – the risk of CNS hemorrhage is compounded by hypertension and thrombocytopenia. Maintaining platelet counts $>50 \times 10^9$/L is strongly recommended until platelet engraftment in all patients with SCD due to their vulnerability to bleed from vasculopathy changes.

> **PRACTICE POINT**
>
> Attention to each of these is very important when planning HCT for SCD. Awareness of the fact that age and severity of disease exacerbate these risks is important.

Transplant-related risks

- BMT from HLA-MSD in children is the gold standard to which transplant outcomes from newer trials are compared.
- Acute and chronic GvHD rates of 20–30% and 10–22%, respectively, are noted following HLA-MSD HCT. Chronic GvHD rates are lower with HLA-MSD (6/6) UCBT; extensive chronic GvHD is rare with MSD UCBT. Methotrexate should be avoided with UCBT.
- GvHD rates and other toxicities are higher following MUD or HI-HCT. The severity of SCD versus the GvHD and mortality risks from HCT influence the decision to pursue alternate donor transplants.
- Immune reconstitution (IR) is most efficient with HLA-MSD HCT. Delayed IR increases susceptibility to infectious complications in especially in alternative donor HCT. Infections are also expected following immunoablative transplants until IR.
- Mixed chimerism has been noted following all transplant approaches. However, RIC or very low intensity conditioning regimens and UCBT tend to predispose more toward mixed chimerism (22% BMT, 37% UCBT, and 27% RIC HCT). Stable mixed chimerism can be compatible with a disease-free state. Generally, patients are asymptomatic and maintain donor erythropoiesis if donor myeloid chimerism is >30%. If donor chimerism is perceived to be unstable, it should be followed every 2–4 weeks and immunosuppression adjusted. Myeloablative and immunoablative regimens benefit from weaning immunosuppression. Very low intensity regimens usually require continued immunosuppression to maintain donor erythropoiesis. If T-cell donor chimerism is preserved and myeloid chimerism is lost, a stem cell boost can be considered. If all donor chimerism is lost, a second transplant will become necessary.
- Graft rejection rates following HLA-MSD HCT are expected to be 2–10%. UCBT has a higher risk of graft rejection.
- Higher rates graft rejection may be expected following alloimmunization against HLA antigens or red cell antigens of donor type – the relationship is ill-defined.

- All patients receiving very low intensity regimen will remain mixed chimera and up to 50% may require continued low dose long-term immunosuppression to maintain donor cells.
- Social aspects – More adults are willing to consider transplant especially after encountering disease complications repeatedly. Fewer children and their families consider HCT due to concern for side effects and the ability to respond well to conservative treatments such as hydroxyurea or red cell transfusion therapy.

PRACTICE POINT

GvHD, graft rejection and mortality rates are low with HLA-MSD HCT supporting consideration of this curative treatment modality in those with a severe form of hemoglobinopathy (primarily Hb SS or Hb Sbthal⁰) that eventually take their toll with age. Adverse effects increase with alternate donor transplants. The pros and cons of transplant should be carefully weighed by patients, caregivers, and families.

Long-term follow up

- Early follow up has revealed persistence of SCD symptoms even after engraftment for several months (new CNS lesions, persistent pain). Pain control is better and opioid use tapers several months after transplant even in adults.
- Long-term follow up has revealed that SCD manifestations are controlled and eventually subside (curative intervention).

- RIC is attractive if organ toxicity is lower and sterility is avoided. Myeloablative HCT results in ovarian failure in 70% of females. Other concerns include organ toxicity and late malignancies.
- There is improvement in QoL and reduction in health care utilization after 1 year post-HCT for MSD (9, 10). The cost for medical care per patient with SCD is estimated at over US$ 460,151 compared to HCT from MSD, which is US$ 112,000–150,000. Health care utilization decreased post-HCT from HLA-MSD HCT. The ultimate goal with HCT would be to abolish the need for inpatient admissions for SCD complications.
- IR is robust in the absence of GvHD and following immunosuppression wean.
- It is not clear if there is an age at which disease sequelae are "too far gone" for improvement. Ongoing adult HCT trials (STRIDE) are designed to answer these questions by comparing transplanted cohorts with patients on continued conservative treatment.
- Transplant may be a better option for those patients unable to access ongoing supportive care (applies to patients returning to countries with sub-optimum care).

PRACTICE POINT

It is important to continue follow up after HCT long-term to track late toxicities, disease related outcomes, and QoL and function. Establishing follow up registries as has been done for malignant disorders can serve this purpose.

Table 27.3 HCT for SCD – Where are we now?

Authors' practice:
Patient related variables:

1. Age – Pediatric transplant experience has been greater; adult transplants are rarely undertaken due to anticipated toxicity. However, with newer protocols, both pediatric and adult transplants can be considered for the "correct" indications with an emphasis on clinical trial enrollment.
2. Indications:
   (i) CNS – Stroke is by far the most important indication because it demonstrates the extent of cerebral vasculopathy. A third of these patients will develop second and third strokes despite regular transfusions. HCT is best performed prior to the establishment of CNS damage resulting in either overt CNS symptoms or deterioration in performance status. High transcranial Doppler velocities that don't abate with transfusions are a risk factor for stroke. Progression of silent stroke despite transfusions – lead to IQ and neurocognitive deterioration
   (ii) Other manifestations based on severity include ACS, pain episodes, priapism/bone/joint disease, nephropathy, retinopathy, etc.
   (iii) Red cell alloimmunization despite the need for chronic transfusion therapy
   In general, the severity of symptoms and quality of life are balanced with donor availability and transplant risks based on the type of transplant. In the presence of a matched sibling donor, HCT can be considered for less severe manifestations due to excellent outcomes. In the unrelated or haploidentical donor setting, established "severe" disease manifestations that progress despite conservative supportive care are worthy of consideration of transplant.
   We discuss transplantation as a treatment modality with all SCD families. Full siblings that do not have the disease are typed as potential donors. Transplant discussions are pursued further in the presence of a HLA-matched sibling. The decision to proceed to transplant is undertaken after mutual agreement between the hematology and transplant teams and the patient and family (as no transplant procedure is without a mortality risk however slight). The reason to be aggressive about such a discussion is that outcomes are best following transplant in the young prior to the development of established disease.
3. Contraindications – these are relative. Undertaking a high-risk transplant in the absence of severe or progressive disease would jeopardize care. Established pulmonary hypertension or liver cirrhosis will jeopardize transplant outcomes. Transplants will not help patients with poor performance status secondary to CNS events or established irreversible lung or cardiac disease. HLA antibodies targeted against donor are a high risk for graft rejection.

(Continued)

Table 27.3 (Continued)

Donor related variables:

Marrow has been the preferred stem cell source though more recent studies have used G-CSF mobilized peripheral blood. UCB has a higher chance of rejection and may require a higher intensity conditioning regimen. Cell dose for cord transplants are critical.

Beyond matched sibling donor transplants, (only 14% of SCD patients are likely to have MSD) all other transplants are to be considered experimental and should be performed in the confines of a study.

We prefer bone marrow for matched sibling donor transplantation. We will supplement it with cord blood cells if they are stored especially in the presence of age and weight discrepancy between donor and recipient.

We have clinical trials open for alternate donor transplants. Patients are enrolled if they have severe disease manifestations, after an extensive discussion regarding pros and cons. In the absence of a sibling donor, the registry is always accessed to identify a HLA-matched unrelated donor (15–20%). Parents or HI siblings are considered next. In each of these situations the risks of mortality, GvHD, infections, and extended hospitalizations are discussed at length prior to proceeding. The alternatives - conservative care are discussed as well.

Preparative regimens:

We currently use RICs for all SCD transplants. We have successfully used immunosuppression with fludarabine/cyclophosphamide and ATG followed by a boost of CD34$^+$ selected cells in an occasional patient with falling myeloid donor chimerism after MSD HCT. If a RIC regimen results in complete graft rejection, MAC may be necessary to ensure achieve engraftment. MAC regimens have a graft rejection rate of approximately 5%. One exception to this approach is when patients are enrolled on formal trials that use prescribed ablative regimens. Another reason would be in the case of infectious complications – since RIC regimens are highly immunoablative, MAC may be preferred in the event of underlying invasive infections. The premise is that reducing intensity will preserve organ function better. Gonadal function is of particular interest. Families are concerned about ovarian failure, decreased sperm production, and sterility following transplant with MAC We have seen no ovarian failure to date with RIC, which is promising, but have no long-term follow up yet to suggest that ovarian and sperm functions are preserved lifelong. Our preferred conditioning regimen for matched sibling donor transplants for SCD is a combination of alemtuzumab, fludarabine, and melphalan when marrow is the stem cell source. The largest experience with matched sibling donor UCBT is with MAC regimens (busulfan, cyclophosphamide, rATG). GvHD prophylaxis for UCBT should include a calcineurin inhibitor and mycophenolate mofetil. Avoiding methotrexate in UCBT has provided better outcomes. Unrelated donor, cord blood, and haploidentical transplants for SCD are experimental and should only be performed on formal trials.

Supportive care pearls:

Seizure prophylaxis, strict hypertension control to within 10% of normal for the SCD patient of the same age, strict fluid and electrolyte balance maintenance, relative isolation during period the period of recovery, good management of thrombocytopenia are all very essential for good outcomes.

Social assessment:

Compliance is key to a chance for a successful outcome. Older children and adolescents often do not realize the importance of compliance. The supportive care team that works with the transplant service does a thorough evaluation and monitors patient compliance closely. Our follow up protocols have been changed to incorporate 2–3 clinic visits in a week early post- transplant.

SUMMARY

Allo-HCT offers a cure for SCD. While the disease poses significant risk for premature morbidity and mortality by affecting vital organs, transplant outcomes are influenced by several factors such as donor source, patient age, disease status, transplant approach, and compliance. Clinical trials continue to determine outcomes of transplant for SCD and pave the way for further improvement. It is the responsibility of the hematology and transplant teams caring for the patient to help with understanding the pros and cons of transplant so an informed decision can be made regarding this treatment modality (Table 27.3). Another curative option under investigation is gene therapy where autologous cells are manipulated to produce normal hemoglobin. These trials are just underway and their utility should be apparent in the coming years.

Selected reading

1. Talano J, Cairo M. Hematopoietic stem cell transplantation for sickle cell disease: state of the science. *Eur J Haematol.* 2015;**94**(5):391–399.

2. Locatelli F, Kabbara N, Ruggeri A, Ghavamzadeh A, Roberts I, Li C, et al. Outcome of patients with hemoglobinopathies given either cord blood or bone marrow transplantation from an HLA-identical sibling. *Blood.* 2013;**122**(6): 1072–1078.

3. King A, Kamani N, Bunin N, Sahdev I, Brochstein J, Hayash R, et al. Successful matched sibling donor marrow transplantation following reduced intensity conditioning in children with hemoglobinopathies. Am J Hematol. 2015.

4. Vermylen C, Cornu G, Ferster A, Brichard B, Ninane J, Ferrant A, et al. Hematopoietic stem cell transplantation for sickle cell anemia: the first 50 patients transplanted in Belgium. *Bone Marrow Transplant.* 1998;**22**(1):1–6.

5. Bernaudin F, Socie G, Kuentz M, Chevret S, Duval M, Bertrand Y, et al. Long-term results of related myeloablative stem-cell transplantation to cure sickle cell disease. *Blood.* 2007;**110**(7):2749–2756.

6. Panepinto J, Walters M, Carreras J, Marsh J, Bredeson C, Gale R, et al. Matched-related transplantation for sickle cell disease: report from the Center for International Blood and Transplant Research. *Br J Haematology.* 2007;**137**: 479–4785.

7. Walters M, Patience M, Leisenring W, Rogers Z, Aquino V, Buchanan G, et al. Stable mixed hematopoietic chimerism after bone marrow transplantation for sickle cell anemia. *Biol Blood Marrow Transplant.* 2001;**7**(12):665–673.

8. Locatelli F, Kabbara N, Ruggeri A, Ghavamzadeh A, Roberts I, Li C, et al. Outcome of patients with hemoglobinopathies given either cord blood or bone marrow transplantation from an HLA-identical sibling. *Blood.* 2013;**122**(6): 1072–108.

9. Lucarelli G, Isgrò A, Sodani P, Marziali M, Gaziev J, Paciaroni K, et al. Hematopoietic SCT for the Black African and non-Black African variants of sickle cell anemia. *Bone Marrow Transplant.* 2014;**49**(11):1376–1381.

10. Dedeken L, Lê P, Azzi N, Brachet C, Heijmans C, Huybrechts S, et al. Haematopoietic stem cell transplantation for severe sickle cell disease in childhood: a single centre experience of 50 patients. *Br J Haematol.* 2014;**165**(3): 402–408.

11. Hsieh M, Fitzhugh C, Weitzel R, Link M, Coles W, Zhao X, et al. Nonmyeloablative HLA-matched sibling allogeneic hematopoietic stem cell transplantation for severe sickle cell phenotype. *JAMA.* 2014;**312**(2):48–56.

12. Bhatia M, Jin Z, Baker C, Geyer M, Radhakrishnan K, Morris E, et al. Reduced toxicity, myeloablative conditioning with BU, fludarabine, alemtuzumab and SCT from sibling donors in children with sickle cell disease. *Bone Marrow Transplant.* 2014;**49**(7):913–920.

13. Horan J, Haight A, Dioguardi J, Brown C, Grizzle A, Shelman C, et al. Using fludarabine to reduce exposure to alkylating agents in children with sickle cell disease receiving busulfan, cyclophosphamide, and antithymocyte globulin transplant conditioning: results of a dose de-escalation trial. *Biol Blood Marrow Transplant.* 2015;**21**(5): 900–905.

14. Krishnamurti L, Kharbanda S, Biernacki M, Zhang W, Baker K, Wagner J, et al. Stable long-term donor engraftment following reduced-intensity hematopoietic cell transplantation for sickle cell disease. *Biol Blood Marrow Transplant.* 2008;**14**(11):1270–128.

CHAPTER 28

Hematopoietic cell transplant in thalassemia

Emanuele Angelucci[1] and Federica Pilo[2]

[1] Unità Operativa Ematologia. IRCCS Azienda Ospedaliera Universitaria San Martino - IST - Istituto Nazionale per la Ricerca sul Cancro, Genova, Italy

[2] Unità Operativa di Ematologia e Centro Trapianti. Ospedale Oncologico di Riferimento Regionale "Armando Businco", Cagliari, Italy

Introduction

β thalassemia major (here referred as thalassemia) is characterized by a genetic defect leading to ineffective erythropoiesis and hemolysis. Thalassemia patients develop a severe long life anemia requiring chronic red blood cell transfusion therapy (transfusion dependent thalassemia = TDT). In TDT, anemia and transfusion related iron overload are finally fatal in a few years if not adequately treated. In recent decades, improvement in thalassemia medical therapy (transfusion and chelation) has been dramatic, leading, in the industrialized world, to a predicted survival of at least four to five decades.

Rationale for allo-HCT

The rational basis of allogeneic hematopoietic cell transplantation (allo-HCT) in thalassemia consists of substituting the thalassemic hematopoietic clone with a normal clone capable of effective erythropoiesis. This cellular replacement therapy is not limited to the diseased erythropoietic compartment, but leads to the replacement of the entire hematopoietic system, that is, including immune system. Nevertheless, it is an efficient way to obtain a long-lasting, probably permanent, clinically effective correction of chronic hemolytic anemia, thus avoiding transfusion requirements and associated complications (i.e., iron overload).

Expected results of transplantation for thalassemia

Since the early 1980s, more than 4000 such transplants have been performed worldwide in several centers with excellent and reproducible results as reported in Table 28.1. A recent survey of the Hemoglobinopathy Registry of the European Group for Blood and Marrow Transplantation (EBMT) demonstrated excellent "real world" results for patients transplanted after January 1, 2000.

Indications for allo-HCT in thalassemia

On a theoretical point of view all patients affected by TDT are candidates for allo-HCT. For obvious reasons, no randomized prospective trial comparing results of transplantation versus medical therapy has been performed (nor is it likely that such a randomized study comparing these approaches or to gene therapy will ever be done). Therefore, the choice to undergo a curative but potentially life-threatening transplant is basically to be taken on an individual basis. In this decision process, several aspects have to be taken in consideration (Figure 28.1).

Risk factors for outcomes with allo-HCT in thalassemia

HCT for thalassemia was started and developed by the Pesaro group in the 1980s and early 1990s. The Pesaro experience (more than 1000 transplants regarding thalassemia performed in a single center) has been the cornerstone of this development. This experience has clearly indicated patient status at time of transplantation as the critical factor predicting outcome.

Three risk factors significantly impacting transplant outcome have been identified in patients aged 16 or

Clinical Manual of Blood and Bone Marrow Transplantation, First Edition. Edited by Syed A. Abutalib and Parameswaran Hari.
© 2017 John Wiley & Sons Ltd. Published 2017 by John Wiley & Sons Ltd.

younger. All of them were iron overload related, see Table 28.2.

These three factors stratify patients into three classes of risk:

1 No factor: low risk.
2 One or two factors: intermediate risk.
3 Three risk factors: high risk.

Pesaro results (1980s to early 1990s)

Early on, overall survival (OS) and thalassemia free survival (TFS) were significantly different in the three groups treated by the same conditioning regimen (oral busulfan 14 mg/kg plus Cyclophosphamide 200 mg/kg): 94 and 87% in the low-risk group, 84 and 81% in the intermediate-risk group, and 70 and 58% in the high-risk group, respectively. The difference was almost entirely due to the transplant-related mortality (TRM) which approached the 50% in the high-risk group. For this reason, intensity of the conditioning was changed in the high-risk group. In the 1990s, with the new, less intensive conditioning (oral Busulfan 14 mg/kg plus cyclophosphamide 120–160 mg/kg), TRM significantly dropped in high-risk patients to 18% but with an increment of the recurrence of thalassemia rate to >20%.

In older adult patients (≥17 years), this risk classification was not applicable, likely because at that time it was not possible to have patients older than 16 years with a long life on regular chelation therapy. In this group of patients, in the 1990s, TRM rate was 30–35% even with the use of the previously mentioned reduced dose of cyclophosphamide.

Lessons from the Pesaro experience

Life-long control of anemia and iron overload are the main factors determining allo-HCT outcome. The liver is the "window" to assess patient condition so a complete liver evaluation is recommended during initial assessment of allo-HCT. These same criteria have also been validated in an HLA-matched unrelated (MUD) transplant setting.

Table 28.1 Results of allo-HCT with HLA-MSD in patients with thalassemia.

Age Group	Overall Survival	Thalassemia Free Survival
Children (<18 years)	82–96%	74–86%
Adults (≥18 years)	80%	76%

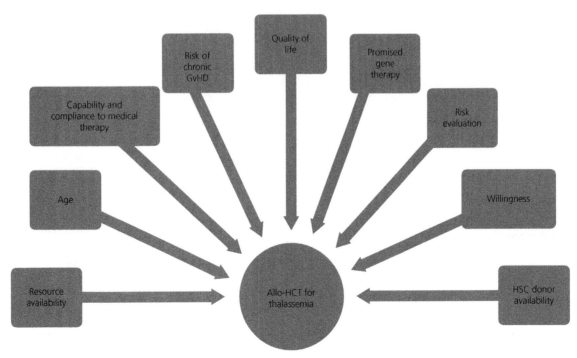

Figure 28.1 Factors that must be considered for individual decision making about allo-HCT for thalassemia. (Angelucci et al., Hematology Am Soc Hematol Educ Program 2010. Reproduced with permission).

Table 28.2 Pesaro risk factors for allo-HCT in thalassemia.

1 Quality of chelation received for the entire life span before transplantation	Regular vs irregular
2 Hepatomegaly	≤2 cm from the costal arch vs >2 cm
3 Liver fibrosis at pre-transplant liver biopsy	Absent vs present

Current results with allo-HCT in thalassemia

In the last decade, improvements in our understanding of iron overload, iron metabolism, and iron chelation therapy have led to improved iron status at transplantation, subsequently improving results according to the Pesaro risk definition. Also, modern transplantation approaches have contributed to the better results obtained today as demonstrated by several groups (see Table 28.1).

Adult patients (≥18 years)
After 2000, transplantation experience in adult patients has been limited with fewer than 100 patients transplanted. Even here, results are improved but TRM (approximately 20%) remains significant.

> **PRACTICE POINTS**
>
> Allo-HCT should be offered as soon as possible in patients with transfusion dependent thalassemia
> Transplant-related risk factors should be evaluated according to the Pesaro risk score. Adequate transfusions/chelation regimen is the major issues to be evaluated before deciding to perform transplant. Allo-HCT in adult patients has a higher risk of complications. Adult patients should be transplanted only in well-experienced transplant centers.

HLA-matched sibling cord blood transplant

A large, international study retrospectively comparing cord blood to bone marrow recipients has recently been completed. Analyses showed that OS, TFS, acute, and chronic graft-versus-host disease (GvHD) were 95, 88, 20, and 12%, respectively, for BM recipients (n = 389), and 96, 81, 10, and 5%, respectively for CB recipients (n = 70). The availability of an adequate number of total nucleated cells (TNCs) (i.e., > 3.5 × 10^7/kg) needs to be taken into account before the procedure.

Beyond HLA-MSD and HLA-matched sibling CB units

Non-HLA-identical family donor
The experience of transplantation from HLA-mismatch relatives is limited and the results are inferior to those obtained with an HLA-identical sibling (MSD and sibling UCB) as donor. Recent experiences using $\alpha\beta^+$ T- and B-cells depleted PBHC are promising but the experience is still very limited.

HLA-matched unrelated donor (MUD)
Transplantation from an HLA-MUD offers results comparable to those obtained in HLA-MSD if stringent criteria of immunogenetic compatibility – based on high-resolution HLA typing – are respected. In this setting it is crucial to achieve extended haplotype identity (i.e., identity from locus HLA-A to locus HLA-DQ on the same chromosome). A study has demonstrated that the risk of thalassemia recurrence after MUD-HCT is associated with the presence of non-permissive HLA-DPB1 mismatches in the GvD direction.

The limited use of MUD transplant suggests caution in using this procedure outside very experienced and dedicated centers. The use of unrelated CBT in transfusion dependent thalassemia has not been explored in well-designed clinical trials. Inconsistent data are reported by today limited literature. Even in the unrelated CB setting the critical point remains the number of nucleated cell infused.

> **PRACTICE POINTS**
>
> Transplantation from an HLA mismatched family member in thalassemia is an experimental procedure to be conducted in the contest of a well-designed controlled trial transplantation from an HLA-MUD is an option to be performed in expert centers. Very stringent compatibility criteria must be used. Unrelated cord blood transplantation must be performed in the context of well-controlled experimental clinical trials in centers with specific cord blood programs. Accepted and experimental donor approaches to allo-HCT are summarized in Table 28.3.

Pretransplantation assessment

Liver biopsy permits an accurate evaluation of fibrosis, iron, and chronic hepatitis with very limited risk of complications. Modern technologies (e.g., liver magnetic resonance imaging, liver transient elastography) offer the possibility of avoiding a liver biopsy; however, these technologies are not always available. The fibroscan has the potential to substitute of liver biopsy in diagnosing cirrhosis and fibrosis. Stage A cirrhosis (compensated) is not a contraindication to allogeneic transplantation. Positivity for hepatitis B and C virus is similarly not a contraindication to transplant nevertheless serologic tests for these infections should be performed. Hepatitis C virus (HCV) eradication can be considered prior to transplantation using available short-term highly effective treatments.

Should a spleenectomy be performed?

Many thalassemia patients have splenomegaly. Hypersplenism can complicate the post-transplant course by increasing the duration of cytopenia and the need for platelet and red blood cell transfusions. In a single, unconfirmed study these adverse post-transplant changes were minimized when spleenectomy was performed pre-transplant, although this procedure was also associated with a shortening in overall survival. Additional experience with this procedure is required before it can be routinely recommended. *Streptococcus pneumoniae* and *Neisseria meningitides* vaccination is recommended if spleenectomy is to be performed.

What about cardiac status?

Cardiac evaluation should include a 12 lead EKG, 24-h Holter monitor, and resting echocardiogram. More accurate diagnostic tests, such as cardiac T2* magnetic resonance imaging, can identify cardiac iron deposition and reductions in cardiac contractility in asymptomatic patients. However, these early alterations do not have a statistically significant influence on transplant outcome. A previous episode of heart failure does not represent an absolute contraindication to allo-HCT.

Endocrine assessment

A complete endocrine evaluation should be performed in patients older than 10 years of age to detect possible deficiencies induced by iron deposition in the pituitary, thyroid, and pancreas. This includes thyroid function tests, growth hormone releasing hormone stimulation test for hypothalamic-anterior pituitary function, and a fasting blood glucose. Sperm bank storage is recommended in male patients with normal semen analyses. The preservation of the ovarian parenchyma is now technically possible and feasible, and may be appropriate for some patients with thalassemia. The preservation of embryos obtained after *in vitro* fertilization is possible but is limited by law and ethical issues in several countries.

Sibling with thalassemia minor

Patient and donor hemoglobin synthesis (or genetic status) must be studied to identify the genetic status of the patient and of the donor (normal, thalassemia minor). A sibling with thalassemia minor can be an optimal bone marrow donor since the post-transplant course is similar to that from a normal donor, except for mild, asymptomatic, anemia, and microcytosis.

Transplant management

The transplantation approach for a nonmalignant disease is much different from transplantation in malignancies. In the former setting, the detrimental immunologic proprieties (i.e., GvH disease) of the engrafted hematopoietic cells are not balanced by an anti-malignancy effect. This characteristic must be always considered in determining the risk/benefit ratio and therapeutic decision such as the kind and intensity of the conditioning regimen, GvHD prophylaxis, source of hematopoietic cell, and adoptive post-transplant therapies.

The biological aspects of allogeneic transplantation in thalassemia are different from those for hematologic malignancies for the reasons presented in Table 28.4.

Outcome of graft source other than bone marrow in an HLA-MSD setting

The lack of a requirement for graft versus malignancy effect is the most likely reason for the predominant use of bone marrow as the graft source (Table 28.4). The use of PB instead of bone marrow as graft has been proposed to prevent graft failure given higher number of T-cells in the PB. Four studies report this type of transplant in

Table 28.3 Accepted and experimental donor approach to allo-HCT in thalassemia.

HLA-identical sibling	Accepted
HLA-identical sibling cord blood	Accepted
HLA-MUD HCT	Accepted
HLA-matched unrelated cord blood HCT	Experimental
HLA-mismatch related donor transplant	Experimental

Table 28.4 Specific aspect of allo-HCT in thalassemia to be considered in selection of graft and condition regimens.

No need to eradicate a malignant clone
Graft-versus-tumor effect is not required
Thalassemia patients have not received previous chemotherapy
Immunological system is not impaired

Table 28.5 Suggested conditioning regimens and GvHD prophylaxis regimens.

Risk Category	Conditioning Regimen	GvHD Prophylaxis
Low-risk	Busulfan iv. 3.2 mg/kg/day day −9, −8, −7, −6 Cyclophosphamide 50 mg/kg/day Day −5, −4, −3, −2 For unrelated transplants: ATG (dose 2 or 10 mg/kg depending from commercial product) day −5, −4, −2.	Cyclosporine 5 mg/kg iv in two divided doses. (oral cyclosporine on discharge) Methotrexate 10 mg/m^2 iv day +1, 7 mg/m^2 iv day +3, +6, + 11.
High-risk and adult patients	Thiotepa 8 mg/kg/day day −6 Treosulfan 14 g/m^2/day day −5, −4, −3. Fludarabine 40 mg/m^2/day day −5, −4, −3, −2 For unrelated transplants: ATG (dose 2 or 10 mg/kg/day depending from commercial product) day −5, −4, −2.	Cyclosporine 5 mg/kg iv in two divided doses. (oral cyclosporine on discharge) Methotrexate 10 mg/m^2 iv day +1, 7 mg/m^2 iv day +3, +6, + 11.

thalassemia. Overall, 886 patients receiving PB grafts have been described with substantially the same conclusions: the procedure is feasible in high-risk patients. One study showed some advantages of graft from PB but three studies showed an increased risk of chronic graft-versus-host disease (GvHD).

Myeloablative condition (MAC) regimen is preferred

Oral busulfan has been replaced by intravenous busulfan (BU) combined with cyclophosphamide (CY) in myeloablative dosages. The addition of azathioprine, hydroxyurea and fludarabine to the BU-CY regimen made an important contribution to improving the results in high-risk patients (high-risk Pesaro group and adults).

Over the last decade, new conditioning regimens for thalassemia patients have been introduced with improved results such as treosulfan associated with thiotepa and fludarabine.

To overcome TRM and morbidity, especially in high-risk Pesaro group and adult patients, reduced intensity conditioning (RIC) regimens have been tested. Although transplant-related toxicity was minimal, many patients showed only transient and incomplete engraftment. This is probably due to the expanded hematopoietic system in thalassemia patients. For this reason, the increased reliance on immunologic effects

that is required to sustain engraftment requires a prudent approach to the wider use of this regimen, and few experiences have been reported so far (see Table 28.5).

PRACTICE POINTS

A MAC regimen without irradiation should always be used. In case of BU-containing regimen, intravenous formulation should be used. RIC regimens are under investigation, to be used only in the context of clinical trials.

GvHD prophylaxis: Regimen and duration

The preferred GvHD prophylaxis in the majority of published studies of allo-HCT from MSDs consisted of cyclosporine and low-dose short-course methotrexate (4 doses intravenous (IV) on days +1, +3, +6, and +11 post-transplantation). The addition of ATG to this regimen has been used by few groups in HLA-identical sibling transplant recipients (MSD and sibling CBT) but is especially used in those transplanted from an unrelated volunteer or an HLA-partially matched relative. In this nonmalignant disease setting GvHD prophylaxis is usually maintained up to 1 year after transplantation with a slow cyclosporine tapering.

Follow-up evaluation post-transplant

Interpretation of chimerism and its implications

Early transient chimerism. Early (up to day 60 after transplant) chimerism is a risk factor for thalassemia recurrence in patients receiving bone marrow-derived grafts. An "early" engraftment greater than 90% is required for a high probability to obtain stable either full or mixed chimerism. This finding can be interpreted as a requirement for a "bulk" engraftment effect that is necessary to achieve a sustained, long-term engraftment (with either full or persistent mixed chimerism). How to manage this situation or how to manage declining donor chimerism is still the subject of intense debate, because the risk/benefit ratio of adoptive immunotherapy in these circumstances is controversial and the impact of host recovery is not well understood.

Late, persistent, chimerism. It has been demonstrated by different groups that a significant group of patients (approximately 11%) develop long-term, stable mixed chimerism after transplantation. Mixed chimeric patients, despite a limited (even 20%) engraftment, achieve a functioning graft status characterized by normal hemoglobin level, no red blood cell transfusion requirement, no iron increment, and a limited, not clinically relevant, erythroid hyperplasia. Because thalassemia is not a malignant disease, mixed chimerism is not a clinical problem per se.

This phenomenon is likely due to the selective advantage of the erythroid lineage cells derived from the transplanted graft that, despite constituting the minority of the marrow cells, are capable of providing a normal number of circulating red cells bearing normal hemoglobin. In these patients, it has been demonstrated a predominant erythroid engraftment in the peripheral blood while the proportion of erythroid precursors (burst forming unit erythroid colonies) and nucleated cells of donor origin in the bone marrow were equivalent.

Immunologically, mixed chimera patients had normal lymphoid subset distribution, normal response to mitogens stimulation, normal response to allogeneic antigens, and normal cytotoxicity activity. In animal models, mixed chimera is associated with reduced susceptibility to GvHD, probably through a mechanism of central tolerance with negative selection of host-reactive donor T-cells.

Thus, in chimeric patients, the genetic disease is under a substantially complete clinical control, without achieving complete eradication of the thalassemic hematopoietic clones.

Mixed chimera remains an extremely interesting and fascinating biological observation, which is not immediately applicable as a target for future medical treatments.

PRACTICE POINTS

Early mixed chimerism is a risk factor for thalassemia recurrence. Late-stable chimerism can occur in a significant percentage of patients and led to clinical control of the disease if allogeneic nucleated cells constitute at least 20% of the bone marrow cells.

Follow-up of chimerism

Chimerism should controlled before day 60. In patients with mixed chimera, chimerism should be checked at least every 3–6 months up to the second year of follow-up. After this time point wider interval can be considered. In patients with full engraftment (100% donor cells), no routine chimerism control is necessary after the second year.

Second transplant

A second transplant can be proposed to patients starting at least 2 years after the first transplant. However, second transplants are associated with higher rates of thalassemia recurrence and mortality and, under standard conditions, is not recommended in a nonmalignant disease.

Other important management aspects after allo-HCT

Post-transplant care should take into account:
1 Transplant-related complication (usual transplant follow-up).
2 Thalassemia related complication follow-up.

Follow-up should be performed in strict collaboration between a transplant physician and an hemoglobinopathies expert physician.

Iron overload: Still an issue

There is no reason to expect that transplant will eliminate the excess iron acquired during years of thalassemia. Persistence of tissue iron overload can cause significant morbidity and mortality,

Progression of liver disease to cirrhosis has been documented in some patients in the years after allo-HCT. Thus, iron removal by phlebotomy or chelation is indicated in all transplanted thalassemia patients who have evidence of iron overload. All patients with a hepatic iron concentration within the range associated with complications (i.e., 3–15 mg/g dry weight) should be treated for iron overload. Patients with a greater degree of iron overload (hepatic iron concentration exceeding 15 mg/g dry weight) should be intensively treated.

Because of the presence of normal erythropoiesis following successful transplantation, phlebotomy is the preferred mechanism to remove excess iron. Phlebotomy is safe, inexpensive, and highly efficient. Phlebotomy can be started once engraftment is sustained.

The general phlebotomy protocol that we use consists of the following steps:

- 6 mL/kg of blood is withdrawn every 14 days.
- Phlebotomy is not performed if the hemoglobin is <9.5 g/dL or the systolic blood pressure is <85–90 mmHg.
- Laboratory testing includes a complete blood count before each phlebotomy, liver and kidney function testing at baseline and then every 3 months, and serum ferritin every 2 months.

In transplanted thalassemia undergoing phlebotomy iron can be completely removed (serum ferritin concentration <100 ng/mL). At this point, patients are free from iron overload and no maintenance therapy is required. Duration of treatment is directly correlated with the magnitude of the iron overload, and ranges from a few months to several years.

In the majority of transplanted thalassemia patients, reduction in or normalization of the iron pool results in marked improvement in serum levels of liver enzymes and in the histological activity index. Patients with early cardiac involvement, characterized by systolic and/or diastolic dysfunction, show complete regression of these subclinical cardiac abnormalities after iron depletion.

Although very well tolerated in the majority of patients, phlebotomy can lead to some, usually mild, adverse effects (mild and spontaneously reversible thrombocytopenia and anemia, low blood pressure).

In patients with high iron levels who cannot be treated with phlebotomies, daily subcutaneous administration of deferoxamine can reduce iron stores. Two oral iron chelators, Deferiprone and Deferasirox have been used in iron-overload patients with thalassemia major but only Deferasirox has been tested after transplantation. Reported cases of deferiprone-induced neutropenia raise concern for its use in the post-transplant setting. Limited experience has been developed with Deferasirox without evidence of significant side effects. Advantages of treatment with Deferasirox consists on possibility of an early start (early suppression of the "toxic free iron forms"), home, oral, therapy with very limited hospital access, and the possibility to treat anemic patients. Of course, any cost issue does not favor Deferasirox therapy (see Table 28.6).

Chronic hepatitis and liver fibrosis

Hepatitis C virus infection is common in thalassemia patients, particularly in those transfused before second generation ELISA tests became available for detecting

Table 28.6 Iron overload – Treatment after allo-HCT.

Phlebotomy 6 ml/kg whole blood every 14 days
Deferoxamine 20–40 mg/kg is a valid alternative to phlebotomy for heavily iron loaded patients
Deferasirox 10–20 mg/kg (once day oral administration) is efficacy and safe but still limited experience (7–14 mg/kg with the new formulation already released in few countries)

HCV in donated blood. Chronic HCV infection is associated with chronic hepatitis, cirrhosis, and, in some patients with cirrhosis, hepatocellular carcinoma. Preliminary observations have also suggested that removal of excess iron and treatment of chronic HCV infection would be most effective in preventing (and in some instances even reversing) liver fibrosis and cirrhosis thus preventing hepatocellular carcinoma. New, recently developed very efficient therapy could clearly facilitate HCV treatment.

Endocrine dysfunction

Hypogonadism is the most common endocrine disorder in medically treated patients with thalassemia major, involving >50% of the patients. The two major risk factors for hypogonadism in transplanted thalassemics are iron overload and the conditioning regimen. In a series involving 50 thalassemia patients transplanted before puberty (mean age 11 years), 40% entered puberty normally despite the usual presence of clinical and hormonal evidence of hypogonadism.

Preliminary observations of young children transplanted in the early phase of thalassemia indicate a good prognosis for growth and fertility. Several normal and spontaneous paternity/maternity 3–12 years after allogeneic transplantation have been reported. Impaired glucose tolerance and diabetes mellitus are common complications of iron overload. They do not appear to be worsened by transplantation.

PRACTICE POINTS

Follow-up should be performed in strict collaboration between a transplant physician and an expert physician in hemoglobinopathies. Iron removal by phlebotomy and/or chelation is indicated in all transplanted thalassemic patients with iron overload. Preventing progression of liver damage to cirrhosis must be a primary goal (e.g., removal of excess iron and treatment of HCV infection). Hypogonadism is the most common endocrine disorder in medically treated patients with thalassemia major. Impaired glucose tolerance and diabetes mellitus are common complications of iron overload.

Table 28.7 The who, when, and how of allo-HCT for thalassemia.

Authors' practice:

A. *PATIENT FACTORS:*

All patients affected by transfusion dependent thalassemia are potential candidate to allogeneic hemopoietic cell transplantation. However, in absence of randomized clinical trial comparing transplantation to medical therapy decision is individualized.

Age:

Excellent results have been reported in pediatric patients with a widely reproduced OS and TFS of 82–96% and 74–86%, respectively. Less satisfactory results have been reported in adult patients (OS and TFS of 80 and 76%, respectively). However, in adult patients, experience in the last decade after understanding iron pathophysiology and implementation of modern chelation treatment is limited.

Risk factors for transplant outcome:
B. *DISEASE FACTORS:*

Even if a recent large retrospective registry study showed decreasing outcome result after the age of 14 years of age is not a risk factor per se in pediatric patients. Iron overload and tissue derived iron overload have been demonstrated to be significant risk factor for transplant outcome. Thus, long life optimal transfusion and chelation therapy is the key for a successful transplant. For patients belonging to the Pesaro low risk category, a >90% of transplant success is predicted.

C. *DONOR EVALUATION:*

A thalassemia minor can be an optimal allo-HCT donor.
Source of graft: Bone marrow or cord blood (HLA-identical sibling) derived cell are preferred. Peripheral blood graft should be avoided
Large experience has been reported with HLA-identical sibling transplantation. A HLA-MUD at all A, B, C, DRB1 loci using high-resolution typing can be considered as donor in the absence of HLA-identical sibling (either MSD or cord blood).
Alternative donor: **HLA-matched** unrelated umbilical cord blood, haploidentical, or antigen-mismatched donors are experimental approaches to be considered with caution.

D. *CONDITIONING THERAPY AND TRANSPLANT MANAGEMENT:*

The transplantation approach for a nonmalignant disease is much different from transplantation in malignancies. This characteristic must be always considered in determining the risk/benefit ratio and therapeutic decision such as the kind and intensity of the conditioning regimen, GvHD prophylaxis, source of hemopoietic graft and adoptive post-transplant therapies (Table 28.4).
In pre-transplant work up all the possible consequence of transfusion therapy must be checked.
Fully myeloablative regimens without radiotherapy is the standard in all patients (Table 28.5).

E. *POST-ALLOTRANSPLANT THERAPY:*

Early mixed chimerism is a risk factor for thalassemia recurrence.
Late-stable chimerism led to clinical control of the disease if allogeneic nucleated cells constitute at least 20% of the bone marrow cells.
Long-term follow-up after successful transplant should be performed in strict collaboration between a transplant and an hemoglobinopathy expert physician.
In case of thalassemia recurrence, a second transplant is usually not recommended.

Long-term health-related quality of life

A recent cross-sectional quality of life study has been recently performed in over 100 thalassemics who had undergone transplantation in the 1980s and 1990s, mainly in Pesaro. The long-term health-related quality of life (QoL) of transplanted thalassemic patients was similar to that of the general population and better respect to a matched thalassemia population receiving transfusion and chelation therapy. Mental health, education level, employment status, marital status, living arrangements, and birth rate were compatible with normal living patterns. As expected, presence of comorbidities (osteoporosis, impaired thyroid function, major fertility issues, amenorrhea, liver disease, hypertension) at the time of the survey and those living alone had worse QoL total scores.

Development of chronic GvHD and an older age at the time of transplantation were important factors for impairment of QoL.

> **PRACTICE POINTS**
>
> The long-term health-related QoL of transplanted thalassemic patients was similar to that of the general population.

Selected reading

1. Angelucci E, Matthes-Martin S, Baronciani D et al. Hematopoietic stem cell transplantation in thalassemia major and sickle cell disease: indications and management recommendations from an international expert panel. *Haematologica* 2014; **99**: 811–820.

2. Angelucci E, Muretto P, Nicolucci A et al. Phlebotomy to reduce iron overload in patients cured of thalassemia by bone marrow transplantation. *Italian Cooperative Group for Phlebotomy Treatment of Transplanted Thalassemia Patients Blood* 1997; **90**: 994–998.

3. Angelucci E. Hematopoietic stem cell transplantation in thalassemia. Hematology Am Soc Hematol Educ Program 2010; 456–462.

4. Baronciani D, Angelucci E, Potschger U, et al. Hemopoietic stem-cell transplantation in thalassemia: A Report from European Society for Blood and Bone Marrow Transplantation Hemoglobinopathy Registry, 2000–2010. *Bone Marrow Transplantation* 2016; **51**(4): 536–541.

5. Bertaina A, Merli P, Rutella S et al. HLA-haploidentical stem cell transplantation after removal of αβ+T and B cells in children with malignant disorders. *Blood* 2014; **124**: 822–826.

6. Locatelli F, Kabbara N, Ruggeri A et al. Outcome of patients with hemoglobinopathies given either cord blood or bone marrow transplantation from an HLA-identical sibling. *Blood* 2013; **122**: 1072–1078.

7. Lucarelli G, Galimberti M, Polchi P et al Bone marrow transplantation in patients with thalassemia. *N Engl J Med* 1990; **322**: 417–421.

CHAPTER 29

Fanconi anemia

Flore Sicre de Fontbrune[1], Jean Soulier[2], and Regis Peffault de Latour[1]

[1] Hematology Transplant Unit, Saint-Louis Hospital, APHP, and National French Reference Center for Bone Marrow Failure, Paris, France

[2] Hematology Laboratory, Saint-Louis Hospital, APHP, University Paris Diderot; and INSERM U944/CNRS UMR7212, University Institute of Hematology, and National French Reference Center for Bone Marrow Failure, Paris, France

Introduction

Fanconi anemia (FA) is caused by a genetic defect in one of the genes of a common DNA repair signaling pathway, the FA/BRCA biological pathway. Seventeen FA genes have been identified: all but one (FANCB located on the chromosome X) are autosomic and responsible for recessive diseases.

FA is characterized by different clinical stages related to age:
- In early childhood, mainly physical signs are present and variable,
- Bone marrow failure usually appears between 5 and 15 years,
- During the second and third decades, myelodysplastic syndromes, acute myeloblastic leukemia, as well as solid tumors develop.

The FA/BRCA biological pathway dysfunction is characterized by an exquisite sensitivity to agents causing DNA interstrand crosslinks (including some chemotherapies and radiotherapy).

Allogeneic hematopoietic cell transplantation (allo-HCT) is the only curative therapy when patients developed bone marrow failure or hematological malignancies, however it is associated with a high risk of severe toxicities and do not prevent solid tumors occurrence. All allo-HCT procedures, especially the conditioning regimen, have to be adapted to the FA patient.

Until the late 1990s, allo-HCT was essentially performed during the first or second decades. Due to the increased recognition of the disease heterogeneity, the improvement of supportive care and the progress in allo-HCT in FA (especially with unrelated donors), a significant number of allo-HCTs are actually performed during adulthood in FA patients.

Historical perspective of allo-HCT in FA

The first transplant in FA was performed in the 1970s. Early in the 1980s, it became evident that allo-HCT in FA was associated with unacceptable toxicities when performed with the same conditioning regimen than other bone marrow failure. The link with the chemosensitivity to alkylating agent and radio sensitivity of FA patient cells was rapidly identified, and adapted conditioning regimen with low-dose cyclophosphamide with or without low-dose radiotherapy have been proposed since 1983. In HLA-matched related donor HCT, it allows engraftment in the majority of patients with low early toxicity. However, the long-term follow-up of these protocols revealed high incidence of chronic GvHD in these patients with a significant impact on the long-term overall survival. Notably FA patients with chronic GvHD experienced more frequent and earlier second solid cancers. The use of T-cell depletion (TCD) was concomitantly reported to have a positive impact on overall survival.

In 1997, the use of fludarabine in FA conditioning regimen was first reported. During the last decade, a lot

---

Clinical Manual of Blood and Bone Marrow Transplantation, First Edition. Edited by Syed A. Abutalib and Parameswaran Hari.
© 2017 John Wiley & Sons Ltd. Published 2017 by John Wiley & Sons Ltd.

of small unicentric studies have reported a favorable outcome after fludarabine based conditioning regimens with or without *in vivo* TCD. Finally, the use of fludarabine based conditioning regimen was demonstrated to be associated with a better overall survival (OS) in HLA-matched related donor (MRD) allo-HCT in large retrospective studies. The estimated 5 years OS is actually over 90% in this setting. The main studies are summarized in Table 29.1 and 29.2.

Until the last decade, outcome of matched unrelated donor allo-HCT remained poor with an estimated OS of 30% at 5 years despite the use of reduce intensity conditioning regimens. This was mainly due to the high incidence of primary and secondary graft failure (20–25%) and the mortality associated with acute and chronic GvHD in this setting. However, new conditioning regimen combining low-dose cyclophosphamide, low-dose TBI, fludarabine, and *in vivo* or *in vitro* TCD improved engraftment rate and decrease TRM. Most recent studies including patient transplanted from 2000 report OS ranging from 70 to 95%. The main studies are summarized in Tables 29.1 and 29.3. Excellent outcome with haploidentical donor have been recently report with similar conditioning regimen and T depleted PBSC but the cohort of patients is small precluding conclusion.

Allo-HCT for FA patients: Appropriate candidate and timing

Allo-HCT is recommended in case of bone marrow failure when transfusions are required as the number of red cell and platelets transfusion before allo-HCT has been demonstrated to have an impact on OS after transplant. Clonal evolution (myelodysplastic syndrome or leukemia) is also an indication of allo-HCT, whereas the appearance of cytogenetic abnormalities alone is not considered yet as a formal indication. However, the risk of hematological malignancies is higher in patients with than without cytogenetic abnormalities (excepted for +1q and del 20q) and these patients have to be followed carefully with regular marrow aspirations (especially when 3q, 7q, and 21q/RUNX1 abnormalities are identified).

Younger age of the recipient (<10 years) at the time of transplant has been reported to be a positive prognostic factor; however, in patients with *moderate* AA that do not required transfusion or G-CSF, a watch and wait attitude could be reasonably chosen if a careful follow-up is feasible.

PRACTICE POINTS

- Bone marrow aspiration with cytogenetic analysis has to be performed at least yearly in patients not transplanted, with a special attention to 3q, 7q and 21q/RUNX1 abnormalities.
- Androgens should be avoided before transplant, as well as long-term G-CSF use.

What is the consensus on conditioning regimen and GvHD prophylaxis for allo-HCT in patients with FA?

Conditioning regimens should be modified in FA patients to avoid toxicity, graft failure, and acute and chronic GvHD.

- Low-dose cyclophosphamide (20–40 mg/kg) associated with fludarabine with or without *in vitro/in vivo* TCD could be recommended based on the recently published series.
- Low-dose TBI (2–3 Gy) is recommended by some authors when the risk of graft failure is high (with unrelated donor notably).
- The choice of *in vitro* or *in vivo* TCD is actually a matter of debates: however, in the largest retrospective study, *in vitro* TCD was associated with a higher rate of graft failure.
- Based on the risk of extensive chronic GvHD, bone marrow should be used preferentially as hematopoietic graft.
- GvHD prophylaxis is usually based on cyclosporine associated or not with mycophenolate mofetil. Short course methotrexate should not be used due to the high rate of mucositis.

PRACTICE POINTS

- Fludarabine and low-dose cyclophosphamide based regimens are recommended.
- *In vitro* or *in vivo* TCD is recommended to avoid chronic graft-versus-host disease in unrelated donor transplantation (and for some authors should also be added in related donor transplantation).
- Low-dose TBI is recommended in some centers in unrelated donor allo-HCT due to the high rate of graft failure.
- Bone marrow is preferred graft source.

Table 29.1 Studies analyzing outcomes of HLA-match related donor transplantation in FA.

Author	N	Disease at HCT	Donor	Conditioning	Graft Failure	cGvHD	TRM	OS	Comments and Practice Implications
Benajiba (2004–2013)	20	AA 90% Chr abn 10%	MRD (BM 80%, CB 20%)	Flu 90, Cy 40*, ATG	0	25%	5%	2 y: 95%	Excellent outcome.
Ayas (1995–2011)	94	AA 89% MDS/AML 11%	MRD 94% MMRD 6%	Cy 60* + ATG or Cy + TBI + ATG or Cy 40* + Flu + ATG	4.3%	8.5%	na	10 y: 86%	Fludarabine based CR associated with better OS (92%), lower graft failure. Lower cGvHD in non-TBI group.
Pasquini (1991–2001)	148	AA 95% AML 5%	MRD (BM)	TBI + Cy +/- ATG, Cy +/- Bu/flu +/- ATG	na	18% in TBI CR and 24% in non-TBI	Early 3%	5 y: 78% in TBI and 81% in non-TBI	CMV + recipients, age >>10 y, androgens prior allo-HCT, and GvHD associated with worse OS.
Farzin (1987–2003)	35	AA 86% Chr abn 9% MDS 5%	MRD (BM 91% or CB)	Cy 20* + TAI + ATG or Cy 40* + TBI + ATG	6%	12%	Early 6%	10 y: 89%	Low cGvHD CI with high dose ATG.
Socié (1981–1996)	50	AA 90% MDS 10%	MRD (BM 92% or CB)	Cy 40* and TAI	8%	70%	2%	4 y 74% and 8 y 58%	cGvHD and > 20 blood products before allo-HCT associated with worse OS.

Abbreviations: TRM, Treatment related mortality; OS, Overall survival; cGvHD, chronic graft-versus-host disease; AA, Aplastic anemia; MDS, Myelodysplastic syndrome; Chr abn, chromosomal abnormalities; AML, Acute myeloid leukemia; MRD, Matched Related Donor; MMRD, MisMatched Related Donor; BM, Bone marrow; CB, Cord blood; PBHC, Peripheral blood hematopoietic cell; Cy, Cyclophosphamide; Flu, Fludarabine; Bu, Busulfan; ATG, Anti-Thymocyte Globulins; TBI, Total body irradiation; CR, conditioning regimen; y, year(s).

* indicate cyclophosphamide dosage in mg/kg

Table 29.2 Studies analyzing outcomes of HLA-matched related and HLA-unrelated donor transplantation in FA.

Author	N	Disease at HCT	Donor	Conditioning	Graft Failure	cGvHD	TRM	OS	Comments and Practice Implications
Peffault (1972–2010)	795	AA 93% MDS/AML 7%	MRD (59%) URD (41%)	Various	11%	19%		5 y 65% 10 y 52% 20 y 36%	AA, no ex vivo TD and flu CR associated with engraftment. MRD, graft after 2000, and MRD associated with OS. CI of secondary malignancies in long-term survivor is 34% at 20 y (RF = PBHC, cGvHD, age > 10 y and clonal evolution).
Locatelli (1989–2005)	64		MRD 44%, URD 40%, MMRD 11% (BM 81%, CB 10 % or TD-PBHC 9%)	Flu, Cy +/– TBI	4%	26%	8y: 33% (MRD: 14%)	8y: 67% (87% in MRD & 40% in URD). OS with & without flu: 86 and 59%	Flu CR and MRD associated with better OS.
Gluckman (1978–1994)	199	AA	MRD 76% URD 24% (BM)	TBI/LFI+Cy 15–25* +/– ATG or Cy 100* +/– ATG	MRD: 8% URD: 24%	MRD 44% and URD 46%	na	2 y: 66% in MRD and 29% in URD	Age <10 y, low-dose Cy, and LFI associated with better OS.

Abbreviations: TRM, Treatment related mortality; OS, Overall survival; cGvHD, chronic graft-*versus*-host disease; AA, Aplastic anemia; MDS, Myelodysplastic syndrome; Chr abn, chromosomal abnormalities; AML, Acute myeloid leukemia; MRD, Matched related donor; URD, Unrelated donor; MMRD, MisMatched related donor; TD-, T-cell depleted-; BM, Bone Marrow; CB, Cord blood; PBHC, Peripheral blood hematopoietic cell; Cy, Cyclophosphamide; Flu, Fludarabine; ATG, Anti-thymocyte globulins; TBI, Total body irradiation; CR, conditioning regimen; y, year(s); RF, Risk factors.
* indicate cyclophosphamide dosage in mg/kg

Table 29.3 Studies analyzing outcomes of HLA-matched unrelated or HLA-mismatch related donor transplantation.

Author (Inclusion Period)	N Total	Disease at HCT	Donor	Conditioning	Graft Failure	cGvHD	TRM	OS	Comments and Practice Implications
Macmillan (1995–2012)	130	AA 92% MDS/AML 8%	URD & MMRD (TD-BM or CB)	Cy 40*, TBI (6.5, 4 or 3 Gy), ATG +/- Fluda	na	10%	na	5 y: 58% 10 y: 57%	Fludarabine in conditioning associated with OS. 5 y OS = 94% in Cy, Flu, ATG, TBI 3 Gy
Chaudhury (1995–2005)	18	AA 44% MDS 22% AML 34%	URD & MMRD (TD-PBHC or BM)	Cy 40*, TBI 4.5 Gy, ATG/campath	0	5%	Day 100: 65% in non- and 24% in fluda based CR		Androgens prior to HCT associated with worse OS
Wagner (1990–2003)	98	AA 77% MDS 14% AML 7%	URD (TD-BM and BM)	Non-flu (53%) and flu based (47%) with Cy +/- TAI/TBI +/- ATG	na	31%	3 y: 47% in flu and 81% in non-fluda	3 y: 52% in flu and 13% in non-flu	Non-flu CR, CMV+ recipients, age >10 y, > 20 blood products before HCT associated with worse OS
Guardiola (1985–1998)	69	AA 84% MDS 12% AML 4%	URD (BM)	Cy 20–40, TBI/TAI +/- ATG	Primary 20% & secondary 19%	42%	3 y: 33%		CMV+ recipients, female donor, malformations, and androgens before HCT are associated with worse OS

Abbreviations: TRM, Treatment Related Mortality; OS, Overall Survival; GvHD, Graft-versus-Host Disease; AA, Aplastic Anemia; MDS, Myelodysplastic Syndrome; AML, Acute Myeloid Leukemia; URD, Unrelated Donor; MMRD, MisMatched Related Donor; TD-, T-cell depleted-; BM, Bone Marrow, PBHC, Peripheral Blood Stem Cell; Cy, Cyclophosphamide; Flu, Fludarabine; ATG, Anti-Thymocyte Globulins; TBI, Total body irradiation; CR, conditioning regimen; y, year(s).
* indicate cyclophosphamide dosage in mg/kg

Hematologic malignancies in FA patients: Should chemotherapy be performed before allo-HCT?

Conventional HCT in patients with clonal abnormalities is associated with higher graft failure and a 25% risk of relapse. There are a few detailed reports on chemotherapy before transplant in FA with myelodysplastic syndromes and acute myeloid leukemia. Most of them are associated with grade III–IV non-hematological toxicities and/or persistent aplasia and the response rate seems low. A strategy of sequential chemotherapy with cytarabine and fludarabine followed by fludarabine based reduced intensity conditioning have been recently published with an excellent outcome (2 years OS: 100%). This strategy could be proposed when blast excess is observed. The role of demethylating agents has not been evaluated neither has targeted therapy been. Mains studies are summarized in Table 29.4.

> **PRACTICE POINTS**
> - Chemotherapy is associated with high rate of extra-hematological toxicities and persistent bone marrow failure in FA patients with hematological malignancies.
> - Sequential strategy with chemotherapy and RIC could be proposed when marrow blast count is over 10% before transplant.

Long-term follow-up after allo-HCT in FA patients: Challenges?

- FA is associated with an exceptionally high rate of solid tumors that are mainly reported during the third and fourth decades.
- After allo-HCT, relative risk of solid tumors is increased by a factor 4. This is incompletely explained by the extension of the risk period in this subgroup of patients cured for their hematopoietic disease. Notably, solid tumors occur at a younger aged after allo-HCT and more frequently in patients that have experienced chronic GvHD.
- The commonest solid tumors are head and neck squamous cell carcinoma, vulvar carcinoma, and skin carcinoma. Human papilloma virus is suspected to play a role in some case (vulvar, anal, and cervical tumors); however, the preventive role of HPV vaccine is not yet demonstrated.

- FA allo-HCT recipients should frequently be evaluated by specialists (especially head and neck tumors specialists and gynecologist) familiar with FA. Owing to the high sensibility of FA tissue to chemotherapy and radiotherapy, thus surgical resection of localized tumors is the only available efficient therapy in this subgroup of patient.

> **PRACTICE POINTS**
> - Solid tumors are responsible of the high rate of delayed mortality after allo-HCT in FA patients.
> - Head, neck, vulvar, and cervical tumors are the more frequent.
> - Screening of tumors by specialists is essential to allow early diagnosis and surgical cure.
> - Chemotherapy and radiotherapy dosage should be adapted to the FA tissue sensitivity.

High yield points

- Allo-HCT is the only curative therapy for hematological disease in FA patients (bone marrow failure and clonal evolution such as AML and MDS).
- Conditioning regimens based on fludarabine, low-dose cyclophosphamide associated with *in vivo* or *in vitro* TCD allowed a dramatic improvement both with matched related and unrelated donors during the last decade.
- Best results are obtained in patients before clonal evolution and before 20 blood-product infusions.
- The role of chemotherapy before allo-HCT in patients with clonal evolution and blast excess is not elucidated yet.
- Solid tumors are the main challenge in long-term survivors after allo-HCT, especially when chronic GvHD occurs.
- Careful screening to allow early diagnosis of surgically curable tumors is actually the only curative option.
- Whether new conditioning regimens without radiotherapy and but using *in vivo/in vitro* TCD will decreased the incidence of solid tumors is actually unknown due to shorter follow-up of these studies.

Follow-up before and after allo-HCT

The authors propose the algorithm in Figure 29.1 for FA patients.

Table 29.4 Transplantation in FA patients with chromosomal abnormalities or hematological malignancies.

Author	N	Disease at allo-HCT	Donor	Conditioning	Graft failure	cGvHD	TRM	OS	Comments & practice implications
Talbot (2006–2011)	6	AML 5 MDS 1	URD (BM 3 & CB 3)	Flu 150 mg/m² cytarabine 10 g/m² followed by Flu 120 mg/m² Cy 40* ATG and TBI 2 Gy	0	17%	0	2y: 100%	No relapse and no TRM.
Mitchell (1988–2011)	20	AML 12 MDS 8 T ALL 1	MRD 2 MMRD 1 URD 12 CB 6 (TD-BM)	Bu + Flu + Cy + ATG or TBI + Flu + Cy + ATG (chemotherapy in 8 before allo-HCT)	5%	19%	na	5 y: 33%	Chemotherapy before HCT: failure in 67%, grade 3 to 4 toxicities in 75%. Relapse in 24% post allo-HCT.
Ayas (1985–2007)	113	Chr abn 48% MDS 40% AML 12%	MRD 74% URD 26% (BM 75%, PBHC 12%, CB 13%)	Radiation based 60%, flu based 27%. ATG in 50%	24%	23%		5 y: 55% (chr abn 67% and MDS/AML 43%)	OS is better in patients younger than 14 y, with MRD, and only chr abn.

Abbreviations: TRM, Treatment related mortality; OS, Overall survival; cGvHD, chronic graft-*versus*-host disease; AA, Aplastic anemia; MDS, Myelodysplastic syndrome; Chr abn, chromosomal abnormalities; AML, Acute myeloid leukemia; T ALL, T-cell Acute lymphoblastic leukemia; MRD, Matched related donor; URD, Unrelated donor; MMRD, MisMatched related donor; TD-, T-cell depleted-; BM, Bone marrow; CB, Cord blood; PBHC, Peripheral blood hematopoietic cell; Cy, Cyclophosphamide; Flu, Fludarabine; ATG, Anti-thymocyte globulins; TBI, Total body irradiation; CR, conditioning regimen; y, year(s); RF, Risk factors.
* indicate cyclophosphamide dosage in mg/kg

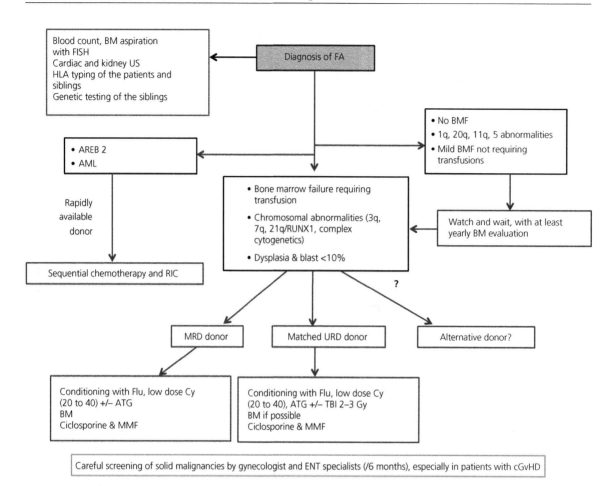

Figure 29.1 Algorithm for FA patients. Abbreviations: FA, Fanconi anemia; BM, Bone marrow; FISH, Fluorescence in situ hybridization; US, Ultra-Sonography; BMF, Bone marrow failure; AREB2, Refractory anemia with blast excess 2; AML, Acute myeloid leukemia; RIC, Reduced Intensity conditioning; MRD, Matched related donor; URD, Unrelated donor; BM, Bone marrow; ATG, Anti-thymocyte globulins; Cy, Cyclophosphamide; Flu, Fludarabine; TBI, Total body irradiation; MMF, Mycophenolate Mofetil; cGvHD, chronic GvHD.

Selected reading

1. Gluckman E, Auerbach AD, Horowitz MM, Sobocinski KA and Gale RP. Bone marrow transplantation for Fanconi anemia. *Blood*, 1995;**86**(7):2856–2862. PMID:7670120.
2. Locatelli F, Zecca M, Pession A, Morreale G and Messiona C. The outcome of children with Fanconi anemia given hematopoietic stem cell transplantation and the influence of fludarabine in the conditioning regimen: a report from the Italian pediatric group. *Haematologica*, 2007;**92**(10):1381–1388. PMID:18024375
3. Peffault de Latour R, Procher R, Dalle JH, Aljurf M and Dufour C. Allogeneic hematopoietic stem cell transplantation in Fanconi anemia: the European group for Blood and Marrow Transplantation experience. *Blood*, 2013;**122**(26):4279–4286. PMID:24144640
4. Ayas M, Siddiqui K, Al-Jefri A, El-Solh H and Al-Seraihy A. Factors affecting the outcome of related allogeneic

hematopoietic transplantation in patients with fanconi Anemia. *BBMT*, 2014;**20**(10):1599–1603. PMID: 24960628.
5. MacMillan ML, DEFor TE, Young JA and Wagner JE. Alternative donor hematopoietic stem cell transplantation for Fanconi Anemia. *Blood*, 2015;**125**(24):3798–3804. PMID:25824692.
6. Socié G, Devergie A, Girinski T, Piel G and Gluckman E. Transplantation for Fanconi's anaemia: long-term follow-up of fifty patients trasnplanted from a sibling donor after low-dose cyclophosphamide and thoraco-abdominal irradiation for conditioning. *BJH*, 1998;**103**(1):249–255. PMID 9792317
7. Guardiola P, Pasquini R, Dokal I, Ortega JJ and Gluckman E. Outcome of 69 allogeneic stem cell transplantations for Fanconi anemia using HLA-matched unrelated donors: a study on behalf of the European Group for Blood and Marrow Trasnplantation. *Blood*, 2000; **95**(2):422–449. PMID:10627445
8. Chaudhury S, Auerbach AD, Krnan NA, Small TN and Boulad F. Fludarabine-based cytoreductive regimen

and T-cell-depleted grafts from alternative donors for the treatment of high-risk patients with Fanconi anaemia. *BJH*, 2008; **140**(6):644–655. PMID:18302713.

9. Pasquini R, Carreras J, Pasquini MC, Camitta BM and Wagner JE. HLA-matched sibling haematopoietic stem cell trasnplantation for fanconi anemia: comparison of irradiation and nonirradiation containing regimens. *BBMT*, 2008;**14**(10):1141–1147. PMID:18804044.

10. Benajiba L, Salvado C, Dalle JH, Jubert C and Peffault de Latour R. HLA-matched related donor HSCT in Fanconi anemia patients conditioned with cyclophosphamide and fludarabine. *Blood*, 2015;**125**(2):417–418. PMID:25573976

11. Ayas M, Saber W, Davies SM, Harris RE and Gale RP. Allogeneic hematopoietic cell transplantation for fanconi anemia in patients with pretransplantation cytogenetic abnormalities, myelodysplastic syndrome, or acute leukemia. *JCO*, 2013;**31**(13):1669–1676. PMID:23547077

12. Mitchell R, Wagner JE, Hirsch B, DeFor TE and MacMillan ML. Haematopoietic cell transplantation for acute leukaemia and advanced myelodysplastic syndrome in Fanconi anaemia. *BJH*, 2014;**164**(3):384–395. PMID: 24172081.

13. Talbot A, Peffault de Latour R, Raffoux E, Buchbinder N and Socié G. Sequential treatment for allogeneic hematopoietic stem cell transplantation in Fanconi anemia with acute myeloid leukemia. *Haematologica*, 2014;**99**(10):e199–200. PMID:25085358.

14. Rosenberg PS, Socié G, Alter BP and Gluckman E. Cancer incidence in persons with Fanconi Anemia. *Blood*, 2005;**105**(1):67–73.

15. Wagner JE, Eapen M, MacMillan ML, Harris RE and Auerbach AD. Unrelated donor bone marrow transplantation for Fanconi anemia. *Blood*, 2007;**109**(5):2256–2262. PMID 17038525.

CHAPTER 30

Immunodeficiency disorders

Jennifer A. Kanakry and Dennis D. Hickstein

Experimental Transplantation and Immunology Branch, National Cancer Institute, National Institutes of Health, Bethesda, MD, USA

Introduction

Primary immunodeficiency diseases (PIDs) are a heterogeneous group of diseases that are hallmarked by an increased susceptibility to malignancy, infection, autoimmunity, atopy, and immune dysregulation. Thus, these diseases are often associated with significant morbidity and early mortality. To date, over 200 PIDs have been phenotypically, genetically, and molecularly described, and this number will continue to grow with the wider use of sophisticated genetic testing. As most PIDs are due to defects in cells of hematopoietic origin, allogeneic blood or marrow hematopoietic cell transplantation (allo-HCT) is a potentially curative approach for many of these diseases.

- Allo-BMT has the potential to reverse the manifestations of PIDs that are due to defects in hematopoietic cells
- For many PIDs, allo-HCT is the only potentially curative therapy available
- Some PIDs are very rare and/or newly described and the role of allo-HCT remains an area of active clinical research

Allo-HCTs for PID were first successfully performed in 1968 using HLA-matched sibling donors (MSDs), one in a child with X-linked, severe combined immune deficiency (SCID) and another in a child with Wiskott–Aldrich syndrome (WAS). At present, over 2,500 patients with PID have undergone allo-HCT, the majority of which are for the most common PIDs – SCID, WAS, and chronic granulomatous disease (CGD). While it is well established that allo-HCT can cure many patients with PIDs but many important questions remain regarding the optimal timing of transplant, conditioning approaches, the use of alternative donors, graft-versus-host disease (GvHD) prevention, and the approach to infectious complications remain the topics of ongoing clinical research.

Much has changed in the field over the past 50 years, including the following:
- High-resolution HLA typing
- Successful use of alternative donors, including HLA-haploidentical donors
- Improvements in GvHD prophylaxis
- Recognition that successful engraftment depends on adequate immunoablation of the host immune system, rather than myeloablation, with a shift to reduced-intensity or non-myeloablative conditioning strategies
- Advances in supportive care and the management/treatment of infectious complications

> **PRACTICE POINT**
>
> Allo-HCT is the treatment of choice for PIDs that are associated with significant morbidity and mortality related to immune defects.

> **PRACTICE POINT**
>
> Allo-BMT clearly has the potential to definitively correct defects within hematopoietic cells; the ability of allo-HCT to influence affected non-hematopoietic cells is much less certain (Table 30.1).

Clinical Manual of Blood and Bone Marrow Transplantation, First Edition. Edited by Syed A. Abutalib and Parameswaran Hari.
© 2017 John Wiley & Sons Ltd. Published 2017 by John Wiley & Sons Ltd.

Table 30.1 Overview of the role of allo-HCT for various PIDs. The table is not meant to be comprehensive, but rather give a general outline of the categories of PIDs where allo-HCT may or may not have efficacy, as well as special considerations for PIDs where other therapies exist, the phenotype is mild, or significant non-hematopoietic involvement limits the potential for full phenotype reversion with allo-HCT.

Categories of PIDs where allo-HCT is potentially curative	Examples of PIDs where allo-HCT may correct some, but not all, disease manifestations	Examples of PIDs where allo-HCT is unlikely to be curative because the defect is predominantly in cells of non-hematopoietic lineage	PIDs where effective, less risky therapies are available
Severe combined immunodeficiencies	**GATA2** – may not reverse lymphedema, hearing loss, vascular abnormalities (seen in some patients)	**Complement deficiencies** (possible exception: C1q deficiency) – proteins of the complement system are largely synthesized by hepatocytes	**Defects of vitamin B12 and folate metabolism** – vitamin supplementation may be sufficient
Combined immunodeficiencies less severe than SCID • WAS • CD40 ligand deficiency • MagT1 deficiency • DOCK8 deficiency • Activated PI3k-δ	**Short telomere syndromes/PIDs associated with DNA repair defects** – patients remain at high risk for solid tumor malignancies, radiosensitivity	**Immunodeficiency with multiple intestinal atresias** – often die at young age due to severe atresias	**Predominantly antibody deficiencies** – may be asymptomatic or only need immunoglobulin replacement
Defects of phagocyte number and/or function • Leukocyte adhesion deficiency • Chronic granulomatous disease • GATA2 deficiency	**NEMO** – colitis due to persistent defect in intestinal epithelial cells	**Type 1 interferonopathies** – progressive encephalopathy	**DiGeorge syndrome with complete athymia** – may benefit more from thymus transplant than allo-HCT
Diseases of severe immune dysregulation/familial hemo-phagocytic lymphohistiocytosis	**Cartilage hair hypoplasia** – skeletal issues/growth failure unaffected by allo-HCT	**Epidermodysplasia verruciformis** – major lineage affected is keratinocytes	**Auto-inflammatory disorders** – targeted blockade of inflammatory cytokines may be effective
Defects of innate immunity	**Familial HLH syndromes with hypopigmentation** – albinism not corrected		**Autosomal dominant hyper IgE syndrome** – multidisciplinary supportive care and immunomodulating agents may result in long-term survival for many

Timing – When do the benefits outweigh the risks?

SCID is a neonatal emergency, now typically diagnosed at birth through newborn screening initiatives. Aside from cases where enzyme replacement or gene therapy may be reasonable alternatives, SCID patients should undergo allo-HCT without delay, irrespective of HLA compatibility. Early intervention with allo-HCT before the onset of infection has unequivocally been associated with superior outcomes as compared to allo-HCT beyond a few months of age. At present, over 90% of SCID patients are cured by allo-HCT using HLA-matched related donors and outcomes with alternative donors are continuing to improve.

Other PIDs often do not manifest at birth. Some are characterized by a more progressive decline in immune function, with signs of the disease later in life. Patients often might not be diagnosed with PID until they have shown themselves to be vulnerable to a constellation of unusual infections, malignancies, autoimmunity, and atopy. Even non-hematologic, syndromic features that are characteristic of some PIDs may only become clinically apparent over time, or may be absent in certain patients. Importantly, the presence of a PID mutation does not directly predict the phenotype and severity of the disease. Genetic anticipation over generations can occur, such as in some of the telomere maintenance diseases, among others. Determining appropriate candidates for allo-HCT and the best time to transplant each individual patient remains a challenge; it is both difficult to subject a patient with few disease manifestations to the risks of transplant and difficult to successfully transplant a patient who has already has significant organ damage, active infections, or malignancy.

Compared to the more extensive experience with transplanting SCID, WAS, and CGD, there is less experience with allo-HCT for the rarer PIDs and outcomes can be variable. The growing knowledge of the natural history of many of these rare PIDs can help to inform decisions about transplant timing. In some cases, more conservative management without allo-HCT is sufficient to result in good disease control and long-term survival. Among transplanted PID patients, those with milder phenotype, absence of infection, better organ function, and younger age at the time of transplant often have better outcomes. For those with familial hemophagocytic lymphohistiocytosis (HLH), allo-HCT outcomes are best if patients are transplanted prior to the development of HLH and, among those who develop HLH, better when hemophagocytosis is controlled prior to transplant.

- Information regarding the natural history of specific PIDs, as well as allo-HCT outcomes across different platforms, will help inform risk/benefit analyses and decisions regarding the role and timing of transplant in these diseases.

> **PRACTICE POINT**
>
> Pre-transplant evaluations should include screening for active infection, uncontrolled autoimmunity, malignancy, viral reactivation, nutritional status, and organ dysfunction so that efforts can be made to optimize these factors prior to transplant if the clinical situation allows.

What are key differences between allo-HCT for PID and allo-HCT for malignancy?

1 GvHD is not beneficial

At the time of allo-HCT, most PID patients do not have an active hematologic malignancy and thus the success of the procedure does not depend upon an effective graft-*versus*-tumor (GvT) effect. By extension, PID patients derive no benefit from GvHD. As T-cells are central to the development of GvHD, removing or manipulating the T-cell composition of the graft can modulate GvHD risk. Various approaches to *ex vivo* or *in vivo* T-cell depletion (TCD) of grafts can be associated with very low rates of GvHD, making these approaches particularly promising for the transplantation of PID patients, where relapse of a hematologic malignancy is typically not a concern. However, it is important to note that some approaches to TCD are associated with high rates of infection, delayed immune reconstitution, graft failure, EBV-posttransplantation lymphoproliferative disorder (EBV-PTLD), and transplant-related mortality (TRM). More recent strategies that either selectively deplete T-cell subsets or "add-back" critical cell populations show the most promise for preventing GvHD while minimizing infectious complications and improving immune reconstitution. Some examples of selective depletion of T-cell subsets include *in vivo* depletion of alloreactive T-cells using high-dose post-transplantation cyclophosphamide or *ex vivo* T-cell receptor αβ/CD19 depletion. Both of these approaches are aimed at leaving cells critical for immune reconstitution, antiviral immunity, and engraftment in the graft, while largely depleting cells that mediate GvHD. CD34+ stem cell selection followed by add-back or after allo-HCT adoptive transfer of natural killer cells, mesenchymal stem cells, regulatory T-cells (Treg), or virus-specific cytotoxic T-cells are other approaches which may improve the balance between effective GvHD prevention and favorable immune reconstitution. Some of these approaches have been associated with very low rates of the complications seen with non-selectively T-cell depleted grafts, including EBV-PTLD, lethal infections, graft failure, and TRM.

- Allo-HCT approaches that have lower GvHD risk can be associated with increased risks of infection, graft failure, and delayed immune reconstitution.
2 Mixed/split chimerism may result in cure
   Unlike allo-HCT for hematologic malignancies where full donor chimerism is necessary, PID may be cured with mixed and/or split chimerism. Furthermore, mixed chimerism has been associated with lower rates of acute and chronic GvHD. Thus, for many PIDs, achieving mixed donor chimerism may be not only sufficient to cure the disease, but beneficial with respect to minimizing complications such as GvHD after allo-HCT.

Donor Selection – What to do when there is no HLA-matched sibling

An HLA-matched sibling remains the preferred allo-HCT donor given the low risk of GvHD and high rates of engraftment. As only ~25% of patients requiring allo-HCT have an HLA-matched sibling, this has historically been a major barrier in the field. Furthermore, in the case of PIDs, one must be careful to make sure that any related donor is not affected by the immunodeficiency, a task which becomes more difficult if the mutation is not identified. For patients without an unaffected, HLA-MSD, alternative donor options include unrelated donors from registries, HLA-haploidentical related donors, and umbilical cord blood units. Alternative donors make allo-HCT available to virtually any patient who requires the procedure, but can be associated with higher rates of GvHD, graft failure, and TRM. Much progress has been made with the use of alternative donors and some current approaches to alternative donor allo-HCT yield outcomes that approximate those with HLA-matched related donos.

If multiple alternative donors are available, additional factors to consider are donor age, blood type, availability for initial and future donations, viral serologies, parity, and the presence of anti-HLA donor-specific antibodies. If multiple HLA-haploidentical related donors are available, the degree of mismatch of the non-shared haplotype can be considered. Additional considerations include the avoidance, when possible, of female donors for male recipients, given the increased risk of GvHD due to alloreactivity against the HY minor histocompatibility antigen. In the future, non-HLA factors, such as killer cell immunoglobulin-like receptor ligand mismatch and others, may factor into decisions regarding donor selection.

- While HLA-MSD are preferred, advances in allo-HCT have resulted in comparably favorable outcomes for recipients of alternative donor grafts

> **PRACTICE POINTS**
>
> Patients with PIDs associated with significant morbidity and mortality risk should be considered for allo-HCT even when a HLA-MSD is not available. Related donors for PID patients should be carefully screened for the immunodeficiency, ideally through mutational testing when available.

Conditioning intensity

Whereas myeloablation prior to allo-HCT for an aggressive and/or untreated hematologic malignancy may achieve better disease control and afford the transplanted immune system time to exert the necessary GvT effect for cure, myeloablative conditioning in PID patients without active hematologic malignancy may only serve to increase both the toxicities of allo-HCT without added benefit. Exceptions do exist, as some PIDs (ex: GATA2 deficiency) can be associated with clonal myeloid processes, including myelodysplastic syndrome or frank acute myeloid leukemia. Reduced-intensity approaches that result in mixed/split chimerism may not be adequate for GATA2 patients and others who are at risk for relapse of an underlying myeloid malignancy. However, myeloablation is associated with increased risk of short- and long-term toxicities, which can include veno-occlusive disease, mucositis, infection, infertility, growth retardation, cardiopulmonary dysfunction, secondary malignancies, and TRM. When myeloablation is used, busulfan/fludarabine may be preferable to busulfan/cyclophosphamide given the lower risk of these toxicities.

Quite simply, the effectiveness of allo-HCT for PID depends largely on the efficient and adequate replacement of a dysfunctional immune system with a normal, healthy immune system. Sufficient immuno-depletion is necessary to achieve this, while full myeloablation may not be in most circumstances. Allo-HCT approaches that can safely and effectively replace the immune system while inflicting minimal toxicity are therefore likely to improve outcomes for PID patients. Thus, the recent application of less intensive conditioning approaches to allo-HCT for PID has been associated with improved outcomes in many settings, particularly among patients with significant comorbidities, organ dysfunction, or active infection, where TRM with myeloablative conditioning has been historically high. Nonetheless, reducing the intensity of conditioning for these diseases has not been without struggles related to mixed/split chimerism and graft failure, discussed in more detail in the next section.

- There are no prospective, randomized studies comparing myeloablative conditioning to reduced-intensity conditioning (RIC) for PIDs.

• The decision regarding the intensity of conditioning should be based on several factors, including the underlying PID and its disease manifestations, patient comorbidities and organ dysfunction, risk of short- and long-term toxicities, and the potential benefits or drawbacks of mixed/split chimerism after transplant.

> **PRACTICE POINT**
>
> To reduce the toxicity of allo-HCT, there is a focus in the field on immunodepletion through RIC, rather than myeloablation, to facilitate successful engraftment. Patients with PIDs associated with DNA repair/telomere maintenance defects should receive conditioning regimens that minimize their exposure to radiation and other DNA damaging agents, as these patients are more sensitive to the cytotoxic effects of such therapies and are at higher risk for long-term complications such as malignancy.

Chimerism and cure: How much is enough?

Not all patients with PID require full donor chimerism across all cell lineages to be cured; split or mixed chimerism may sufficiency correct the immune defect in many cases. Some PIDs can be cured when split donor chimerism is achieved, where only particular cell lineages are effectively replaced by donor cells. In SCID patients, unconditioned, HLA-MSD allo-HCT can result in engraftment of donor T-cells, leading to vast improvement in the immunodeficiency but lifelong dependence on immunoglobulin replacement due to the absence of engrafted donor B-cells. Patients with IPEX syndrome (immune dysregulation, polyendocrinopathy, enteropathy, X-linked) can be cured when Treg cells are of donor origin, even if other cell subsets remain or revert to recipient-derived cells. Mixed donor chimerism, even at low levels, can lead to phenotype reversion in some PIDs. In patient cases where mixed chimerism persists and appears stable, immunologic assays to assess if the immune defect has been corrected may be helpful in determining whether mixed chimerism is sufficient. In sum, the degree of donor chimerism necessary for phenotype reversion is quite variable across the range of PIDs and may even vary across patients with the same genetic defect.

Mixed chimerism is not necessarily a stable state and may be a harbinger of graft rejection. Establishing tolerance between the graft and the host is important both to prevent GvHD, as well as a host-versus-graft reaction and subsequent graft rejection. However, maintaining host tolerance of donor cells in a mixed chimeric state may require ongoing immunosuppression, which defeats in part the objective of allo-HCT for PID. Correlating changes in donor chimerism percentage as they relate to the intensity of post-allo-HCT immunosuppression, as well as changes that occur around the time of immunosuppression cessation or withdrawal, may be critical pieces of information to better assess donor-host tolerance and inform decisions regarding the role of further immunosuppression and/or donor cell infusion in improving chimerism and preventing graft rejection. While donor lymphocyte infusion can be used to boost donor chimerism, the risk of GvHD makes such interventions unappealing in the setting of allo-HCT for PID.

Other complications can result from mixed/split chimerism. There is the potential for residual host lymphocytes to cause hemophagocytosis, cytopenias due to donor-directed alloantibody production, or other transplant-related immune complications. Donor lymphocytes can also mediate autoimmunity after allo-HCT. Some PIDs, such as WAS, are classically regarded to require the achievement of full donor chimerism to avoid after allo-HCT autoimmune complications and complete phenotype reversion. Myeloid chimerism <50% has been associated with failure to correct the thrombocytopenia and bleeding diathesis in WAS patients. In a retrospective, multicenter study, 8% of WAS patients with full donor chimerism developed post-allo-HCT autoimmune complications, while 72% of WAS patients with mixed/split donor chimerism developed these complications. A more refined evaluation of lineage-specific chimerism and its relationship to immune complications after allo-HCT is necessary to understand this complex phenomenon.

Figure 30.1 diagrams a conceptual view of how chimerism relates to graft failure, GvHD, post-transplant autoimmunity, infection risk, and cure of the underlying immunodeficiency.

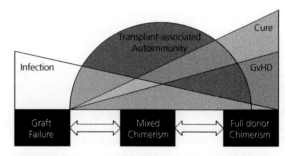

Figure 30.1 The relationship between donor chimerism and complications of allo-HCT, including GvHD, infection, and transplant-associated autoimmunity. Low levels of donor chimerism may result in cure of some PIDs, while other PIDs require full donor chimerism for cure. Mixed chimerism may be an unstable state that can convert to full donor chimerism or progress to graft failure, depending on the balance between the donor and host immune systems.

- In patients with mixed/split chimerism that appears sufficient to reverse the disease phenotype, close follow-up remains necessary to ensure the stability of the chimeric state and allow early intervention should there be signs of secondary graft failure.
- Mixed chimerism is associated with lower rates of GvHD.
- Mixed chimerism may be ameliorated after allo-HCT with modulation of immunosuppression and/or donor cell infusions. However, donor cell infusions that contain significant numbers of T-cells are associated with a risk of GvHD.

Infectious issues

Infection remains a major cause of morbidity and death in PID patients undergoing allo-HCT, despite significant advances in the prophylaxis, early detection, and treatment of infection. Full immune reconstitution after allo-HCT takes time, is influenced by the maturity and breadth of immunity in the transplanted graft as well as the allo-HCT platform, and can be further delayed if patients have poor graft function or require ongoing immunosuppression for GvHD. Even bacterial infections can occur late after transplant, particularly when re-vaccination must be delayed or antibody responses are impaired. Intravenous immunoglobulin G may be given after allo-HCT for hypogammaglobulinemia to provide some protection against infection. Viral infections due to reactivation or episodic exposure remain significant risks both early and late after allo-HCT, although reactivation of HSV and VZV is lessened by the use of prophylactic acyclovir. Routine monitoring for viral reactivation after allo-HCT with quantitative PCR allows pre-emptive treatment for the reactivation of certain viruses, such as cytomegalovirus (CMV) and adenovirus, resulting in decreased morbidity and TRM. Serial monitoring also allows for interventions such as the tailoring or reduction of immunosuppression, when possible, if patients show signs of clinically significant viral reactivation or high levels of proliferation of Epstein–Barr virus-infected B-cells. Ongoing improvements in the technology to engineer virus-specific cytotoxic T-cells have markedly improved therapeutic options for patients with viral infections after allo-HCT. Opportunistic or unusual infections should be considered in allo-HCT patients, even late after transplant, particularly among those with delayed immune reconstitution.

The role of infection in modulating the risk for complications such as GvHD and graft failure is an area of active research. Post-transplant infections, particularly viral reactivation, may also have a large impact on the T-cell repertoire and diversity that develops after allo-HCT. Additionally, anecdotal experience suggests that pre-allo-HCT infections may initially worsen or flare after allo-HCT before improving, seeming to represent an immune reconstitution syndrome akin to that seen in HIV patients upon starting antiretroviral therapy.

- Reactivation of latent viruses is fairly common after allo-HCT, but elevated viral copies in the urine or blood may not always predict disease. Effective therapies are often lacking and available pharmacologic therapies can be associated with significant toxicities. However, monitoring for viral reactivation after allo-HCT and pre-emptive therapy, when clinically indicated, can reduce the morbidity and mortality associated with infections such as CMV and adenovirus.
- Virus-specific cytotoxic T-cell therapy has shown significant promise in addressing the issues of viral complications after allo-HCT.
- The relationship between infections and post-allo-HCT immune reconstitution/repertoire diversity, graft failure, and GvHD risk are complex and areas of active research.

PRACTICE POINTS

Opportunistic infections can occur late after allo-HCT, particularly if immune reconstitution is slow, immunosuppression is prolonged, or prophylaxis is prematurely stopped.

High yield points

- Allo-HCT is potentially curative for a wide range of PIDs, some of which have only been recently described and for which the role of allo-HCT is still being defined.
- Avoiding GvHD is paramount to the success of transplants for PID, as these patients do not need the GvT effect that might accompany GvHD.
- Alternative donors are increasingly being used in allo-HCT for PID and are a reasonable donor source if paired with an allo-HCT platform that (1) carries a low risk of graft failure and GvHD and (2) is associated with favorable, brisk immune reconstitution.
- In general, PID patients do best if they enter transplant with no active infections, minimal end-organ damage, and few comorbidities. However, the upfront risks of allo-HCT must be weighed against the projected future risks of living with an uncorrected PID (Figure 30.2).
- RIC reduces the toxicities of allo-HCT, making the procedure less risky and available even to those with organ dysfunction, but can be associated with mixed/split chimerism.
- Mixed/split chimerism may be sufficient to cure some PIDs, but may result in autoimmunity, dependence on immunoglobulin replacement, or secondary graft failure in some PIDs.

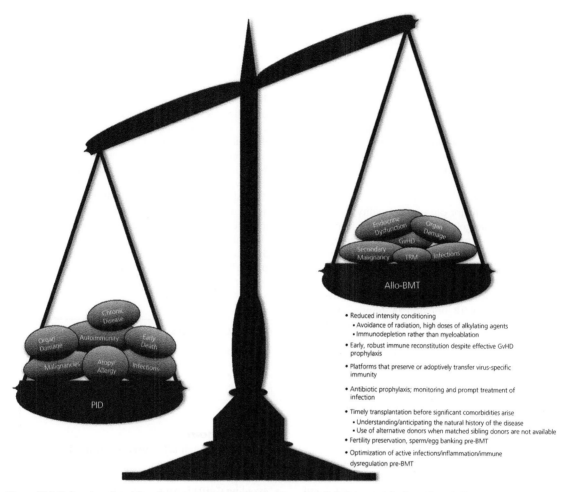

Figure 30.2 Balancing the risks of an uncorrected primary immunodeficiency with the risks of allo-HCT. With the interventions listed on the right (see bullet points in figure), the risks of allo-HCT can be lessened, shifting the balance in favor of pursuing allo-HCT for PIDs that carry the potential for high morbidity and mortality.

Selected reading

1. Spinner MA, Sanchez LA, Hsu AP, et al. GATA2 deficiency: a protean disorder of hematopoiesis, lymphatics, and immunity. *Blood.* 2014;**123**(6):809–821.

2. Pai SY, Logan BR, Griffith LM, et al. Transplantation outcomes for severe combined immunodeficiency, 2000–2009. *N Engl J Med.* 2014;**371**(5):434–446.

3. Ouachee-Chardin M, Elie C, de Saint Basile G, et al. Hematopoietic stem cell transplantation in hemophagocytic lymphohistiocytosis: a single-center report of 48 patients. *Pediatrics.* 2006;**117**(4):e743–750.

4. Bertaina A, Merli P, Rutella S, et al. HLA-haploidentical stem cell transplantation after removal of alphabeta+T and B cells in children with nonmalignant disorders. *Blood.* 2014;**124**(5):822–826.

5. Grossman J, Cuellar-Rodriguez J, Gea-Banacloche J, et al. Nonmyeloablative allogeneic hematopoietic stem cell trans-

plantation for GATA2 deficiency. *Biol Blood Marrow Transplant.* 2014;**20**(12):1940–1948.

6. Bartelink IH, van Reij EM, Gerhardt CE, et al. Fludarabine and exposure-targeted busulfan compares favorably with busulfan/cyclophosphamide-based regimens in pediatric hematopoietic cell transplantation: maintaining efficacy with less toxicity. *Biol Blood Marrow Transplant.* 2014;**20**(3):345–353.

7. Cuellar-Rodriguez J, Freeman AF, Grossman J, et al. Matched related and unrelated donor hematopoietic stem cell transplantation for DOCK8 deficiency. *Biol Blood Marrow Transplant.* 2015;**21**(6):1037–1045.

8. Gungor T, Teira P, Slatter M, et al. Reduced-intensity conditioning and HLA-matched haemopoietic stem-cell transplantation in patients with chronic granulomatous disease: a prospective multicentre study. *Lancet.* 2014;**383**(9915):436–448.

9. Marsh RA, Vaughn G, Kim MO, et al. Reduced-intensity conditioning significantly improves survival of patients with hemophagocytic lymphohistiocytosis undergoing allogeneic

hematopoietic cell transplantation. *Blood*. 2010;**116**(26): 5824–5831.

10. Slatter MA, Rao K, Amrolia P, et al. Treosulfan-based conditioning regimens for hematopoietic stem cell transplantation in children with primary immunodeficiency: United Kingdom experience. *Blood*. 2011;**117**(16):4367–4375.

11. Neven B, Leroy S, Decaluwe H, et al. Long-term outcome after hematopoietic stem cell transplantation of a single-center cohort of 90 patients with severe combined immunodeficiency. *Blood*. 2009;**113**(17):4114–4124.

12. Qasim W, Cavazzana-Calvo M, Davies EG, et al. Allogeneic hematopoietic stem-cell transplantation for leukocyte adhesion deficiency. *Pediatrics*. 2009;**123**(3):836–840.

13. Lawler M, McCann SR, Marsh JC, et al. Serial chimerism analyses indicate that mixed haemopoietic chimerism influences the probability of graft rejection and disease recurrence following allogeneic stem cell transplantation (SCT) for severe aplastic anaemia (SAA): indication for routine assessment of chimerism post SCT for SAA. *Br J Haematol*. 2009;**144**(6):933–945.

14. Moratto D, Giliani S, Bonfim C, et al. Long-term outcome and lineage-specific chimerism in 194 patients with Wiskott–Aldrich syndrome treated by hematopoietic cell transplantation in the period 1980–2009: an international collaborative study. *Blood*. 2011;**118**(6): 1675–1684.

15. Pai SY, Logan BR, Griffith LM, Buckley RH, Parrott RE, Dvorak CC, et al. Transplantation outcomes for severe combined immunodeficiency, 2000–2009. *New England Journal of Medicine*. 2014;**371**(5):434–446.

CHAPTER 31

Inherited metabolic disorders

Jaap Jan Boelens[1,3] and Robert F. Wynn[2]

[1] *University Medical Center Utrecht, Pediatric Blood and Marrow Transplantation Program, Utrecht, The Netherlands*

[2] *Royal Manchester Children's Hospital, Department of Hematology/BMT, Manchester, UK*

[3] *Laboratory Translational Immunology, University Medical Center Utrecht, Utrecht, the Netherlands*

Introduction

The inborn errors of metabolism (IEM) are a diverse group of diseases arising from genetic defects, including deficiencies in the production of the lysosomal enzymes (Lysosomal Storage Disease, LSD) and abnormalities of peroxisomal function. Lysosomal enzymes are hydrolytic and catalyze the degradation of specific substrates within the acidic environment of lysosomes. Peroxisomes are subcellular organelles primarily involved in lipid metabolism. Roughly, these diseases are characterized by devastating systemic processes that may affect bone integrity, growth, and development, cardiopulmonary status, the airway, hearing and vision, neurologic, and cognitive function. In severe phenotypic disease with little residual enzyme activity there is typically onset in infancy or early childhood with subsequent rapid deterioration and early death. Allogeneic-hematopoietic cell transplantation (allo-HCT) has shown to be a treatment option for a selected group of patients with an IEM. Timely diagnosis and immediate referral to a "specialist in IEM," along with discussion on these patients in a multidisciplinary team, including a transplant-physician, are essential steps. Treatment recommendations are based on: the disorder; its phenotype including age at onset, rate of progression, severity of clinical signs and symptoms; family values and expectations; and the risks and benefits associated with available therapies such as allo-HCT.

Interest in allo-HCT for IEM is driven by:

1 Timely diagnosis and immediate referral to an IEM specialist
2 Cell source used in transplantation
3 Donor chimerism and post-HCT enzyme levels
4 Management of the post-transplant residual disease burden by this multidisciplinary team and its other applied therapies.

Allogeneic-HCT in IEM: What is the rationale and how did we get here?

The demonstration of the principal of "cross correction" established that the accumulation of substrate in the cells of patients with lysosomal enzyme deficiencies could be reduced in the presence of cells producing the missing enzyme. With this as a rationale, allo-HCT was explored in numerous lysosomal diseases, including Mucopolysaccharidosis type-1, Hurler phenotype (MPS-1H), and the inherited lysosomal leukodystrophies; in particular, metachromatic leukodystrophy (MLD), X-linked adrenoleukodystrophy (X-ALD), and globoid cell leukodystrophy (GLD; or Krabbe's disease). HCT has since become the standard of care in a selected group of disorders (e.g., MPS-1H, early X-ALD) and since the first HCT in an MPS-1H patient, over 2000 patients with an IEM have been transplanted (Figure 31.1).

Treatment recommendations may vary significantly, even within a particular diagnosis. These decisions reflect the type of disorder, its predicted phenotype, the extent of disease progression, family values and expectations, and the risks and benefits associated with available therapies. Allo-HCT for IEM is performed using donor-derived hematopoietic stem cells obtained from bone marrow (BM), growth factor mobilized peripheral blood (PB), and in the last decade predominantly from umbilical cord blood (CB). Allogeneic HCT has become much safer due to the availability of better-matched cords, enhanced techniques for HLA matching, improved preparative regimens, and supportive care. At this point, for patients with non-malignant disease such as IEM, transplant related complications such as infections and graft-versus-host disease (GvHD), are relatively low, especially for chronic GvHD.

Clinical Manual of Blood and Bone Marrow Transplantation, First Edition. Edited by Syed A. Abutalib and Parameswaran Hari.
© 2017 John Wiley & Sons Ltd. Published 2017 by John Wiley & Sons Ltd.

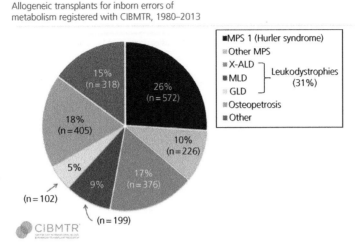

Figure 31.1 Since the early 1980s, over 2000 allo-HCT in IEM have been performed. Here the distribution of the various diseases/disease-groups is shown (CIMBTR database 2013).

Which diseases to transplant?

Although HCT has proven to influence the natural course of a variety of IEM significantly not all diseases of phenotypes profit from allo-HCT. The currently accepted IEM diagnoses (and optional or investigational diagnosis) being treated with allo-HCT are described in Table 31.1.

All transplant decisions are based on a balance of risk and potential benefits. There is a greater opportunity for benefit in patients with a milder phenotype and/or in those patients that are earlier in the course of their disease. Much of the morbidity associated with the disease itself is not reversed by allo-HCT, except organomegaly in the LSDs. Treatment of the central nervous system (CNS) with transplant is, we believe, primarily mediated by the engraftment of donor-derived microglial cells in the brain. As it takes several months to replace sufficient microglia with those derived by the donor, there is a delay in any significant benefits of transplant to the CNS. Diseases affecting the brain that are rapidly progressive are therefore more difficult to treat with transplantation (e.g., infantile GLD). As results of allo-HCT improve and its risks are thereby reduced, then it is appropriate to consider whether diseases of milder phenotype might be considered for allo-HCT, as the alternative is weekly 4–6 hour infusions of enzyme. This might include milder LSD currently managed with enzyme replacement therapies (ERT), such as Hurler–Scheie, attenuated MPSII, or MPSVI.

Much of the literature describing outcomes with allo-HCT in any particular disease is outdated: for example, it is said that HCT is ineffective in MPSII (Hunter), but such a statement is derived from allo-HCT experience in symptomatic children using sibling donor grafts. The outcomes may be different in those same patients had it been performed earlier and using an *unrelated* CB donor, where enzyme delivery would have been optimized as shown in some recent studies. Thus, some of these HCT questions must be re-evaluated in this modern era. Collaboration between centers for these re-evaluations is of utmost importance since these diseases are rare and sometimes even ultra-rare.

The role of allo-HCT is a selected group of LSD and cerebral-adrenoleukodystrophy (C-ALD) is well established and are discussed in more detail next. Its role in other metabolic disease is less clear. Furthermore, there is some evidence that it has a role in mitochondrial disease and benefits have been reported in MNGIE (Mitochondrial Neurogastrointestinal Encephalomyopathy) and recently some other mitochondrial diseases, as well as in GSD (Glycogen Storage Disease) Type Ib (discussed in a recent review).

Are outcomes of HCT in IEM satisfying and how can we further optimize the outcomes?

Here we describe the outcomes of the most frequently transplanted diseases: MPS-1 (27%) and Leukodystrophies (31%): see also Figure 31.1.

Hurler syndrome, MPS-1H

Hurler syndrome (MPS IH), the most severe phenotype of alpha-L-iduronidase deficiency, is an autosomal recessive disorder characterized by progressive

Table 31.1 The currently accepted IEM diagnoses being treated with allo-HCT. Inborn errors of metabolism for which allogeneic hematopoietic cell transplantation may be indicated.

Disorder	Enzyme/Protein	Indication	Comments
Mucopolysacchararidoses			
Hurler (MPS IH)	alpha-L-iduronidase	Standard	ERT first-line therapy
Hurler/Scheie (MPS IH/S)	alpha-L-iduronidase	Option	ERT first-line therapy
Scheie (MPS IS)	alpha-L-iduronidase	Option	Only early or asymptomatic
Hunter: Severe (MPS IIA)	Iduronate-2-sulfatase	Investigational	ERT first-line therapy
Hunter: Attenuated (MPS IIB)	Iduronate-2-sulfatase	Option	ERT first-line therapy
Maroteaux-Lamy (MPS VI)	Arylsulfatase B	Option	
Sly (MPS VII)	Beta-glucuronidase	Option	
Leukodystrophies			
X-ALD, cerebral	ALD protein	Standard	Not for advanced disease
MLD: Early infantile	Arylsulfatase A	No	Gene-therapy trial open (Milan)
MLD: late-infantile/Juvenile	Arylsulfatase A	Option/Standard	Only early or asymptomatic
MLD: Adult onset	Arylsulfatase A	Standard	Neonate, screening diagnosis, or second case
GLD: Early onset	Galactocerebrosidase	Standard	in known family; not for advanced disease
GLD: Late onset	Galactocerebrosidase	Option	
Glycoprotein metabolic and miscellaneous disorders			
Fucosidosis	Fucosidase	Option	In known family
Alpha-mannosidosis	alpha-Mannosidase	Option	Neonate, screening diagnosis, or second case
Aspartylglucosaminuria	Aspartylglucosaminidase	Option	ERT first-line therapy
Farber	Ceraminidase	Option	Limited benefit of ERT
Tay-Sachs: Early onset	Hexosaminidase A	No	ERT available
Tay-Sachs: Juvenile	Hexosaminidase A	Option	ERT first-line therapy
Sandhoff: Early onset	Hexosaminidase A & B	No	Only early or asymptomatic
Sandhoff: Juvenile	Hexosaminidase A & B	option	May be viewed as Standard
Gaucher I (non-neuronopathic)	Glucocerebrosidase	Unknown	Not in advanced disease
Gaucher II (acute neuronopath)	Glucocerebrosidase	Option	
Gaucher III (subacute neuronopathic)	Glucocerebrosidase	Unknown	
Pompe	Glucosidase	Unknown	
Niemann Pick: Type A	Acid sphingomyelinase	Investigational	
Niemann Pick: Type B	Acid sphingomyelinase	Unknown	
Niemann Pick: Type C	Cholesterol trafficking	Option	
Wolman Syndrome	Acid lipase	Option	
Multiple sulfatase deficiency	Sulfatases	Investigational	
MNGIE (mitochondrial neurogastrointestinal encephalomyopathy)	Thymidine phosphorylase	Option	

This table does not include diseases where allo-HCT is not indicated/contra-indicated.

- Standard: Allo-HCT applied routinely. Considerable published research evidence from registries and institutions demonstrates efficacy. Delayed diagnosis and/or advanced disease may preclude transplant for individual patients.
- Option: Allo-HCT is effective but other therapy is increasingly considered first choice. Or, insufficient published evidence for allo-HCT to be considered Standard.
- Investigational: Possible *a priori* reason for allo-HCT. Further published evidence needed to support the use of allo-HCT in clinical practice.

accumulation of glycosaminoglycans (GAGs). Hurler and other phenotypes of MPS I - Scheie (MPS IS, attenuated) and Hurler–Scheie (MPS IH/S, intermediate) represent a continuous clinical spectrum. Accumulation of GAGs results in progressive, multi-system dysfunction associated with premature death. Over 600 allo-HCTs have been performed worldwide for children with MPS IH since 1980 (EBMT/CIBMTR registry), making it the most commonly transplanted IEM (Figure 31.1).

Allo-HCT for children with MPS IH has been shown to increase life expectancy and improve clinical manifestations of disease. Allo-HCT must be performed early in the disease course as some disease related complications, including neurologic deterioration, are irreversible. Donor cell engraftment after allo-HCT has resulted in the rapid reduction of obstructive airway symptoms and hepatosplenomegaly. Hearing, vision, and linear growth improve in most cases. Hydrocephalus is either prevented or stabilized and the otherwise expected cardiovascular pathology is altered beneficially after HCT. Although cerebral damage already present before allo-HCT appears to be irreversible, successful transplant is able to prevent progressive psychomotor deterioration and permit continued neuro-development.

International collaborative studies identified predictors for graft-failure associated with poor "event free survival"-rates, including T-cell depleted grafts and reduced intensity conditioning, while busulfan with therapeutic drug monitoring (targeting to a myeloablative exposure) appeared to be a predictor for higher "event free survival" in comparison to prior experiences. These data has led to an EBMT transplant protocol/guideline (*EBMT/EHA Handbook* 2008 and 2012). These guidelines included a standardized busulfan (Bu)/cyclophosphamide (Cy) conditioning regimen and the use of CB as a preferred graft source, second only to non-carrier matched sibling BM. This transplant protocol with well-matched grafts resulted in a significant improved engrafted survival rate of over 90% in larger experienced allo-HCT-centers specialized in transplanting MPS patients, who also have standardized long-term follow up programs. Recently the conditioning was modified to Bu with pharmacokinetic monitoring: targeting to myeloablative busulfan exposure) + fludarabine (*EBMT/EHA Handbook* 2012). Recent conditioning comparisons (Bu-Cy vs Flu-Bu) suggest similar allo-HCT outcomes but with reduced toxicity.

Over the past decade, unrelated CB has been used with increasing frequency as a graft source for allo-HCT in children with an IEM. CB offers several advantages over BM or PB including reduced time to HCT, greater tolerance for HLA-mismatch, lower incidence and severity of GvHD, and reduced likelihood of transmitting viral infections. Recent collaborative studies suggest that the highest EFS rates are achieved in patients receiving an identical matched sibling donor or an identical (6/6) unrelated cord blood, followed by 5/6 matched CB or 10/10 matched unrelated donor. Interestingly, almost all CB recipients had full-donor chimerism associated with normal enzymes levels, while mixed-chimerism was more frequently seen in HLA-matched sibling and HLA-MUD donors. It is also important to recognize that most matched sibling donors are carriers, influencing post-transplant enzyme levels. Lower enzyme levels appear to be important for long-term outcomes, including neurocognitive outcomes. This issue is currently being analyzed in an international long-term outcome study,

which may further refine donor selection for clinical practice.

Survival of MPS-1H patients has significantly improved last decade; however, major limitation remain, as surviving patients continue to have substantial morbidity due to "residual disease burden"; primarily musculoskeletal features that often require orthopedic surgical interventions. Use of improved and reduced toxicity allo-HCT techniques at an earlier age and the achievement of full-donor-chimerism with normalization of enzyme activity may enhance outcomes. Newborn screening may prove a major step forward in early identification of individuals with MPS IH.

Leukodystrophies

Globoid Cell Leukodystrophy: GLD; or Krabbe disease (incidence 1:100.000), is a recessive disorder caused by defects in the galactocerebrosidase (GALC). Over 80% of cases of GLD manifest in infancy, characterized by irritability, poor feeding, and progressive loss of motor function; the majority of these patients die before 2 years of age. Generally accepted there is no role for HCT in symptomatic patients with the classic infantile phenotype (80% have this phenotype). However, if patients are identified very early in life, either due to a positive family history or through newborn screening, allo-HCT alters the course of the disease. However, despite HCT, significant gross motor changes are still be observed post-HCT, while cognitive function is relatively spared. The relative contribution of peripheral demyelination to motor-related dysfunction is difficult to assess, although it is clear that nerve conduction abnormalities are present in GLD. The later onset forms of GLD progress less quickly, providing a greater opportunity for allo-HCT. Later onset forms of GLD may not only be stabilized, but can potentially improve following allo-HCT (reviewed recently).

Metachromatic Leukodystrophy (MLD): Metachromatic leukodystrophy, also recessive in inheritance (1 in 40,000) is caused by defect in the arylsulfatase A (ARSA) gene. Sulfatides accumulate in myelin producing cells, resulting in both central and peripheral demyelination. ARSA testing is important in establishing the diagnosis, pseudodeficiency states exist in which measured ARSA levels are low, but no sulfatides are present in the urine. Urine sulfatide testing is therefore important to confirm the diagnosis of MLD. The clinical manifestations of MLD is categorized based on age of onset: late infantile (younger than 2 years), juvenile (3–16 years), and adult forms. The late infantile form is the most common form resulting in progressive motor dysfunction with loss of the ability to walk, stand, and sit, dysarthria, swallowing difficulties, an inability to handle secretions, and early death (<4 years of age). There is no role for allo-HCT in symptomatic late infantile MLD. Patients with late infantile disease that proceeded to allo-HCT pre-symptomatically achieved some stabilization of disease but still in most/all severe motor difficulties were observed due to peripheral nerve dysfunction. The asymptomatic infantile group is also the target of recent gene-therapy initiatives and has the capacity to deliver more enzyme than standard allo-HCT. First evidence of efficacy has been shown recently. In attenuated form of the disease a greater opportunity exists to impact the disease process with allo-HCT. Patients with juvenile disease transplanted while still asymptomatic been reported to attain better outcomes. The adult form of MLD (20% of cases), which can become apparent as late as the seventh decade, have less motor findings, but may be emotionally labile and have difficulties in executive function, progressive dementia, psychosis, and difficulties with substance abuse. Although limited data available there is a role for allo-HCT for adult-onset disease (reviewed recently).

Adrenoleukodystrophy (ALD): In 1976 it was demonstrated that very long chain fatty acids (VLCFAs) accumulate in the brain and adrenal tissue of patients with ALD. The inability to degrade VLCFA is due to mutations in the ABCD1 gene, encoding a peroxisomal membrane protein. ALD is X-linked in inheritance (1 in 17,000) and has a highly variable clinical manifestations of the disease despite a conserved genotype. The most severe phenotype of ALD is the cerebral form (C-ALD; 35–40%) of individuals with ALD by age 20. Cerebral ALD is an acute, inflammatory, demyelinating condition. In almost all (95%) of cases, C-ALD is associated with progressive neurologic deterioration and ultimately death within several years. C-ALD is rare before 4 years of age but with a median age of 7 years old. Since the first report by Patrick Aubourg on the beneficial effect of HCT in a boy with early-stage C-ALD in 1990 additional experience has established allo-HCT as the standard of care for early C-ALD. Until now the exact mechanism of the effect remains elusive, but it is thought that the chemotherapy and immune suppression associated with HCT controls the neuro-inflammation. It has been hypothesized that donor microglial cells provide support to the ALD oligodendrocyte. The Loes MRI scoring system, provides a numeric score based on the number of areas of the brain with evidence of demyelination. Loes score is a predictor for survival, with higher mortality rates in advanced patients: those with higher scores (>9) have worse outcomes. Unfortunately, most patients are not diagnosed as having C-ALD until they develop clinically evident neurologic changes, thus are having already advanced disease. Recently there is some early evidence that mortality with allo-HCT in advanced patients with C-ALD may be less using a reduced intensity regimen and anti-oxidative therapy, but with significant residual disease burden. Furthermore, an intriguing question regarding the role of HCT in ALD is

whether allo-HCT alters the natural history adrenomyeloneuropathy (AMN), a late onset ALD disease complication. Adrenomyeloneuropathy affects the spinal cord, is non-inflammatory, and results in slow progression of motor-related limitations beginning in the third decade of life. Recently, early reported success of gene therapy (autologous gene-transduced HCT) has been published and a second trial recently has started.

PRACTICE POINT

Earlier allo-HCT and using a conditioning regimen and (non-carrier) donors that achieve full-donor chimerism are predictors for better outcomes. We have summarized this in Table 31.2, based on over 20 years of single center and collaborative studies. In the upcoming decade, with evolving therapies like gene-therapy, this table may need further updates.

When to do allo-HCT?

It is clear that, in IEM, the outcomes (either transplant outcomes and late outcomes) are superior in patients in whom transplant is performed early. This has been demonstrated for several diseases including Hurler, MLD, C-ALD, and Krabbe. It will likely hold true for other (ultra-rare) IEM for which allo-HCT has a role.

Newborn screening is emerging as an option for these disorders; previously the median age at transplant for Hurler is ~16 months of age, as most children are diagnosed based on clinical signs and symptoms. The age at transplant will likely be significantly reduced as neonatal screening is implemented (which is agreed on in some countries; e.g., the Netherlands). The test(s) need to be specific, cost-effective, be able to identify disease-causing mutations, and be able to offer a reliable prediction of the phenotype to minimizing anxiety and uncertainty in families. Of course, the introduction of such screening should be prospectively evaluated in a standardized manner to evaluate the benefits of intervention.

In C-ALD, as discussed above, intervention with HCT should only offered when demyelination is documented based on MRI changes. Neonatal screening for ALD has already begun in New York, and will likely expand in the near future (including the Netherlands). This will allow boys to be identified early, providing them the best chance for performing allo-HCT quickly as cerebral disease is identified and allowing detection of adrenal failure so that life-saving hormone replacement therapy can be given. Currently, allo-HCT is not performed in boys without documented MRI changes because of the risk associated with allo-HCT, and due to our inability to

Table 31.2 The current state of allo-HCT practice in IEM.

	What do we know *now* about the transplant?	How *might* the transplant change?
When to transplant?	1 As soon as possible after diagnosis in LSD, e.g. Hurler 2 With early MRI change in X-ALD	1 After neonatal screening diagnosis of LSD 2 All asymptomatic X-ALD boys once longer term benefits of allo-HCT established
Which diseases to transplant?	1 Certain LSD – paradigm disorder – MPSI Hurler 2 X-ALD	1 As HCT is safer it is offered to attenuated (milder) phenotype disease of MPSI since superior efficacy 2 In place of disorders currently managed with ERT since more efficacious and more cost effective, e.g. MPSVI 3 Other metabolic disorders, e.g. mitochondrial disease
How to transplant?	1 Full intensity conditioning including targeted busulfan 2 Umbilical cord blood donor ("wild type")	1 Reduced intensity and reduced toxicity regimens that permit blood and CNS engraftment 2 Gene modified autologous blood stem cell therapy (with increased enzyme delivery)
Complimentary therapies	1 Pre-transplant ERT in LSD to improve tolerability of procedure	1 Abbreviated ERT to aid engraftment and reduce allo-antibody 2 Post-transplant ERT to optimise patient outcomes after transplant 3 Other complimentary therapies delivered in parallel to transplant, e.g. substrate reduction therapy, stop codon read-through

identify those who will ultimately develop cerebral disease. This paradigm is likely to change when evidence proves that allo-HCT alters the course of AMN, as discussed previously.

PRACTICE POINT

Earlier transplantation (in course of disease or life) will have significant impact on the outcomes (either transplant outcomes and late outcomes).

How to transplant a patient with an IEM?

Engraftment has been shown to require myeloablative conditioning (MAC), most commonly utilizing full dose targeted busulfan. In dedicated, experience centers, transplanting patients with IEM, the engrafted survival rates are above 90–95% using busulfan-based MA. If, in upcoming years protocols can be developed with even further reduction of the toxicity associated with equivalent engraftment as the current MAC protocols this will be advantageous, especially when this will give benefits in regards to fertility and more normal endocrine function after allo-HCT. Agents such as treosulfan are considered to be less toxic, there is data that clearly suggests that busulfan may provide superior microglial engraftment (essential for earlier and higher delivery of the missing enzyme in the brain). The replacement of cyclophosphamide for fludarabine combined with exposure-targeted busulfan has proven to be as effective (including absence of mixed chimerism, which is also more frequently seen in treosulfan-based regimens) but significantly less toxic. Based on current literature the recommended conditioning regimen and cell source hierarchy is described in Table 31.3.

The enzyme dose delivered by allo-HCT is important in patient's "late outcomes" from transplant as currently performed. Children that are engrafted from donors with high enzyme levels need less orthopedic surgery and grow better. Several lines of evidence suggest that autologous cells that are gene-modified to express the deficient enzyme may further improve outcomes compared to wild type donor. Furthermore, gene therapy has the capacity to enhance enzyme secretion not only by increasing the gene copy number but also by re-regulating gene expression so that it occurs in monocytic and other mature blood cells. As the enzyme level has shown to be a predictor for long-term outcomes (e.g., skeletal disease) higher enzymes achieved with gene-therapy my influence the long-term outcomes positively in the future.

Biffi and colleagues have demonstrated clinical benefit to such an approach in infantile MLD. Whether gene therapy is superior to allo-HCT needs to be determined after longer-term follow up. Several other similar gene-therapy approaches that are quite close to the clinic (e.g., MPS-3, MPS-1). In addition to improving enzyme delivery gene therapy may reduce transplant risk since autologous cells should allow accelerated immune reconstitution and eliminate GvHD as a

Table 31.3 Donor hierarchy and conditioning.

A Graft source hierarchy in lysosomal storage diseases and peroxisomal disorders:		
1 Identical-SIB (HLA-MSD; not carriers)		
2 UD (10/10)* = Unrelated Cord Blood (UCB: 6/6)		
3 UCB (5/6)		
4 UCB (4/6) = mismatched-UD (non-T-depleted)		
5 UCB (3/6) = HAPLOIDENTICAL (not recommended)		
○ UD (10/10) may be bypassed depending on institutional preference or because of time.		
○ For UD: BM preferred cell source		
○ Cell dose for UCB: 5–6/6 match: >3.0×10^7 NC/kg and/or 2×10^5 CD34$^+$/kg, 4/6-match >5×10^7 NC/kg and/or >3×10^5 CD34$^+$/kg. Matching according to intermediate resolution criteria (low resolution on A and B, high resolution on DR)		
6 Unrelated donors are regarded as non-carriers of the mutation		
B Serotherapy:		
- id-SIB:	no	
- UCB	ATG (Thymoglobuline)* 4 × 2.5 mg/kg	(day –9 to –6)
- UD:	either Campath-1H 3 × 0.3 mg	(day –9 to –7)
	or ATG (Thymoglobuline)* 4 × 2.5 mg/kg	(day –4 to –1)
	*ATG dose for 15–30 kg: 3 × 2.5 mg/kg and for > 30 kg 2 × 2.5 mg/kg (start day –9)	
C Conditioning:		
- SIB/UCB/UD:	Busulfan weight-based dosing (IV: day –5 to –2) with therapeutic drug monitoring AUC 90 mg*h/L (range 85–95) cumulative over 4 days (AUC in uM*min = 22, range 20.5–23.5) Fludarabine 160 mg/m^2 (day –5 to –2)	
D GvHD-prophylaxis:		
- SIB:	CsA (+ MTX: 10 mg Msq; day +1, +3, and +6)	
- UD (BM):		
- with Campath-1H	CsA	
- with ATG:	CsA + MTX (10 mg Msq; day +1, +3, and +6)	
- UD (PBHC) UD/ Mismatched-UD (BM)	CsA + MMF (30 mg/kg: stop day +28 in case no GvHD)	
- UCB:	CsA + Prednisone 1 mg/kg (until day +28, taper in 2 wks)	
CsA-trough level: 200 ug/L		
Tapering GvHD-prophylaxis:		
- SIB/UD:	CsA until day +50. Then taper 20% per week	
- UCB:	CsA until + 6 month. Then taper in 3 month	

complication. Of course, the efficacy of such an approach should be prospectively evaluated against conventional therapies especially in terms of safety and long-term and stable gene expression. For C-ALD similar lentiviral mediated genetic therapy of autologous hematopoietic cells has been performed. Preliminary data are encouraging (with only short term follow up) and needs to be confirmed in longer-term follow up studies and in more patients.

> **PRACTICE POINT**
>
> Currently the best (>90% engrafted survival rates) are reached using busulfan-based myeloablative conditioning combined with fludarabine (as reduced toxicity) or cyclophosphamide (Table 31.3). In the future, autologous gene-modified hematopoietic transplants may replace conventional allo-HCT.

Are there alternative treatment options for patients with an IEM?

In addition to supportive care of disease manifestations and allo-HCT alternative therapies are increasingly available for these conditions. The spectacular clinical and financial success of Cerezyme® (Imiglucerase, Genzyme) for the treatment of Gaucher disease has led to the development of similar therapies for other LSDs. Fabry disease, mucopolysaccharidoses I, II, VI, and Pompe disease all have licensed ERT and many more enzymes are in various stages of clinical development. Like all medical treatments this approach has several limitations; not all patients are suitable for treatment, some organs or tissues (e.g., lung, liver, spleen) are more amenable to correction then others (e.g., skeletal, CNS). In addition, there are problems gauging efficacy in this group of highly variable disorders. Furthermore, there is a burden of weekly (or even more frequent) infusions, development of (neutralizing) antibodies to the recombinant proteins and the impermeability of the central nervous system to intravenous ERT, which makes ERT not an effective treatment option for patients with CNS disease. This has resulted in stimulation of the development of alternative therapies using oral small molecules acting as either inhibitors of substrate accumulation or as chaperones to misfolded proteins. With this approach, or combined strategies it is hoped that there is some or better effect on CNS disease, but all are too early to concluded anything.

As already discussed, gene therapy approaches have translated from the laboratory to the clinic; the first trials are accruing patients in C-ALD and MLD. In near future, trials in other LSDs will also start: for example, MPS-3, MPS-1.

PRACTICE POINT

In patients with an IEM with CNS disease currently allo-HCT is the only effective treatment for CNS disease (in selective group of diseases). In the future, gene therapy may be an attractive and possible more effective alternative.

Adjuvant therapies to allo-HCT

Intravenously administered enzyme does not cross the blood brain barrier (BBB), so ERT is not able to prevent CNS deterioration. However, it is hypothesized that ERT prior to allo-HCT can improve the somatic performance of the child and decrease the probability of HCT-related complications influenced by the accumulation of storage material. The combination of ERT and HCT for MPS IH children has been evaluated in single and multi-center studies and found that although ERT was well tolerated, the combination of ERT and allo-HCT did not affect rates of survival, engrafted survival, or HCT-associated morbidity within the entire cohort. However, patients in a very poor clinical condition, especially those with cardiac dysfunction, may improve significantly on ERT, making them eligible for allo-HCT. Currently, many transplant centers are administering ERT to MPS IH patients prior to allo-HCT and continuing it until either start of the conditioning or achievement of donor-derived engraftment.

PRACTICE POINT

There is no evidence in MPS IH that peri-transplant ERT influences the outcomes; neither positively nor negatively. However, for those in a very poor clinical condition significant improvement can be seen with ERT, which may provide a better opportunity for a good outcome. More extensive analysis of the role of ERT remains to be confirmed.

High yield points

- Myeloablative conditioning has been required for sustained donor cell engraftment in patients with IEM. This is best achieved with exposure-targeted busulfan in combination with immune suppressive drugs (Fludarabine or Cyclophosphamide) and serotherapy (e.g., ATG: anti-thymocyte globulin/ Campath).
- In recent years engrafted survival rates have significantly improved and in experienced centers might be expected to be as high as 90%.
- CB as a donor cell source gives better chimerism than BM or PB after myeloablative conditioning.
- The primary goal of allo-HCT is optimizing the functional outcomes of these patients, and their "quality of life (QoL)." However, once donor-derived engraftment is achieved, there is no means to deliver additional enzyme, and so achieving additional benefit is limited. However, there are variables that can be addressed to increase efficacy of therapy, including:
  - *Age at transplant.*
  - *Levels of enzyme delivered to recipient tissue* by engrafted donor leucocytes. In the future, the use of gene-therapy protocols may result in supra-normal enzyme levels, which may have an impact on the long-term outcomes of these patients.
  - *Phenotype of disease.*

Selected reading

1. Fratantoni JC, Hall CW, Neufeld EF. Hurler and Hunter syndromes: mutual correction of the defect in cultured fibroblasts. *Science.* 1968;**162**(3853):570–572.

2. Boelens JJ, Aldenhoven M, Purtill D, et al. Outcomes of transplantation using various hematopoietic cell sources in children with Hurler syndrome after myeloablative conditioning. *Blood.* 2013;**121**(19):3981–3987.

3. Aldenhoven M, Wynn RF, Orchard PJ, et al. Long-term outcome of Hurler syndrome patients after hematopoietic cell transplantation: an international multicenter study. *Blood.* 2015;**125**(13):2164–2172.

4. Boelens JJ, Orchard PJ, Wynn RF. Transplantation in inborn errors of metabolism: current considerations and future perspectives. *Br J Haematol.* 2014.

5. Aldenhoven M, Boelens JJ, de Koning TJ. The clinical outcome of Hurler syndrome after stem cell transplantation. *Biol Blood Marrow Transplant.* 2008;**14**(5):485–498.

6. Boelens JJ, Bierings M, Wynn RF. *HSCT Hand Book EBMT/ESH 2012*: HSCT for children and adolescents. 2012;1–14.

7. Bartelink IH, van Reij EML, Gerhardt CE, et al. Fludarabine and exposure-targeted busulfan compares favorably with busulfan/cyclophosphamide-based regimens in pediatric hematopoietic cell transplantation: maintaining efficacy with less toxicity. *Biol Blood Marrow Transplant.* 2014;**20**(3):345–353.

8. Aldenhoven M, Jones SA, Bonney D, et al. Hematopoietic cell transplantation for mucopolysaccharidosis patients is safe and effective: results after implementation of international guidelines. *Biol Blood Marrow Transplant.* 2015;**21**(6):1106–1109.

9. Escolar ML, Poe MD, Provenzale JM, et al. Transplantation of umbilical-cord blood in babies with infantile Krabbe's disease. *N Engl J Med.* 2005;**352**(20):2069–2081.

10. Biffi A, Montini E, Lorioli L, et al. Lentiviral hematopoietic stem cell gene therapy benefits metachromatic leukodystrophy. *Science.* 2013;**341**(6148):1233158–1233158.

11. Miller WP, Rothman SM, Nascene D, et al. Outcomes after allogeneic hematopoietic cell transplantation for childhood cerebral adrenoleukodystrophy: the largest single-institution cohort report. *Blood.* 2011;**118**(7):1971–1978.

12. Cartier N, Hacein-Bey-Abina S, Bartholomae CC, et al. Hematopoietic stem cell gene therapy with a lentiviral vector in X-linked adrenoleukodystrophy. *Science.* 2009;**326**(5954):818–823.

13. Bartelink IH, Boelens JJ, Bredius RGM, et al. Body weight-dependent pharmacokinetics of busulfan in paediatric haematopoietic stem cell transplantation patients: towards individualized dosing. *Clin Pharmacokinet.* 2012;**51**(5):331–345.

CHAPTER 32

Aplastic anemia and paroxysmal nocturnal hemoglobinuria

Andrew C. Dietz and Michael A. Pulsipher

Pediatric Hematology, Oncology, & Blood and Marrow Transplantation, Children's Hospital Los Angeles, University of Southern California, Los Angeles, CA, USA

Introduction

Acquired AA is a rare bone marrow failure disorder with an estimated annual incidence of two cases per million and with over 600 new cases in the United States each year. There is a biphasic distribution of onset with peaks occurring between 10 and 25 years of age and over 60 years of age. Patients present with infection, bruising, pallor, and fatigue due to cytopenias in at least two of the three key components of blood: red cells, white cells, or platelets. Aplastic anemia is considered *very severe* if the ANC is less than 200 cells per microliter, *severe* (SAA) if less than 500, and *moderate* if those criteria are not met. The majority of cases are thought to be related to autoimmune destruction of marrow microenvironment or hematopoietic stem cells; accordingly, the disease can be treated and often cured by either immune suppression or marrow replacement through allogeneic hematopoietic cell transplantation (allo-HCT).

Diagnostic approach: Differentiating between toxic damage and inherited marrow failure

Working through the differential diagnosis of SAA is important to first ensure there is not a reversible process caused by a toxic exposure or infectious etiology. Malignant or genetic marrow disorders are also possible. When performing a marrow examination to follow-up on peripheral cytopenias, it is important to look for:

1 Bone marrow cellularity- hypocellularity is observed in AA (Table 32.1)

2 Signs of malignancy
3 Myelodysplasia morphologically or by clonal cytogenetic abnormalities detected through fluorescence *in-situ* hybridization (FISH) or karyotype
4 Cells associated with infiltrative marrow disorders, such as Gaucher cells.

Additionally, a comprehensive history and physical exam should be performed to ensure the patient does not have constitutional AA as a presenting sign of an inherited bone marrow failure syndrome, which can occur in 15–20% of cases. If there is anything out of the ordinary, appropriate screening tests and genetic analysis should be performed (Tables 32.1 and 32.2). However, a number of patients with an inherited syndrome will present with no associated findings. Pediatric patients with SAA should be screened for Fanconi anemia (see Chapter 29) using chromosomal breakage testing (DEB or other appropriate) and screening for dyskeratosis congenita with telomere length by flow-FISH should also be considered, as these patient populations cannot tolerate conventional chemotherapy and radiation doses used during allo-HCT.

PRACTICE POINT

All patients meeting diagnostic criteria for SAA should be worked up for malignancy, myelodysplasia, or presence of an inherited bone marrow failure syndrome before starting treatment for SAA. HLA typing of siblings should be initiated immediately in order to quickly move to allo-HCT if appropriate.

Clinical Manual of Blood and Bone Marrow Transplantation, First Edition. Edited by Syed A. Abutalib and Parameswaran Hari.
© 2017 John Wiley & Sons Ltd. Published 2017 by John Wiley & Sons Ltd.

Table 32.1 Can I call this SAA?

Yes	No or Needs Further Workup
<ul><li>Bone marrow cellularity <25%</li><li>Bone marrow cellularity <50% with <30% residual hematopoietic cells</li><li>At least two out of three:<ul><li>Severe neutropenia</li><li>Severe thrombocytopenia</li><li>Anemia with severe reticulocytopenia</li></ul></li></ul>	<ul><li>Toxic exposure as cause of marrow suppression, such as pesticides, arsenic, benzene, or ionizing radiation</li><li>Drug exposure as cause of marrow suppression, such as chloramphenicol, carbamazepine, felbamate, phenytoin, quinine, or others</li><li>Malignant or infiltrative cell population</li><li>Clonal cytogenetic abnormality tested on marrow</li><li>Family history suggestive of inherited syndrome (see Table 32.2)</li><li>Medical history or exam suggestive of inherited syndrome (see Table 32.2)</li><li>Chromosomal breakage to clastogens (Fanconi anemia; Chapter 26)</li><li>Very low *leukocyte* telomere length on flow-FISH (dyskeratosis congenita)</li><li>Decreased serum trypsinogen/isoamylase or reduced stool elastase (Schwachman–Diamond syndrome)</li><li>Elevated *RBC* adenosine deaminase (Diamond–Blackfan anemia)</li><li>Genetic testing consistent with any inherited syndrome including, but not limited to, those listed above as well as congenital amegakaryocytic thrombocytopenia</li></ul>

Table 32.2 History and exam features suggestive of inherited bone marrow failure syndromes.

History or Exam Feature	Associated Syndrome
Abnormal or missing thumbs and/or radius	Fanconi anemia
Metaphyseal chondrodysplasia and/or narrow chest	Schwachman–Diamond syndrome
Café-au-lait spots	Fanconi anemia
Reticular skin pigmentation	dyskeratosis congenita
Hypo/hypertelorism or small eyes	Fanconi anemia
Dystrophic fingernails or toenails	dyskeratosis congenita
Oral leukoplakia	dyskeratosis congenita
Abnormal head	Schwachman–Diamond syndrome, Fanconi anemia
Developmental delay	Fanconi anemia
Hypospadius or cryptorchidism	Fanconi anemia, dyskeratosis congenita
Cardiac anomalies	Fanconi anemia, dyskeratosis congenita
Horseshoe kidney	Fanconi anemia
Personal or family history of pulmonary fibrosis	dyskeratosis congenita
Personal or family history of liver fibrosis or cirrhosis	dyskeratosis congenita
Small or fatty pancreas with exocrine pancreatic insufficiency	Schwachman–Diamond syndrome
Osteopenia in a young patient	Schwachman–Diamond syndrome, dyskeratosis congenital
Severe dental abnormalities	Schwachman–Diamond syndrome
Unusual cancers, such as squamous cell carcinoma of the head, neck, vulva, or cervix	Fanconi anemia, dyskeratosis congenita
Unusual response to treatment, such as severe toxicity or prolonged pancytopenia	Fanconia anemia, dyskeratosis congenita

Treatment options for SAA

Best treatment option for younger patients: HLA-matched sibling allo-HCT

Allo-HCT from a HLA-matched sibling donor (MSD) is the standard of care for younger, newly diagnosed patients with long-term survival rates exceeding 90% in patients under the age of 20 years and around 76% for patients older than 20 years. Conditioning regimens typically consist of cyclophosphamide and serotherapy with either antithymocyte globulin (ATG) or alemtuzumab. GvHD prophylaxis generally consists of a calcineurin inhibitor with or without methotrexate.

> **PRACTICE POINT**
>
> Allo-HCT from HLA-MSD is first line therapy for younger, newly diagnosed patients with SAA.

What if the patient does not have a HLA-MSD or is not a candidate for allo-HCT?

Because only 25% of siblings will be HLA matched, most patients (70–80%) will not have sibling donors. Immunosuppressive therapy (IST) is the front-line treatment for SAA patients who lack HLAS-MSD or are not candidates for allo-HCT. Treatment consists of cyclosporine (CSA) and ATG, with horse ATG showing superiority over rabbit ATG. Important outcomes after IST therapy:

1 Hematopoietic response rate ranges are between 55 and 75%
2 Up to 20–40% of patients eventually relapse
3 An additional 10–20% develop secondary clonal disease, with repeated trials of IST increasing that risk
4 It typically takes 2–4 months following initiation of IST therapy before a response is seen
5 Patients typically remain on CSA for a minimum of 6–12 months, with some centers stopping at that point and other centers using prolonged taper schedules
6 The addition of mycophenolate, sirolimus, and other medications has not improved outcomes over horse ATG with cyclosporine
7 Eltrombopag, a thrombopoietin mimetic agent, has recently been approved for patients refractory to other approaches due to achievement of hematologic response in at least one cell lineage in 40% of patients, half of whom achieved trilineage response. Clonal cytogenetic abnormalities were observed in 19% of patients and dysplasia in 5%. This medication is currently being investigated in combination with CSA/ATG for newly diagnosed patients.

When patients fail or relapse after IST

Repeat courses of IST are possible, either with ATG and CSA, or with agents such as alemtuzumab. A second course of IST works about 30% of the time if patients fail up-front treatment, and more often if patients relapse after stopping or tapering CSA. This is the point in the treatment algorithm where consideration is given for allo-HCT, even if there is no available HLA-MSD. Over the last two decades, there have been significant advances in the use of allo-HCT, with improvements in outcomes using HLA-matched unrelated donors (MUD), as shown in Figures 32.1 and 32.2, likely due to:

1 Use of leuko-depleted blood products
2 Limitation of transfusions to minimize alloimmunization and iron overload
3 Use of antimicrobial prophylaxis and empiric therapy, particularly antifungal
4 Better tissue typing of recipient and donors resulting in better HLA-matching
5 Effective reduction in intensity of conditioning regimens
6 Movement of patients to transplantation quickly after failure of IST

The incorporation of fludarabine and serotherapy with reduction of cyclophosphamide and reduction or elimination of TBI has been trialed now in multiple countries with studies starting to show improved overall survival (OS) and decreasing rates of graft failure as well as acute and chronic GvHD (Table 32.3). It has become the standard of care to offer a HLA-MUD allo-HCT to patients that are refractory or relapse after IST when a HLA-MSD is not available.

No studies in adults have supported up-front HLA-MUD transplant, but some pediatric retrospective studies have examined outcomes with this approach compared to IST and HLA-MSD transplants. HLA-MUD transplants were found to be comparable to HLA-MSD transplant strategy and there was a suggestion of improved outcomes compared to IST approach. This has led to questions about the use of up-front HLA-MUD transplantation, at least in pediatrics, if a donor can be available in a timely fashion. This strategy is now being studied in both Europe and the United States.

> **PRACTICE POINT**
>
> HLA-MUD transplantation is the standard of care for patients that are refractory or relapse after IST if they lack HLA-MSD. HLA-MUD transplantation is being studied as an up-front treatment option in children.

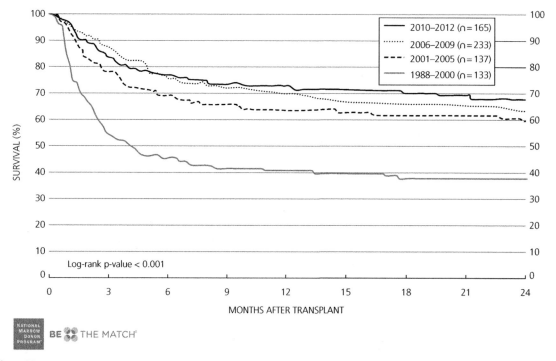

Figure 32.1 Improvements over time in HLA-MUD allo-HCT for SAA in adults.

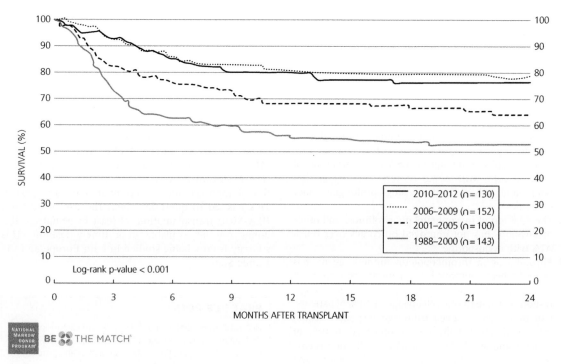

Figure 32.2 Improvements over time in HLA-MUD allo-HCT for SAA in pediatrics.

Table 32.3 HLA-MUD transplants in SAA*.

Study (year)	N	Conditioning	Median Age	GF%	aGvHD %	cGvHD %	OS %
Bacigalupo (2010)	100	Flu/Cy/ATG±TBI	20	17	18	27–50	75 (5 y)
Kang (2010)	28	Flu/Cy/ATG	13	0	46	35	68 (3 y)
Yagasaki (2010)	31	Various	9	3	37	27	94 (5 y)
Samarasinghe (2012)	44	Flu/Cy/Alem	8	0	32	7	95 (5yr)
Chen (2013)	22	Various	6	9	23	29	96 (5yr)

*Some studies include HLA-mismatch unrelated donors

Is it appropriate to use a HLA-mismatched unrelated donor (MMUD)?

There is practice variation in this area. A number of the studies listed in Table 32.3 that examined unrelated donor transplants include a portion of patients receiving HLA-MMUD transplantation. Often it can be hard to separate these out due to small numbers. Some providers consider them together as an option. However, other providers are worried about the increased rates of GvHD and decreased OS that has been reported with HLA-MMUD compared to HLA- MUDs and would consider alternative options first.

What about patients who fail multiple attempts at immune suppression and don't have HLA-MUD: Do they have transplantation options?

Historically, success with cord blood and haplo-identical transplantation has been poor, with OS rates less than 60% and high rates of graft failure as well as both acute and chronic GvHD. Newer optimized reduced-intensity regimens with fludarabine, lower doses of both cyclophosphamide and TBI, and ATG have shown outcomes similar to standard HLA-MUD in small studies and are being investigated in larger multicenter trials.

> **PRACTICE POINT**
>
> Transplantation with HLA-mismatched unrelated, cord blood, or HLA-haplo-identical donors should ideally be performed in the context of a clinical trial given that the disease is rare, and trials are needed to demonstrate improved outcomes using these sources.

A word about paroxysmal nocturnal hemoglobinuria

Paroxysmal Nocturnal Hemoglobinuria (PNH) is a rare acquired problem with stem cells that can often be associated with bone marrow failure and in more severe forms can also be associated with:
1 Hemolytic anemia
2 Thrombosis
3 Smooth muscle dystonia
4 Renal failure
5 Arterial and pulmonary hypertension
6 Recurrent infections.

PNH typically results from a mutation in the x-linked gene phosphatidylinositol glycan class A (PIG-A) whereby cells lack two important complement regulatory proteins CD55 and CD59. There is a non-malignant clonal expansion where PNH cells have a conditional survival advantage in the setting of an autoimmune attack. This may underpin the relationship between PNH and bone marrow failure where PNH clones can be detected in up to 60% of all AA cases and 20% of all low-risk myeslodysplasia (MDS) cases. PNH can be diagnosed with flow cytometry using fluorescent aerolysin (FLAER), where clones <1% can be detected.

There are three forms of PNH:

1 **Classical**
  a No evidence of bone marrow failure
  b Presents with symptoms mentioned above
  c Risk of transformation to MDS is 5%
  d Risk of transformation to AML is 2.5%
  e Can be treated with eculizumab, a monoclonal antibody that blocks the activation of terminal complement C5
  f Allo-HCT, while the only curative therapy, is only recommended in countries where eculizumab is not available or in patients who do not respond to eculizumab therapy

2 **Associated with AA**
  a Typically, PNH clones are <10% and while some hemolysis may be seen, usually patients are clinically asymptomatic
  b Treatment of PNH is based on treatment of underlying bone marrow failure process, and allo-HCT is often indicated with reduced-intensity preparative regimens
  c No need for eculizumab therapy before or after transplantation unless there are major clinical symptoms associated with an expanding clone

3 **Subclinical**
  a Small clone size, typically <1%
  b No hemolysis and otherwise clinically asymptomatic
  c No treatment needed
  d Monitor for clonal expansion or disease evolution every 6–12 months

How should SAA patients be followed after therapy?

SAA Patients treated with IST

For those patients that do not undergo transplantation, bone marrow morphology should be assessed again at 6 and 12 months after treatment and then yearly thereafter to monitor for clonal evolution, especially if any cell lines begin to decrease. Additionally, frank recurrence of pancytopenia warrants repeat marrow examination immediately to exclude clonal evolution.

SAA patients treated with allo-HCT

A unique aspect of transplantation for SAA is the occurrence of late secondary graft failure, reported as late as 10 years post-transplantation. Therefore, the patient should continue to be followed closely by a transplant or hematology clinic for many years.

Beyond the first few years, many patients will transition to a transplantation survivorship clinic. Fortunately, as a result of the reduced-intensity conditioning used and the generally limited previous therapy, the late effects of transplantation seen in this patient population are typically less than those transplanted for malignant conditions. In fact, most patients will go on to live healthy and lives without impact on educational attainment or fertility and only very minimal risk of late complications.

However, continued and consistent evaluation is warranted for late effects that have been described in a limited portion of this patient population. These issues are typically found more in patients that received unrelated or alternative donor transplantation and include:

1 Secondary malignancy
2 Osteonecrosis
3 Cardiovascular problems
4 Stroke
5 Seizures
6 Renal failure
7 Fertility problems
8 Gonadal failure
9 Growth failure
10 Cataracts
11 Hypothyroidism
12 Depression
13 Anxiety
14 Post-traumatic stress

> **PRACTICE POINT**
>
> SAA patients treated for IST can develop late clonal evolution and should have counts followed for the first two decades after therapy. Most patients transplanted for SAA will have limited late effects due to the use of reduced-intensity condition regimen, however, continued follow-up in a survivorship clinic is warranted to identify those patients at highest risk.

High yield points

1 During workup for SAA, HLA typing should be initiated immediately; malignancy including myelodysplasia, toxin or medication exposure, and inherited bone marrow failure syndromes should be excluded prior to definitive therapy for AA.
2 Standard of care first line therapy in younger, newly diagnosed patients is a HLA-MSD transplant.
3 Standard of care for some patients who are refractory or relapsed after IST is a allo-HCT from HLA-MUD.
4 Transplantation with HLA-MMUD, cord blood, or HLA-haploidentical donors should ideally be performed in the context of a clinical trial.
5 Patients should continue to be followed long term due to the risks of late secondary graft failure, graft-versus-host disease, and the potential for late effects.
6 Given the difference in outcomes according to age, different algorithms exist for pediatric and adult patients (Figures 32.3 and 32.4).

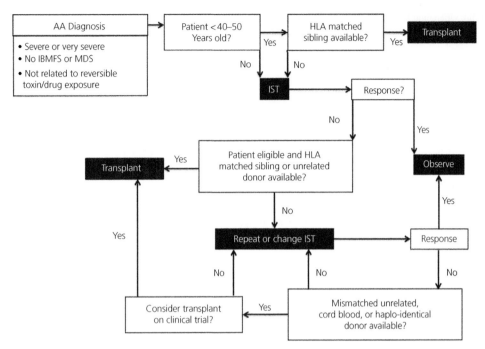

Figure 32.3 Treatment algorithm for adult patients with SAA.

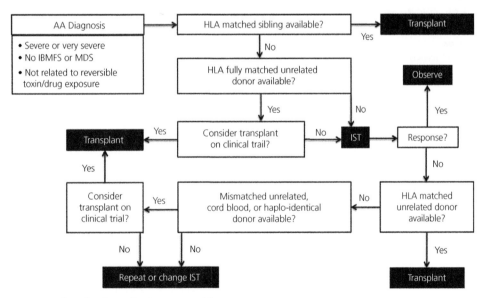

Figure 32.4 Treatment algorithm for pediatric patients with SAA.

Table 32.4 Who, when, and how of allo-HCT for aplastic anemia

Author's Practice:

A PATIENT FACTORS

Age:
Patients under age 40–45 are considered better candidates for allo-HCT; patients over this age are typically treated with IST first.
Performance Status and Comorbidity:
Patients should not have an inherited bone marrow failure syndrome, as there are unique issues with this population in terms of comorbidities and risk of toxicity.
Transplantation is much higher risk in patients with uncontrolled infection or significant organ toxicity. While reduced-intensity conditioning is used, these patients may not qualify for transplantation until these issues are under control.

B DISEASE FACTORS
Newly Diagnosed:
Younger patients with an available HLA-MSD would be offered transplantation as front-line therapy. Pediatric patients with a quickly available HLA-MUD could be offered transplantation as front-line therapy in the context of a clinical trial.
Refractory to Immunosuppression Therapy:
Patients with a HLA-MUD would be offered transplantation. Patients without a HLA-MUD could be considered for a clinical trial using alternative donor sources.
Relapse after Immunosuppression Therapy:
Patients with a HLA-MUD would be offered transplantation. Alternatively, a second course of immunosuppression can be attempted according to patient preference. Patients without a HLA-MUD could be considered for a clinical trial using alternative donor sources.
Clonal Evolution:
All patients with clonal evolution without significant co-morbid conditions should be offered allo-HCT. Those with advance MDS or AML may benefit from chemotherapy prior to allo-HCT.

C DONOR EVALUATION
Ideal Donor:
HLA-matched sibling or unrelated donor matched at all A, B, C, DRB1 using high resolution typing.
Alternative Donor:
Single-allele HLA-mismatched unrelated, mismatch umbilical cord blood, and HLA-haplo-identical donors could be used for patient without other options, especially if clinical trials studying these approaches are available.

D CONDITIONING
Should be Reduced-Intensity:
HLA-MSD – cyclophosphamide with ATG
HLA-MUD – fludarabine, low dose cyclophosphamide, low dose TBI, and ATG
* OR *
fludarabine, cyclophosphamide, and alemtuzumab
Alternative Donor – should be in the context of a clinical trial

E POST-TRANSPLANTATION FOLLOW-UP
All patients should continue to be followed in a transplant or hematology clinic for late secondary graft failure. Any patients with GvHD should continue to be followed in a transplant clinic. Subsequently all patients should transition to a transplant survivorship clinic for monitoring of late effects from the transplantation process.

Selected reading

1. Desmond R, Townsley DM, Dumitriu B et al. Eltrombopag restores trilineage hematopoiesis in refractory severe aplastic anemia that can be sustained on discontinuation of drug. *Blood*. 2014 Mar 20;123(12):1818–1825. PMID: 24345753.

2. Bacigalupo A, Socie G, Lanino E, et al. Fludarabine, cyclophosphamide, antithymocyte globulin, with or without low dose total body irradiation, for alternative donor transplants, in acquired severe aplastic anemia: a retrospective study from the EBMT-SAA Working Party. *Haematologica*. Italy. 2010;95:976–982.

3. Kang HJ, Shin HY, Park JE, et al. Successful engraftment with fludarabine, cyclophosphamide, and thymoglobulin conditioning regimen in unrelated transplantation for severe aplastic anemia: A phase II prospective multicenter study. *Biol Blood Marrow Transplant* 2010;16(11): 1582–1588.

4. Yagasaki H, Takahashi Y, Hama A, et al. Comparison of matched-sibling donor BMT and unrelated donor BMT in children and adolescent with acquired severe aplastic anemia. *Bone Marrow Transplantation* 2010;45(10): 1508–1513.

5. Samarasinghe S, Webb DKH. How I manage aplastic anaemia in children. *Br J Haematol*. 2012 Apr;157(1):26–40.

6. Chen J, Lee V, Luo CJ, et al. Allogeneic stem cell transplantation for children with acquired severe aplastic anemia; a retrospective study by the Viva-Asia Blood and Marrow Transplantation Group. *Br J Haematol*. 2013;162(3): 383–391.

7. Buchbinder D, Nugent DJ, Brazauskas R, Wang Z, Aljurf MD, Cairo MS, et al. Late effects in hematopoietic cell transplant recipients with acquired severe aplastic anemia: A report from the late effects working committee of the center for international blood and marrow transplant research. *Biol Blood Marrow Transplant*. 2012 Dec;18(12):1776–1784.

8. Devalet B, Mullier F, Chatelain B, Dogne JM, Chatelain C. Pathophysiology, diagnosis, and treatment of paroxysmal nocturnal hemoglobinuria: A review. *Eur J Haematol*. 2015 Mar;95(3):190–198.

9. Eapen M, Horowitz MM. Alternative donor transplantation for aplastic anemia. *Hematology ASH Education Program*. 2010: 43–46.

10. National Marrow Donor Program: Be The Match (US). Severe Aplastic Anemia and Other Marrow Failure Syndromes. [Internet] Available from: https://bethematchclinical.org/transplant-indications-and-outcomes/disease-specific-indications-and-outcomes/severe-aplastic-anemia-and-marrow-failure/(accessed January 2017).

11. Scheinberg P, Young NS. How I treat acquired aplastic anemia. *Blood*. 2012 Aug 9;120(6):1185–11896.

CHAPTER 33

HIV infection and transplantation

Nitya Nathwani, Stephen J. Forman, and Amrita Krishnan

City of Hope National Medical Center, Duarte, CA, USA

Introduction

In the era of highly active antiretroviral therapy (HAART) therapy, the lifespans of HIV-infected patients have improved considerably. The incidence of opportunistic infections and AIDS-related syndromes in these individuals have decreased. HIV-infected individuals have an increased tendency to develop malignancy for a variety of reasons, and in part due to impaired cellular immunity. These malignancies are an important cause of mortality in these individuals, especially since these patients are living longer. Among the non-Hodgkin lymphoma (NHL) group, the incidence of systemic NHL, central nervous system (CNS) lymphoma, and primary effusion, or body cavity lymphoma are increased in this population. There has also been an increase in HIV related Hodgkin lymphoma, usually Epstein–Barr virus (EBV) positive, probably related to immune stimulation resulting from higher CD4$^+$ cell counts; see Table 33.1.

AIDS-related lymphomas (ARL) are often characterized by:

1 Clinically aggressive behavior
2 Advanced HIV with a low CD4$^+$ cell count and high viral load
3 B symptoms (fevers, drenching night sweats, weight loss >10% from baseline in the past 6 months)
4 Extranodal presentation with gastrointestinal, liver, lung, CNS, and bone marrow involvement
5 Advanced stage disease
6 Unusual locations such as soft tissue and body cavities

Evaluation of a suspected patient with HIV lymphoma

1 Complete history and physical
2 Biopsy of the affected lymph node or organ involved
3 Bone marrow aspiration and biopsy
4 Imaging: CT scans with FDG-PET may identify the most metabolically active site with the prospective highest yield for biopsy
5 Upper and lower endoscopy if suspected gastrointestinal involvement
6 CNS evaluation with neuroimaging and cerebrospinal fluid (CSF) examination if suspected CNS involvement. CSF analysis should include cell count, cytology, protein, glucose, and flow cytometry. In HIV-associated PCNSL, positive EBV by PCR on CSF is diagnostic.
  Risk factors associated with CNS involvement:
  a Bone marrow involvement
  b Involvement of more than two extranodal sites with elevated LDH
  c Burkitt's histology
  d Paranasal sinus involvement
  e Paraspinal involvement
  f Testicular involvement

PRACTICE POINT

A fine needle aspiration is inadequate for diagnosis. A core biopsy at the minimum, but preferably an excisional biopsy is required for accurate diagnosis. Corticosteroids may interfere with biopsy interpretation, so it is preferable to obtain tissue diagnosis prior to starting empiric corticosteroids.

Clinical Manual of Blood and Bone Marrow Transplantation, First Edition. Edited by Syed A. Abutalib and Parameswaran Hari.
© 2017 John Wiley & Sons Ltd. Published 2017 by John Wiley & Sons Ltd.

Table 33.1 Cancers with increased risk in patients infected with HIV.

AIDS defining malignancies (as defined by the CDC)	Kaposi sarcoma B-cell NHLs (see Table 33.2) Cervical cancer
Non-AIDS defining malignancies	Lung cancer Hodgkin lymphoma Skin cancer Head and neck cancers Hepatocellular cancer Colorectal cancer Testicular seminomas Renal cell carcinoma Conjunctival cancer Esophageal cancer Sarcomas

Table 33.2 Incidence of AIDS-related B-cell NHLs.

Systemic NHLs	~80%
• Diffuse large B-cell lymphoma	• ~75%
• Burkitt's lymphoma	• ~25%
• Indolent B-cell lymphoma	• <10%
• Plasmablastic lymphoma	• <5%
Primary CNS lymphoma	~15%
Primary effusion or body cavity lymphoma	<5%

Treatment principles

In the pre-HAART era, the standard treatment for AIDS associated NHL was low dose chemotherapy. It was thought that patients would be unable to tolerate intensive chemotherapy due to the underlying immunodeficiency. In the post-HAART era, patients were treated more aggressively due to improved hematologic reserve in patients on HAART. Patients are now treated in a similar way to non-HIV NHL patients. Their remission rates and median survival with aggressive combination chemotherapy and HAART is similar to their HIV negative counterparts.

Choice of therapy depends on the stage and subtype of NHL. HAART is an important treatment component, but it remains controversial whether to give HAART concurrently with chemotherapy or to temporarily hold antiretroviral therapy during chemotherapy due to potential drug interactions. The commonest subtype of NHL, diffuse large B-cell lymphoma (DLBCL), is treated similarly to the HIV negative population. Limited stage disease is usually treated with chemotherapy and involved field radiation (IFRT). Advanced stage disease, which is more common, is treated with combination chemotherapy. The most widely used regimen uses a combination of rituximab with cyclophosphamide, adriamycin, vincristine, and prednisone (R-CHOP). Abbreviated R-EPOCH (rituximab, etoposide, vincristine, adriamycin, cyclophosphamide, prednisone) has also shown durable remissions.

Consequently, more aggressive therapies such as high dose chemotherapy (HDCT) and autologous hematopoietic cell transplantation (AHCT) have been studied in the HAART era with encouraging results.

AHCT

There are various preparative regimens used for AHCT in AIDS lymphoma. The ideal regimen should be able to eradicate the malignancy, have no mortality, and manageable toxicity. Unfortunately, no such treatments exist. Drugs are chosen that have no overlapping toxicities except for the hematologic toxicity. In NHL, frequently used agents include cytarabine, cyclophosphamide, etoposide, carmustine (BCNU), and melphalan. HAART should be continued during conditioning, although myelosuppressive medications such as azidothymidine should be avoided, and drug interactions need to be carefully considered.

How did we get here?

AHCT has been the standard treatment for HIV negative patients with relapsed NHL since the landmark PARMA trial published by Philip et al. in the *New England Journal of Medicine* in 1995. In this trial, patients with relapsed chemosensitive aggressive NHL were treated with two cycles of DHAP (dexamethasone, cisplatin, and cytarabine) and if responsive, randomly assigned to get either DHAP for four additional cycles or high dose chemotherapy with BEAC (BCNU/carmustine, etoposide, cytarabine, and cyclophosphamide) followed by AHCT. The results of this study demonstrated an overall survival (OS) benefit of 53 versus 32% (p = 0.038) in favor of the high dose chemotherapy arm.

AHCT in HIV-positive patients was pioneered by the French in the pre-HAART era, and the first patient reported was a 40-year-old male with HIV related NHL who was able to undergo successful mobilization and engraftment, but did poorly due to several opportunistic infections from uncontrolled HIV.

What are the data with AHCT in HIV associated lymphoma?

This is summarized in Table 33.3. In the post-HAART era, AHCT was considered feasible, with manageable infectious issues, and no apparent adverse consequences related to HIV. The bulk of the data suggested that HIV should not preclude lymphoma patients from undergoing AHCT. Infection prophylaxis and close monitoring of immune recovery is important in these patients.

Discrepancy between studies

The discordant outcomes are likely due to variations in:
1 Patient selection:
   a Differences in chemotherapy sensitive versus chemotherapy refractory disease between studies.
   b Number of lines of prior therapy.
   c Disease status at the time of AHCT.
   d Different eligibility criteria: for example, some studies excluded CNS disease and bone marrow involvement, while others allowed these patients.
   e Histology: for example, the proportion of patients with NHL versus HL differed among studies, the latter typically having a better prognosis.
   f Different IPI risk groups
2 Conditioning regimens employed (e.g., different dose intensities of busulfan based conditioning, radiation *versus* non-radiation based regimens, BEAM vs CBV)
3 Length of follow-up
4 HIV control: some studies required stricter control of the underlying HIV than others
5 Year of transplant.

Ideally, treatment should be administered in the context of randomized prospective multicenter clinical trials, but given the rarity of the disease and the challenges in conducting randomized trials in this unique population of patients that often require urgent treatment, this approach is difficult.

Which patients are suitable candidates for AHCT?

This depends primarily on patient and disease specific risk factors. In general, patients should have an adequate performance status, organ function testing, and no active infections. The underlying HIV infection needs to be under control, ideally with an undetectable viral load. In general, patients should have chemotherapy sensitive disease as the outcomes in patients with chemotherapy refractory disease are poor. Our approach is outlined in Table 33.4.

Allogeneic transplantation in HIV

These immunologic effects of allogeneic hematopoietic cell transplantation (allo-HCT) could be particularly valuable in the treatment of HIV infection. Allogeneic stem cell transplantation (allo-HCT) is more challenging than AHCT in HIV-infected individuals due to the need for chronic immunosuppression in an already immunocompromised patient. There is limited data on allo-HCT in HIV.

Allo-HCT in HIV

History

Early reports in the pre-HAART era from Johns Hopkins showed no significant regimen-related toxicity, or engraftment issues, but the patient succumbed to relapsed lymphoma at day +47. At autopsy, no evidence of HIV, either by culture, or PCR was found in tissue specimens, raising the fascinating question "could allogeneic transplant be a path to treat HIV infection?"

Data for allo–HCT in HIV infected individuals: Where do we stand?

There was a report of two HIV-positive patients who received nonmyeloablative (NMA) transplants at the Fred Hutchinson Research Center with HLA-matched peripheral blood grafts, one from a HLA-matched sibling and the other from an HLA-matched unrelated donor, following fludarabine and 200 cGy TBI conditioning, with cyclosporine, and mycophenolate mofetil as GvHD prophylaxis. HAART was continued. HIV RNA remained undetectable and no HIV related infections occurred. The first patient died from GvHD. The second patient continues beyond 180 days post-transplant. Interestingly, both patients' and donor cells expressed wild-type CCR5 co-receptor, and not the CCRΔ32 allele that is linked with resistance to HIV infection.

The largest study was a retrospective series through the CIBMTR of 23 HIV-positive patients undergoing myeloablative (87%) or NMA (13%) HLA-matched sibling donor (n = 19) or HLA-matched unrelated donor (n = 4) allo-HCT between 1987 and 2003. In 21 out of 23 patients, the indication for allo-HCT was a malignant hematologic disorder, and in the remaining two patients, transplantation was for a non-malignant hematologic disorder. The cumulative incidence of grades 2–4 acute GvHD was 30% at 100 days and chronic GvHD was 28% at 2 years. At a median follow-up of 59 months, the OS at 2 years was 30%. Non-relapse mortality was high at in 9 out of 23 patients (39%), mostly related to pulmonary toxicity (6 out of 9 patients). Survival was better in patients who underwent

Table 33.3 Results of autologous transplant in individual with HIV infection and lymphoma.

Author	N total N auto	Trial Setting	Conditioning regimen	TRM	OS	PFS	Comments and Practice Implications
Krishnan et al.	20/20	NHL and HL, high-risk IPI in CR1, or chemosensitive relapse	carmustine, etoposide, Cy, or FTBI, etoposide, Cy	5%	85%	85% at 32 months	less advanced lymphoma, chemotherapy refractory patients disqualified; engraftment times comparable to HIV negative patients, median was 11 days; poor tolerance of HAART during transplant period; low TRM; low incidence of opportunistic infections; underlying HIV disease did not deteriorate as a result of the transplant; CD4+ cell counts recovered to pre-transplant levels by one year in all patients; superior disease free survival in this series may be mediated in part by well controlled HIV infection.
Spitzer et al.	27/20	NHL and HD not in CR, or chemosensitive relapse	busulfan-cyclophosphamide	5%	74.4%	49.5% at 6 months	multi-institutional trial; well tolerated regimen with substantial anti-tumor activity; favorable DFS and OS; favorable immune reconstitution; no deaths from infection; CD4+ cell counts recovered to baseline levels by day+260;
Gabarre et al.	14/14	relapsed or refractory NHL or HL	various including BEAM/busulfan/ high dose Cy/Cy-thiotepa/TBI	0	36%	29% at 49 months	AHCT is feasible with respect to CD34+ cell cell harvesting, engraftment, and adverse events, but long term results are disappointing; all patients here did not have chemosensitive disease.

Author	N total N auto	Trial Setting	Conditioning	TRM	OS	PFS	Comments and Practice Implications
Re et al.	50/27	primary refractory or relapsed NHL or HL with chemosensitive disease	BEAM	0	75%	75%	no significant HIV-associated infections noted; infectious risk in patients on effective HAART was similar to patients without HIV who underwent AHCT; only lymphoma response significantly affected OS after transplantation; median OS of all 50 eligible patients was 33 months (OS 50%); low CD4+ cell count, marrow involvement, and poor performance status independently affected survival.
Balsalobre et al.	68/68	retrospective analysis from EBMTcenters,multi-institutional; NHL and HL	BEAM and variants	7.5%	61%	56% at 32 months	on multivariate analysis, chemotherapy resistant disease, and not attaining complete remission predicted poorer progression free survival and OS; disease control with chemotherapy at the time of AHCT predicts a more favorable result.
Krishnan et al.	58/29	Case series of HIV positive and negative NHL	CBV or BEAM	11%	75%	76% at 24 months	29 patients with HIV positive NHL were matched with HIV negative NHL controls with respect to sex, time to AHCT, year of transplant, histology, age, disease status, number of prior regimens, and conditioning regimen; higher proportion of poor risk HIV positive NHL patients; causes of death in the HIV-positive cohort were mostly from relapsed lymphoma, and not infection; disease status at the time of transplant was the only clear predictor of outcome.

Table 33.4 Who, when, and how of autologous HCT for AIDS NHL

Authors' practice:

A *PATIENT FACTORS:*
Age:
AIDS- related lymphomas typically affect younger patients. There is no upper limit for age in determining eligibility for AHCT in AIDS lymphoma and "biologic age" is more important than chronologic age.

Performance Status (PS) and Comorbidity:
AHCT is feasible with low TRM in those with good PS. We typically exclude patients with Karnofsky performance status (KPS) <70. The minimum KPS is greater than or equal to 60%. An ECOG performance status ≤2 is an alternative measure.

We typically exclude patients with renal failure (creatinine clearance or GFR < 60 mL/min)

We typically exclude patients with cardiac dysfunction with an ejection fraction below 50%. On occasion, we may allow an ejection fraction > 40% if BEAM conditioning is used with Cardiology clearance, but in general, a minimum ejection fraction of ≥50% is required when using chemotherapy regimens with known cardiac toxicity (e.g., cyclophosphamide-based regimens) or (TBI)-based conditioning regimens.

Adequate pulmonary function defined as FVC and DLCO of > 50% of predicted is required.

Adequate liver function defined as total bilirubin less than or equal to two times the upper limit of normal (unless the patient has Gilbert's disease) and AST/ALT less than or equal to 2.5 times the upper limit of normal. If hepatic function is abnormal due to underlying malignancy the patient may be approved for HCT. Patients with cirrhosis are excluded. Active viral hepatitis is excluded.

Patients with active bacterial, fungal, or viral infections are excluded

Patients with dementia or degenerative or demyelinating diseases of the CNS are excluded.

Malignancy other than lymphoma, unless (1) in complete remission and more than 5 years from last treatment, or (2) cervical/anal squamous cell carcinoma *in situ*, or (3) superficial basal cell and squamous cell cancers of the skin.

Uncontrolled comorbid medical illnesses including coronary artery disease, hypertension and/or diabetes are excluded.

Patients with psychosocial dysfunction that precludes the ability to give informed consent and/or places the patient as high-risk for non-compliance with medical treatment and follow-up care post-HCT are excluded

Patients with evidence of myelodysplasia on bone marrow examination are excluded due to the risk of developing secondary AML

B. *DISEASE FACTORS:*
Relapsed AIDS-related lymphoma (NHL or HL) demonstrating chemosensitivity
HIV viremia should be controlled (responding to HAART therapy), and no opportunistic infections

C. *DONOR EVALUATION:*
Not applicable

D. *CONDITIONING THERAPY:*
We typically use one of the following two regimens:

CBV (cyclophosphamide, carmustine and etoposide).

Day	Treatment
−8	Admission to hospital. Begin Levetiracetam
−7	Carmustine (150 mg/m² Adjusted BSA) IV
−6	Carmustine (150 mg/m² Adjusted BSA) IV
−5	Carmustine (150 mg/m² Adjusted BSA) IV
−4	Etoposide (60 mg/kg Adjusted BW) IV
−3	Rest Day
−2	Cyclophosphamide (100 mg/kg Ideal BW) IV
−1	Rest Day
0	Reinfusion of G-CSF primed CD34⁺ cells
+5	G-CSF 5 mcg/kg/day IV

BEAM (carmustine, etoposide, cytarabine, melphalan)

Day	Treatment (All chemotherapy based on Adjusted Body Weight)
−8	Admission to hospital. Begin Levetiracetam
−7	Carmustine (150 mg/m²) IV

Table 33.4   (Continued)

-6	Carmustine (150 mg/m²) IV
-5	Ara-C 200 mg/m² Q12 h IV; Etoposide 200 mg/m² IV
-4	Ara-C 200 mg/m² Q12 h IV; Etoposide 200 mg/m² IV
-3	Ara-C 200 mg/m² Q12 h IV; Etoposide 200 mg/m² IV
-2	Ara-C 200 mg/m² Q12 h IV; Etoposide 200 mg/m² IV
-1	Melphalan 140 mg/m² IV
0	Reinfusion of /G-CSF primed CD34⁺ cells
+5	G-CSF 5 mcg/kg/day IV
E POST ALLOTRANSPLANT THERAPY: Not applicable	

allo-HCT after 1996 when HAART use became widespread. Thus, reduction of transplant related mortality (TRM) and control of HIV infection together are central to the success of allo-HCT in this population.

Allo-HCT in hematologic malignancies: Moving forward

Prospective trials are needed to study allo-HCT further in this population. There is an ongoing prospective multicenter Phase II study being conducted by the CTN (#0903) to look at the safety and feasibility of this procedure in 15 patients with chemotherapy sensitive hematologic malignancies.

Allo-HCT for HIV infection
Allo-HCT has the exciting potential to control or "cure" the HIV infection. HIV-1 enters host cells by binding to a CD4 receptor on T-cells and then interacting with either CCR5 or the CXC chemokine receptor (CXCR4). Homozygosity for a 32-bp deletion (delta 32) in the CCR5 allele confers natural resistance to infection with CCR5 tropic HIV strains (R5 HIV) because of the lack of CCR5 cell-surface expression.

A case report from Germany, the "*Berlin experience*" describes a 40-year-old patient with a 10-year history of HIV who underwent allo-HCT in February 2007 for relapsed AML from an HLA-matched unrelated donor who was homozygous for the CCR5 delta 32 allele. It appears that he has remained off HAART and had no evidence of HIV disease for over 4 years post-transplant. The study suggests that CCR5Δ32/Δ32 HCT has probably led to a cure of HIV infection in this patient.

However, a similar approach was unsuccessful in additional patients, and in one patient, a CXCR4-tropic HIV-1 variant rebounded rapidly after transplantation. This co-receptor switch is a viral escape mechanism, and

although speculative, viral control may be improved if HAART therapy is not discontinued.

An experience of two patients on HAART with HL and HIV, heterozygous for the CCR5Δ32 mutation, who underwent allo-HCT from donors with wild-type CCR5+ cells with reduced intensity conditioning, demonstrated loss of detectable HIV-1 which correlated temporally with full donor chimerism, development of GvHD, and a sustained reduction in the HIV-1 peripheral reservoir. This suggestion of a therapeutic effect on the HIV reservoir could change the natural history of HIV.

Gene therapy for HIV infection
The risk to benefit ratio of allo-HCT is inappropriately high to recommend it in the absence of an underlying malignancy for which it is warranted as therapy. It cannot be proposed as a treatment strategy for the majority of HIV-infected patients who can live long healthy lives with the use of HAART. Homozygosity for the delta 32 mutation is only found in a minority of the population, so it is not possible to find such HLA-matched donors for the majority of patients. Preferably, one would hope to incorporate the benefits of transplantation of cells with the CCR5 mutation without the hazards of allo-HCT. One potential way to achieve this would be to transplant autologous grafts that were genetically modified to express antiretroviral genes to resist infection by the HIV virus. We have performed trials at the City of Hope using this approach with a lentivirus-based system, and the concept is that engraftment of these cells will lead to HIV resistance and elimination of the HIV reservoir. Future trials will address how to augment engraftment of the genetically modified CD34⁺ cells with planned interruption of HAART to demonstrate the functionality of these genetically modified cells. It is thought that a combination of approaches may be necessary to achieve a cure.

Selected reading

1. Frisch M, Biggar RJ, Engels EA, Goedert JJ. Association of cancer with AIDS-related immunosuppression in adults. *JAMA*. 2001 Apr 4;**285**(13):1736–1745. PubMed PMID: 11277828. Epub 2001/04/13. eng.

2. Shiels MS, Koritzinsky EH, Clarke CA, Suneja G, Morton LM, Engels EA. Prevalence of HIV Infection among U.S. Hodgkin lymphoma cases. *Cancer Epidemiol Biomarkers Prev*. 2014 Feb;**23**(2):274–281. PubMed PMID: 24326629. Pubmed Central PMCID: PMC3946161. Epub 2013/12/12. eng.

3. Philip T, Guglielmi C, Hagenbeek A, Somers R, Van der Lelie H, Bron D, et al. Autologous bone marrow transplantation as compared with salvage chemotherapy in relapses of chemotherapy-sensitive non-Hodgkin's lymphoma. *N Engl J Med*. 1995 Dec 7;**333**(23):1540–1545. PubMed PMID: 7477169. Epub 1995/12/07. eng.

4. Krishnan A, Molina A, Zaia J, Smith D, Vasquez D, Kogut N, et al. Durable remissions with autologous stem cell transplantation for high-risk HIV-associated lymphomas. *Blood*. 2005 Jan 15;**105**(2):874–878. PubMed PMID: 15388574. Epub 2004/09/25. eng.

5. Balsalobre P, Diez-Martin JL, Re A, Michieli M, Ribera JM, Canals C, et al. Autologous stem-cell transplantation in patients with HIV-related lymphoma. *J Clin Oncol*. 2009 May 1;**27**(13):2192–2198. PubMed PMID: 19332732. Epub 2009/04/01. eng.

6. Woolfrey AE, Malhotra U, Harrington RD, McNevin J, Manley TJ, Riddell SR, et al. Generation of HIV-1-specific CD8+ cell responses following allogeneic hematopoietic cell transplantation. *Blood*. 2008 Oct 15;**112**(8):3484–3487. PubMed PMID: 18698002. Pubmed Central PMCID: PMC2569185. Epub 2008/08/14. eng.

7. Gupta V, Tomblyn M, Pedersen TL, Atkins HL, Battiwalla M, Gress RE, et al. Allogeneic hematopoietic cell transplantation in human immunodeficiency virus-positive patients with hematologic disorders: a report from the center for international blood and marrow transplant research. *Biol Blood Marrow Transplant*. 2009 Jul;**15**(7):864–871. PubMed PMID: 19539219. Pubmed Central PMCID: PMC2881828. Epub 2009/06/23. eng.

8. Allers K, Hutter G, Hofmann J, Loddenkemper C, Rieger K, Thiel E, et al. Evidence for the cure of HIV infection by CCR5Delta32/Delta32 stem cell transplantation. *Blood*. 2011 Mar 10;**117**(10):2791–2799. PubMed PMID: 21148083. Epub 2010/12/15. eng.

9. Henrich TJ, Hu Z, Li JZ, Sciaranghella G, Busch MP, Keating SM, et al. Long-term reduction in peripheral blood HIV type 1 reservoirs following reduced-intensity conditioning allogeneic stem cell transplantation. *J Infect Dis*. 2013 Jun 1;**207**(11):1694–1702. PubMed PMID: 23460751. Pubmed Central PMCID: PMC3636784. Epub 2013/03/06. eng.

10. Zaia JA, Forman SJ. Transplantation in HIV-infected subjects: is cure possible? *Hematology Am Soc Hematol Educ Program*. 2013;**2013**:389–393. PubMed PMID: 24319209. Epub 2013/12/10. eng.

11. Spitzer TR, Ambinder RF, Lee JY, Kaplan LD, Wachsman W, Straus DJ, et al. Dose-reduced busulfan, cyclophosphamide, and autologous stem cell transplantation for human immunodeficiency virus-associated lymphoma: AIDS Malignancy Consortium study 020. *Biol Blood Marrow Transplant*. 2008 Jan;**14**(1):59–66. PubMed PMID: 18158962. Epub 2007/12/27. eng.

12. Gabarre J, Marcelin AG, Azar N, Choquet S, Levy V, Levy Y, et al. High-dose therapy plus autologous hematopoietic stem cell transplantation for human immunodeficiency virus (HIV)-related lymphoma: results and impact on HIV disease. *Haematologica*. 2004 Sep;**89**(9):1100–1108. PubMed PMID: 15377471. Epub 2004/09/21. eng.

13. Re A, Michieli M, Casari S, Allione B, Cattaneo C, Rupolo M, et al. High-dose therapy and autologous peripheral blood stem cell transplantation as salvage treatment for AIDS-related lymphoma: long-term results of the Italian Cooperative Group on AIDS and Tumors (GICAT) study with analysis of prognostic factors. *Blood*. 2009 Aug 13;**114**(7):1306–1313. PubMed PMID: 19451551. Epub 2009/05/20. eng.

CHAPTER 34

Engraftment and graft failure: Assessment and practical considerations

Yogesh Jethava[1], Madan Jagasia[2], Mohamed Mohty[3], and Bipin N. Savani[2]

[1] Divison of Hematology and Oncology, University of Arkansas for Medical Sciences, Little Rock, AR, USA

[2] Hematology and Stem Cell Transplantation Section, Division of Hematology/Oncology, Department of Medicine, Vanderbilt University Medical Center and Veterans Affairs Medical Center, Nashville, TN, USA

[3] Department of Haematology, Saint Antoine Hospital, Paris, France

Introduction

The unique ability of hematopoietic progenitor cells to circulate/traffic from bone marrow to blood is responsible for engraftment of hematopoietic stem cells (HSC) after hematopoietic cell transplant (HCT). This chapter will review the assessment of engraftment after allogeneic HCT, factors contributing toward graft failure and the management of graft failure.

Engraftment assessment

Neutrophil engraftment is generally defined as an absolute neutrophil count $>0.5 \times 10^6$ mm^3 on 3 consecutive days. However, platelet engraftment is variably characterized and platelet count of at least 20, 50, or 100×10^6 mm^3 sustained for 7 days without transfusion support have been considered platelet engraftment. Red cell engraftment is defined as hemoglobin of 8 gm/dl without transfusion support. CD34+ cells in the graft appear to be critical for recovery of hematopoiesis.

The term "chimera" designates an organism whose body contains cell populations derived from different individuals. Chimerism testing is used to assess the relative proportion of donor hematopoietic cells contributing to hematopoiesis. Chimerism status following HCT will depend upon the disease for which transplant was undertaken, the conditioning intensity and graft-versus-host disease prophylaxis (GvHD). Regular analysis of chimerism to monitor successful engraftment is useful to identify early graft rejection and early relapse.

Methods for chimerism analysis

In this section, we will discuss the various methods for performing chimerism analyses.

Table 34.1 summarizes the various methods and their pitfalls.

Fluorescence in situ hybridization (FISH) analysis

The FISH technique utilizes sex-specific probes and allows the rapid screening of a large number of cells with high sensitivity (true positives) rates. FISH using a Y-specific probe or dual-color X/Y probes, is efficient and useful in the sex-mismatched transplant setting. The various X and Y-specific FISH probes used are satellite sequences of DXZ1, DXZ3 for the X chromosome and DYZ1, DYZ3 for the Y chromosome. These probes hybridize to their complementary chromosomal locations at interphase nuclei and provide a quick read out of the proportion of donor and recipient cells in the sex-mismatched donor setting.

Limitations: This is a time consuming procedure, because it requires 300 or more cells to be examined (in order to exclude low degrees of mosaicism).

Short tandem repeats (STRs) (microsatellites: STR, VNTR)

The most commonly used technique for chimerism analysis utilizes amplification of distinguishing polymorphic DNA sequences of recipient and donor by polymerase chain reaction (PCR). In this technique, DNA microsatellites, also known as STRs, comprising of 2–8 base pairs located on genome from donor and recipient are amplified using PCR. These STRs from donor and recipient are used as distinctive polymorphic markers for quantitative assessment of donor and recipient hematopoiesis after allogeneic transplants. A similar

Table 34.1 Chimerism detection methods: Advantages and disadvantages.

Technique	Sensitivity (%)	Advantages	Disadvantages
Erythrocyte phenotyping	1	Simple, accurate, and sensitive technique	Less informative and blood transfusion can lead to confusion.
FISH	1–10	Screen large number of cells, low false positivity rate	Restricted to sex-mismatched HCT. More sample size needed.
Cytogenetics	NA	Very effective in cases of CML for monitoring Ph+ve cells	Only dividing cells evaluated, less sensitive, high false positivity rates.
STR-PCR	0.1	Informative study and independent of sex or HLA mismatch	Low sensitivity due to same primer competition for both minor and major cell population

technique using variable number tandem repeats (VNTRs) has also been used but the PCR technique most widely used is STR-PCR. STR-PCR based chimerism analysis in the peripheral blood can be performed using either total leukocytes or using leukocyte subsets (CD3, CD33, CD56 sorted cells). The PCR based total leukocyte chimerism in peripheral blood is less sensitive compared to leukocyte subset analysis or lineage specific chimerism. Hence flow cytometry or immunomagnetic bead separation is used for specific leukocyte subset separation with chimerism analysis performed on specific subsets/lineages. The sensitivity of leukocyte subset chimerism test is 0.1–0.01%, that is, one to two logs higher than analysis of total leukocyte preparations.

> **PRACTICE POINT**
>
> STR-PCR based chimerism analysis of lineage specific individual leukocyte subsets is more specific and permits the assessment of impending relapse with higher sensitivity.

Red cell phenotypes (RCP)

Complete red cell phenotyping of patient and donor performed using different antigens is a reliable and simple method of erythrocyte chimerism analysis: A, B, C, c, E, D, K, Fy^a, Jk^a, Jk^b, M, N, S, and s. The advantages of RCP assay are that, they are easy to perform and sensitive. This technique was particularly used to determine the engraftment in chronic myeloid leukemia (CML). However, it has limitations and the results can be misleading or un-interpretable due to conditions such as pure red cell aplasia (PRCA), hemolytic situations, or repeated transfusions.

> **PRACTICE POINT**
>
> RCP is not used in current practice for the assessment of chimerism.

Restriction fragment length polymorphism (RFLP)

RFLP analysis is based on the differences in the presence or absence of cutting sites on DNA for restriction endonucleases in patients and donors.

DNA studies using RFLP can easily detect donor–recipient chimerism at the 5–10% level and under optimal conditions at the 0.1–1% level.

> **PRACTICE POINT**
>
> RFLP is more sensitive than cytogenetics; however, it is technically challenging and supplanted by STR-PCR.

Cytogenetic markers

Rarely used in modern clinical practice for chimerism analysis. Generally, this involves sex chromosome specific marker analysis limited to sex-mismatched donor–recipient pairs or Philadelphia chromosome marker in CML.

Some of the techniques are:
1 Y-chromosome-specific markers
2 X-chromosome-specific markers
3 X–Y chromosome-based amelogenin marker
4 Amplification refractory mutation system (ARMS)
5 Image processing and restriction endonuclease in situ digestion (IPA-REISD2)

> **PRACTICE POINT**
>
> Cytogenetic markers are not used in clinical practice.

> **PRACTICE POINT**
>
> STR analysis of lineage specific leukocyte subsets by PCR is most commonly used method of chimerism analysis.

How to select suitable STR markers for chimerism analysis

The accuracy and reliability of quantitative chimerism analysis in post-transplant samples is affected by:

1 Homozygosity/heterozygosity of STR alleles between donor and recipient,
2 Shared alleles between donor and recipient,
3 The positional relationship between alleles.

The international consortium called "EuroChimerism (EUC) consortium" has established criteria facilitating selection of appropriate STR markers for chimerism testing. The EUC group has developed a common descriptive nomenclature for allelic configurations termed the RSD (Recipient-Shared-Donor) code. This code displays optimal allele constellations and helps the laboratory personals in rapid, accurate, and reproducible chimerism analysis. It is mandatory for the laboratory to have CLIA (Clinical Laboratory Improvement Amendments) certification in the USA.

Which cells are used for chimerism/engraftment analysis?

CD3+ and CD33+ cells representing T-cells and myeloid cells respectively are routinely used for chimerism assessment. Studies in pediatric acute lymphoblastic leukemia (ALL) patients have shown the importance of monitoring CD3+ and CD56+ natural killer (NK) cells. Patients displaying mixed chimerism in CD3+ and CD56+ cells between days +14 and +35 appear to have a very high risk of graft rejection. Recipient chimerism in T-cells below 50% indicated a very low risk of rejection (1.4%), while high levels of recipient chimerism (>90%) both in T- and NK-cells were associated graft loss in the majority of patients (90%) despite therapeutic interventions. Recipient chimerism >50% in T-cells and ≤90% in NK-cells defined an intermediate risk group in which timely donor lymphocyte infusion (DLI) frequently prevented rejection. Early analysis of T- and NK-cell chimerism can therefore be instrumental in the risk assessment and therapeutic management of imminent graft rejection.

PRACTICE POINTS

Cells used for chimerism analysis: CD3+, CD33+, and rarely, CD56+ cells.

Chimerism time points:
- We recommend peripheral blood leukocyte subset chimerism to be performed on D30, D60, D100, D180, and yearly afterwards.
  Definitions of Chimeric Situations:
- Full donor chimerism: all cells or >95 % of cells are of donor origin
- Mixed or partial chimerism: a proportion of cells of recipient origin is detected
- Transient mixed chimerism: recipient cells (typically <10%) detected in the first 6 months post-HCT; after which full donor chimerism is established

- Stable mixed chimerism: persistence of mixed profile with a proportion recipient cells detected post-HCT that remain constant over time
- Progressive mixed chimerism: mixed chimerism with recipient cells increasing over time

Chimerism and reduced-intensity conditioning

Since the advent of non-myeloablative and RIC allografts, serial chimerism analysis has assumed greater importance. As conditioning intensity is reduced, recipient cell persistence is common as myeloablation is not intended. Thus, a period of mixed chimerism is common following transplants using non-myeloablative or RIC. This is expected to be transient since over time donor T-cells, NK-cells, and myeloid cells will proliferate and lead to full donor chimerism. Loss of donor chimerism or progressive mixed chimerism in this setting is a cause for concern. On the other hand, complete donor chimerism may not be necessary for the correction of nonmalignant disorders.

Detection of imminent leukemia relapse post-transplant by chimerism analysis

The relapse of disease after allogeneic HCT can be identified by detection of previously present molecular, cytogenetic, or immunophenotypic markers. For example, the markers on myeloid cells such as CD34, CD7 and CD56, and CD34; CD19 in B-cell precursor ALL can be used during follow up after transplantation. Similarly, cytogenetic abnormalities such as 5q, -7, inv3, and molecular abnormalities such as FLT3, NPM, DNMT3A, c-kit may be present in acute myeloid leukemia (AML). Reappearance of these molecular, cytogenetic, and immunophenotypic markers after allogeneic transplant, reveal persistence or reappearance of autologous leukemic cells.

In patients who do not have specific markers, chimerism testing can be used for identifying impending relapse. The reappearance of MC in the CD33 compartment suggests persistence or reappearance of autologous allelic patterns within myeloid cell subsets that might harbor leukemic cells. Occasionally the only observation made before hematological relapse is loss of chimerism and or graft rejection. Graft rejection is associated with loss of graft-versus-leukemia effect and therefore early relapse. These results provide basis for early intervention such as DLI.

Graft failure

Graft failure remains one of the most important causes of morbidity and mortality after allogeneic HCT.

Primary graft failure

Graft failure was defined as >95% recipient CD3$^+$ or CD34$^+$ cells at any single time after engraftment, re-infusion of donor cells because of permanent loss of neutrophils (<0.5×10^9/L) and/or platelets <30×10^9/L or >50% recipient CD3$^+$ cells and treatment with DLI.

Secondary graft failure

Patients meeting the criteria for initial engraftment but subsequently developing loss of a previously functioning graft defined by at least two cytopenic lines are considered to have late or secondary graft failure. Table 34.2 shows some of the factors associated with graft failure.

Major risk factors for graft failure
Major histocompatibility complex (MHC) disparity between recipient and donor

HLA mismatched allogeneic transplants, degree of HLA mismatch, and low resolution HLA typing is associated with higher incidence of graft failure. Recipient derived NK-cells surviving the preparative regimen can also eliminate the graft through the mechanism of "missing-self recognition," provided that the recipient: expresses the specific KIR, leading to a KIR/KIR-ligand mismatch in the host-versus-graft direction.

Sensitization caused by blood transfusions or pregnancy

Prior history of extensive blood transfusions and pregnancy results in sensitization to histocompatibility antigens leading to an increased risk of rejection. In sensitized patients, donor-specific antibodies that recognize major and minor histocompatibility antigens on the donor cells are formed, which are considered cause of rejection. Patients with non-malignant blood disorders, such as aplastic anemia and thalassemia major, who have been treated with multiple transfusions before transplant, had rejection rates in the range of 5–60% in earlier transplant series.

Red cell antibody mediated

ABO incompatibility and the presence of ABO antibodies against donor red cells are found in approximately 20–30% of the HLA- matched HCT. Major ABO incompatibility in the transplant setting is defined by the presence of isohem-agglutinins in the recipient plasma against the donor RBCs. For example, recipient is O blood group and donor is A blood group. In this case, the recipient will have anti-A and anti-B in the plasma, which will be directed against donor A, making it major ABO mismatch. While some studies have shown that ABO incompatibility has no influence on the engraftment, a large series (n=224) by Remberger et al. suggests that major ABO incompatibility was associated with increased incidence of graft failure.

PRACTICE POINT

In patients with prior significant transfusion history or in the presence of a known HLA mismatch, we recommend checking HLA antibody titer in the recipient serum for the detection of donor-specific antibodies. It has been indicated that donor-specific antibody(ies) against CD34$^+$/VEGFR-2+ may also be involved in graft failure after allo-HCT.

Table 34.2 Factors associated with graft failure.

Quantitative progenitor issues:
- Low cell yield (e.g., CD34$^+$)
- Presence of splenomegaly
- Iron overload and Inherited diseases of erythropoiesis (i.e., thalassemia)
- Acquired marrow failure diseases (i.e., myelodysplastic syndrome, myelofibrosis, severe aplastic anemia)
- Presence of marrow involvement with disease

Immunologic issues:
- Donor and recipient HLA disparity
- Donor and recipient ABO disparity
- Manipulation of the graft (i.e., T-cell depletion, CD34$^+$ cell selection)
- Prior transfusion history
- Adequate post-transplantation immunosuppressive medication
- Reduced-intensity conditioning regimen with residual host effector cells
- Presence of acute or chronic graft-versus-host disease

Viral infections:
- Cytomegalovirus, HHV-6, HHV-8, parvovirus
- HHV, human herpesvirus
- BK virus
- Influenza

Miscellaneous:
- Drugs such as ganciclovir, valganciclovir, cidofovir
- Bactrim, allopurinol

Preparative regimen and post-transplant immunosuppression

The transplant preparative regimen can affect the graft failure rate. Higher graft failure rate is associated with non-myeloablative transplantation. Adequate immunosuppression with myeloablative conditioning, results in effective eradication of host immune cells, resulting in better engraftment.

Graft failure rates can vary considerably and even when the same class of drugs are used for the conditioning. For example, randomized study of fludarabine versus cladrabine plus busulfan and low-dose TBI as conditioning for allogeneic HCT was prematurely stopped since the cladrabine arm was associated with higher rates of graft failure. RIC is generally associated with MC, which can persist for several months after allo-HCT. Low levels of donor T-cell chimerism is predictive of graft failure rates. Studies have demonstrated that 50% patients had graft failure if donor T-cell chimerism level was below 25% by day 30 post-transplantation, compared with 4%, where it was between 51 and 75% by this time. Similarly, post-transplant T- and NK-cell chimerism at days 14 and 28 after transplant were important predictors of graft failure. There is an array of transplant conditioning regimens that consider patient- and donor-specific factors and experimental and clinical studies are required to better understand how an alteration in a preparative regimen impacts the incidence of graft failure. Significant percentages of patients receiving alemtuzumab based conditioning require DLI to ensure full donor engraftment.

Occasionally $CD34^+$ selected donor cell boost and donor leukocyte infusion can be used for conversion to full donor engraftment. It has been suggested that prolonging immunosuppressive medications up to 100 days results in stable donor engraftment especially so in RIC and TCD transplants.

Low progenitor cell dose in the graft

The data regarding the predictive value of BM nucleated cells and graft failure is not consistent. Most studies have demonstrated that minimum numbers of progenitor cells are requires for successful engraftment. A high total nucleated cell (TNC) dose and a high $CD34^+$ cell dose correlates with faster engraftment of neutrophils in recipients of a marrow graft while a higher $CD34^+$ cell dose correlates with faster platelet engraftment in PBSC graft recipients. Threshold doses to prevent graft failure are difficult to define since the dose requirement is modified by conditioning intensity, T-cell dose, graft source, and the underlying disease. Generally for myeloablative allo-HCT, 5×10^7 TNCs/kg from a peripheral blood (PB) graft is considered an adequate dose, while cell doses less than 3×10^7 TNCs/kg from PB graft are associated with an increased incidence of graft failure.

Cell dose is critically important in cord blood transplantation.

Viral infections

In the setting of bone marrow failure, post allogeneic transplant, it is recommended to check CMV, HHV6, and parvovirus B19. HHV-6 has been shown to latently infect early bone marrow progenitor cells. *In vitro* studies have demonstrated that HHV-6 infection of bone marrow progenitor cells causes suppression of granulocyte-macrophage proliferation, erythroid, and megakaryocyte cell lines. Parvovirus infection causes PRCA by attaching to P antigens on erythrocytes causing direct destruction of pro-erythroblasts. The aplasia associated with B19 parvovirus often produces a characteristic morphologic finding of giant pro-erythroblasts in the bone marrow.

Table 34.3 summarizes investigations in to graft failure.

Treatment of graft failure

Treatment of the underlying cause- decrease in chimera and/or bone marrow failure or both?

The most important strategy is to treat the underlying cause. This includes, optimization of post-transplant immunosuppression, management of CMV, HHV6, and parvovirus disease, management of graft-versus-host disease (GvHD), withholding (or changing) myelosuppressive drugs such as gancyclovir and treatment of sepsis.

Changes in immune suppression

Suboptimal immune suppression in the immediate post-transplantation period, especially in RIC transplants, can increase the risk of early graft failure. Immunosuppression should be monitored very stringently and therapeutic levels of immunosuppression should be maintained to

Table 34.3 Summary of investigations for graft failure.

PB leukocyte subset chimerism
Viral studies:
- CMV PCR
- Adenovirus PCR
- HHV6 PCR
- BK virus PCR
- Influenza testing
- EBV PCR
- Parvovirus PCR

Bone marrow studies:
- Chimerism for $CD3^+$, $CD33^+$ cells
- Bone morrow analysis

Miscellaneous tests:
- Serum EPO levels
- Serum iron/TIBC/Ferritin levels
- Vitamin B12 levels.

support the engraftment by inhibiting HvG reactions. It is unclear whether early withdrawal of immunosuppressive drug in patients with MC hastens the graft loss. Further studies are required to define how an alteration in post-transplantation immune suppression will affect engraftment and graft failure.

Cellular-based approaches

CD34+ selected cells from the same or different donor: Second HCT

A second HCT from the same donor or an alternative donor is used especially in patients with primary graft failure or acute graft rejection associated with profound trilineage aplasia. Patients with primary or secondary graft rejection should be prepared for a second allograft using a higher immunosuppressive conditioning regimen including lymphotoxic agents, such as fludarabine, cyclophosphamide, ATG, and/or alemtuzumab. A single dose of total body irradiation (200–400 cGy) can be also considered in order to optimize the immunosuppression of the recipient. In the majority of patients with secondary graft failure and autologous reconstitution, a fully myeloablative regimen should be employed in order to eradicate recipient hematopoiesis.

There are no conclusive data for supporting the choice of using either the same donor of the first allograft or an alternative donor; however, in patients with an immune mediated graft rejection, the use of alternative donor, whenever possible, is recommended. CD34+ selected cell "boosts" following G-CSF mobilization, without conditioning regimen prior to infusion, can be a valid option in order to improve a poor graft function in patients with complete donor chimerism or predominance of donor hematopoiesis.

PRACTICE POINTS

Factors to consider for second transplant:

- Should the same or a different donor be used?
- Should bone marrow or granulocyte colony-stimulating factor-mobilized blood be used?
- When is a CD34+ selected boost *versus* an unmanipulated graft preferred?
- Should a preparative regimen be used? If so, which one?
- Is post-second-transplantation immunosuppressive medication necessary?
- What is the role of DLI for converting partial chimerism?

DLI

DLI is a form of adoptive immunotherapy to induce graft-versus-leukemia (GvL) activity in RIC allogeneic transplant recipients. The efficacy of this approach depends upon the type of disease and the dose of infused CD3+ lymphocytes. Encouraging results have been observed in CML and indolent lymphomas; however, the response is generally limited in florid relapse of AML or ALL, and the patients are at risk of severe GvHD or marrow aplasia.

RIC and prophylactic DLI

DLIs have also been performed in patients with hematological malignancies with residual disease or mixed chimerism after RIC HCT. In the event of falling CD3+ chimersim <90% and falling CBC, we recommend considering prophylactic DLI infusions. We recommend starting at lower doses of DLI, such as 1×10^6 and then gradually increasing the dose of DLI. In acute leukemia, the smaller doses of DLI may not be effective and large doses are required. It is well documented that DLIs can induce severe, sometimes fatal GvHD. In order to minimize severe side effects, and potentiate the GvL effect, several approaches have been investigated. These include setting a limit of T-cell dose, selective depletion of certain T-cell subsets, insertion of suicide genes or chimeric receptors into effector cells or activation of donor T-cells *ex vivo*. The use pre-DLI chemotherapy, granulocyte colony-stimulating factor-mobilized PB CD34+ cells and post-DLI immunosuppression has been suggested as a regimen to lower GvHD risk; however, the cumulative incidence of acute GvHD is still substantial.

PRACTICE POINTS

- DLI is effective in converting mixed chimerism to full donor chimerism.
- DLI is effective for disease control in indolent lymphomas and CML but effective only in 15–20% of AML patients.

Mesenchymal stromal cells

Mesenchymal stromal cells (MSCs) are pleuripotent precursors that can be isolated from several human tissues (including bone marrow, cord blood, fat tissue); they are capable of differentiation in to several mesenchymal lineages (i.e., osteoblasts, chondrocytes, and adipocytes among others). Increasing interest in this heterogeneous population of cells stems from their immune-modulatory properties on virtually all cell types involved in the immune response.

At present, MSCs are mainly used, in clinical trial setting, for the treatment of acute GvHD unresponsive to first-line therapies. However, it was shown that MSCs contribute to the formation of the so-called hematopoietic stem cell *niche*, having a crucial role in hematopoietic stem cell homeostasis and development, as well as in the differentiation of the hematopoietic system. Moreover, several animal studies have shown that *in vivo* infusion of human MSCs may promote engraftment of hematopoietic progenitors. This has been replicated in humans in the setting of HLA-haploidentical transplants. In a pilot study on six patients with poor hematopoietic recovery, Meuleman et al. infused MSCs at a dose of 1×10^6/kg of recipient weight, without hematopoietic CD34$^+$ cell boost or reconditioning: two of them displayed rapid hematopoietic recovery. In view of this available evidence, some authors recommend the use of MSCs as first-line treatment for graft failure after allogeneic HCT.

PRACTICE POINT

This is an investigative approach to be considered as a part of clinical trial.

Selected reading

1. Bader P, Kreyenberg H, Hoelle W, Dueckers G, Handgretinger R, Lang P, et al. Increasing mixed chimerism is an important prognostic factor for unfavorable outcome in children with acute lymphoblastic leukemia after allogeneic stem-cell transplantation: possible role for pre-emptive immunotherapy? *Journal of Clinical Oncology: Official Journal of the American Society of Clinical Oncology.* 2004 May 1;**22**(9): 1696–1705.
2. Lion T. Summary: reports on quantitative analysis of chimerism after allogeneic stem cell transplantation by PCR amplification of microsatellite markers and capillary electrophoresis with fluorescence detection. *Leukemia.* 2003 Jan;**17**(1):252–254.
3. Lion T, Daxberger H, Dubovsky J, Filipcik P, Fritsch G, Printz D, et al. Analysis of chimerism within specific leukocyte subsets for detection of residual or recurrent leukemia in pediatric patients after allogeneic stem cell transplantation. *Leukemia.* 2001 Feb;**15**(2): 307–310.
4. Thiede C, Bornhauser M, Oelschlagel U, Brendel C, Leo R, Daxberger H, et al. Sequential monitoring of chimerism and detection of minimal residual disease after allogeneic blood stem cell transplantation (BSCT) using multiplex PCR amplification of short tandem repeat-markers. *Leukemia.* 2001 Feb;**15**(2):293–302.
5. Choi SJ, Lee KH, Lee JH, Kim S, Chung HJ, Lee JS, et al. Prognostic value of hematopoietic chimerism in patients with acute leukemia after allogeneic bone marrow transplantation: a prospective study. *Bone Marrow Transplantation.* 2000 Aug;**26**(3):327–332.
6. Remberger M, Watz E, Ringden O, Mattsson J, Shanwell A, Wikman A. Major ABO blood group mismatch increases the risk for graft failure after unrelated donor hematopoietic stem cell transplantation. *Biology of Blood and Marrow Transplantation: Journal of the American Society for Blood and Marrow Transplantation.* 2007 Jun;**13**(6):675–682.
7. Meuleman N, Tondreau T, Ahmad I, Kwan J, Crokaert F, Delforge A, et al. Infusion of mesenchymal stromal cells can aid hematopoietic recovery following allogeneic hematopoietic stem cell myeloablative transplant: a pilot study. *Stem Cells and Development.* 2009 Nov;**18**(9):1247–1252.

CHAPTER 35

Immune reconstitution and tolerance

Ludovic Belle and William R. Drobyski

Medical College of Wisconsin, Milwaukee, WI, USA

Introduction

Hematopoietic cell transplantation (HCT) remains the only curative treatment option for many patients with hematological malignancies and genetic disorders. Recipients can receive either an autologous or allogeneic graft, which is often dependent upon the primary disease for which transplantation is contemplated. One of the major goals of transplantation is the development of a fully functional immune system. Patients undergoing allogeneic hematopoietic cell transplantation (allo-HCT), in particular, have the highest rate of transplant-related mortality (TRM) due to complications that can result from immunodeficiencies or immune dysregulation that occurs as a consequence of the procedure. These include, but are not limited to, infections, graft-versus-host disease (GvHD), autoimmune disorders, and secondary malignancies. Recovery of a fully functional immune system is thus critical for HCT success and improving immune reconstitution is of great clinical interest (Figure 35.1 and Table 35.1). This chapter will focus on immune reconstitution following allo-HCT since immune recovery is more complicated in this setting due to the underlying HLA disparity between the donor and the recipient.

When and how are the different immune components reconstituted?

Homing and engraftment

Homing of hematopoietic stem cells (HSCs) into the bone marrow (BM) is a multistep process, which occurs during the first hours following transplantation (and no longer than 2 days) and involves multiple cytokines, chemokines, and other proteins. Circulating HSCs roll and adhere to blood vessel walls by binding to VCAM-1, E-, and P-selectin. HSCs then migrate across the blood/BM into specialized BM HSC niches located in the extravascular space of the endosteal region and periarterial sites. After their firm adhesion in these niches, HSCs are able to proliferate and begin the process of differentiation. Short-term engraftment is carried out by differentiated progenitors, while only HSCs are responsible for durable long-term multi-lineage engraftment. Patients are usually transplanted with a minimum of 2×10^6 CD34$^+$ cells/kg, although higher numbers of CD34$^+$ cells have been associated with more rapid hematologic engraftment.

Innate immunity

The innate immune system includes several cell populations, such as neutrophils, monocytes, natural killer cells (NK-cells), and dendritic cells (DCs) that recognize and eliminate pathogens without prior priming or antigen presentation.

Neutrophils, monocytes, and macrophages

Following myeloablative conditioning, recipients undergo a profound period of pancytopenia typically spanning several weeks, depending on the HSC source. Patients receiving conditioning with reduced intensity regimens (RIC) tend to have more abbreviated periods of neutropenia due to the reduction in the intensity of conditioning regimen, which mitigates the neutropenic interval. In either setting, however, infections are the main complication and the duration of neutropenia influences both the risk and spectrum of infectious complications. Neutrophils are the first granulocyte population to reach normal numbers. On average, it takes approximately 14 days after peripheral blood (PB) HCT, 21 days following bone marrow transplantation

Clinical Manual of Blood and Bone Marrow Transplantation, First Edition. Edited by Syed A. Abutalib and Parameswaran Hari.
© 2017 John Wiley & Sons Ltd. Published 2017 by John Wiley & Sons Ltd.

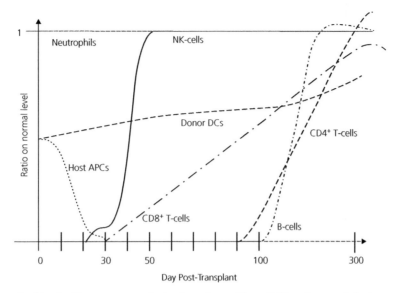

Figure 35.1 Representative kinetic of immune reconstitution in patients without GvHD, relapse, or infections.

(BMT) and 30 days after umbilical cord blood transplantation (UCBT). Qualitatively, their functional capabilities, which include chemotaxis, phagocytosis, superoxide production, and bacterial killing, remain abnormal very early after HCT, but progressively normalize by 2 months post-transplantation. GvHD prophylaxis, with agents such as methotrexate that function as an anti-metabolite, can delay neutrophil recovery. Monocyte and macrophage reconstitution follows the same kinetic pattern as neutrophil recovery.

NK-cells

NK-cells are the first lymphocyte subpopulation to return to normal levels following allo-HCT and usually take 1–2 months to normalize. They may represent up to 80% of total lymphocytes early after transplantation. Rapid recovery of NK-cells is due to expansion of CD56^{bright} cytokine-producing NK-cell subpopulations with low expression of CD16 and KIR molecules and high levels of the inhibitory receptor CD94:NKG2A. However, this relative expansion typically declines within the first year post-transplantation due to recovery of other lymphocyte populations. About 6 months post-transplantation, KIR expression begins to reach normal levels on donor NK-cells, corresponding to a mature NK-cell phenotype with CD56^{dim} and CD16$^+$ expression.

Newly generated donor-derived NK-cells are fully functional and retain their ability to kill KIR-incompatible target cells, such as recipient leukemic cells *in vitro*. Indeed, NK-cell recovery has been associated with a strong graft-versus-leukemia (GvL effect). High numbers of NK-cells early after transplant correlate with

increased remission rate, OS, and decreased pathogen infections in hematologic malignancies. Finally, NK-cells have been demonstrated to impair GvHD development and to support allo-engraftment in animal models, through killing of residual host antigen-presenting cells (APCs) and T-cells.

DCs

Even though donor DCs can be detected in the blood within the first weeks after allo-HCT, total number of DCs may be subnormal for more than 1-year post-transplantation. While more than 80% of total DCs are from donor origin in PB, up to 70% of tissue DCs may be of host origin (this state may persist up to 1 year post-transplantation). The function of newly generated DCs remains unclear, but some studies suggest that DC function may be impaired.

DCs can be divided into two subpopulations: (1) myeloid DCs (mDCs) and (2) plasmacytoid DCs (pDCs), an IFN-α secreting population that stimulates CD4$^+$ and CD8$^+$ T-cells. mDCs secrete mainly IL-12 and IL-15 in response to bacterial components such as peptidoglycans, lipopolysaccharide (LPS) or flagellin, and extracellular bacterial DNA. On the other hand, pDCs are specialized in innate antiviral immune responses by producing type I interferons (mainly IFN-α and IFN-β) upon exposure of intracellular TLR9 and TLR7 to DNA- and RNA-viruses. mDCs are known to be the conventional DCs that infiltrate peripheral tissues while pDCs migrate directly from the blood into lymphoid organs. Finally, mDCs are also considered professional APCs with high MHC class II and co-stimulatory molecule

Table 35.1 Immune system recovery following HCT.

Cell Type	Time Necessary for Recovery	Subsets	Repertoire	Functionality	Origin		Implication in HCT Outcomes
Neutrophils	Weeks. Depends on HSC source	–	–	Normal phagocytosis and oxidative burst by 1 months	D		Bacterial/Fungal Infection prevention
Monocytes/Macrophages	Weeks to months	–	–	Normal by 1 months to 1 year	Tissue: R Blood: D		GvHD
NK-cells	Within 1st Month	CD56^{bright} recovers first, followed by CD56^{dim}	–	Functional	D		GvL effect
Dendritic cells	In blood: Within 1st Month. In tissues: By 6 months	Higher mDCs/pDCS ratio during 1st year post-transplant	–	Not Studied	D/R		GvHD, GvT effect
B-cells	Months to years. Later if GvHD	Naïve B-cells precede the memory subset	Skewed toward nonsomatically mutated VDJ genes	Normal IgM production; Low IgG/IgA production; low antibody response to vaccine	D		GvHD, particularly chronic GvHD
CD4$^+$ T-cells	Years	1–5 years for memory/effector; Years for Naïve	Oligoclonal during first year	Suboptimal early and late post-transplant, worse with GvHD	D		GvHD, GvT effect, Bacterial/Fungal Infection prevention
CD8$^+$ T-cells	Months	Within 6 months for memory subsets; Years for naïve	Oligoclonal during first year	Subnormal early, normalizes later	D		GvHD, GvT effect, Bacterial/Fungal Infection prevention
Regulatory T-cells	Years – but earlier than conventional CD4$^+$ T-cells	–	Not Studied	Normal *in vitro* suppressive activity by 2 months	D		GvHD prevention

expression, while pDCs have lower MHC and co-stimulatory molecule expression levels.

Recovery of DCs can also be predictive of GvHD development and OS. Low total DC counts at engraftment after allo-HCT have been associated with poor OS, increased relapse, and increased GvHD incidence. A study by Mohty et al. showed that low (0.725 cells/μL, as reported in the original study) pDCs and mDCs counts using RIC, at 3 months post-transplant, were associated with severe acute GvHD (aGvHD). On the other hand, high pDC counts were associated, in RIC and BM graft studies, with increased chronic GvHD (cGvHD) incidence and increased relapse.

Finally, the GvHD prophylaxis regimen may impair DC recovery since calcineurin inhibitors and rapamycin suppress antigen presentation and co-stimulatory molecule expression, while glucocorticoids inhibit maturation and activation of DCs, as well IL-12, TNF-α, and IL-1β secretion.

PRACTICE POINTS

Despite data highlighting the role that DCs play in the biology of allogeneic hematopoietic stem cell transplantation, DC levels are not typically assessed, primarily due to the fact that it has been unclear as to how the results would modify clinical decision-making.

Adaptive immunity

The adaptive immune response is more complex than the innate response and is comprised of both B-cells and T-lymphocytes that mediate antigen-specific immune responses and have the capacity to establish a compartment of memory cells that allows for more robust and accelerated recognition of antigens to which these cells were previously exposed.

B-cells

B-cell reconstitution is typically slow post-transplantation and reflects normal ontogeny. Naïve B-cells, generated in the BM, migrate into secondary lymphoid structures to become activated when they encounter an antigen, often presented by CD4+ T-cells or DCs. Maturation of activated B-cells then requires interactions with T-cells to undergo isotype switching allowing for IgG, IgA, or IgE expression.

B-lymphocytes are usually undetectable during the first 2 months following HCT. Cell numbers rise slowly until reaching a normal PB level. However, reconstitution is not complete during at least the first 2 years in most patients. Early following allo-HCT, the majority of detectable B-lymphocytes are donor-derived naïve B-cells (IgM+ IgD+) with very few

memory B-cells. Memory B-cell development can take up to 5 years. IgM production recovers first, by 2–6 months, followed by IgG secretion with normal levels observed between 3 and 18 months post-transplantation. IgA production recovers last and can take up to 3 years to reach normal adult production levels. Notably, recipient-derived immunoglobulin production can be observed for several months and years following HCT, even if detectable B-cells are from donor origin. Therefore, immunoglobulin production in the early stage of B-cell reconstitution may not be indicative of donor B-cell recovery. This recipient production can be due to radio- and/or chemoresistance of recipient plasma cells and may persist for up to 2 years. Recipient-derived immunoglobulin production disappears faster in patients diagnosed with GvHD, suggesting elimination of persistent recipient plasma cells by the graft. Finally, the B-cell repertoire is often restricted following HCT due to a decreased ability to undergo isotype switching. B-cells with hypermutated genes are therefore often missing during the first year. This could be explained in part by impaired T-cell reconstitution, since naïve B-cell maturation requires CD4+ T-cell signaling. Both B-cell number and repertoire recovery can be further delayed due to the development of GvHD and/or its therapy. For example, slower B-cell reconstitution is frequently observed in chronic GvHD patients.

The extent to which B-cells fully reconstitute has important clinical implications. Low B-cell numbers, 6 months after following T-cell depleted HCT in adult patients receiving myeloablative conditioning, have been associated with decreased OS, increased relapse, and graft failure, while low numbers at day + 80 post-HCT following allo-HCT correlated with an increased risk of infections. Decreased levels of immunoglobulins, lack of memory B-cells, impaired isotype switching and loss of complexity in the B-cell repertoire also render patients vulnerable to encapsulated bacteria (*Streptococcus pneumonia*, *Haemophilus influenza*). Moreover, these decreased B-cell functions result in reduced responses to vaccines. The response to protein antigens recovers faster (within 1–2 years) than against polysaccharide antigens (≥2 years following HCT) and responses to protein recall antigens tend to recover faster than to protein neo-antigens.

Finally, B-cells have been shown to contribute to the pathogenesis of both acute and chonic GvHD. Direct demonstration of the role of B-cells in GvHD pathogenesis has been reported in murine studies. Indeed, B-cell depletion results in a decreased incidence of aGvHD. Paradoxically, B-cells can also play a protective role in GvHD by controlling naïve T-cell differentiation into effector T-cells and inhibiting the proliferation of these cells, via IL-10 secretion. Furthermore, administration of anti-CD20 mAb immediately after HCT or before the appearance of serum autoantibodies (targeting host tissue, such as anti-nuclear, anti-mitochondrial, anti-smooth muscle, anti-cardiolipin, anti-liver-kidney microsomal, anti-DNA, anti-neutrophil cytoplasmic, and anti-thyroid antibodies) was able to prevent the induction of cGvHD by depleting donor B-cells and protecting the host thymus. Indeed, thymocyte production was restored in anti-CD20 mAb-treated mice compared to the isotype-treated control group, and reached similar yields and percentages to the BM control group. Thymic epithelial cell numbers were also increased and were similar to that observed in the BM group.

In clinical studies, while rituximab, given during conditioning, reduced the incidence and severity of acute GvHD, post-HCT rituximab administration failed to reduce GvHD incidence. Indeed, a CIBMTR-based study found lower rates of aGvHD in patients who had received rituximab in the 6 months prior to allo-HCT. Similarly, a retrospective study found that rituximab before allogeneic HCT was associated with complete elimination of acute GvHD grades III–IV. However, other groups have reported relatively high incidences of aGvHD after allo-HCT with peri-transplant rituximab. Moreover, both recipient and donor B-cells may participate in cGvHD pathogenesis by priming donor T-cells, producing allo- or autoantibodies and secreting pro-inflammatory cytokines. The production of autoantibodies in cGVHD is thought to be due to the large amounts of B-cell-activating factor (BAFF) present after transplantation in patients with cGVHD. Finally, *in vivo* depletion of B-cells by rituximab reduced the incidence of cGVHD and improved the disease in approximately 66% of patients with steroid-refractory cGVHD.

PRACTICE POINTS

Clinical studies are ongoing to determine whether targeting of B-cell populations in patients with chronic GvHD will attenuate disease severity, but there have been no randomized clinical trials to support this approach yet.

T-cells

T-cell recovery following HCT is achieved via two different pathways: (1) homeostatic peripheral expansion (HPE) and (2) thymopoiesis.

Early post-transplantation period relies on homeostatic peripheral expansion

HPE is an alternative expansion pathway for T-cell development achieved through rapid cell division of mature T-cells. This process is mediated by cytokines,

such as IL-7 and IL-15, and inhibited by regulatory T-cells (Tregs) and TGF-β. HPE is the more predominant mechanism of donor T-cell recovery early after HCT. Elevated IL-7 and IL-15 levels facilitate the homeostatic expansion of transplanted T-cells, inducing a shift from a naïve to a memory phenotype. Indeed, most of the T-cells observed following HCT are generated from mature T-cells contained in the graft, resulting ultimately in a more limited T-cell repertoire. Indeed, the T-cell receptor (TCR) repertoire resulting from HPE tends to be more restricted, skewed, and oligoclonal. Differences are also observed between CD4+ and CD8+ T-cells since HPE results in faster recovery of memory and effector CD8+ than CD4+ T-cells. Memory/effector CD8+ counts typically normalize after 6 months post-HCT whereas memory and effector CD4+ T-cell counts often remain low for at least 1 year, leading to an inversion of the CD4/CD8 ratio. Finally, this mature T-cell compartment, generated from HPE, is primarily responsible for modulating allo-engraftment, GvHD, the GvL effect and the response to infections (see next).

Thymopoiesis recovery is delayed after HCT: Why and how do I monitor its recovery?

The thymus is the primary site for T-cell development (Figure 35.2). During thymopoiesis, T-cell progenitors, generated in the BM, migrate to the thymus for maturation. This process includes (1) acquisition of the TCR, generated through recombinant rearrangement of VDJ regions ensuring TCR repertoire diversity, and (2) positive and negative selection. Measurement of thymopoiesis is assessed by TCR rearrangement excision circles (TRECs), which are episomal DNA circles generated from the spliced DNA circles remaining after VDJ recombination. They are not replicated during cell division and thereby serve as a marker for recent thymic emigrants. High frequencies of recent emigrant cells are indicative of robust thymopoiesis, whereas lower frequencies of TRECs is evidence of impaired thymic function and higher peripheral T-cell expansion (i.e., HPE). Use of TCR spectratyping can be performed to assess the breadth of the TCR repertoire, which is another indicator of effective T-cell reconstitution. Unfortunately, this technique is still not routinely available.

Thymopoiesis is severely impaired after HCT, resulting in low newly generated T-cell output. Indeed, naïve T-cell counts are typically reduced, reflected by low TREC levels during the first 3–6 months post-transplant. This is particularly true for older patients in whom reconstitution is impaired due to the involution of the thymus. When thymopoiesis remains impaired, CD4+ and CD8+ numbers can remain low (less than 200 cells/mm^3) for several years (>5 years for CD4+).

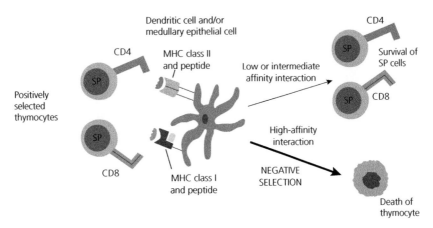

Figure 35.2 Deletion as the mechanism of central tolerance in T-cells. Thymocytes expressing a TCR with high affinity for self-MHC class I or II plus self-peptide are deleted (negatively selected) as a consequence of interacting with thymc dendritic cells and/or medullary epithelial cells. Thymocytes expressing a TCR with lower affinity for self-MHC class I or II plus self-peptide survive. Source: Coico 2015. Reproduced with permission of John Wiley & Sons.

Clinical factors and thymus recovery

Several factors influence thymopoiesis following allo-HCT. First, the thymus involutes with age resulting in a loss in the ability to generate naïve T-cells (identified as CD45RA+CD45RO−CCR7+CD62L+), which induces a repertoire skewed toward effector/memory T-cells. Data also suggest each successive decade of the patient reduces the rate and potential for thymus renewal. The thymus is also damaged in HCT recipients by exposure to cytotoxic drugs or radiation, and GvHD. For example, use of RIC is associated with enhanced CD4+ T-cell recovery and TCR repertoire diversity, even if it also reduces IL-7 and IL-15 cytokine levels. Furthermore, the graft source also influences immune recovery kinetics since it determines availability of functional T-cell progenitors that can go through thymopoiesis. Recipients receiving UCBT have higher TREC frequencies than patients receiving adult BM grafts. This probably can be explained by higher frequencies of progenitors in cord blood grafts. Graft manipulation also influences T-cell recovery since patients receiving a PB HCT recover normal peripheral T-cell counts more quickly, while recipients treated with a T-cell depleted graft experience a delay in T-cell reconstitution. The degree of mismatch between donor and recipient also affects T-cell recovery since transplantation with partially matched or unrelated donors induces delayed T-cell reconstitution with skewed repertoires and low TREC frequencies. Finally, GvHD can adversely affect thymic function as alloreactive donor T-cells can directly damage the thymus impeding the generation of naïve T-cells. Therefore, protection of the thymus from injury and enhancing thymic function, are important goals in ensuring that the thymic-dependent pathway

is optimized. Without recovery of this process, T-cell reconstitution and TCR repertoire diversity can be impaired indefinitely.

Regulatory T-cells (Tregs) in allo-HCT: Clinically or only laboratory relevant?

Tregs, identified as CD4+ or CD8+ FoxP3+ T-cells, are critical for both central and peripheral tolerance (see section later). This T-cell subset can be divided into thymically derived Tregs (termed "natural Tregs"; nTregs) and peripherally derived Tregs (referred to as "induced Tregs"; iTregs). Tregs exert their suppressive functions (Figure 35.3) through different mechanisms such as (1) modulation of APC activity through Treg engagement of co-stimulatory receptors on the DC surface, leading to weak or abrogated signals to naïve/effector T-cells; (2) cytokine deprivation, cyclic AMP-mediated inhibition, and adenosine receptor (A2A)-mediated immunosuppression; (3) competition for critical cytokines, such as IL-2, or direct disruption of effector cell engagement with APCs; (4) direct cytotoxic effects through the production of Granzyme B and Perforin and consequent apoptosis of effector T-cells or APCs; and (5) production of inhibitory cytokines, including IL-10, IL-35, and TGF-β. Other mechanisms, like CTLA-4, adenosine generation by CD39 and CD73, and GITR, also help Tregs to maintain immune homeostasis.

A recent paper by Socié's research group describes Treg reconstitution after allo-HCT and observed correlations with acute and chronic GvHD. Total Treg, naïve Treg and memory Treg reconstitution were delayed after HCT and remained below the normal range for up to 2 years after HCT compared to healthy controls. Total

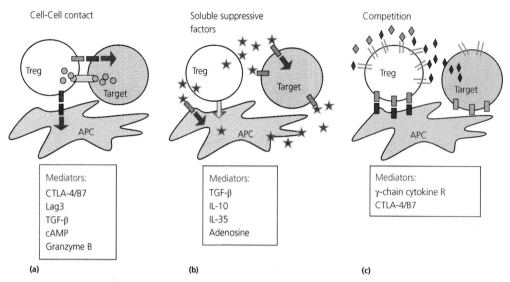

Figure 35.3 Mechanisms of regulatory T-cell (Treg) suppression. (a) Cell–cell contact. Tregs may suppress target cells via direct interaction of receptor–ligand pairs on Tregs and target cells; delivery of suppressive factors via gap junctions including cyclic adenosine monophosphate (cAMP); direct cytolysis; membrane-bound suppressive cytokines such as transforming growth factor-β (TGF-β); and/or indirectly via modulating the APC through cell–cell contact, possibly through reverse signaling via Treg–cytotoxic T-lymphocyte antigen-4 (CTLA-4) engagement of B7 on dendritic cells. (b) Soluble suppressive factors. Tregs can directly secrete interleukin-10 (IL-10), TGF-β and IL-35 or induce APCs to secrete such factors. Expression of CD73/CD39 by Tregs facilitates the local generation of adenosine that can down-modulate immune function. (c) Competition. Tregs may compete for some cytokines that signal via receptors that contain the common γ-chain (IL-2, IL-4, and IL-7). Additionally, they may compete for APC costimulation via constitutive expression of CTLA-4. Arrow indicates an inhibitory signal. Source: Sojka 2008. Reproduced with permission of John Wiley & Sons.

Treg reconstitution after HCT was mostly due to an increase in memory Tregs. RIC, PB HCT, and recipient age (<25 years) were associated with a better short-term reconstitution. Naïve Treg long-term reconstitution was mainly influenced by recipient age. Prior aGvHD impaired Treg and CD4 reconstitution. Finally, no correlation was observed between Treg numbers and frequencies with the occurrence of cGvHD.

Identification of Tregs as suppressors of activation and proliferation of conventional T-cells (identified as CD4$^+$ or CD8$^+$ CD25$^-$ FoxP3$^-$ T-cells) has led to great interest into how these cells might be involved in GvHD pathogenesis and tolerance development. In murine models, depletion of Tregs has been associated with an increase in GvHD mortality. Conversely, the adoptive transfer of Tregs along with the marrow graft reduces GvHD mortality in recipient mice. In clinical studies, the infusion of Tregs has been shown to be safe and may result in reduced GvHD incidence and, improved immune recovery, although randomized clinical trials have yet to be done, In fact, one murine study has suggested that adoptive transfer of Tregs led to the (1) abrogration

of GvHD, (2) preservation of thymic and peripheral lymph node architecture, and (3) accelerated donor lymphoid reconstitution of a diverse TCR-Vbeta repertoire. Furthermore, a small clinical study in 28 patients has also suggested that the adoptive transfer of Tregs after haploidentical HCT prevents GvHD, while promoting lymphoid reconstitution, improving immunity to opportunistic pathogens, and not abrogating the GvL effect.

How does tolerance develop after HCT?

T-cell tolerance is achieved via two mechanisms: (1) Central tolerance consists of the elimination of self-reactive T-cells during thymopoiesis and (2) Peripheral tolerance with elimination and/or tolerization of self-reactive mature T-cells in the periphery.

Central tolerance: Development of central tolerance takes place within the thymus. Lymphoid precursors migrate from the BM to the thymus and where they undergo a differentiation process characterized by the rearrangement of the TCR (see above) and the subsequent expression of both CD4 and CD8 cell surface markers, which are regulated by factors such as IL-7 and Notch-1. Double-positive thymocytes then undergo positive selection, which involves recognition of the MHC-self-peptide complex. More than 95% of thymocytes do not have specificity for an MHC ligand and will subsequently die. The small proportion that binds to an MHC ligand with mild avidity then continues the differentiation process to become single positive CD4+ or CD8+ T-cells. Negative selection is the second step in intra-thymic T-cell tolerance and eliminates autoreactive T-cell clones for self-antigens presented by hematopoietic cells and thymic epithelial cells. High affinity for self-antigens results in elimination of thymocytes by Fas-dependent apoptosis, while low affinity binding allows survival and maturation of thymocytes. The autoimmune regulator (AIRE) was recently described as an important transcriptional regulator of T-cell negative selection. It is expressed on thymic epithelial cells and promotes self-tolerance by inducing transcription of tissue-specific antigens in the thymus. Absence of AIRE results in restricted self-antigen expression on thymic epithelial cells, leading to severe autoimmune disease.

While mature donor T-cells (see the HPE section) present in the graft are responsible for GvHD development and recipient T-cells that survive conditioning mediate graft failure, T-cells that are generated through thymopoiesis in recipient *do not* cause GvHD or graft rejection. Indeed, precursors bearing receptors for self-antigens will be eliminated by clonal deletion. If central tolerance is not effective, autoreactive T-cells can emerge from the thymus and these cells have, in animal models, been shown to be able to cause GvHD.

Peripheral tolerance: The development of peripheral tolerance is responsible for inhibition of mature autoreactive T-cells (see the HPE section). Different mechanisms exist and include clonal deletion by apoptosis, induction of anergy, development of regulatory and suppressor cells, activation-induced cell death, and clonal exhaustion. Clinical studies have revealed that inflammatory mediators and GvHD prophylaxis agents (such as calcineurin inhibitors) can interfere with the development of tolerance.

What are the different strategies to enhance immune reconstitution following transplantation?
Enhancement of T-cell recovery by strengthening thymic recovery
Keratinocyte growth factor
Keratinocyte growth factor (KGF, also called palifermin, Kepivance, Biovitrum; Amgen) belongs to the fibroblast growth factor family and mediates epithelial cell proliferation and differentiation in the gut, skin, and thymus.

Non-hematopoietic stromal cells are the main source, while in the thymus fibroblasts, mesenchymal stem cells and thymocytes (after the double negative stage) also produce KGF. KGF acts as a protective and tropic molecule and augments thymocyte proliferation and maturation. Administration of KGF before conditioning and after transplantation resulted in improved thymopoiesis and peripheral T-cell numbers in several animal models. Moreover, KGF-treated GvHD mice showed preservation of the thymic environment with normal thymic function. Enhancement of thymopoiesis and T-cell recovery was also observed in a non-humane primate transplantation model. However, clinical studies have not yet confirmed the efficacy of KGF on recipient thymopoiesis. In patients who underwent allo-HCT, KGF did not increase transplantation toxicity in allo-HCT recipients. However, this molecule failed to reduce aGvHD incidence, while OS, engraftment, and hematopoietic recovery were unchanged. Finally, long-term follow-up of these patients failed to reveal significant differences in infection risk, cGvHD incidence or long-term survival.

Androgen blockade
Age-related atrophy of the thymus is correlated with increased circulating amounts of sex steroids. Sex hormone blockade has been demonstrated to enhance thymic function, resulting in increased naïve T-cell output. Interestingly, restoration of B-cell production was also observed. The Boyd group recently published a small clinical HCT study, which reports that TREC numbers, TCR repertoire recovery and naïve CD4+ and CD8+ T-cell numbers were increased in the luteinizing hormone-releasing hormone agonist-treated patients early after allo-HCT. Improved T-cell function was also observed. However, larger clinical studies are needed.

The combination of KGF with sex hormone blockade was also tested on recipients undergoing allo-HCT with a myeloablative conditioning regimen. Higher thymopoiesis with a broader TCR repertoire and decreased homeostatic peripheral T-cell proliferation were observed in treated mice.

Growth hormone
Neuroendocrine hormones influence several immunologic responses. Growth hormone (GH) seems to exert its beneficial effects through promotion of pluripotent HSC or common lymphoid precursor migration to the thymus. GH-deficient mice experience defective cellular immunity and thymus atrophy, which is reversible with GH administration. Furthermore, GH administration increases thymocyte numbers in allo-HCT recipient mice.

> **PRACTICE POINT**
>
> Recombinant GH (genotropin, Pfizer) is currently being evaluated in patients undergoing UCBT.

Notch-based cultured systems

Notch1 activation is essential for BM-derived multipotent progenitors that seed the thymus, and for proliferation and further progression of early thymocytes along the T-cell lineage. Dysregulated activation of Notch1 significantly contributes to the generation of T-cell acute lymphoblastic leukemia. Moreover, blockade of Notch1 signaling resulted in partial inhibition of thymocyte differentiation and accumulation of precursors within the thymus.

The OP9-DL1 *in vitro* T-cell development system allows production of large numbers of highly purified T-cell precursors, generated by incubating HSCs with the BM stromal cell line OP9, transduced with the Notch ligand Delta-like 1 (OP9-DL1). Using this approach, T-cell reconstitution was enhanced and anti-tumor activity was preserved in pre-clinical HCT murine models. Furthermore, when CB progenitors expanded *ex vivo* in the presence of Notch ligand were infused in 10 patients receiving a myeloablative preparative regimen for stem cell transplantation, the time of neutrophil recovery was substantially shortened. In another clinical study, transfer of cultured T-cell precursors with allo-HSCs increased thymic cellularity and chimerism, as well as enhanced peripheral T- and NK-cell reconstitution compared with recipients receiving allo-HSCs only.

Interleukin-7

IL-7 has been demonstrated to be important for T-cell development and promotes both thymic- dependent and independent pathways. Non-hematopoietic stromal cells are the major source of IL-7, while the IL-7R is expressed on several developing lymphocyte subsets. IL-7 improves thymopoiesis by enhancing immature thymic progenitor proliferation. Its beneficial effect on T-cell reconstitution remains controversial in both murine and human studies. Enhanced proliferation of immature thymic progenitors, lymphocytes, and homeostatic proliferation of circulating T-cells were observed in some murine HCT models. However, treatment with IL-7 in a non-human primate HCT model led to an increase in CD4+ cell counts, explained by peripheral expansion rather than thymic production, with development of GvHD-like disease in the gut.

In clinical trials, IL-7 produced a marked dose-dependent increase in circulating CD3+, CD4+, and CD8+ T-cell numbers. IL-7 administration disproportionately increased naïve and central memory cells, leading to an overall increase in TCR diversity. In the light of these observations, IL-7 treatment seems to induce thymus-independent T-cell growth in naïve and central memory population with increased TCR diversity.

Interleukin-15

IL-15 induces T-, B-, and NK-cell proliferation through a multi-domain receptor containing the IL-15Rα, IL-2Rα and the IL-2Rγ chain. This molecule has showed the potential to enhance immunity for immunotherapy and tumor vaccination. Moreover, it was recently observed that IL-15 could improve T-cell engraftment in mice. Administration of IL-15 following BMT improved peripheral memory CD8+ T- and NK-cell expansion by promoting proliferation and decreasing apoptosis by increasing intracellular Bcl-2 levels. Enhanced T- and NK-cell functions were also observed. While the GvL effect was increased, GvHD was aggravated in some, but not all, allo-HCT recipient mice.

> **PRACTICE POINT**
>
> There are no clinical trials evaluating IL-15 for HCT currently ongoing.

Interleukin-22

IL-22 belongs to the IL-10 family and is mainly produced by Th17 and innate lymphoid cells (ILCs). This interleukin has been shown to have a role in promoting antimicrobial immunity at mucosal surfaces and in the maintenance of epithelial integrity. A murine study reported that thymic injury, as a consequence of irradiation, induced IL-23 production by thymic DCs, which in turn promoted IL-22 production by thymic ILCs. IL-22 then was able to promote the survival and proliferation of thymic epithelial cells, leading to regeneration of the stromal microenvironment and enhanced thymopoiesis. More importantly, recombinant IL-22 administration in sub-lethally irradiated mice resulted in improved thymic recovery. Together, these findings suggest a role for IL-22 in thymic recovery.

Table 35.2 shows a number of the strategies to improve immune reconstitution.

> **PRACTICE POINT**
>
> The safety of IL-22 administration is currently being evaluated in healthy volunteers.

Table 35.2 Strategies to improve immune reconstitution.

Treatment	Benefits	References
Sex Steroids inhibition	↑ lymphoid progenitors in BM, thymopoiesis, repair of thymic damage, peripheral T-cell expansion/survival/function	(Kelly et al. 2008, Sutherland et al. 2008)
KGF administration	↑ thymopoiesis, repair of thymic damage, peripheral T-cell expansion/survival/function	(Rossi et al. 2002, Seggewiss et al. 2007)
Recombinant GH administration	↑ thymopoiesis, lymphoid progenitor homing, peripheral immune responses	(Knyszynski et al. 1992, Chen et al. 2003)
IL-7 administration	↑ thymopoiesis, peripheral T-cell expansion/survival/function	(Rosenberg et al. 2006, Sportes et al. 2008)
IL-15 administration	↑ thymopoiesis, peripheral T-cell expansion/survival/function, GvL effect	(Lin et al. 2006, Sun et al. 2006)
Notch-based culture system	↑ T-cell lineage committed precursors, T-cell reconstitution, GvT effect, NK-cell activity, engraftment of CD34⁺ hematopoietic cells	(Schmitt and Zuniga-Pflucker 2002, Zakrzewski et al. 2006, Delaney et al. 2010)
IL-22	↑ thymopoiesis,	(Dudakov et al. 2012)

SUMMARY

1 Allo-HCT offers the opportunity for successfully treating malignancies and immune disorders.

2 Delayed immune reconstitution remains one the major limitations.

3 Clinical studies have highlighted that:

  a The innate immune system recovers faster

  b Adaptive immune reconstitution can be hampered for years

  c B-cell recovery reflects their ontogeny

  d T-cell reconstitution derives from both thymic-dependent and thymic-independent pathways

4 Both murine pre-clinical models and small clinical studies have highlighted some promising molecules, such as IL-7, IL-15, IL-22, KGF, the Notch-based culture system, GH, and sex hormone blockade.

5 Carefully designed randomized clinical studies are needed to determine whether any of these approaches can augment immune reconstitution in humans and reduce morbidity and mortality from infectious complication and transplant-related morality.

Selected reading

1. Bosch, M., F. M. Khan and J. Storek (2012). "Immune reconstitution after hematopoietic cell transplantation." *Curr Opin Hematol* **19**(4): 324–335.

2. Gress, R. E., S. G. Emerson and W. R. Drobyski (2010). "Immune reconstitution: how it should work, what's broken, and why it matters." *Biol Blood Marrow Transplant.* **16**(1 Suppl): S133–137.

3. Mackall, C., T. Fry, R. Gress, K. Peggs, J. Storek, A. Toubert, et al. (2009). "Background to hematopoietic cell transplantation, including post transplant immune recovery." *Bone Marrow Transplant.* **44**(8): 457–462.

4. Seggewiss, R. and H. Einsele (2010). "Immune reconstitution after allogeneic transplantation and expanding options for immunomodulation: an update." *Blood.* **115**(19): 3861386–3861388.

5. Velardi, E., J. A. Dudakov and M. R. van den Brink (2013). "Clinical strategies to enhance thymic recovery after allogeneic hematopoietic stem cell transplantation." *Immunology Letters.* **155**: 31–35.

6. Williams, K. M. and R. E. Gress (2008). "Immune reconstitution and implications for immunotherapy following haematopoietic stem cell transplantation." *Best Pract Res Clin Haematol.* **21**(3): 579–596.

7. Zakrzewski, J. L., A. A. Kochman, S. X. Lu, T. H. Terwey, T. D. Kim, V. M. Hubbard, et al. (2006). "Adoptive transfer of T-cell precursors enhances T-cell reconstitution after allogeneic hematopoietic stem cell transplantation." *Nat Med* **12**(9): 1039–1047.

8. Mohty, M., B. Gaugler, C. Faucher, D. Sainty, M. Lafage-Pochitaloff, N. Vey, et al. (2002). "Recovery of lymphocyte and dendritic cell subsets following reduced intensity allogeneic bone marrow transplantation." *Hematology* **7**(3): 157–164.

9. Olson, J. A., D. B. Leveson-Gower, S. Gill, J. Baker, A. Beilhack and R. S. Negrin (2010). "NK-cells mediate reduction of GVHD by inhibiting activated, alloreactive T-cells while retaining GVT effects." *Blood* **115**(21): 4293–4301.

10. Perales, M. A., J. D. Goldberg, J. Yuan, G. Koehne, L. Lechner, E. B. Papadopoulos, et al. (2012). "Recombinant human interleukin-7 (CYT107) promotes T-cell recovery after allogeneic stem cell transplantation." *Blood* **120**(24): 4882–4891.

11. Alpdogan, O., J. M. Eng, S. J. Muriglan, L. M. Willis, V. M. Hubbard, K. H. Tjoe, et al. (2005). "Interleukin-15 enhances immune reconstitution after allogeneic bone marrow transplantation." *Blood* **105**(2): 865–873.

12. Alpdogan, O. and M. R. van den Brink (2012). "Immune tolerance and transplantation." *Semin Oncol* **39**(6): 629–642.

13. Levine, J. E., B. R. Blazar, T. DeFor, J. L. Ferrara and D. J. Weisdorf (2008). "Long-term follow-up of a phase I/II randomized, placebo-controlled trial of palifermin to prevent graft-versus-host disease (GvHD) after related donor allogeneic hematopoietic cell transplantation (HCT)." *Biol Blood Marrow Transplant* **14**(9): 1017–1021.

14. Lin, S. J., P. J. Cheng, D. C. Yan, P. T. Lee and H. S. Hsaio (2006)."Effect of interleukin-15 on alloreactivity in umbilical cord blood." *Transpl Immunol* **16**(2): 112–116.

15. Sutherland, J. S., L. Spyroglou, J. L. Muirhead, T. S. Heng, A. Prieto-Hinojosa, H. M. Prince, et al. (2008). "Enhanced immune system regeneration in humans following allogeneic or autologous hemopoietic stem cell transplantation by temporary sex steroid blockade." *Clin Cancer Res* **14**(4): 1138–1149.

CHAPTER 36

Donor lymphocyte infusion

David C. Halverson and Daniel Fowler

Experimental Transplantation and Immunology Branch, National Cancer Institute, National Institutes of Health, Bethesda, MD, USA

What is the rationale for donor lymphocyte infusions (DLIs)?

DLI may be given:
1 To treat overt disease recurrence or progression after allogeneic cell transplantation.
2 As pre-emptive therapy in minimal residual disease or high risk disease.
3 To promote further donor engraftment in recipients with mixed donor chimerism.
4 As treatment of uncontrolled post-transplant viral infections (not discussed here).
5 As treatment for a post-transplant lymphoproliferative disorder (PTLD, not discussed here).

What factors should be considered in deciding to proceed with a DLI?

Figure 36.1 represents a suggested decision making algorithm for considering a DLI. In addition to having one of the indications listed above, additional important considerations can help to estimate the risk and benefit of pursuing a DLI in any given patient.
1 *Graft-versus-tumor (GvT) susceptibility*: Clinical experience has suggested that malignant diseases have varying susceptibilities to GvT effects. These generalizations have come from indirect observations of the relationship in any particular malignancy between the development of chronic GvHD and lower rates of relapse. Alternatively, more direct evidence of GvT effects can be inferred in most diseases by a direct response of some relapsed patients to DLI.

Collective clinical experience to date has led to the following generalization about inherent GvT susceptibility: CML>low grade NHL>high grade NHL>HD>MM>AML>ALL. As the field of allogeneic transplant is constantly evolving concerning conditioning intensity, donor types, graft manipulation, and peri-transplantation care of patients, caution should be exercised interpreting the continued validity of these generalizations with newer approaches.
2 *Transplant recipient GvHD status*: New or worsening GvHD has been a limiting side effect of DLI. In general, patients with active acute or chronic GvHD requiring ongoing immunosuppression have been considered inappropriate candidates for DLI. Patients with a history of past severe GvHD must be considered high risk for GvHD recurrence after DLI and may warrant immunosuppression concurrent to DLI. These generalizations may also change as post-transplant adoptive T-cell therapies increasingly involve manipulation of the infused cell products to increase specificity of targeting (chimeric antigen receptor transfection) or lower the risks of subsequent GvHD (alloreactive depletion or subset enrichment).
3 *Primary disease status*: In general, DLIs are more likely to be successful in eradicating minimal amounts of disease. To this end, DLIs may be more effective after cytoreductive therapies. This possible benefit has to be weighed against the potential toxicities of the cytoreductive therapies and their potential alteration of the recipient's immunologic and target tissue environments. Whether the amount of disease is simply a surrogate marker for higher risk biology or directly compromises the effectiveness of a DLI has not been adequately studied.

Clinical Manual of Blood and Bone Marrow Transplantation, First Edition. Edited by Syed A. Abutalib and Parameswaran Hari.
© 2017 John Wiley & Sons Ltd. Published 2017 by John Wiley & Sons Ltd.

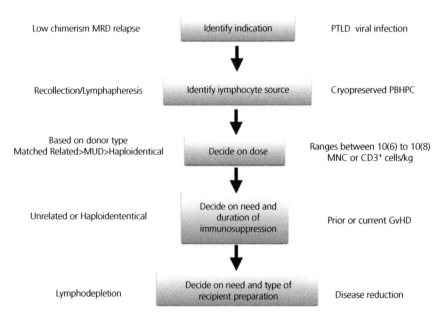

Figure 36.1 DLI decision-making algorithm.

How are donor lymphocytes collected?

The lymphocytes used as a DLI may be either newly acquired from the donor by additional lymphapheresis or can be in an aliquot of mobilized peripheral blood hematopoietic progenitor cells (PBHPC) not used in the original transplant. Mobilized PBHPC, although enriched for stem cells, still contain mostly lymphocytes.

PRACTICE POINT

Our practice has been to preferentially use donor lymphocytes taken by lymphapheresis. This avoids the potential immunologic effects of the G-CSF mobilization procedure (Type II cytokine profile skewing and modulation of regulatory T-cells). In addition, many of our protocols involve T-cell manipulations (CAR transfection, activation, cytokine profile skewing) that are best performed on steady state donor lymphocytes. If part of the reason for DLI is less than optimal myeloid engraftment, then the use of a mobilized CD34⁺ enriched product as the DLI may be helpful.

How is a DLI administered?

The cells comprising a DLI can be either fresh or previously cryopreserved. No benefits, other than avoiding

DMSO toxicities and some obligate cell loss, are known to exist for one approach *versus* the other. It is not mandatory to use a central line to administer DLI. In general, the volume of a DLI will be small in the 25–50 cc range. Premedication, as used for any blood product, is a matter of choice. Febrile reactions or side effects from the DMSO used in cryopreservation are rare. Outpatient administration is feasible and customary. Coordination with the blood bank, storage facility, and clinical unit are crucial to ensure the administration of a viable product.

What is an optimal dose of CD3⁺ cells?

The dose is usually expressed as a number of mononuclear cells (MNC) or CD3⁺ cells (T-cells) per kilogram of the recipient's weight. The doses actually given in any particular study have varied widely and been chosen arbitrarily as little concrete data has been available to guide this decision. Historically, the dose range for DLI has been between 10^6 and 10^8 MNC or CD3⁺ cells/kg of recipient body weight. The type of donor-recipient relationship has been the variable most often used to justify giving higher or lower doses within this range, with progressively lower doses for HLA-matched -related, -unrelated, and HLA-haploidentical donor sources respectively. DLI in the context of cord blood transplantation (CBT) is not currently feasible, although attempts at expanding cord blood T-cells *ex vivo* have been reported and are currently being studied. Several studies have suggested that higher doses of lymphocytes, especially beyond 1×10^8/kg, are correlated with higher risks of subsequent GvHD without improving responses. This relationship has been inconsistent in the literature. The development of GvHD has, unfortunately, been highly correlated with subsequent anti-tumor effects in most series and the morbidity and mortality associated tends to blunt the overall survival (OS) benefit.

> **PRACTICE POINT**
>
> Our practice has been to limit unmanipulated CD3⁺ cell dose to 1×10^8/kg in HLA-matched related DLI, 1×10^7/kg in HLA-matched unrelated DLI, and 1×10^6/kg in HLA-haploidentical DLI.

Frequency of DLIs?

Usually, a single DLI is given. Some clinicians have proposed and tested varying schemes of dose escalation, primarily for CML but no such approach has become a standard. The number of DLIs any patient will receive is usually limited by one of the following factors: (1) the number of donor products available, (2) the subsequent occurrence of GvHD, (3) a response, or (4) progression of the disease despite the DLI. There certainly is a role for considering repeated DLI using an increased dose if response is absent or inadequate and GvHD has not occurred. It is important that the results of each DLI be evaluated after a period of at least 3–4 weeks has elapsed and usually in the absence of any immunosuppression before deciding if additional DLI is either necessary or safe.

Should the DLI be preceded by disease specific therapy?

The decision to use disease specific therapy depends on the disease burden, the likelihood of a meaningful response, and the growth kinetics of the patient's disease. A theoretically important consideration is that DLI after toxic chemotherapy may increase the risks of subsequent GvHD in much the same fashion as GvHD is more prevalent after more intense transplant conditioning regimens. Thus, the decision to use disease reduction prior to any DLI must be individualized based on disease and patient considerations.

> **PRACTICE POINT**
>
> We reserve disease specific therapy prior to DLI for those patients in which relapse kinetics are rapid or disease burden is either high or bulky. In general, toxic, or prolonged anti-neoplastic therapies just prior to DLI may result in more problems from delay and overlapping toxicities than benefit. The availability, likelihood of response, and likely durability of any response to disease specific therapy are important variables to consider.

Is there a role for recipient lymphodepletion prior to DLI?

DLI is functionally a type of adoptive T-cell therapy. In other allogeneic and autologous settings, lymphodepletion of the recipient before adoptive T-cell therapies appears to enhance their activity. This is felt to be mediated through the creation of a homeostatic environment skewed toward T-cell proliferation and activation. This concept has been referred to as "making space" but is more accurately represented as increasing homeostatic T-cell cytokines (IL-7, IL-12, IL-15) by removing cytokine sinks that theoretically allows more free cytokines to be available to the newly infused T-cells.

> **PRACTICE POINT**
>
> Our practice has been to strongly consider the use of lymphodepletion prior to our experimental DLIs and we prefer relatively T-cell specific and gentle methods such as a combination of pentostatin and low dose oral cyclophosphamide. Practically, this provides for an augmented homeostatic environment and potentially the abrogation of existing tolerance. More research is needed to define the optimal regimen and situation for pre-DLI lymphodepletion.

Should the recipient be on immunosuppression at the time of DLI?

Historically, DLI was given without immunosuppression. The concurrent use of immunosuppression is a decision based on perceived risk of not inducing GvHD. The prophylactic agent, dose, and length of therapy have not been defined in a systematic way and remain a clinical judgment. Temporary immunosuppression with cyclosporine, tacrolimus, or sirolimus can add a margin of safety but their possible impairment of a desired GvT reaction remains an undefined risk.

PRACTICE POINT

Our preference is to strongly consider a short course (7–14 days) of calcineurin inhibitor during DLI, in patients at higher risk of GvHD (prior GvHD, HLA-matched unrelated donor, or toxic preceding cytoreductive therapy). These agents' blunt T-cell responses without compromising subsequent T-cell number or function after they are discontinued. There is no current standard in the use of immunosuppressive therapy in patients who are at low risk for GvHD (especially those with no prior GvHD and with matched sibling donors).

How long does it take for a DLI to work?

This varies by disease but is best characterized in the treatment of CML relapse. In this setting, GvT can be a slow and prolonged process taking up to a year. More typically, because other diseases are not as chronic or slow in their manifestations of relapse, some effect of a DLI should be evident within 30 days. In general, as with all allogeneic immunological processes, a minimum of 21 days and an absence of immunosuppression should be allowed before assessing for the ultimate positive or negative effects of a DLI.

What are the side effects of DLI?

Historically, GvHD after DLI was felt to occur at higher rates than seen with initial allogeneic hematopoietic cell transplant (allo-HCT), in the range of 40–60%.

This rate, though, should be considered a variable influenced by underlying disease, donor type, prior GvHD history, use of prophylaxis, presence and type of manipulation, and lymphocyte dose. As these have variables have changed rapidly in practice, the reported rates of GvHD after DLI have varied widely. This is demonstrated in Table 36.1, which includes the pooled rate of post-DLI GvHD data by disease from a recent meta-analysis and Table 36.2 includes GvHD data from a variety of noteworthy studies of DLI. Unfortunately, no consistent strategy has been found that avoids post-DLI GvHD while preserving the desired GvT.

Post-DLI marrow aplasia with cytopenias was described with some regularity after DLI for CML and likely reflected a vigorous graft-*versus*-host marrow response in these patients. The presence of a significant amount of host hematopoiesis (malignant or normal) as a part of relapse is a risk factor for a subsequent period of relative host aplasia before donor hematopoiesis can recover. Thus, monitoring for aplasia in these situations is important. Fortunately, the cytopenias are rarely problematic with spontaneous recovery with time and supportive care as the rule. As expected, an aplastic response to DLI is usually correlated with an anti-tumor response.

Practically, the occurrence of alloreactivity (manifested as GvT) after DLI is the desired result of administration. Unfortunately, alloreactivity (manifested as GvHD) lacks clinical predictability and control. Manipulation of both the DLI content (qualitatively and quantitatively) and the host environment they encounter represents a daunting set of variables that future studies will need to address in order to optimize the balance of GvT/GvHD.

Table 36.1 Overview of data with donor lymphocyte infusion.

Disease	Relative Susceptibility to GvL	Complete Response Rates Reported	Acute and Chronic GvHD rate
CML	1	82 (60–90)	55
AML	3	26 (17–55)	60
ALL	4	27 (16–40)	49
Multiple Myeloma	4	26 (19–33)	52
Aggressive NHL	2	44 (33–55)	48
Indolent NHL	1	64 (44–82)	59
Hodgkins	3	37 (20–56)	58
CLL	2	55 (15–92)	77
MDS	3	20 (14–40)	43

* 1 = best response to DLI and 4 = poor response to DLI

Table 36.2 Selected notable publications on DLI.

Citation	Disease	Number of Patients	Donor types	Dose/kg	Result	GvHD	Comment
Kolb HJ, Blood. 1990; 76:2462–2465.	CML	3	MRD	$4.4-7.4 \times 10^8$ MNC	3/3 CR	2/3	First report of successful DLI
Kolb HJ, Blood. 1995; 86(5):2041–2050	AML ALL CML	135	MRD (90%)	$0.1-15 \times 10^8$ MNC	CML=77% AML=29% ALL=0% (CR)	41% (>Grade I)	Established lower expectations for acute leukemias
Anderlini P, Leukemia & Lymphoma. 2012; 53(6): 1239–1241	Hodgkin's	27	MRD (17) MUD (10)	10^7	37% (CR/PR) 20% (4 y OS)	100% of responders	Confirmed modest expectations in Hodgkin's
Peggs et al. (2004)	MM Hodgkins NHL	46	MRD (32) MUD (14)	10^6 to 3×10^8	MM=63% (CR/PR) HL=70% (CR/PR) NHL=30% (CR)	MRD=25% MUD=77%	High rate of GvHD with DLI after MUD correlated with higher cell doses
Najla EJ, Immunotherapy. 2013; 5(5):457–466.	Lymphoid	624 from 39 studies	MRD MUD	NR	ALL=27% CLL=55% MM=26% NHL=52% HL=37% (CR)	ALL=49% CLL=77% MM=52% NHL=59% HL=58%	Meta-analysis. No randomized trials. GvHD pooled acute and chronic. Confirmed GvT range in lymphoid.
Zeidan AM, Biol Blood Marrow Transplant. 2014; 20:314–318	Hematologic	40	Haplo	10^6(80%) 10^5 to 10^8	30% (CR) 20% (DFS at 1 y)	25% (Acute)	Most extensive experience of haplo DLI after post-transplant cyclophosphamide
Bar M, Biol Blood Marrow Transplant. 2013;19: 949–957	Hematologic	225	MRD (171) MUD (41) MM (17)	A=$<10^7$ B=10^7 to $<10^8$ C = $>10^8$	A=47 B=45 C=32 (3 y OS)	A=21 B=45 C=55	Single institution. Most compelling relation of cell dose to outcome.

(Continued)

Table 36.2 (Continued)

Citation	Disease	Number of Patients	Donor types	Dose/kg	Result	GvHD	Comment
Takami A, Biol Blood Marrow Transplant. 2014;20:1785–1790	AML	143	MRD MUD	NR	32% (1 y OS) 17% (2 y OS) 7% (5 y OS)	18% (Acute)	Confirmed poor results with AML in an Asian population
Haines HL, Biol Blood Marrow Transplant. 2015;21:288–292	Non-malignant Mixed chimerism	27	MRD MUD MM	10^6 (0.02 to 20)	56% (>20% increase) 37% (Full)	37% (Acute) 10% (Grade III)	Pediatric Safety in converting MC
Yan CH, Blood. 2012; 119(14): 3256–3662	AML ALL	814 A = 709 (MRD−) B = 49 (MRD+ IL-2) C = 56 (MRD + DLI)	MRD Haplo MUD	$1.9–7.3 \times 10^7$ (CD3+)	A = 18.1% B = 64.4% C = 27.8% (Relapse)	DLI (C) 30.8% (Acute Grade II–IV) 42.9% (Chronic)	Efficacy of pre-emptive DLI based on MRD status.
Peggs et al. (2004)	Hodgkin's	76	MRD (42) MUD (34)	10^6 Mixed Chimera 10^7 to 10^8 (MRD Relapse) 10^6 to 10^7 (MUD Relapse)	Mixed Chimeras 19/22 (86%) Full Chimera 95% DFS No DLI 57% PFS Relapse 19/24 14 CR 5 PR 59% 4 y OS	1/22 Acute 4/22 Chronic (23%) 8/24 Acute 5/24 Chronic (54%)	Unexpectedly strong protection from relapse in group given DLI for MC (5% versus 43%). DLI for relapse with significant GvHD burden correlated with response. Better OS than previously demonstrated.

How effective is DLI?

The complete response (CR) rates for DLI in specific diseases varies widely across the literature and, to date, contains no data from randomized trials. As has often been true of allogeneic transplant itself, the ultimate benefit of DLI is often tempered by the short and long term negative effects associated with GvHD. Unfortunately, response to DLI is heavily correlated to developing acute and chronic GvHD. Most studies lack truly prolonged follow up, but where it is available, ultimate survival benefit is often compromised by late deaths associated with GvHD or complicating infection. Table 36.1 summarizes a recent meta-analysis showing the pooled rates of both CR and GvHD after DLI for the diseases where it has traditionally been utilized.

Limitations of data regarding DLI

As DLI is most often used to treat relapse, the situation in which any DLI is given is necessarily individualized to the needs of a specific patient. This inherent variability has led to inconsistent and widely disparate practices that tend to be institution and investigator specific. As in the case of allogenic transplant itself, randomized trials of DLI have been impeded by the lack of a defined standard of care. Thus, all of the data available remains experiential and retrospective in nature. More definitive answers to the questions in this chapter await a higher level of consensus to allow rationally designed randomized trials.

What are some of the disease specific considerations for DLIs?

CML

Disease most associated with successful use of DLI. It was the first disease relapsed after allo-HCT that was shown to be cured by DLI alone. CR rates of 80% have been consistently reported. The factors that likely account for this include the presence of a specific mutated protein produced by all tumor cells, the ability to monitor minimal residual disease (MRD) and intervene sooner in relapse, and the relapse of the disease into a chronic phase in most cases. A GvT effect resulting in cytogenetic CR in CML is seen at a median of 78 days after DLI, but response can be seen for up to a year after, making patience important. Understanding the more recent experience in treating MRD in CML with DLI has been complicated by the less frequent application of allo-HCT in the tyrosine kinase era as well as the availability of several specific tyrosine kinase inhibitors (TKIs) that are often given concurrently with DLI at relapse.

AML

The use of DLI has been less satisfying in AML. The CR rates reported vary between 17 and 55%. In general, about 25% of patients seem to benefit and this is, once again, highly correlated with inducing GvHD. This lower effectiveness likely is the result of the rapid growth and relapse kinetics of the disease resulting in higher blast variability, more disease at relapse, and shorter time available for GvT effects to work. Most patients in the available series have received further chemotherapy prior to DLI and often are treated in a state of resulting pancytopenia. Whether this is the optimal approach is not clear. Hopes for better future outcomes of DLI in AML may rest on earlier detection of MRD, pre-emptive use of DLI in high risk populations, identification of patient specific AML immunogenic targets, and a better understanding of both recipient, donor, and cell product factors that can be manipulated to increase the chances of success.

ALL

Despite success of DLI in treating relapse in some B-cell malignancies (especially follicular NHL), ALL has been an elusive target for GvT after both initial transplantation and DLI. The reasons for this are not entirely clear. CR rates <20% are commonly reported. As in AML, ALL is usually retreated prior to DLI in hopes of reducing the disease burden. New approaches to DLI in ALL are clearly needed and will likely only come after elucidation of the molecular and genetic mechanisms of apparent resistance of ALL to GvT effects in general.

The newer generation of chimeric antigen receptor (CAR) transfected donor T-cells against B-cell antigens (CD19 and CD22) used as DLI have shown striking activity in relapsed ALL. Unfortunately, toxicities (as cytokine release syndrome) have been significant and many of these patients eventually relapse after a single CAR T-cell DLI. The dosing, role of repetition, newer CAR constructs, and timing of subsequent application of second allo-HCT are all being studied to try to optimize this exciting salvage therapy.

Multiple myeloma

DLI in myeloma has suffered from the same apparent limitations as allo-HCT itself for myeloma with a distinct lack of predictable GvT effects. Malignant plasma cells seem to have a clinically resistant phenotype to many forms of therapy with eventual relapse almost a given even after prolonged remissions. The precise reason for this have not been clearly elucidated but is consistent with the "hard to cure despite being responsive" experience in other low-grade B-cell neoplasms. Despite this curative nihilism, responses can be seen in 10–20% of myeloma patients after DLI, usually corresponding to clinically apparent GvHD. Rarely, some of these responses can be complete and durable.

Low-grade NHL, CLL, and MCL

These neoplasms of more mature B-cells appear to have a more innate susceptibility to GvT effects, and, thus, to DLI. Response in greater than 50% of patients can be expected. There does appear to be higher rates of chronic GvHD after DLI in this population that may account for this higher response in disease.

Aggressive NHL

Although experimentally susceptible to GvT, these lymphomas clinically are difficult to treat with DLI presumably because of their aggressive growth kinetics. The use of additional chemotherapy to reduce disease burden just prior to DLI is usually necessary and can be a successful strategy. Improved results for DLI in these lymphomas remains an elusive goal that will require new strategies to provide more potent or specific GvT (i.e., anti-CD19 or CD22 CAR T-cells, or T-cell check-point inhibition).

Hodgkin's lymphoma

Allo-HCT for HL has been used as a last resort in those patients who fail induction and autologous high dose therapy. HL patients have higher than expected levels of treatment related mortality (TRM) after standard myeloablative transplant approaches likely due to their heavy pretreatment, prior mediastinal radiation, and the underlying immunological aberrations associated with HL. Lower intensity approaches to minimize these toxicities have unacceptably high levels of relapse suggesting that GvT effects were of limited benefit. More recently though, more reports of successful DLI for relapse after reduced intensity hematopoietic cell transplantation have suggested that the situation leading to that conclusion is more complicated than previously thought. A relatively large series of patients treated for mixed chimerism (MC) or relapse after T-cell depleted (alemtuzumab) RIC allo-HCT showed strong evidence for GvT effects with only 5% relapses in the MC group given DLI (versus 43% in full chimeras given no DLI) and responses in 79% of patients treated for relapse with a 4-year OS of 59% in the group. As expected, GvT effects were strongly correlated with the development of post-DLI GvHD.

Nonmalignant diseases

DLI is used exclusively in this setting to convert MC to full chimerism as GvT effects are not relevant. The decision to use DLI for this purpose must be carefully weighed in terms of the clinical need for full chimerism in reversing the disease phenotype and the significant risk of DLI induced GvHD. Most of the literature on DLI in non-malignant diseases is from pediatric series. As there

is no benefit in this population to any level of GvHD, both prophylaxis and early aggressive treatment of GvHD after DLI are paramount. The specific considerations for DLI in these rare diseases are highly disease dependent and are beyond the scope of this chapter.

SUMMARY POINTS

1 There is no randomized data to compare the results of DLI in any disease.

2 DLI to date has been most useful for CML minimal residual disease or relapse but less so for other hematologic malignancies in descending order of response probability: indolent NHL, HL, aggressive NHL, MM, AML, and ALL.

3 Currently, the decision to employ DLI in any specific disease or patient requires consideration of a complex mix of variables and should be done only by an experienced transplant team.

4 Diseases appear to have a wide variability in susceptibility to unmanipulated DLI based on the available retrospective series.

5 Randomized and prospective data concerning DLI dose, DLI composition, DLI timing, DLI manipulations, and host preparation in each disease, donor type, and transplant intensity are required to ultimately improve DLI safety and efficacy.

6 GvHD after DLI remains the biggest obstacle to its successful use but remains strongly correlated to benefit via GvT effects.

7 Current technologies under evaluation, including manipulation of donor lymphocyte specificity, genotype, phenotype, and enrichment of various T-cell subsets hold promise in making DLI more safe and effective across all diseases.

Selected reading

1. Mackinnon S, Papadopoulos EB, Carabasi MH, et al. Adoptive immunotherapy evaluating escalating doses of donor leukocytes for relapse of chronic myeloid leukemia after bone marrow transplantation: separation of graft-versus-leukemia responses from graft-versus-host disease. *Blood.* 1995 Aug 15;**86**(4):1261–1268.

2. Najla El-Jurdi, Tea Reljic, Ambuj Kumar, et al. Efficacy of adoptive immunotherapy with donor lymphocyte infusion in relapsed lymphoid malignancies. *Immunotherapy.* May 2013;**5**(5):457–466.

3. Chang YJ, Huang XJ. Donor lymphocyte transfusions for relapse after allogeneic transplantation: when, if and for whom? *Blood Rev.* 2013;**27**(1):55–62.

4. Peggs KS, Kayani I, Edwards N, et al. Donor lymphocyte infusions modulate relapse risk in mixed chimeras and induce durable salvage in relapsed patients after T-cell-depleted allogeneic transplantation for Hodgkin's lymphoma. *J Clin Oncol.* 2011;**29**:971–978.

5. Haines HL, Blessing JJ, Davies SM, et al. Outcomes of donor lymphocyte infusion for treatment of mixed donor chimerism after a reduced-intensity preparative regimen for pediatric patients with nonmalignant diseases. *Biol Blood Marrow Transplant*. 2015;**21**(2):288–292.

6. Bar M, Sandmaier BM, Inamoto Y, et al. Donor lymphocyte infusion for relapsed hematological malignancies after allogeneic hematopoietic cell transplantation: prognostic relevance of the initial CD3⁺ T-cell dose. *Blood Marrow Transplant*. 2013;**19**:949–957.

7. Ferrara JLM, Reddy P. Cellular therapy for hematology malignancies: allogeneic hematopoietic stem cell transplantation, graft-versus-host disease, and graft versus leukemia effects. *Advances in Stem Cell Research, Stem Cell Biology and Regenerative Medicine*. 2102. Springer Science + Business Media, LLC: 303–366.

8. Frey NV, Porter DL. Graft-versus-host disease after donor leukocyte infusions: presentation and management. *Best Pract Res Clin Haematol*. 2008;**21**(2):205–222.

9. Zeidan AM, Forde PM, Symons H, et al. HLA-haploidentical donor lymphocyte infusions for patients with relapsed hematologic malignancies after related HLA-haploidentical bone marrow transplantation. *Biol Blood Marrow Transplant*. 2014;**20**:314–318.

CHAPTER 37

Diagnosis and treatment of acute graft-versus-host disease

Natasha Kekre[1] and Vincent T. Ho[2]

[1] Blood and Marrow Transplant Program, The Ottawa Hospital and Ottawa Hospital Research Institute, Ottawa, Canada

[2] Dana Farber Cancer Institute, Boston, MA, USA

Introduction

In the first few months following allogeneic hematopoietic cell transplantation (allo-HCT), acute graft-versus-host disease (aGvHD) remains an important cause of morbidity and mortality. Despite advancements in both the prevention and treatment of aGvHD, the mainstay of therapy remains corticosteroids. This chapter will briefly outline the pathophysiology and risk factors of aGvHD, the diagnostic criteria, and finally the therapeutic strategies for aGvHD. The prevention of aGvHD is discussed elsewhere (Chapter 9).

Pathophysiology and risk factors of aGvHD

Do we completely understand the pathophysiology of aGvHD?

The organs classically affected by aGvHD (skin, gastrointestinal mucosa and liver) are often compromised by intense conditioning regimens prior to allo-HCT. This tissue injury leads to increased presentation of host antigens, and permeability/entry of microbial immunostimulatory molecules such as endotoxin. This consequently leads to the recruitment, activation, and expansion of alloreactive donor T-cells in secondary lymphoid tissue. Target organ damage is subsequently mediated by the direct cytotoxic actions of activated donor effector T-cells, which migrate to extra-lymphoid target sites, as well as the actions of local cytokines. The most commonly accepted model of these three phases of aGvHD is depicted in Figure 37.1.

Some important risk factors associated with aGvHD

1 *Donor:* Unrelated donors (particularly HLA mismatched donors), older age, multiparity, gender mismatch (especially female donor to male recipient), prior transfusions, donor-recipient ABO incompatibility, and CMV seropositivity.
2 *Recipient:* Older age, advanced disease stage, CMV seropositivity.
3 *Graft source:* Peripheral blood has a slightly higher risk of aGvHD than bone marrow in a large meta-analysis. Cord blood transplantation appears to be associated with similar aGvHD incidence compared to HLA-matched unrelated donor (MUD) bone marrow transplantation.
4 *Conditioning regimen intensity:* myeloablative conditioning is associated with a higher risk and earlier onset of aGvHD compared to reduced-intensity conditioning (RIC).

Diagnosis and clinical manifestations of aGvHD

How is aGvHD defined?

Although classically thought of as occurring within 100 days from allo-HCT, this is now obsolete especially since aGvHD tends to develop later after RIC transplantation. The current definition is based on clinical signs and symptoms associated with gastrointestinal (GI), cutaneous, and hepatic involvement and can occur at any time after transplant. Clinicians often refer to GvHD that occurs within 14 days of allo-HCT as hyperacute

Clinical Manual of Blood and Bone Marrow Transplantation, First Edition. Edited by Syed A. Abutalib and Parameswaran Hari.

© 2017 John Wiley & Sons Ltd. Published 2017 by John Wiley & Sons Ltd.

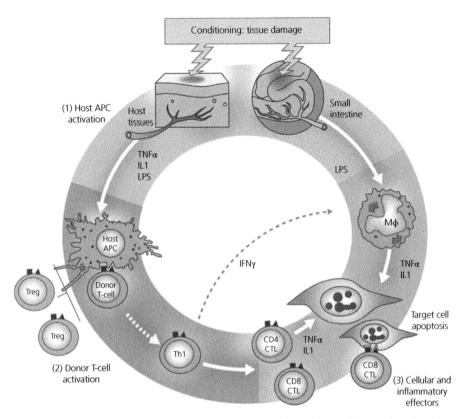

Figure 37.1 Pathophysiology of aGvHD. Progression of aGvHD occurs through three phases: (1) activation of antigen-presenting cells; (2) donor T-cell activation, proliferation, differentiation, and migration; and (3) target tissue destruction. Source: Ferrara 2009.[13] Reproduced with permission of Elsevier.

GvHD and after 100 days as late onset aGvHD. GvHD that develops after 100 days from allo-HCT is often due to the taper of immune suppression agents used for GvHD prophylaxis. If aGvHD symptoms are associated with signs or symptoms of "classic" chronic GvHD, (cGvHD) this is referred to as "overlap syndrome."

What are the chances of getting aGvHD and what is the usual timing?

In one randomized trial that compared two standard pharmacologic approaches (tacrolimus/methotrexate vs cyclosporine/methotrexate) to GvHD prophylaxis after myeloablative allo-HCT, the incidence of grade II-IV aGvHD was 33% in HLA-matched sibling donors (MSD).[1] This is closer to 40–50% in HLA-MUD and even higher with mismatched unrelated donors. In patients with clinically relevant grade II-IV aGvHD, the incidence of any involvement of the gut, skin, or liver was 73, 70, and 44% respectively in this study. The median time to onset of any clinically evident aGvHD is 3 weeks (range 1–14 weeks) in one cohort of over 500 patients.[2]

Clinical manifestations of gastrointestinal GvHD

The GI tract is probably the most commonly involved organ in aGvHD with modern GvHD prophylaxis regimens and is likely to be under diagnosed since many patients with persistent nausea may not undergo upper endoscopy to confirm the diagnosis. Gut only aGvHD was reported in 17% of patients with aGvHD in one randomized study.[1] The staging of lower GI aGvHD is based on the volume of diarrhea. In addition to watery diarrhea, patients with acute GI GvHD can have GI bleeding, abdominal pain, and ileus if it is severe. Upper GI aGvHD is separate and symptoms are very nonspecific including anorexia, nausea, and dyspepsia.

Clinical manifestations of cutaneous GvHD

Skin involvement is another common clinical manifestation of aGvHD, and is the only organ involved in about 15% of patients with aGvHD. It is most commonly associated with a maculopapular rash, often difficult to distinguish from a drug eruption. This rash can be asymptomatic, pruritic, or painful in nature.

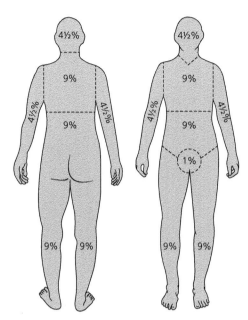

Figure 37.2 Rule of 9's in determining body surface area in cutaneous aGvHD. Adapted from http://medical-dictionary.thefreedictionary.com/rule+of+nines

The staging of acute skin GvHD is based on the total body surface area involved, and can be simply estimated in the clinic using the "rule of 9's" used commonly in burn patients (Figure 37.2). As the rash progresses, it can become more confluent, the erythema can become more intense and painful, and in its most severe form erythroderma and bullae formation can occur.

Clinical manifestations of hepatic GvHD

The liver is the least commonly involved organ in aGvHD, and is rarely observed as the only organ involved (4% of patients with aGvHD), and more commonly manifests concurrently with gut or skin involvement. The clinical diagnosis of liver aGvHD is based on an elevated bilirubin, but patients can often present with a concomitant transaminitis. Presentation with transaminase elevations in the absence of hyperbilirubinemia can also occur. Patients are generally asymptomatic but can have painful hepatomegaly, dark urine, pale stool, edema, and pruritis. In its most severe form, it can lead to fulminant liver failure and complete loss of biliary ducts (so called "vanishing bile duct" syndrome) and hepatic encephalopathy.

What is the differential diagnosis of aGvHD?

1 *Engraftment syndrome:* All of the clinical manifestations of GI, skin, and liver aGvHD can be seen with engraftment syndrome. This occurs around the time of neutrophil engraftment and is often associated with fever without an infectious cause, with or without rash, diarrhea, and peripheral or pulmonary edema. Generally, patients with engraftment syndrome respond very rapidly to corticosteroids and do not require a prolonged taper as needed with GvHD. The timing and rapid resolution of symptoms on corticosteroids can sometimes be the only clue that a patient has engraftment syndrome and not classic or hyperacute aGvHD.

2 *Infection(s):* Patients with diarrhea after allo-HCT should undergo standard stool cultures to rule out infections such as CMV or adenovirus colitis and *Clostridium difficile.* Viral exanthem is on the differential for a patient with a rash after allo-HCT. Infectious causes of liver dysfunction after allo-HCT include hepatic candidiasis and viral hepatitis, which can be diagnosed by blood cultures, PCR, or serology. The viral hepatitides are generally associated with more hepatocyte injury and marked elevations of liver transaminases compared to the more cholestatic presentation seen with liver GvHD.

3 *Drug reaction:* Diarrhea can be a manifestation of drug toxicity especially with high doses of total body irradiation or chemotherapy. Although conditioning regimens can cause diarrhea, this is usually short-lived and should not result in the persistent large volume watery diarrhea that is often seen with acute GI GvHD. Drug eruptions on the skin can be difficult to differentiate from acute skin GvHD. Skin biopsy demonstrating the presence of an eosinophil infiltrate may suggest a drug eruption, although this alone does not rule out GvHD and skin biopsies are often not useful to differentiate drug eruption from GvHD. Clinically, drug eruptions are less likely to affect the palms and soles and the timing of the rash relative to drug administration can help (7–10 days after first exposure or 1–2 days after subsequent exposure).

4 *Hepatic sinusoidal obstructive syndrome (SOS):* Previously known as hepatic veno-occlusive disease (VOD), this is associated with high intensity conditioning regimens and the use of sirolimus as part of GvHD prophylaxis regimens. Generally, SOS occurs within 21 days from allo-HCT, and leads to painful hepatomegaly, jaundice, ascites and/or weight gain. Liver GvHD can be distinguished from SOS by liver biopsy as SOS is associated with obstruction of the sinusoids or central veins, whereas liver GvHD is associated with injury to the bile ducts and portal triads.

Is biopsy necessary in diagnosing aGvHD?

Because the clinical symptoms of aGvHD are non-specific, a biopsy is helpful in making the diagnosis and ruling out other causes, especially in regards to GI GvHD. For example, a biopsy of the colon can show

GvHD features, but also viral inclusions if viral colitis is present. Often the diagnosis can be made with flexible sigmoidoscopy, but occasionally a full colonoscopy is needed. Skin biopsy can be helpful in making the diagnosis of cutaneous aGvHD, but is often not performed as the results are usually non-specific. A 4 mm punch biopsy of the skin can reveal the severity of skin involvement. For hepatic GvHD, a biopsy may be warranted to rule out other causes of liver dysfunction, but this procedure is associated with a risk of bleeding, especially after allo-HCT when patients often have thrombocytopenia. Transjugular liver biopsy may be preferred as it is less invasive and associated with lower risk of post procedural bleeding.

Biopsy findings in aGvHD:

1 **GI:** Crypt cell necrosis with the accumulation of degenerative material in the dead crypts; if severe, there may be areas of complete loss of the epithelium of the gut lining.

2 **Skin:** Lymphocyte exocytosis (presence of lymphocytes in the epidermis), vacuolization of the basal layer of the dermal-epidermal junction and necrotic epidermal cells; if severe, separation of the dermal and epidermal layers.

3 **Liver:** Bile duct degeneration and lymphocytic infiltration of the small bile ducts.

Is radiographic imaging needed in diagnosing aGvHD?

Imaging can sometimes be helpful at determining the extent of GvHD or to rule out other causes of a patient's symptoms. Radiographic imaging may be helpful to demonstrate air or fluid levels if there is an ileus or small bowel wall thickening in GI GvHD, but this is not needed to make the diagnosis. Radiographic imaging is often not helpful to differentiate hepatic GvHD from other causes of liver dysfunction, but findings of gallbladder wall thickening and/or presence of ascites would be more suggestive of gall bladder disease or hepatic SOS. Hepatic ultrasound with Doppler can help differentiate GvHD from SOS as patients with severe SOS will often have reversal of flow in the portal venous system.

Grading aGvHD – Is one classification better than the other?

The currently accepted clinical grading of aGvHD is based solely on clinical signs and symptoms, not on biopsy results. Although there are histologic grades for GI, liver, and skin GvHD on pathology, these do not always correlate with clinical grading. The original clinical grading system for aGvHD was created by Glucksberg et al. over 30 years ago and was revised shortly after.[3] This is still the most commonly used classification system in current GvHD trials.

More recently, a new schema was developed by the International Blood and Marrow Transplant Registry (IBMTR) in 1997. Both classification systems (Table 37.1) have performed similarly in explaining the variability in survival by GvHD grade, but the Glucksberg classification predicted early survival better and the IBMTR classification was associated with less bias and error in determining grades of GvHD.[2] Regardless of these differences, the maximum grade of aGvHD with either score was predictive of survival, whereas timing of onset or progression of aGvHD was not.

PRACTICE POINT

In aGvHD, the diagnosis is generally based on skin, GI, and liver manifestations which often require tissue biopsy. Rash and diarrhea are the most common complaints of a patient with aGvHD, but these symptoms are non-specific and can be associated with engraftment syndrome, infection, or drug toxicity. Tissue biopsy should be considered when GvHD is suspected and there are no contraindications to biopsy. Grading is useful in following patients for response or progression. Maximal aGvHD grade has prognostic implications on survival after allo-HCT.

Treatment of aGvHD

Who does not need systemic therapy for aGvHD?

Patients with grade I (skin only) aGvHD (less than 50% body surface area), may not require systemic therapy. These patients can often respond to topical corticosteroids. If the rash progresses on topical corticosteroids, the potency of it can be increased or topical tacrolimus can be added (although this is not an approved indication for this drug). If patients become more symptomatic or have progression to greater skin involvement or other organ involvement, then systemic therapy should be initiated as quickly as possible.

How should corticosteroids be given for initial therapy of aGvHD?

Corticosteroids continue to be the mainstay of treatment for aGvHD. The route of administration, formulation, and dosing remains variable among transplant physicians. Based on one retrospective review of over 400 patients, the response to corticosteroids alone was 55% at 28 days after starting treatment, but this was only durable in 35% of patients.

In an effort to reduce the side effects associated with higher dose systemic corticosteroids, non-absorbable glucocorticoids have been tested in combination with lower dose corticosteroids as first-line therapy for GI

Table 37.1 Staging and grading of aGvHD.

Individual Organ Staging:

Organ	Skin	Liver	Gastrointestinal
Stage	**Body Surface Area**	**Bilirubin (mg/dL)**	**Diarrhea (mL/day)**
1	Rash < 25%	2–2.9	500–1000 or biopsy-proven upper GI involvement
2	Rash 25–50%	3–6	1000–1500
3	Rash > 50%	6.1–15	1500–2000
4	Generalized erythroderma with bullae	>15	>2000 or severe abdominal pain with or without ileus

For bilirubin in µmol/L: Stage 1 = 34–50. Stage 2 = 51–102, Stage 3 = 103–255, Stage 4 >255

Revised Glucksberg Grading:

Overall Grade	Skin	Liver	Gastrointestinal
I	Stage 1–2	None	None
II	Stage 3 or	Stage 1 or	Stage 1
III	–	Stage 2–3 or	Stage 2–4
IV	Stage 4 or	Stage 4	–

International Bone Marrow Transplant Registry Grading:

Overall Grade	Skin	Liver	Gastrointestinal
A	Stage 1	None	None
B	Stage 2	Stage 1 or 2	Stage 1 or 2
C	Stage 3	Stage 3	Stage 3
D	Stage 4	Stage 4	Stage 4

aGvHD. Smaller studies have demonstrated that the addition of oral beclomethasone or budesonide to systemic corticosteroids for GI GvHD can increase the likelihood of both initial and durable responses. In a phase III randomized controlled trial comparing prednisone alone to prednisone plus oral beclomethasone, there was a trend toward less GvHD-treatment failures with prednisone plus oral beclomethasone at day 50 after initiating therapy, but this was not statistically significant. However, a larger randomized trial failed to show added benefit of oral beclomethasone. The role of oral non-absorbable glucocorticoids in the initial treatment of acute GI GvHD remains undefined, but GI infections, particularly *Clostridium difficile*, should be ruled out first if being used.

The initial dose of corticosteroids for first-line aGvHD treatment has been studied in two prospective trials:

1 Van Lint et al. randomized patients to methylprednisolone at 10 mg/kg/day for 5 days with subsequent taper versus 2 mg/kg/day. The response rate was about 30% in both arms, and rates of progression to grade III–IV aGvHD and overall survival were similar, but there were more infections in the higher dose arm.

2 Mielcarek et al. stratified patients based on grade of aGvHD and then randomized them to standard or low-dose corticosteroids. Patients with grade IIa aGvHD (upper GI symptoms, stool volume <1.0 L/day, and no hepatic dysfunction) were randomized to prednisone at 1 mg/kg/day or 0.5 mg/kg/day. Patients with grade IIB or higher aGvHD were randomized to prednisone at 2 mg/kg/day or 1 mg/kg/day. Although patients with ≥grade IIB aGvHD were more likely to require secondary immune suppression agents, there was no difference in overall survival or progression to grade III–IV aGvHD in either cohort. There was also no difference in corticosteroid related toxicity based on initial steroid treatment.

Only one study has examined the impact of steroid taper on GvHD outcomes. In patients responding to corticosteroids after 14 days of therapy, patients were randomized to a short taper lasting 12 weeks versus a longer taper lasting 21 weeks. The median time to resolution of aGvHD was 42 days with short taper and 30 days with long taper (p = 0.01). The incidence rates of aGvHD reactivation during the taper, chronic GvHD, and infectious and non-infectious steroid-related complications were similar in both groups.

Guidelines for initial steroid therapy in grade II-IV aGvHD:

1 Treat with 1.0–2.0 mg/kg/day prednisone (or equivalent) +/- topical corticosteroids (skin cream or oral non-absorbed corticosteroids), but strongly consider 2 mg/kg/day in patients with grade III–IV aGvHD.
2 Once aGvHD is under good control, taper prednisone by 0.2 mg/kg/day every 5–7 days. Starting the taper within 5 days of corticosteroid initiation is generally not recommended unless there are significant corticosteroid side effects or clinical indications to do so.
3 Taper rates should be slowed after the prednisone dose has been decreased to less than 20–30 mg/day.

Should another drug be added to corticosteroids for initial therapy of aGvHD?

The relatively low durable remission rates to corticosteroids alone have spurred great interest in the use of other systemic agents in conjunction with corticosteroids as initial therapy of aGvHD. Several randomized trials comparing corticosteroids alone to corticosteroids plus a second agent for front-line therapy of aGvHD have been reported. A phase II randomized trial from the Blood and Marrow Transplantation Clinical Trials Network (BMT-CTN) tested the addition of etanercept, denileukin, pentostatin or mycophenolate mofetil (MMF) to corticosteroids as initial aGvHD therapy. The results suggested that the addition of MMF to corticosteroids was associated with the most encouraging GvHD response. However, a follow up randomized phase III trial adding MMF versus placebo to corticosteroids as up-front therapy was terminated prematurely when a futility rule was triggered, and there was no difference in day 56 GvHD response rates or 6 month survival. Similarly, other randomized trials adding ATG, IL-2 receptor antibodies, or infliximab to corticosteroids as initial aGvHD therapy have failed to show a benefit. Table 37.2 summarizes these randomized trials. As such, the current standard of care for initial systemic therapy of aGvHD remains corticosteroids alone.

What should be used when first-line therapy for aGvHD fails?

Corticosteroid refractory aGvHD is generally defined in one of the following ways:
1 Progression after 3 days of corticosteroid therapy
2 No change after 5–7 days of corticosteroid therapy
3 Incomplete response after 14 days of methylprednisolone at 2 mg/kg/day or equivalent

Table 37.2 Summary of randomized controlled trials for first-line therapy of aGvHD.

Study	Study Arms	Mechanism of Study Drug	N	Response Assessment	CR (%)	6 Month OS (%)	Comments
Cahn et al. 1995	Methylpred + CsA	Murine monoclonal antibody against CD25	35	day 20	54	66	Bacterial, viral, or fungal infections were similar in both arms
	Inolimomab + Methylpred + CsA		34	day 20	44	78	
Cragg et al. 2000	Pred	Horse derived antibodies against human T-cells	46	day 42	76*	48	More CMV and pneumonitis in ATG arm
	Horse ATG + Pred		50	day 42	76*	65	
Lee et al. 2004	Corticosteroid	Humanized monoclonal antibody against CD25	49	day 42	49	76	Longer hospital stay in Daclizumab arm
	Daclizumab + Corticosteroid		53	day 42	43	53	
Couriel et al. 2009	Pred	Chimeric monoclonal antibody against TNF-α	28	day 28	54	52	Bacterial, viral, or fungal infections were similar in both arms
	Infliximab + Pred		29	day 28	55	54	
Bolanos-Meade et al. 2014	Pred	IMPDH inhibitor (needed for B- and T-cell growth)	116	day 56	54	73	Higher incidence of leukopenia in the MMF arm
	MMF + Pred		119	day 56	60	72	

Methylpred = methylprednisolone; CsA = cyclosporine A; Pred = prednisone; MMF = mycophenolate mofetil; IMPDH = inosine monophosphate dehydrogenase; CR = complete response; OS = overall survival. CD25 is the interleukin-2 receptor.
* complete and partial response reported together.

This definition is the standard employed in most clinical trials. It should also be noted that in lower GI GvHD, the daily diarrhea volume may not decrease immediately even if the GvHD/inflammatory response is controlled, as reabsorptive function of the colon does not normalize until the intestinal mucosa has healed. As such, more time should be allowed in the evaluation of GvHD response in these lower GI cases before declaring treatment failure.

The American Society of Blood and Marrow Transplantation (ASBMT) has summarized the available data and concluded that there is currently no standard of care for second line treatment of aGvHD. Many single arm trials have shown aGvHD responses for a wide variety of second line agents after corticosteroid failure. However, long term survival in this population remains poor, with 1-year mortality reported to be as high as 80–90%, mostly due to infections. Table 37.3 outlines the currently available second line medications for aGvHD.

What supportive care measures can be used for aGvHD?

There are supportive therapies that can be used for symptom control but more importantly to prevent and treat complications of therapy:

1 Anti-histamines and topical anti-pruritis agents can help manage pruritis in acute skin GvHD.
2 Anti-motility agents and octreotide or other somatostatin analogs can help treat symptoms of diarrhea.
3 GI rest and parental nutrition are often needed in acute GI GvHD. When restarting oral intake, it is imperative to advance slowly, starting with isotonic fluids and advancing every few days as tolerated by the patient.
4 Drugs with GI or hepatic toxicity should be avoided when possible.
5 Infectious prophylaxis should include trimethoprim-sulfamethoxazole or an equivalent to prevent *Pneumocystis jirovecii* pneumonia, acyclovir or an equivalent to prevent herpesvirus reactivation, and prophylaxis against invasive fungal infections with an antifungal agent. Patients with grade III–IV GvHD or significant lower GI GvHD, or those treated with anti-TNF-alpha agents should receive fungal prophylaxis with coverage against invasive molds such as Aspergillus and/or Mucor. Regular monitoring of serum fungal markers such as beta-glucan and galactomannan are recommended. Routine CMV monitoring is imperative and pre-emptive therapy against CMV should be initiated when reactivation occurs. Serum gammaglobulin should be monitored routinely and intravenous gammaglobulin (IVIG) administered to help prevent infections if hypogammaglobulinemia is detected.

What is the prognosis of patients with aGvHD?

Despite the use of first and second line therapies, the mortality associated with aGvHD remains high. This is partially related to the disease itself, but is also due to secondary infections from the immune suppressive nature of the GvHD itself, compounded by the immunosuppressive agents usually employed as treatment. Overall grade of aGvHD correlates with survival after diagnosis of aGvHD (reviewed by Cahn et al.[14]). One caveat is that these patients often have risk factors for aGvHD as previously described, which are independent predictors of mortality in allo-HCT patients.

PRACTICE POINT

Patients with grade II-IV aGvHD require systemic treatment with corticosteroids, at a minimum dose of 1 mg/kg/day. Although about half of patients will respond, these responses are often not durable. When corticosteroids fail, another drug should be initiated. Which drug is used in second line treatment will depend on ease of administration, familiarity of the physician with the drug and clinical trial availability. Patients need to be monitored closely for infectious complications and other toxicities related to the therapies administered.

Summary of diagnosis and treatment of aGvHD

- aGvHD is associated with cutaneous, gastrointestinal and hepatic signs, and symptoms after allo-HCT.
- Tissue biopsy is often required to confirm the diagnosis and rule out other causes of diarrhea in lower GI GvHD, but less useful in skin GvHD. Liver biopsy is encouraged for the diagnosis of hepatic GvHD (cespecially when there is absence of involvement of other organs), however, the risk and morbidity from the biopsy should be considered. A transjugular approach is often favored.
- Engraftment syndrome, infections, drug toxicity, and SOS need to be considered in the differential diagnosis of aGvHD.
- All patients with grade II–IV aGvHD should have systemic corticosteroid treatment initiated as quickly as possible.
- Corticosteroids alone remain the current standard front-line therapy for aGvHD. Second line treatment for aGvHD varies across transplant centers, and there are no clear guidelines regarding which second line agents to choose or the sequence of additional therapies after corticosteroids.

Table 37.3 Drugs used in aGvHD treatment (adapted from ASBMT guidelines).

Drug	Mechanism of Action	Toxicity Concerns	Author Practice
Corticosteroids	Broad anti-inflammatory and lymphocytoxic effects	Hyperglycemia, hypertension, insomnia, labile mood, gastritis, osteopenia, avascular bone necrosis, myopathy, impaired wound healing, secondary adrenal insufficiency.	Standard first-line therapy
Mycophenolate Mofetil (CellCept®, Myfortic®)	Non-competitive inhibitor of IMPDH, the rate limiting step for *de novo* purine synthesis on which lymphocytes depend	Dose related cytopenia and gastrointestinal toxicity. Enteric-coated mycophenolic acid (Myfortic®) may be better tolerated.	Subsequent line therapy, but be wary of GI toxicity in patients with GI aGvHD
Denileukin diftitox (Ontak®)	Recombinant fusion molecule of human IL-2 and diphtheria toxin that binds to the IL-2R-α and triggers apoptosis in activated T-cells	Dose limiting elevation of hepatic transaminases.	Not currently available
Sirolimus (Rapamune®)	Binds to FK-binding protein complex and blocks mTOR, ultimately causing cell cycle arrest in G1	Reversible cytopenia, hypertriglyceridemia, nephrotoxicity (HUS/TMA) and neurotoxicity (TTP). Less common are transaminitis, edema, arthralgias, and non-infectious pneumonitis.	Subsequent line therapy, but be wary of increased liver toxicity and TMA
Infliximab (Remicade®)	Chimeric murine/human monoclonal antibody that binds with high affinity to soluble and membrane-bound TNFα, resulting in clearance of TNFα and T-cells	Anaphylaxis is uncommon, but can occur.	Subsequent therapy, particularly in GI aGvHD, be wary of increased risk of invasive fungal infections
Etanercept (Enbrel®)	Soluble dimeric fusion protein that competes for TNF-α binding and renders it inactive	Generally well tolerated.	Subsequent therapy, particularly in GI aGvHD, be wary of increased risk of invasive fungal infections
Pentostatin (Nipent®)	Nucleoside analog that potently inhibits adenosine deaminase, reducing CD4 and CD8 T-cells, and B-cells and lowering of IgG levels	Myelosuppression, should reduce dose by 50% if ANC <1000 per μL and discontinue if ANC < 500 μL. Reversible transaminitis, renal insufficiency, and neurotoxicity can occur.	Subsequent therapy, uncommonly used due to severe risk of infection
Daclizumab (Zenepax®)	Humanized monoclonal antibody against CD25 (IL-2 receptor) which prevents T-cell proliferation	Well tolerated, anaphylaxis has not been observed.	Not currently available
Basiliximab	Chimeric (murine/human) monoclonal antibody against CD25 (IL-2 receptor) which prevents T-cell proliferation	Anaphylaxis and hypersensitivity reactions have been reported but are not common.	Subsequent line therapy
Horse antithymocyte globulin (ATGAM®)	Antilymphocytic, primarily monomeric IgG, from hyperimmune serum of horses immunized with human thymus lymphocytes	Anaphylaxis is uncommon but skin testing prior to first dose is recommended. Fever and chills common, also thrombocytopenia, leukopenia, and rash. Less common are serum sickness, dyspnea/apnea, arthralgia, chest, back, or flank pain; diarrhea and nausea and/ or vomiting.	Subsequent therapy, uncommonly used due to severe risk of infection

(Continued)

Table 37.3 (Continued)

Drug	Mechanism of Action	Toxicity Concerns	Author Practice
Rabbit antithymocyte globulin (Thymoglobulin®)	Antilymphocytic globulin from hyperimmune serum of rabbits immunized with human thymus lymphocytes	Skin testing is not considered necessary but must monitor closely for anaphylaxis or cytokine release syndrome. Thrombocytopenia and opportunistic infections are common.	Subsequent therapy, uncommonly used due to severe risk of infection
Alemtuzumab (Campath®)	Humanized IgG1monoclonal antibody against CD52 on normal and malignant T- and B-cells, NK-cells, monocytes, macrophages, and some granulocytes	Cytopenias including hemolytic anemia. Most common reactions are rigors and fever and nausea and vomiting. Less common are rash, fatigue, hypotension, urticaria, dyspnea, pruritus, headache, and diarrhea.	Subsequent therapy, uncommonly used due to severe risk of infection
Extracorporeal photopheresis (ECP)	Direct apoptosis of mainly lymphocytes and reinfusion interferes with dendritic cell maturation, cytokine modulation, and expansion of regulatory T-cells	Limited, but includes blood loss from the extracorporeal circuit, hypocalcemia due to anticoagulant, and mild cytopenia.	Subsequent line therapy, particularly in skin aGvHD, and overlap syndrome, be aware of slow time to respond

Source: Martin 2012. Reproduced with permission of Elsevier.

Selected reading

1. Ratanatharathorn V, Nash RA, Przepiorka D, Devine SM, Klein JL, Weisdorf D, et al. Phase III study comparing methotrexate and tacrolimus (prograf, FK506) with methotrexate and cyclosporine for graft-versus-host disease prophylaxis after HLA-identical sibling bone marrow transplantation. *Blood.* 1998;**92**(7):2303–2314.

2. Cahn JY, Klein JP, Lee SJ, Milpied N, Blaise D, Antin JH, et al. Prospective evaluation of 2 acute graft-versus-host (GvHD) grading systems: a joint Societe Francaise de Greffe de Moelle et Therapie Cellulaire (SFGM-TC), Dana Farber Cancer Institute (DFCI), and International Bone Marrow Transplant Registry (IBMTR) prospective study. *Blood.* 2005;**106**(4):1495–1500.

3. Glucksberg H, Storb R, Fefer A, Buckner CD, Neiman PE, Clift RA, et al. Clinical manifestations of graft-versus-host disease in human recipients of marrow from HL-A-matched sibling donors. *Transplantation.* 1974;**18**(4):295–304.

4. Rowlings PA, Przepiorka D, Klein JP, Gale RP, Passweg JR, Henslee-Downey PJ, et al. IBMTR Severity Index for grading acute graft-versus-host disease: retrospective comparison with Glucksberg grade. *British Journal of Haematology.* 1997;**97**(4):855–864.

5. MacMillan ML, Weisdorf DJ, Wagner JE, DeFor TE, Burns LJ, Ramsay NK, et al. Response of 443 patients to steroids as primary therapy for acute graft-versus-host disease: comparison of grading systems. *Biology of Blood and Marrow Transplantation: Journal of the American Society for Blood and Marrow Transplantation.* 2002;**8**(7):387–394.

6. Hockenbery DM, Cruickshank S, Rodell TC, Gooley T, Schuening F, Rowley S, et al. A randomized, placebo-controlled trial of oral beclomethasone dipropionate as a prednisone-sparing therapy for gastrointestinal graft-versus-host disease. *Blood.* 2007;**109**(10):4557–4763.

7. Van Lint MT, Uderzo C, Locasciulli A, Majolino I, Scime R, Locatelli F, et al. Early treatment of acute graft-versus-host disease with high- or low-dose 6-methylprednisolone: a multicenter randomized trial from the Italian Group for Bone Marrow Transplantation. *Blood.* 1998;**92**(7):2288–2293.

8. Mielcarek M, Furlong T, Storer BE, Green ML, McDonald GB, Carpenter PA, et al. Effectiveness and safety of lower-dose prednisone for initial treatment of acute graft-versus-host disease: a randomized controlled trial. Haematologica. 2015.

9. Hings IM, Filipovich AH, Miller WJ, Blazar BL, McGlave PB, Ramsay NK, et al. Prednisone therapy for acute graft-versus-host disease: short- versus long-term treatment. A prospective randomized trial. *Transplantation.* 1993;**56**(3):577–580.

10. Martin PJ, Rizzo JD, Wingard JR, Ballen K, Curtin PT, Cutler C, et al. First- and second-line systemic treatment of acute graft-versus-host disease: recommendations of the American Society of Blood and Marrow Transplantation. *Biology of Blood and Marrow Transplantation: Journal of the American Society for Blood and Marrow Transplantation.* 2012;**18**(8):1150–1163.

11. Alousi AM, Weisdorf DJ, Logan BR, Bolanos-Meade J, Carter S, Difronzo N, et al. Etanercept, mycophenolate, denileukin, or pentostatin plus corticosteroids for acute graft-versus-host disease: a randomized phase 2 trial from the Blood and Marrow Transplant Clinical Trials Network. *Blood.* 2009;**114**(3):511–517.

12. Bolanos-Meade J, Logan BR, Alousi AM, Antin JH, Barowski K, Carter SL, et al. Phase 3 clinical trial of steroids/mycophenolate mofetil vs steroids/placebo as therapy for acute GvHD: BMT CTN 0802. *Blood.* 2014;**124**(22):3221–3227; quiz 335.

13. Cragg L, Blazar BR, Defor T, Kolatker N, Miller W, Kersey J, et al. A randomized trial comparing prednisone with

antithymocyte globulin/prednisone as an initial systemic therapy for moderately severe acute graft-versus-host disease. *Biology of Blood and Marrow Transplantation: Journal of the American Society for Blood and Marrow Transplantation.* 2000;**6**(4a):441–447.

14. Lee SJ, Zahrieh D, Agura E, MacMillan ML, Maziarz RT, McCarthy PL, Jr., et al. Effect of up-front daclizumab when combined with steroids for the treatment of acute graft-versus-host disease: results of a randomized trial. *Blood.* 2004;**104**(5):1559–1564.

15. Couriel DR, Saliba R, de Lima M, Giralt S, Andersson B, Khouri I, et al. A phase III study of infliximab and corticosteroids for the initial treatment of acute graft-versus-host disease. *Biology of Blood and Marrow Transplantation: Journal of the American Society for Blood and Marrow Transplantation.* 2009;**15**(12):1555–1562.

CHAPTER 38

Diagnosis and treatment of chronic graft-versus-host disease

Sabarinath Venniyil Radhakrishnan and Daniel R. Couriel

Division of Hematology and Hematologic Malignancies, Huntsman Cancer Institute, University of Utah, Salt Lake City, UT, USA

Introduction

Chronic graft-versus-host disease (cGvHD) is a major limiting complication and major contributor to morbidity and non-relapse mortality (NRM) from allogeneic hematopoietic cell transplant (allo-HCT). The exact pathophysiology is not well defined, and it can affect almost any organ system. As the mechanisms leading to cGvHD are not completely understood, treatment approaches are mostly based on broadly immunosuppressive strategies, and corticosteroids remain the single most effective therapy. Thus, long-term complications from corticosteroids are almost unavoidably present, and blend into the syndrome of cGvHD in more severe cases.

Diagnostic criteria

Definition and clinical manifestations

cGvHD has been recently redefined by the National Institutes of Health (NIH) Consensus Development Project on Criteria for Clinical Trials in Chronic Graft-*versus*-Host Disease based on clinical manifestations, changing the traditional and rather arbitrary, chronological "beyond Day 100" definition. In this new definition of cGvHD as a syndrome, clinical manifestations of acute GvHD (aGvHD) occurring after 100 days of transplant are considered to be late-onset aGvHD and not cGvHD. In this section, we will focus specifically on the definition of cGvHD, as established by the NIH Consensus.

The diagnosis of cGvHD requires:
- *Diagnostic signs and symptoms*: These are manifestations that establish the diagnosis of cGvHD by themselves, and do not need further testing or any other organ involvement.

- *Distinctive signs and symptoms of cGvHD*: Unlike diagnostic manifestations, these are not sufficient to make a conclusive diagnosis of cGvHD per se; therefore, distinctive manifestations require additional evidence in the form of histopathological documentation, tests like pulmonary function test (PFT), and so on. A more detailed description of the diagnostic and distinctive criteria is provided in Table 38.1.

As per the 2014 Working group consensus definition, cGvHD can be diagnosed by the presence of at least one diagnostic manifestation or the presence of a distinctive manifestation with confirmation by biopsy, laboratory test, or imaging studies and ruling out other causes like infection that may have a similar picture.

In the absence of features fulfilling criteria for the diagnosis of cGvHD, the persistence, recurrence, or new onset of characteristic skin, gastrointestinal tract, or liver abnormalities should be classified as aGvHD regardless of the time after transplantation. The term "overlap syndrome," refers to the presence of one or more manifestation of aGvHD in a patient diagnosed with cGvHD with the above criteria. As this overlap category includes a very heterogeneous group of patients, it has fallen out of favor.

The most common manifestations of cGvHD are cutaneous and mucosal, and their involvement falls into two main categories that can overlap:
- *Lichen Planus-like or lichenoid cGvHD* (Figure 38.1a): This subtype is very similar to primary lichen planus, and manifests with the same type of purplish, flat-topped maculopapular rash. Sicca syndrome with dry eye, dry mucosae, and lichenoid involvement of the oral and vaginal mucosae are very common in these patients
- *Sclerodermatous cGvHD* (Figure 38.1b): In this case fibrosis is the predominant manifestation, and it can be very disabling in severe cases, particularly when hidebound and with joint involvement.

Clinical Manual of Blood and Bone Marrow Transplantation, First Edition. Edited by Syed A. Abutalib and Parameswaran Hari.
© 2017 John Wiley & Sons Ltd. Published 2017 by John Wiley & Sons Ltd.

Table 38.1 Clinical manifestations that define chronic GvHD.

Site	Diagnostic	Distinctive	Both Acute and Chronic GvHD	Others
Skin	Poikiloderma Lichen planus like lesions Morphea and lichen sclerosis like lesions	Depigmentation Papulosquamous lesions Loss of body hair, new onset of scarring or non-scarring alopecia, scaling of skin	Erythema Maculopapular rash pruritis	Ichthyosis Hypo or hyperpigmentation Sweat impairment Keratosis pilaris Grey hair
Nails	None	Dystrophy, longitudinal ridging, brittle nails, onycholysis, symmetrical bilateral nail loss		
Mouth	Lichen planus like lesions	Xerostomia, pseudomembrane, ulcerations, mucoceles, mucosal atrophy	Gingivitis, mucositis, erythema, pain	
Eyes	none	New onset of dry, gritty or painful eyes, keratoconjunctivitis sicca, confluent areas of punctate keratopathy		Blepharitis, photophobia, periorbital hyperpigmentation
GI tract	Esophageal web Stricture or stenosis in the upper to mid 1/3 of the esophagus	None	Anorexia, nausea, vomiting, diarrhea, weight loss	Exocrine pancreatic insufficiency
Liver			Total bilirubin, alkaline phosphatase or ALT 2× upper limit of normal	
Lung	Bronchiolitis obliterans diagnosed by lung biopsy	Air trapping and bronchiectasis on chest CT		Restrictive lung disease and Cryptogenic organizing pneumonia
Genitalia	Lichen planus like and lichen sclerosis like lesions Females: vaginal scarring/stenosis, clitoral/labial agglutination Males: phimosis, urethral scarring/stenosis	Erosions, fissures, and ulcers		
Muscles, fascia, and joints	Fasciitis, joint stiffness and contractures secondary to fasciitis or sclerosis	Myositis or polymyositis		

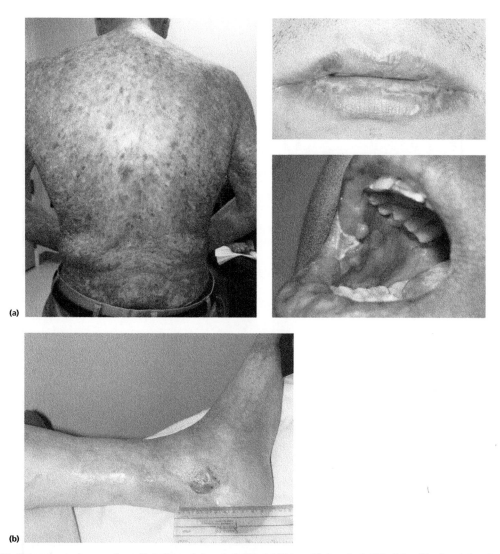

Figure 38.1 Cutaneous and mucosal manifestations of chronic GvHD. (a) Lichenoid chronic GvHD of the skin, lips and oral mucosa. (b) Sclerodermatous chronic GvHD of the skin with complicating ulcer.

GvHD global severity score

Severity of involvement in eight organs are graded in the scoring system including skin, mouth, eyes, gastrointestinal tract, liver, lung, joints/fascia, and genital tract (Table 38.2). Clinical manifestations are only scored if partially or totally attributable to cGvHD. The global score is then calculated including the number of organs and the severity of the involvement in each organ, with the notable exception of the performance score (PS). Of note, asymptomatic manifestations are also included and described, but they do not contribute to the global score.

Severity of cGvHD can be categorized into:
- Mild: one or two organs involved with no more than score 1 plus a lung score of 0
- Moderate: three or more organs involved with no more than score 1 OR lung score 1 OR at least one organ other than the lung with a score of 2
- Severe: At least one organ with a score of 3 OR lung score of 2 or 3

Table 38.2 Scoring of chronic GvHD.

	SCORE 0	SCORE 1	SCORE 2	SCORE 3
PERFORMANCE SCORE: KPS ECOG LPS	☐ Asymptomatic and fully active (ECOG 0; KPS or LPS 100%)	☐ Symptomatic, fully ambulatory, restricted only in physically strenuous activity (ECOG 1, KPS or LPS 80–90%)	☐ Symptomatic, ambulatory, capable of self-care, >50% of waking hours ou of bed (ECOG 2, KPS or LPS 60–70%)	☐ Symptomatic, limited self-care, >50% of waking hours in bed (ECOG 3–4, KPS or LPS <60%)
SKIN† Score % **BSA**				
GvHD features to be secored by BSA:	☐ No BSA involved	☐ 1–18% BSA	☐ 19–50% BSA	☐ >50% BSA

Check all that apply:

☐ Maculopapular rash/erythema
☐ Lichen planus-like features
☐ Sclerotic features
☐ Papulosquamous lesions or ichthyosis
☐ Keratosis pilaris-like GvHD

| **SKIN FEATURES SCORE:** | ☐ No sclerotic features | | ☐ Superficial sclerotic features "not hidebound" (able to pinch) | **Check all that apply:** ☐ Deep sclerotic features ☐ "Hidebound" (unable to pinch) ☐ Impaired mobility ☐ Ulceration |

Other skin GvHD features (NOTscored by BSA)

Check all that apply:

☐ Hyperpigmentation
☐ Hypopigmentation
☐ Poikiloderma
☐ Severe or generalized pruritus
☐ Hair involvement
☐ Nail involvement
☐ Abnormality present but explained entirely by non-GvHD documented cause (specify): _____

(Continued)

Table 38.2 (Continued)

	SCORE 0	SCORE 1	SCORE 2	SCORE 3
MOUTH *Lichen planus-like features present:* ☐ **Yes** ☐ **No**	☐ No symptoms	☐ Mild symptoms **with** disease signs but not limiting oral intake significantly	☐ Moderate symptoms with disease signs **with** partial limitation of oral intake	☐ Severe symptoms with disease signs on examination **with** major limitation of oral intake
☐ *Abnormality present but explained entirely by non-GvHD documented cause (specify):* _____				
EYES *Keratoconjunctivitis sicca (KCS) confirmed by ophthalmologist:* ☐ **Yes** ☐ **No** ☐ **Not examined**	☐ No symptoms	☐ Mild dry eye symptoms not affecting ADL (requirement of lubricant eye drops ≤3 × per day)	☐ Moderate dry eye symptoms partially affecting ADL (requiring lubricant eye drops >3 × per day or punctal plugs), **WITHOUT** new vision impairment due to KCS	☐ Severe dry eye symptoms significantly affecting ADL (special eyeware to relieve pain) **OR** unable to work because of ocular symptoms **OR** loss of vision due to KCS
☐ *Abnormality present but explained entirely by non-GvHD documented cause (specify):* _____				
GI Tract **Check all thai apply:** ☐ Esophageal web/ proximal stricture or ring ☐ Dysphagia ☐ Anorexia ☐ Nausea ☐ Vomiting ☐ Diarrhea ☐ Weight loss ≥5%* ☐ Failure to thrive	☐ No symptoms	☐ Symptoms without significant weight loss* (<5%)	☐ Symptoms associated with mild to moderate weight loss* (5–15%) **OR** moderate diarrhea without significant interference with daily living	☐ Symptoms associated with significant weight loss* >15%, requires nutritional supplement for most caloric needs **OR** esophageal dilation **OR** severe diarrhea with significant interference with daily living
☐ *Abnormality present but explained entirely bv non-GvHD documented cause (specify):* _____				
LIVER	☐ Normal total bilirubin and ALT or AP <3 × ULN	☐ Normal total bilirubin with ALT ≥3 to 5 × ULN or AP ≥3 × ULN	☐ Elevated total bilirubin but ≤3 mg/dL or ALT >5 ULN	☐ Elevated total bilirubin >3 mg/dL
☐ *Abnormality present but explained entirely by non-GvHD documented cause (specify):* _____				

LUNGS**
Symptom score:

☐ No symptoms

☐ Mild symptoms (shortness of breath after climbing one flight of steps)

☐ Moderate symptoms (shortness of breath after walking on flat ground)

☐ Severe symptoms (shortness of breath at rest: requiring O_2)

Lung score:
%FEV1 ☐

☐ FEV1 ≥80%

☐ FEV1 60–79%

☐ FEV1 40–59%

☐ FEV1 ≤39%

Pulmonary function tests
☐ Not performed
☐ *Abnormality present but explained entirely by non-GvHD documented cause (specify):* _____

JOINTS AND FASCIA
P-ROM score
(see below)
Shoulder (1-7): ____
Elbow (1-7): ____
Wrist/finger (1-7): ____
Ankle (1-4): ____

☐ No symptoms

☐ Mild tightness of arms or legs. normal or mild decreased range of motion (ROM) **AND** not affecting ADL

☐ Tightness of arms or legs **OR** joint contractures, erythema thought due to fasciitis, moderate decrease ROM **AND** mild to moderate limitation of ADL

☐ Contractures **WITH** significant decrease of ROM **AND** significant limitation of ADL (unable to tie shoes. button shirts, dress self etc.)

☐ *Abnormality present but explained entirely by non-GvHD documented cause (specify):* _____

GENITAL TRACT
(See Supplemental figure‡)
☐ Not examined

Currently sexually active
☐ Yes
☐ No

☐ No signs

☐ Mild signs‡ and females with or without discomfort on exam

☐ Moderate signs‡ and may have symptoms with discomfort on exam

☐ Severe signs‡ with or without symptoms

☐ *Abnormality present but explained entirely by non-GvHD documented cause (specify):* _____

Other indicators, clinical features or complications related to chronic GvHD (check all that apply and assign a score to severity (0-3) based on functional impact where applicable none – 0, mild -1. Moderate -2. severe – 3)

☐ Ascites (serositis) ____
☐ Pericardial Effusion ____
☐ Pleural Effusion(s) ____
☐ Nephrotic syndrome ____

☐ Myasthenia Gravis ____
☐ Peripheral Neuropathy ____
☐ Polymyositis ____
☐ Weight loss >5%* without GI symptoms ____

☐ Eosinophilia > 500 µl ____
☐ Platelets <100,000/µl ____
☐ Others (specify): ____

(Continued)

Table 38.2 (Continued)

	SCORE 0	SCORE 1	SCORE 2	SCORE 3
Overall GvHD Severity *(Opinion of the evaluator)*	☐ No GvHD	☐ Mild	☐ Moderate	☐ Severe

Photographic Range of Motion (P-ROM)

How effective is aGvHD prophylaxis for cGvHD?

The incidence of cGvHD in T-cell replete HCT continues to be high, despite the use of calcineurin or m-TOR inhibitors with methotrexate for the prevention of aGvHD. Nash et al. noted no difference in the incidence of cGvHD when prophylaxis with a combination of cyclosporine and methotrexate was compared to tacrolimus and methotrexate. cGvHD occurred in 70% of the patients in the cyclosporine arm compared to 78% in the tacrolimus arm at the 2-year follow-up. Inamoto et al. retrospectively studied 456 patients with granulocyte colony stimulating factor (G-CSF) mobilized blood cell allo-grafts and found that there was no difference in the risk of cGvHD (HR 0.89, CI 0.581.38, p value 0.61) between tacrolimus treated vs cyclosporine treated patients. Cutleret al. in an open label, phase 3 multicenter randomized controlled trial (RCT) comparing tacrolimus and sirolimus with tacrolimus and methotrexate did not find any difference in the incidence of cGvHD in 305 patients with HLA-matched sibling transplants (53% vs 45%, P=0.06). In essence there is no evidence to suggest that one aGvHD prophylaxis regimen is better than another one to prevent cGvHD.

How about rituximab for prevention of cGvHD?

Cutler et al. studied the use of prophylactic administration of rituximab in 65 patients in a phase 2 trial. Rituximab (375 mg/m²) was given at 3, 6, 9, and 12 months after transplantation. They observed a significant decrease in the cumulative incidence of both cGvHD and chronic steroid requiring GvHD at 2 years (48 and 31%) compared to control cohorts. This translated into lower treatment related mortality (TRM) at 4 years of 5% compared to 19% in controls. The Stanford group treated 35 high-risk patients with chronic lymphocytic leukemia and mantle cell lymphoma with rituximab (four weekly doses starting on Day 56) after allo-HCT. They observed a cumulative incidence of chronic GvHD at 4 years of 20%. There are no randomized trials yet to address the issue of prophylaxis with rituximab but it seems to be a promising preventive modality especially with B-cell mediated tissue damage as one of the main causative factors for cGvHD.

T-cell depletion for cGvHD

T-cell depletion (TCD) utilizing *in vivo* (e.g., antithymocyte globulin, alemtuzumab) has been associated with a lower incidence of both acute- and chronic-GvHD, although at the expense of a higher rate of relapse. In two studies from Memorial Sloan Kettering Cancer Center, *ex-vivo* TCD was associated with substantially lower rates of acute GvHD (17.3 vs 42.6%), and chronic GvHD (13.5 vs 33.4%) compared to conventional grafts, without any significant impact on relapse.

cGvHD in cord blood transplants and HLA-haploidentical transplants with post cyclophosphamide

Cord blood transplantation (CBT) seems to be associated with a lower incidence of chronic GvHD. A recent study from EBMT shows a cumulative incidence of 32% at 3 years, which is substantially lower than that reported historically for other lo-grafts sources. Likewise, HLA-haploidentical transplantation performed using T-cell replete grafts and post-transplantation cyclophosphamide achieves outcomes that may be equivalent to those of contemporaneous transplantation performed using HLA-matched related donors(MRDs) and HLA-matched unrelated donors (MUDs). In this case, cyclophosphamide is given within a critically narrow window following transplantation to induce immunologic tolerance. These encouraging results of HCT across HLA-barriers with the application of a relatively simple post-transplant intervention is being further studied and compared to CBT in an ongoing Clinical Trial Network multicenter study.

What is the best initial therapy for cGvHD?

The cGvHD severity score helps to direct treatment in cGvHD. In most cases of mild symptomatic cGvHD topical or no therapy can be appropriate. However, in moderate to severe cases of cGvHD systemic immunosuppressive therapy should be considered. Systemic treatment may also be indicated in less severe cases in the presence of factors that predict a poorer outcome, such as thrombocytopenia, raised bilirubin, fasciitis, or if the onset of symptoms occurs when the patient is already on topical corticosteroids.

PRACTICE POINT

Outside of a clinical trial, the best initial treatment for cGvHD is unknown.

Steroids in cGvHD: Dose and schedule?

Steroids are still the standard first line of treatment for cGvHD and no other agent has yet proved superior, alone or in combination with other strategies. The Seattle group proposes the initial dose of 1 mg/kg/day of prednisone to be continued till there is objective evidence of response and to start tapering the alternate day dose by 20–30% every 2 weeks. The dose of 1 mg/kg/day on alternate days is maintained till there is complete resolution of the symptoms and then a similar tapering course of 20–30% every 2 weeks is restarted till there is either exacerbation or recurrence of the disease. At that time the dose should be increased by two levels and administered daily. This is maintained for 2–4 weeks and then changed to alternate day dosing for 3 months before the taper is reinitiated. Once the dose has reached 0.1 mg/kg every other day, this should be maintained for at least 4 weeks before discontinuing treatment. Some patients may require these low doses for a long period of time to prevent recurrence.

Although there is no clear efficacy from adding immunomodulating medications to initial therapy with corticosteroids, the combination with calcineurin inhibitors may serve as a steroid-sparing strategy, potentially decreasing long-term complications such as avascular necrosis of the hip.

Second-line therapy should be considered in patients who fail to adequately respond to steroids, or those who reflare their cGvHD during a steroid taper. The definitions for steroid refractoriness vary according to different authors, but in general, the following situations are indications of second-line therapy:
- Progressive cGvHD after 2 weeks of initiation of steroids
- No or minimal response at 4–6 weeks after initiation of steroids
- Reflare of cGvHD while tapering steroids

PRACTICE POINTS

- Steroids are still the single most effective agent to treat chronic GvHD
- Concurrent use of a calcineurin inhibitor can spare steroid-related toxicity, like avascular necrosis
- Indications for second-line therapy include: progressive cGvHD after 2 weeks of initiation of steroids, no or minimal response at 4–6 weeks after initiation of steroids and reflare of cGvHD while tapering steroids

---

What are the second-line treatment options?

In patients who do not respond to corticosteroids or those with an initial response and a subsequent flare during taper, a second-line therapy is indicated. The objective of second-line therapy is the improvement of GvHD manifestations, as well as a steroid-sparing effect. The best treatment option in these cases is also a clinical trial. In the absence of a clinical study, there are a variety of options. As there is no evidence that any of these options is better than the others, treatment decisions are individualized taking into consideration comorbidities, organs involved, accessibility, compliance, and insurance coverage. In this section, we focus on the most commonly used second-line options for patients with inadequate (response but unable to taper or no response) response to corticosteroids.

Rituximab

Cutler et al. evaluated the benefit of rituximab in the treatment of steroid refractory chronic GvHD. In 21 patients treated with rituximab ($375 \, mg/m^2$, 4 weekly doses and repeated a second cycle if no response) there was an objective response in 70% of patients with two patients achieving a complete response and the improvement was mainly noted in skin and musculoskeletal GvHD. In the GITMO study with rituximab (weekly $375 \, mg/m^2$, median number of four treatments), they reported active control of the disease in 65% of patients and here also the benefits were mainly in skin and musculoskeletal GvHD. Recent work by the Blazar group in a cGvHD murine model may help explain the differential effects of rituximab when used to treat cGvHD. The antibody causes peripheral B-cell depletion, but has no impact on B-cells in the lung, which correlates with the lack of response of bronchiolitis obliterans (BO) to rituximab.

PRACTICE POINT

Rituximab is a reasonable second-line option for steroid refractory cGvHD involving skin, mucosae, and musculoskeletal cGvHD given the few long-term adverse effects and the excellent tolerability.

Extracorporeal photopheresis

ECP is an immunomodulatory therapy in which after apheresis, peripheral blood leukocytes are treated with 8-methoxpsoralen and ultraviolet A light and reinfused back to the patient. The exact mechanism how ECP modulates chronic GvHD is not known but it is believed that the treatment causes apoptosis of the treated leukocytes that leads to a tolerogenic response. In the only multicenter RCT that has been done to assess the efficacy of ECP, Flowers et al. randomized patients to either ECP plus conventional treatment or to conventional treatment alone. Patients in the study group received 12 weeks of ECP; three times during week 1 and then twice weekly on consecutive days during weeks 2–12. The control arm was allowed to cross over to ECP after 12 weeks if there was no improvement of symptoms. The primary end point of the study was the improvement in the Vienna total skin score (TSS) at 12 weeks. Even though there was a trend in the reduction in TSS at 12 weeks (−14.5% vs −8.5%) in the ECP arm it was not significant. Similarly, 25% of the ECP treated patients had a 50% or greater reduction in the steroid dose compared to 12.8% in the control arm. It was thought that the lack of statistical significance was due to the utilization of early study endpoints in a chronic disease like skin GvHD. In a follow-up of this study, Greinix et al. studied the patients in the control arm that crossed over to the ECP arm. They found that at 24 weeks, 31% patients achieved either a complete or partial response in skin GvHD and 33% achieved a ≥50% steroid dose reduction. In a large retrospective analysis of ECP done at MD Anderson Cancer Center, Couriel et al. evaluated 71 patients; all patients were initiated with 2–4 treatments per week and then tapered down to one treatment per week when they achieved partial response and then placed on maintenance regimen of two treatments every 2 weeks. They observed an overall response rate of 61% and a complete response in 14 patients. The responses were seen in GvHD of the skin, liver, oral mucosa, and eye. Sixty-seven percent of patients with sclerodermatous cGvHD had an objective response to ECP. Even though the number of patients with BO were small, 54% patients responded to ECP with most of them having at least a partial response with significant tapering of steroids. The median time to response to treatment varied with the organ involved however, over a median of 46 days. The response to treatment was not sustained and there was a cumulative incidence of progression of 40% after initial response. ECP is well tolerated and adverse effects are usually mild and do not need discontinuation of treatment. The requirement for blood or platelet transfusion or catheter-associated infections were also less than 5%. Skin, liver and GI GvHD has consistently shown improvement with ECP but the benefit in lung GvHD appears to vary in different studies, possibly related to the heterogeneity in the severity of BO at the time of initiation of ECP. Taken together, given the low toxicity and the good response to most manifestations of GvHD it should be strongly considered in patients with steroid refractory GvHD.

> **PRACTICE POINT**
>
> ECP is one of the most widely used second-line treatments for cGvHD, and responses have been observed in both cutaneomucosal and visceral forms.

Imatinib and dasatinib

Transforming growth factor-β (TGF-β) and platelet derived growth factor-receptor (PDGF-R) pathways have been proposed to play a role in the fibrotic process associated with cGvHD. This has led to the use of imatinib as it blocks both these pathway. Olivieri et al. in a phase II prospective study assessed the effects of imatinib (starting dose of 100 mg/day with escalation to 400 mg/day) in steroid refractory GvHD. Of the 39 patients that were evaluated at 6 months, 51% patients showed a partial response as per NIH criteria. They also showed that the patients with improvement at 6 months after starting imatinib had a 3-year OS of 94% compared to only 58% in the non-responders. The responses were seen in the GI, lung along with skin. In a retrospective analysis of 39 patients with sclerodermatous steroid-resistant GvHD, de Masson et al. reported that imatinib improved skin sclerosis in only 30% of the patients and led to stability of disease in another 31% but caused worsening in 39% at an average duration of treatment of 13 ± 10 months. In another prospective phase II study of 20 patients including children and adults with steroid refractory sclerotic skin cGvHD treated with imatinib, there was a partial response in 36% and stable disease in 50% of the patients at 6 month of treatment. In patients intolerant or resistant to imatinib, dasatinib has been used for the treatment of sclerotic skin GvHD. In a small series of three patients, Duarte et al. used dasatinib and reported a partial response in all three of them and good tolerability of the agent. The response was also sustained with a median follow-up of almost 2 years.

Taken together, it seems that imatinib at best has a partial response in some patients and these effects have been mostly seen in skin. Imatinib is not well tolerated at the full adult dose of 400 mg and adverse effects include cytopenias, fatigue, myalgia, fluid retention; therefore, the recommended initial dose is 100–200 mg/daily.

> **PRACTICE POINT**
>
> Sclerodermatous cGvHD showed modest responses to imatinib and dasatinib. The high cost of these drugs may limit their use too.

Sirolimus

Couriel et al. conducted a phase II trial of sirolimus combined with tacrolimus and methylprednisolone in patients with steroid-resistant cGvHD. Thirty-five patients who developed GvHD after Day 100 post-transplant were studied, and had an ORR of 63%, and responses were predominantly cutaneomucosal. Major adverse events related to the combination of tacrolimus and sirolimus were hyperlipidemia, renal dysfunction, and cytopenias. Four patients had thrombotic microangiopathy (TMA) and 27 (77%) had infectious complications. A similar activity and concerning toxicity profile for the combination of sirolimus and tacrolimus was reported by Johnston et al.

Mycophenolate mofetil (MMF)

Although extensively used as second-line therapy for cGvHD, there is very little information on efficacy and steroid-sparing effect. Busca et al. reported a small series of patients treated with MMF, with an overall response rate of 60%, mainly cutaneomucosal, and in cases without sclerodermatous involvement.

Bortezomib

Given the possible role of B-cells in the pathophysiology of cGvHD and based on benefits observed in murine model of cGvHD, Pai et al. conducted a single institution intra patient dose escalation study starting at $0.2\,mg/m^2$ subcutaneously weekly and increased every 2 weeks by $0.2\,mg/m^2$ until toxicity in steroid refractory cGvHD. Of the 10 patients enrolled in the study, six were able to receive more than 60% of the scheduled doses. Of the six patients that received, five had a partial response to treatment, but only half of the patients could complete the scheduled 6 months' therapy.

Is there a role for cellular therapy in prevention or treatment of cGvHD?

Other than ECP, two forms of cellular therapy that are currently undergoing clinical trials for the management of cGvHD, include IL-2 induced T-regulatory cells (Tregs) and mesenchymal stem cells (MSCs)

Treg-cells: Do they really work in cGvHD?

Di Ianni et al. studied the efficacy of Tregs in 28 HLA-haploidentical transplants. Conditioning regimen included total body irradiation (TBI) with 8Gy, thiotepa, fludarabine, and cyclophosphamide and donor Treg infusion at Day 4. Only two of the 26 evaluable patient developed

grade II or more aGvHD and at a median follow-up of 11.2 months none of the patients developed cGvHD. Koreth et al. (NEJM) treated 29 patients with steroid refractory cGvHD with daily low dose subcutaneous IL-2 for 8 weeks of the 12-week study period. Of the 23 patients that were evaluated at the end of the 12-week period, 12 had a partial response and 11 had stable disease with no progression of cGvHD. IL-2 was continued in responding patients and most of them showed sustained improvement in symptoms and none showed progression of cGvHD. There was an average eight-fold increase in the level of Tregs with IL-2 infusion.

Mesenchymal stem cells

MSCs have potent anti-inflammatory effects and are studied in acute- and chronic- GvHD. Weng et al. treated 19 patients with steroid refractory cGvHD after HLA-matched related donor transplants with mesenchymal stem cells. Out of 19 patients, 14 had severe grade cGvHD by NIH criteria. Patients received a median dose of $0.6 \times 10^6/kg$ cells and the median number of treatments received was two. The ORR was 73.7% with a median time to best response of 233 days. Because the study population is small it is difficult to differentiate if the improvement was limited to certain organs or sites. Skin, oral mucosa, liver, GI tract, and eyes had good response rate to treatment. Ten of the 14 surviving patients were able to either completely go off immunosuppressants or were able to taper down the steroids to 0.1 mg/kg. This single center study shows promising results, but also highlights the difficulties with harvesting adequate cells in a timely manner and the need to be freshly harvested from cultures, thus limiting its applicability.

Supportive care

Monitoring for cGvHD

Comprehensive assessment of the organs that could be affected by GvHD should be done using the NIH GvHD consensus guidelines, and is summarized on Table 38.3.

Prevention of infections

As cGvHD is per se immunosuppressive, and is treated with prolonged immunosuppressive therapy, patients are prone to infections. Infections are the major cause of

Table 38.3 Monitoring recommendations in recipients of allogeneic hematopoietic cell transplantation.

Summary of Monitoring Recommendations*	
Parameter	Minimum Frequency (months) During Systemic Immunosuppressive Therapy
Interval history with symptom assessment (including psychosocial symptoms) and medication review	3
Physical examination (by healthcare provider)	
General	3
Photographic ROM	3–6
Skin surveillance for secondary malignancy	6–12
Weight:	
Adults	3
Children	1–3
Height:	
Adults	12
Children	3–6
Nutritional assessment†	
Adults	3–6
Children	1–6
Tanner score (children and adolescents)	6–12
Developmental assessment (children and adolescents)	3–6
Laboratory monitoring	
Complete blood counts with differential	3
Chemistry panel including renal and liver function tests	3
Therapeutic drug monitoring	3
IgG level (until normal and independent of replacement)	1–3‡
Lipid profile (during treatment with corticosteroids or sirolimus).	6
Iron indices (if red cell transfusions are required or if iron overload has been documented previously)	6–12
Pulmonary function tests (PFT)	3–6
Endocrine function evaluation, e.g., thyroid function tests, bone densitometry (if an abnormal result might change clinical management), calcium levels, 25-OH vitamin D	12
Subspecialty evaluations	
Ophthalmology	3–12
Dental assessment and oral cancer surveillance, including soft and hard tissues examination (radiographs as indicated); culture, biopsy or photographs of lesions (as clinically indicated); and professional dental hygiene.	6
Dermatology with assessment of extent and type of skin involvement, biopsy, or photographs (as clinically indicated).	12*
Gynecology for vulvovaginal involvement (as clinically indicated).	3–12
Physiotherapy with assessment of ROM (if joint limitation is present).	3–12
Neuropsychological testing (as clinically indicated).	12

Adapted from Carpenter PA et al. *Biol Blood Marrow Transplant* 2015; **21**(7): 1167–1187.

* These recommendations are for patients with chronic GvHD on systemic immunosuppressive therapy

† Assessment can be done by health care provider with referral to nutritionist as needed

‡ This is dependent on IgG levels and need for replacement

death in this patient population. Antibiotic prophylaxis against pneumocystis should be given for at least 6 months post-transplantation and until after discontinuation of all systemic immunosuppressive therapy. Patients on corticosteroids should also receive antibiotic prophylaxis against encapsulated bacteria until steroid discontinuation. Intravenous gamma globulins (IVIG) should be considered for patients who have recurrent sinus and pulmonary infections and an IgG level <400 mg/dl more than 90 days after transplant. Some centers monitor IgG levels and administer IVIG routinely in cGvHD even though there is no data to show improved outcome.

Primary antifungal prophylaxis with mold active agents posaconazole or voriconazole is usually prescribed for patients with cGvHD on corticosteroids. If the patient had a fungal infection before HCT, mold active antifungals are usually started since the beginning of the transplant.

Antiviral prophylaxis to prevent herpes simplex virus (HSV) and varicella zoster virus (VZV) infection are usually prescribed to all patients, irrespective of the existence of cGvHD. Cytomegalovirus (CMV) infection risk depends on the serological status of the donor and recipient. If both the donor and the recipient are seronegative then there is no need for prophylaxis or CMV monitoring. If there is a history of CMV infection or disease then weekly CMV viremia testing should be done and pre-emptive treatment initiated if there is viremia. If there is no previous history of CMV infection then viremia can be tested every 1–4 weeks and pre-emptively treated upon seroconversion

Vaccinations against encapsulated organisms should be given with T-cell dependent vaccines as early as 3–6 months after transplant. Vaccination with trivalent influenza vaccine should be given to all recipients and their contacts. No live vaccines should be given for at least 2 years post-transplant.

Does treatment of cGvHD increase relapse-related mortality?

The beneficial effects of allo-HCT are mostly based on the graft-versus-tumor (GvT) effect. Boyiadzis et al. reported on the impact of cGvHD on late relapses in 7489 patients after MAC regimens for the CIBMTR. cGvHD was associated with a higher TRM and inferior OS in all leukemias; there was a protective effect against late relapse in chronic myeloid leukemia, but this was absent for all the other types of leukemias and MDS. Another CIBMTR study by Weisdorf et al. studied the impact of cGvHD and GvT using a 1-year landmark to differentiate the effects of acute- and chronic-GvHD. In patients receiving MAC allo-HCT, the incidence of relapsed disease was lower in patients with acute- and chronic-GvHD, but the TRM was high. The overall

effect was higher treatment failure and lower OS. In patients receiving RIC HCT, the results were similar. After surviving 1-year, in patients who underwent MAC HCT, GvHD did not provide any benefit in preventing disease recurrence, and there was a significant increase in TRM leading again to decrease in OS in these patients. When a similar comparison was done in 1-year survivors of RIC HCT, relapse rates were significantly lower in patients with acute- and chronic-GvHD but had higher TRM leading to an decrease in OS. In a retrospective study of 2656 patients by Inamoto et al., cGvHD was associated with decreased disease recurrence but there was no difference in the OS, suggesting once again that the survival benefit from GvT was negated by the TRM from GvHD. They further reported that there was no difference in late disease recurrence beyond 18 months after HCT in patients who are on immunosuppressive therapy compared to those where this was discontinued.

In another CIBMTR report, Lee et al. showed that the presence of cGvHD was associated with fewer relapses but more TRM. In this study, the benefit of a GvT was limited to the group of patients with milder cGvHD, where OS and DFS were similar, or better, than those of patients without cGvHD. Once again, in patients with more severe forms of cGvHD, TRM negated the potential benefits of the GvT effect and a lower recurrence rate.

Altogether, these findings emphasize that delaying or reducing treatment of moderate to severe cases of cGvHD in order to preserve its associated GvT effect and lower recurrence rate, may not be in the best interest of the patient.

> **PRACTICE POINT**
>
> Treat moderate to severe cGvHD as soon as the diagnosis is established, using the NIH Consensus Criteria for diagnosis and scoring.

Selected reading

1. Jagasia MH, Greinix HT, Arora M, et al. National Institutes of Health Consensus Development Project on criteria for clinical trials in chronic graft-versus-host disease: I. The 2014 Diagnosis and Staging Working Group report. *Biol Blood Marrow Transplant* 2015; **21**(3): 389–401 e1.
2. Nash RA, Antin JH, Karanes C, et al. Phase 3 study comparing methotrexate and tacrolimus with methotrexate and cyclosporine for prophylaxis of acute graft-versus-host disease after marrow transplantation from unrelated donors. *Blood* 2000; **96**(6): 2062–2068.
3. Cutler C, Logan B, Nakamura R, et al. Tacrolimus/sirolimus vs tacrolimus/methotrexate as GvHD prophylaxis after

matched, related donor allogeneic HCT. *Blood* 2014; **124**(8): 1372–1377.

4. Flowers ME, Martin PJ. How we treat chronic graft-versus-host disease. *Blood* 2015; **125**(4): 606–615.

5. Cutler C, Miklos D, Kim HT, et al. Rituximab for steroid-refractory chronic graft-versus-host disease. *Blood* 2006; **108**(2): 756–762.

6. Flowers ME, Apperley JF, van Besien K, et al. A multicentre prospective phase 2 randomized study of extracorporeal photopheresis for treatment of chronic graft-versus-host disease. *Blood* 2008; **112**(7): 2667–2674.

7. Greinix HT, van Besien K, Elmaagacli AH, et al. Progressive improvement in cutaneous and extracutaneous chronic graft-versus-host disease after a 24-week course of extracorporeal photopheresis – results of a crossover randomized study. *Biol Blood Marrow Transplant* 2011; **17**(12): 1775–1782.

8. Couriel DR, Hosing C, Saliba R, et al. Extracorporeal photochemotherapy for the treatment of steroid-resistant chronic GvHD. *Blood* 2006; **107**(8): 3074–3080.

9. Couriel DR, Saliba R, Escalon MP, et al. Sirolimus in combination with tacrolimus and corticosteroids for the treatment of resistant chronic graft-versus-host disease. *Br J Haematol* 2005; **130**(3): 409–417.

10. Johnston LJ, Brown J, Shizuru JA, et al. Rapamycin (sirolimus) for treatment of chronic graft-versus-host disease. *Biol Blood Marrow Transplant* 2005; **11**(1): 47–55.

11. Koreth J, Matsuoka K, Kim HT, et al. Interleukin-2 and regulatory T-cells in graft-versus-host disease. *N Engl J Med* 2011; **365**(22): 2055–2066.

12. Weng JY, Du X, Geng SX, et al. Mesenchymal stem cell as salvage treatment for refractory chronic GvHD. *Bone Marrow Transplant* 2010; **45**(12): 1732–1740.

13. Carpenter PA, Kitko CL, Elad S, et al. National Institutes of Health Consensus Development Project on criteria for clinical trials in chronic graft-versus-host disease: V. The 2014 Ancillary Therapy and Supportive Care Working Group Report. *Biol Blood Marrow Transplant* 2015; **21**(7):1167–1187.

14. Weisdorf D, Zhang MJ, Arora M, Horowitz MM, Rizzo JD, Eapen M. Graft-versus-host disease induced graft-versus-leukemia effect: greater impact on relapse and disease-free survival after reduced intensity conditioning. *Biol Blood Marrow Transplant* 2012; **18**(11): 1727–1733.

15. Inamoto Y, Flowers ME, Lee SJ, et al. Influence of immunosuppressive treatment on risk of recurrent malignancy after allogeneic hematopoietic cell transplantation. *Blood* 2011; **118**(2): 456–463.

CHAPTER 39

Prevention and treatment of infection

Corrado Girmenia[1], Gian Maria Rossolini[2], and Claudio Viscoli[3]

[1] Dipartimento di Ematologia, Oncologia, Anatomia Patologica e Medicina Rigenerativa, Azienda Policlinico Umberto I, Sapienza University of Rome, Rome, Italy

[2] Dipartimento di Biotecnologie Mediche, University of Siena, Siena; Dipartimento di Medicina Sperimentale e Clinica, University of Florence, Florence; SOD Microbiologia e Virologia, Azienda Ospedaliera Universitaria Careggi, Florence, Italy

[3] University of Genoa (DISSAL), IRCCS S. Martino – IST, Genoa, Italy

Introduction

Infections are frequent and life threatening complications after hematopoietic cell transplant (HCT). The risk of severe infection in the early post-transplant period is lower in autologous (auto-HCT) compared to allogeneic HCT (allo-HCT). In addition, the risk of infection continues to be high even after neutrophil engraftment in allo-HCT recipients. This is due to protracted defects in cell-mediated immunity and occurrence of acute or chronic graft-versus-host disease (GvHD) requiring immunosuppressive therapy (Figure 39.1). The modification of the infectious risk in the HCT populations is not only the direct result of the changes in the transplant strategies but also of the global epidemiology of the hospital and community-acquired infections.

Prevention of bacterial infections

Antibacterial agents and vaccines are the cornerstones in the prevention of bacterial diseases, however, the infection-control team should also consider the prevention of transmission of pathogens. Health care workers and persons in contact with HCT recipients should routinely follow appropriate hand hygiene practices to avoid exposing recipients to bacterial pathogens. Additional precautions for patients colonized with certain high-risk pathogens should ensue and instructions with regard to visitors, pets, and plants are crucial aspects in the overall prevention of bacterial infections in HCT recipients (Table 39.1).

Antibacterial prophylaxis: Challenge in the era of multi-resistance

The European Conference on Infection in Leukemia (ECIL) and Infectious Diseases Society of America (IDSA) guidelines recommend prophylaxis with fluoro-quinolones in HCT recipients during the engraftment period until recovery from neutropenia (Table 39.2). Prophylaxis with fluoroquinolones is recommended both in auto-HCT and allo-HCT; however, several experiences in the autologous setting showed a less evident impact on hospital length of stay, duration of fever, and duration of antibacterial treatment, raising the question of a revision in the antimicrobial prevention strategies at least in lower-risk auto-HCT populations (i.e., auto-HCT in multiple myeloma).

An important issue concerning prophylaxis is antibiotic resistance. The alarm over the emergence of resistant bacteria or *Clostridium difficile* infection as a result of the expansive use of fluoroquinolones has been raised. Although actually the phenomenon of quinolone-resistance does not seem to be a contraindication to the use of these drugs in prophylaxis during neutropenia, the epidemiology of resistant isolates among gram-negative bacilli (i.e., carbapenem-resistant enterobacteria (CRE), multi-drug-resistant (MDR)-XDR non-fermenting gram-negative bacteria) should be carefully monitored and the proficiency of the practice of antibacterial prophylaxis periodically re-evaluated according to the epidemiological evolution or antibiotic-resistances.

In the last few years, the emerging phenomenon of infections by MDR gram-negative bacteria, such as CRE, which frequently cause invasive infections starting from the colonized intestinal tract, has also raised the question

Clinical Manual of Blood and Bone Marrow Transplantation, First Edition. Edited by Syed A. Abutalib and Parameswaran Hari.
© 2017 John Wiley & Sons Ltd. Published 2017 by John Wiley & Sons Ltd.

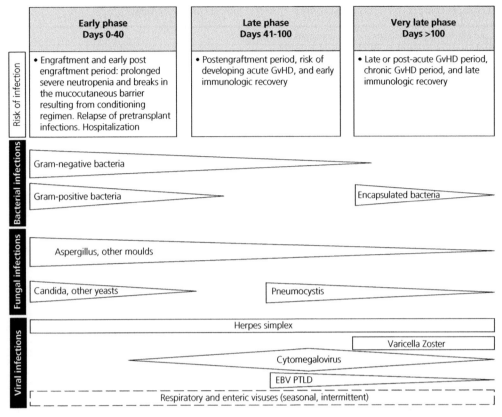

	Early phase **Days 0-40**	**Late phase** **Days 41-100**	**Very late phase** **Days >100**
Risk of infection	• Engraftment and early post engraftment period: prolonged severe neutropenia and breaks in the mucocutaneous barrier resulting from conditioning regimen. Relapse of pretransplant infections. Hospitalization	• Postengraftment period, risk of developing acute GvHD, and early immunologic recovery	• Late or post-acute GvHD period, chronic GvHD period, and late immunologic recovery

Bacterial infections
- Gram-negative bacteria
- Gram-positive bacteria
- Encapsulated bacteria

Fungal infections
- Aspergillus, other moulds
- Candida, other yeasts
- Pneumocystis

Viral infections
- Herpes simplex
- Varicella Zoster
- Cytomegalovirus
- EBV PTLD
- Respiratory and enteric visuses (seasonal, intermittent)

Figure 39.1 Typical infections during different phases after allogeneic HCT recipients.

of reconsidering the use of selective digestive decontamination with oral non-absorbable antibiotics. Although digestive decontamination with oral gentamicin or oral colistin in carriers of CRE that are susceptible to these agents might be considered, in view of the small experience in hematologic populations and of the need of further data about safety (risk for resistance selection) there is poor evidence to support this practice.

Prevention of bacterial infections after PMN engraftment

Patients undergoing allo-HCT are at increased risk of sepsis caused by encapsulated bacteria (*Streptococcus pneumoniae*, *Haemophilus influenzae*, and meningococci) due to functional asplenia and impaired B-cell immunity, particularly in patients with chronic GvHD (cGvHD) and in those with low IgG levels, therefore prophylaxis against these infections is advised. Penicillins (penicillin V or amoxicillin, adult 250–500 mg q12h, although 500 mg q24h may be more realistic if compliance is a particular problem) are the drugs of choice; in case of penicillin allergy, clarithromycin 250 mg q12h orally (reduce the dose for children) can

be considered. It should be initiated at 3 months after allo-HCT and be continued until at least 1 year after transplant or until immunosuppressive therapy has been discontinued in patients with cGvHD. Patients should receive prophylaxis regardless of prior administration of pneumococcal vaccines. A vaccine schedule including pneumococcal, *Haemophilus influenzae* type B, and meningococcal vaccines has been well established (Table 39.3).

Prevention of fungal infections

The risk of invasive fungal disease (IFD) is variable in the HCT population according to the characteristics of the patient, the underlying disease, the donor, the graft source, and the type of conditioning regimen. It may vary in between patients and in the same patient along the transplant course. The incidence of IFDs is very low (less than 1%) after auto-HCT from mobilized peripheral blood cells, and primary antifungal prophylaxis is generally not indicated in this setting (fluconazole primary prophylaxis, 400 mg QD, may be considered in patients

Table 39.1 Precautions needed for HCT patients colonized by certain antibiotic-resistant bacteria.

Bacteria and Mechanism of Resistance	Precautions and Comments
Methicillin-resistant *Staphylococcus aureus* (MRSA), vancomycin-intermediate *Staphylococcus aureus* (VISA)	MRSA colonization in HCT recipients generally does not represent an increased risk to develop post-transplantation invasive complications. There is insufficient evidence at present to recommend routine screening of all HCT recipients for MRSA or the use of topical or systemic antimicrobial therapy for patients with asymptomatic MRSA colonization. Colonization and infection by VISA in HCT recipients is anecdotal and outside of local epidemics screening is not required. However, contact precautions should be adopted for MRSA and VISA colonized or infected patients.
Vancomycin-resistant enterococci (VRE)	VRE colonization in HCT recipients is frequently observed but there is no clear correlation between VRE colonization and post-transplantation severe infections in the HCT setting. VRE screening is not required but it may be considered in the context of epidemiological survey. However, contact precautions should be adopted for VRE colonized patients.
Carbapenem-resistant enterobacteria (CRE)	In transplant centers located in settings with known significant CRE spread, monitoring of colonization is strongly recommended as part of the microbiological pre-transplant evaluation, prior to hospital admission. In patients not colonized, weekly post-transplant monitoring is indicated in the event of CRE isolation from other patients in the same unit. Patients with post-transplant intestinal complications, in particular, GvHD, should undergo fecal culture including examination for CRE. A rectal swab should be repeated in patients who were not colonized and are re-hospitalized for post-transplant complications. Patients who are colonized or infected with CRE, as well as those with a previous history of CRE, should be housed in single rooms and placed on contact precautions. If single rooms are not available, the patient may be cohorted. Patients entering the transplant unit should be considered as potentially colonized and managed accordingly, until proven otherwise. In cases with a high suspicion of colonization by resistant pathogens, three consecutive negative culture or molecular test results separated by ≥48h each may presumably be required to exclude CRKp colonization. In addition to patient cohorting, staff cohorting should be considered.
Multi-drug-resistant (MDR) and extensively-drug-resistant (XDR) non-fermenting gram-negative bacteria (i.e., *Pseudomonas aeruginosa*, *Acinetobacter* spp., *Stenotrophomonas maltophilia*)	The above infection-control strategy for CRE should be considered also for MDR and XDR non-fermenting gram-negative bacteria
Clostridium difficile infection (CDI)	Patients with CDI should be placed on contact precautions for the duration of illness. All Health Care Workers (HCWs) who have contact with a *C. difficile*-infected patient or the patient's environment should don gloves and gowns before entering the patient's room. If there is evidence of ongoing transmission of *C. difficile* despite implementation of the basic prevention practices described above, HCT centers should consider maintaining contact precautions even after diarrhea has resolved and until hospital discharge. During nosocomial CDI outbreaks, HCT centers should work closely with their Infection Prevention and Control staff to ensure implementation of appropriate control measures. The following practices are *not* recommended for prevention of *C. difficile* transmission: • Performing routine stool surveillance cultures or toxin assays for *C. difficile* among asymptomatic patients or HCWs, even during outbreaks; • Culturing HCWs' hands for *C. difficile*; • Treating asymptomatic *C. difficile* carriers to prevent clinical infection.

with severe mucositis). On the contrary, the risk of IFDs along a prolonged period after transplant (until one year) is variably high (between 4 and 20%) after allo-HCT and antifungal prophylaxis is indicated.

Prevention strategies are based on environmental precautions and antimicrobial treatment. While there is a general agreement in the role of High Efficiency Particulate Air (HEPA) filtration with positive pressure for the control of airborne filamentous fungal infections during hospitalization, the indication of pharmacological prophylaxis is still debated. The distribution of IFDs in the various post-transplant phases changed over the years as a result of changing indication to transplant and transplant procedures. In epidemiological studies on populations transplanted in the previous decades, the vast majority of IFDs were documented late after engraftment and were generally associated with occurrence of GvHD. In more recent experiences,

Table 39.2 European Conference on Infection in Leukemia (ECIL) and Infectious Diseases Society of America (IDSA) guidelines on antibacterial prophylaxis in neutropenic hematology and hematopoietic cell transplant subjects.

Guideline	Recommendation and Grading
ECIL	An oral fluoroquinolone should be used Levofloxacin: 500 mg daily (AI) Ciprofloxacin: 500 mg bid (AI) Norfloxacin: 400 mg bid (BI) (less effective than Ciprofloxacin) Ofloxacin: 200–300 mg bid,(BI) (less tested than Ciprofloxacin in randomized controlled trials and at variable daily doses, lower activity against *P. aeruginosa* and less effective than Ciprofloxacin)
IDSA	Fluoroquinolone prophylaxis should be considered for high-risk patients with expected prolonged and profound neutropenia (ANC <100 cells/mm³ for >7 days) (BI). A systematic strategy for monitoring the development of fluoroquinolone resistance among gram-negative bacilli is recommended (A-II). Addition of a gram-positive active agent to fluoroquinolone prophylaxis is generally not recommended (A-I)

Table 39.3 Vaccination schedule employed after allo-HCT at the Department of Hematology of the Policlinico Umberto I of Rome, Italy.

	Recommended Vaccines	
Months after HCT	**HCT recipient's age < 7 years**	**HCT recipient's age > 7 years**
4 to 6	• Influenza, inactivated (yearly)	• Influenza, inactivated (yearly)
6	• I Esavalent (tetanus, diphtheria, polio inactivated, pertussis, Hepatitis B, *Haemophilus influenzae* B) • I Pneumococcal (13 valent conjugated, PCV 13)	• I Tetravalent (tetanus, diphtheria, polio inactivated, pertussis) • I Hepatitis B • I *Haemophilus influenzae* B • I PCV 13
7	• I Meningococcus B • II PCV 13	• I Meningococcus conjugated C/ACWY • II PCV 13
8	• II Esavalent • III PCV 13	• II Tetravalent • II Hepatitis B • II *Haemophilus influenzae* B • III PCV 13
9	• I Meningococcus conjugated C/ACWY	• I Meningococcus B
10	• II Meningococcus B	• II Meningococcus conjugated C/ACWY
11	• II Meningococcus conjugated C/ACWY	• II Meningococcus B • Human Papilloma Virus in females (11–45 years)
14	• III Esavalent • IV PVC 13	• III Tetravalent • III Hepatitis B • III *Haemophilus influenzae* B • IV PCV 13
>24	• Evaluation for I measles, mumps, rubella, varicella if immunosuppressive therapy discontinued	• Evaluation for I measles, mumps, rubella, varicella if immunosuppressive therapy discontinued • Hepatitis A, in endemic areas • In patients without chronic GvHD a V dose with the 23-valent pneumococcal polysaccharide vaccine (PPSV23) to broaden the immune response might be given after 1 year from the IV PCV 13
>26	• II measles, mumps, rubella, varicella if lack of response to I dose	• II measles, mumps, rubella, varicella if lack of response to I dose

a large number of cases of IFD, mainly invasive aspergillosis, occurred during the early post-transplant period. The high rate of IFD documented in this early phase after transplant was related to the high number of patients who had one or more conditions associated with a significantly increased risk of early IFD. These risk factors are an IFD within the 6 months prior to transplant, an active acute leukemia at the time of transplant, a graft from a donor other than identical sibling. In the late and very late phases after transplant, acute GvHD (aGvHD) and cGvHD represent the major predisposing factors, respectively. However, GvHD is a heterogeneous syndrome which may significantly differ according to stem cell source, type of donor, and GvHD prophylaxis and the dynamic evolution of GvHD, with a consequent variable risk of IFD. The risk for IFD in patients with grade II–IV aGvHD not followed by extensive cGvHD is low (<3%) in patients transplanted from a HLA-matched related donor and high (>10%) in those transplanted from an alternative donor. When aGvHD is followed by cGvHD the risk is high regardless of the donor type (very high with unrelated donor). Finally, the rate of IFDs in patients with cGvHD not preceded by aGvHD (also called *de novo* cGvHD) is relatively low (<4%) in all types of transplant.

How to plan an antifungal prophylaxis strategy

In the planning of an antifungal prophylaxis strategy in different patients and in the same patient in different post-transplant phases the first step is represented by the definition of risk according to the time after transplant.

- Three time periods should be distinguished in allo-HCT: an early phase (from day 1 to 40), a late phase (from day 41 to 100) and a very late phase (after day 100) (Figure 39.1). The three phases reflect the risk of IFD being associated with neutropenia (early), with aGvHD and the early immune recovery (late) and with late aGvHD or cGvHD together with late immunologic recovery (very late).
- Patients could be stratified in those not requiring antifungal prophylaxis (low risk), those requiring a *Candida*-active prophylaxis (standard risk) and those requiring a prophylaxis active against both yeasts and filamentous fungi (high risk).

The second step, after the level of risk is defined, is represented by the choice of the antifungal drug. The ECIL (www.kobe.fr/ecil/telechargements2013/ECIL5antifun galprophylaxis%2020062014Final.pdf) and the GITMO produced the most recent guidelines on primary antifungal prophylaxis in allo-HCT (Tables 39.4 and 39.5).

Table 39.4 ECIL 2013 guidelines on primary antifungal prophylaxis in allogeneic HCT recipients.*

Transplant Condition	Recommendation and Evidence Grading
Pre-engraftment, low risk for molds	Oral or IV Fluconazole (400 mg q.d.) AI Itraconazole (200 mg i.v. followed by oral solution 200 mg b.i.d.) BI Voriconazole (200 mg b.i.d. oral) BI Posaconazole oral solution (200 mg t.i.d), delayed release tablet (300 mg/24 h) BII Micafungin (50 mg q.d. iv) BI Caspofungin/anidulafungin, no data Polyenes i.v. CI Aerosolized liposomal AmB plus fluconazole CIII
Pre-engraftment, high risk for molds	Oral or IV Fluconazole AIII, against Itraconazole (200 mg i.v. followed by oral solution 200 mg b.i.d.) BI Voriconazole (200 mg b.i.d. oral) BI Posaconazole oral solution (200 mg t.i.d), delayed release tablet (300 mg/24 h) BII Micafungin (50 mg q.d. iv) CI Caspofungin/anidulafungin, no data Polyenes i.v. CII Aerosolized liposomal AmB plus fluconazole BII
High-risk acute- and chronic GvHD	Oral or IV Fluconazole AIII, against Itraconazole (200 mg i.v. followed by oral solution 200 mg b.i.d.) BI Voriconazole (200 mg b.i.d. oral) BI Posaconazole oral solution (200 mg t.i.d), delayed release tablet (300 mg/24 h) AI Micafungin (50 mg q.d. iv) CII Caspofungin/anidulafungin, no data Polyenes i.v. CII Aerosolized liposomal AmB plus fluconazole, no data

Table 39.5 GITMO 2014 recommendations for primary antifungal prophylaxis in allogeneic HCT recipients.

Level of risk for IFD	Criteria for the Definition of the Level of Risk			PAP Recommended
	Early phase after HCT (day 0–40)	Late phase after HCT (day 41–100)	Very late phase after HCT (day >100)	
High risk	• Active acute leukemia at the time of transplant (AII); • CB transplant (AII); • grade III–IV aGvHD after any type of transplant (AII); • HCT from MMRD or UD and one or more of the following additional risk factors: grade II aGvHD, steroid dose >2 mg/kg/day for at least one week, CMV disease, recurrent CMV infection, prolonged neutropenia (PMN <500/microliter for more than 3 weeks), iron overload (BIII); • Steroid refractory/dependent aGvHD after any type of HCT (AIII).	• Grade III–IV aGvHD after any type of HCT (AII). • HCT from MMRD or UD and one or more of the following additional risk factors: Grade II aGvHD, steroid dose >2 mg/kg/day for at least one week, CMV disease, recurrent CMV infection, recurrent neutropenia (PMN <500/microliter for more than 1 week) (BII) • Steroid refractory/dependent aGvHD after any type of transplant (AIII).	• persistent or late onset grade III–IV aGvHD (AII). • persistent or late onset steroid refractory/dependent aGvHD after any type of HCT (AII). • persistent or late onset grade II aGvHD after transplant from MMRD or UD (BIII). • Extensive cGvHD when preceded by an aGvHD (AII).	• Mold active PAP is recommended. • Posaconazole in GvHD (AI) (TDM advised for oral solution) • Voriconazole (BI) (TDM advised) • Liposomal Amphotericin B (CIII) • Caspofungin (CIII) • Micafungin (CIII) • Aerosolized amphotericin B plus fluconazole (CIII)
Standard risk	All remaining patients not included in the high-risk category (AI).	All remaining patients not included in the high-risk category (BII).	Limited cGvHD who receive only a non-steroid immunosuppression and cGvHD without previous history of aGvHD (BII).	Candida-active PAP is recommended Fluconazole (AI) Voriconazole (BI) Itraconazole(BI) Micafungin (BI)
Low risk	No patient may be considered at low risk for IFD during this phase.	No patient may be considered at low risk for IFD during this phase.	Absence of any type of GvHD and no steroid therapy (AII).	No PAP is recommended.

PAP = primary antifungal prophylaxis; CB = cord blood; MMRD = mismatched-related donor; UD = unrelated donor; aGvHD = acute graft-versus-host disease; cGvHD = chronic graft-versus-host disease; CMV = cytomegalovirus; TDM = therapeutic drug monitoring.

Secondary antifungal prophylaxis

An evidence-based approach to secondary antifungal prophylaxis (SAP) in patients with a previous IFD and requiring HCT remains a challenging issue. Most of experiences show that duration of post-transplant neutropenia, status of the underlying disease, and length of antifungal therapy pre-transplant represented determinant factors for progression or reactivation of IFD despite SAP. While SAP in patients with a resolved infection is able to minimize the risk of relapse after transplant, patients with an active/not resolved IFD at the time of transplant continue to be at risk of a potentially fatal reactivation. Generally, the same antifungal drug used in the treatment of a pre-transplant IFD is recommended although several factors, including toxicity and drug-drug interactions, should be considered in the choice.

Prophylaxis of *Pneumocystis* pneumonia

Prophylaxis of *Pneumocystis* pneumonia (PCP), caused by *P. jirovecii* is recommended in all allo-HCT recipients and selected auto-HCT recipients (including those affected by multiple myeloma or lymphoma, have undergone auto-graft manipulations as CD34+ selection, or have recently received purine analogs) from engraftment until 6 months after HCT or longer in patients who continue to receive immunosuppressive therapy.

The preferred regimen for PCP prophylaxis is trimethoprim-sulfamethoxazole. The optimal dosage has not been defined in HCT patients. Several regimens may be used [double-strength (160/800 mg) tablet orally daily; or one single-strength (80/400 mg) tablet orally daily; or one double-strength tablet orally three times/week] and all appear efficacious. Atovaquone (750 mg twice daily or 1500 mg once daily, orally), dapsone (50 mg orally two times/day; or 100 mg orally daily), and monthly aerosolized pentamidine (300 mg every 3–4 weeks by Respirgard II™ nebulizer), may be used in patients who cannot tolerate trimethoprim-sulfamethoxazole. However, none is as effective as trimethoprim-sulfamethoxazole for PCP prophylaxis; therefore, every effort should be made to administer trimethoprim-sulfamethoxazole. Use of either trimethoprim-sulfamethoxazole or dapsone as PCP prophylaxis is contraindicated in patients with known G6PD deficiency, and alternative therapy should be sought. At present, aerosolized pentamidine or atovaquone are recommended options.

Prevention of viral infections in HCT patients

Several viral infections may occur in HCT recipients, but only for herpesviruses and hepatitis B virus (HBV) prophylactic strategies have been defined, while vaccine schedules for several viral infections have been standardized (Table 39.2). Both herpesviruses and HBV infections after HCT generally constitute reactivations of viruses.

Prophylaxis of herpesvirus diseases

Following allo-HCT the risk for Herpes Simplex Virus (HSV) reactivation is approximately 80%, for cytomegalovirus (CMV) is 50–80% and for varicella zoster virus (VZV) is 20–50%, among seropositive recipients without prophylaxis. Epstein–Barr Virus (EBV) is associated with post-HCT lymphoproliferative disease (EBV-PTLD) particularly in high-risk conditions such as unrelated and mismatched HCT, use of T-cell depletion, and EBV serology mismatch between the donor and the recipient (increased risk for seronegative patients with a seropositive donor).

Prevention of HSV
- Primary HSV infection after HCT is unusual, and antiviral chemoprophylaxis is thus not recommended in HSV-seronegative patients. On the contrary, prophylaxis with an HSV-active agent, such as acyclovir, (from 5 to 10 mg/kg thrice i.v. daily; from 200 mg thrice to 800 mg twice orally daily) or valacyclovir, (500 mg once or twice orally daily), should be offered to all HSV-seropositive auto-HCT and allo-HCT recipients.
- Prophylaxis should be given for a prolonged period. In HCT patients with frequent recurrent HSV infections or those with GvHD, acyclovir prophylaxis can be continued for up to 1 year.

Prevention of VZV
- Seronegative HCT recipients are at high risk of varicella after a face-to-face contact of 5 min or more with a person with varicella or intimate contact (touching or hugging) with a person with *Herpes zoster*. Patients residing in the same household, or in hospital in the same room or adjacent beds in a large ward where there is a contagious person are also at risk.
  - Passive immunization with i.v. varicella zoster specific immunoglobulins (at a dose of 0.2–1 ml/kg) or i.v. normal immunoglobulin (300–500 mg/kg) should be given as soon as possible after exposure (<96 h) to VZV-seronegative patients.
  - In VZV-seropositive patients the risk of a new infection after exposure is low but not insignificant, therefore some experts suggest to use passive immunization with immunoglobulins also in these cases.
  - The efficacy of antiviral agents for post-exposure prophylaxis in recipients of HCT is uncertain, but uncontrolled experiences seem to suggest that prophylaxis may reduce the incidence of varicella and its severity. The use of antimicrobial prophylaxis after exposure may be particularly indicated if immunoglobulin administration in not possible starting during 3–21 days after exposure.

- Although most HCT recipients are VZV-seropositive, they are at risk of virus reactivation for a prolonged period after transplant. Therefore, for VZV-seropositive patients, prophylaxis with oral acyclovir (800 mg twice daily; for children: 20 mg/kg twice daily) or valacyclovir (500 mg once or twice daily) is recommended for 1 year, or longer in the presence of GvHD requiring immunosuppressive therapy.

Prevention of CMV

- In the overall strategy of the CMV infection control the selection of the donor according to his/her serological status is crucial not only for the risk of a CMV infection but also for the transplant-related mortality.
  - CMV-seronegative patients receiving graft from a CMV-seronegative donor (D–/R–) have a very low risk of primary infection if CMV safe blood products are used.
  - Approximately 20–40% of seronegative or seropositive recipients transplanted from a seropositive donor (D+/R–; D+/R+) develop primary CMV infection.
  - The risk of CMV reactivation is particularly high (up to 80%) and recurrence is frequent until several months from HCT when a seropositive recipient is transplanted from a seronegative donor (D–/R+).
- The preventive strategies for CMV disease include chemoprophylaxis, preemptive therapy or treatment of symptomatic CMV infection. A preemptive antiviral strategy based on the serial monitoring of CMV (usually quantitative PCR, but also pp65antigen) represents the most widely used approach. CMV monitoring (once or twice a week) is performed during the period at risk (at least until day +100) and either gancyclovir or foscarnet are the drugs of choice.
  - Viral load thresholds are difficult to establish because of differences in assay performance and testing material (whole blood versus plasma), and variability in predicting viral disease according to degree of immunosuppression and types of transplant.
  - The initial viral load, the viral dynamic (doubling time), the ongoing immunosuppressive therapy, and the type of donor are generally considered for the start of a preemptive CMV therapy.
- The frequency of CMV reactivation in auto-HCT recipients is high, but the risk of evolution to overt CMV disease is very low, therefore routine surveillance in these patients is unnecessary and prophylaxis or serial CMV monitoring not recommended. However, subgroups of auto-HCT patients including those receiving CD34+-selected auto-grafts and prior treatment with fludarabine or other purine analogs are at high risk of acquiring CMV disease: therefore, they should be monitored similar to allo-HCT recipients.

Antiviral chemoprophylaxis may be an alternative to preemptive therapy:

- Intravenous gancyclovir prophylaxis is an effective strategy for the prevention of CMV disease in subgroups of high-risk allo-HCT patients, but toxicity concerns, the increasing risk of late CMV reactivation and the potential for resistance to gancyclovir among CMV hamper its unselected prophylactic use.
- High doses of acyclovir (10 mg/kg i.v. thrice daily) or valacyclovir (2 g orally thrice daily) can be used, however, this approach must be combined with serial CMV monitoring and preemptive therapeutic intervention.

Prevention of HHV-6 and HHV-8

Given the low risk of HHV-6 and HHV-8 diseases and the toxicity of the available antiviral drugs, chemoprophylaxis of such viral infections is not recommended.

Prevention of EBV

There is no effective antiviral prophylaxis against EBV and monitoring EBV reactivation (quantitative PCR) in high-risk patients is used to allow preemptive treatment with rituximab in association to the reduction of immunosuppression.

Prophylaxis of HBV reactivation

Reactivation of hepatitis B is a well-characterized syndrome associated to the reappearance or rise of HBV DNA in the serum of a patient with previously inactive or resolved HBV infection and is frequently accompanied by reappearance of early or late hepatic disease activity. In immunocompromised patients, reactivation of HBV has been reported not only in HBsAg-positive patients, but also in a proportion of HBsAg-negative patients with anti-HBc (with or without anti-HBs) antibodies.

- In HBsAg-positive recipients an anti-HBs negative donor should be vaccinated before graft collection. On the contrary, transplantation of a HBsAg-negative patient with graft from an HBsAg-positive donor is associated with a high risk of transmission, but few patients develop aggressive acute infection or chronic hepatitis B.
- Prophylaxis with nucleoside analogs decreases the incidence of HBV reactivation and the frequency of clinical hepatitis and death from HBV-associated liver injury in patients undergoing HCT. Initiating therapy once reactivation has occurred appears to be ineffective.
- Although there are several oral agents approved for the treatment of chronic hepatitis B (lamivudine, adefovir, entecavir, tenofovir, telbivudine), the published experience in prevention and treatment of HBV reactivation following chemotherapy is almost entirely limited to lamivudine (100 mg daily). Such therapy should start before starting transplant and should continue until 6–12 months after immune

suppression discontinuation. A major concern with prolonged use of lamivudine is the possibility of viral breakthrough following the emergence of resistance mutations particularly in patients with active infection and during prolonged administrations. In HBsAg-positive patients and in those requiring prolonged antiviral prophylaxis entecavir and tenofovir are more attractive candidates given their high potency and extremely low resistance rates.

Treatment of infections in HCT recipients

Infectious complications in HCT recipients are frequently characterized by nonspecific clinical presentation and fever may be the only clinical sign. Considering the importance of an early treatment, particularly in patients with severe neutropenia or undergoing intensive immunosuppression, a targeted choice of the antimicrobial drugs is frequently preceded or replaced by an early empiric or preemptive approach in which antibacterial, antifungal, and antiviral treatments may be sequentially administered. While a targeted therapy in patients with a microbiologically documented infection is easy to choose, the timing, and the type of empirical or preemptive treatments, based on the clinical and laboratory suspicion, are difficult to define. In the next paragraphs, we will discuss the empirical/preemptive antimicrobial strategies usually applied in the HCT setting. We invite the readers to refer to the international (ECIL, IDSA) guidelines for further details on the treatment of documented bacterial, fungal, and viral infections. In consideration of the emerging epidemiology of MDR gram-negative bacterial infections we will limit the description of tailored strategies to this setting.

Neutropenic fever in HCT recipients
Fever in a high-risk neutropenic transplant patient should be considered a medical emergency and the following indications should be used:
- Empiric broad spectrum antibacterial therapy should be initiated within 60 minutes of triage after blood cultures have been obtained and before any other investigations have been completed. It is generally administered intravenously in a hospital setting.
- Monotherapy with an anti-pseudomonal beta-lactam agent (preferably piperacillin-tazobactam, but also third/fourth generation cephalosporins or meropenem) is recommended, and other antimicrobials (aminoglycosides, fluoroquinolones, and/or glycopeptides) may be added to the initial regimen if antimicrobial resistance is suspected or proven.

- Clinical response and culture and susceptibility results should be monitored closely, and therapy should be adjusted in a timely fashion in response to this information.
- In the event of a persistent fever (3–5 days) despite broad spectrum antibiotics, a further diagnostic work-up for bacterial and fungal infections should be performed. Markers of viral infection (i.e. CMV PCR) should be also considered.
- Antifungal therapy may be empirical (fever-driven), preemptive (diagnostic-driven strategy) or targeted (pathogen-driven) according to the results of the diagnostic work-up. (Figure 39.2). Empiric antifungal therapy cannot be a remedy of an inadequate diagnostic strategy and a diagnostic work-up should be always performed in patients with persistent fever.

Fever in non-neutropenic HCT recipients
The therapeutic approach to suspected infections after engraftment in non-neutropenic HCT patients should follow some rules conventionally applied in neutropenic patients but with some substantial differences.
- An accurate clinical evaluation that takes into account infectious and non-infectious causes of fever should be implemented. In this setting fever is not considered a medical emergency requiring an immediate empirical treatment in clinically stable patients but should be considered a trigger for a diagnostic-driven approach.
- In allo-HCT patients with GvHD and/or undergoing immunosuppressive therapy, particularly with steroids, any suspect of an infectious complication, frequently represented by fever, should be followed by an aggressive diagnostic work-up shared with the microbiology laboratory and radiology. Invasive diagnostic procedures (i.e., bronchoalveolar lavage, biopsies) frequently are crucial in guiding an appropriate therapy.

New perspectives in the choice of antibacterial therapy in an era of emerging infections by MDR and XDR gram-negative bacteria.

The emergence of XDR gram-negative bacteria potentially unsusceptible to the conventional antibiotic treatments with beta-lactamase protected penicillins, cephalosporins, carbapenems and fluoroquinolones raises the challenging problem of the choice of the empiric antibacterial therapy of post-transplant febrile neutropenia. A key issue of the treatment of infections by XDR gram-negative bacteria is represented by the need of the use of non-conventional agents such as colistin/polymyxin B, tigecycline, and fosfomycin as the only remaining treatment options.

Treatment definition   **Approach definition**

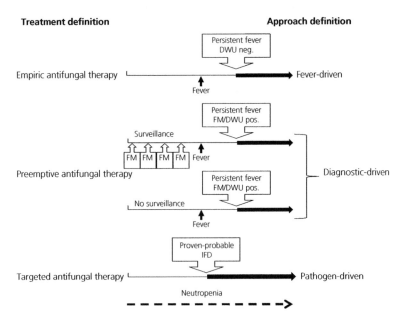

FM: fungal marker; IFD: invasive fungal disease; DWU: diagnostic work-up

➤ (FM + CT + other exams) Antifungal therapy

Figure 39.2 Antifungal strategies in neutropenic patients after HCT.

These agents should be preferably used in combination with other agents that remain active *in vitro* (such as gentamicin or amikacin, or carbapenems if a certain, although reduced, in vitro activity remains), because of suboptimal efficacy (e.g., tigecycline) and risk of resistance selection (e.g., colistin, fosfomycin). The use of these drugs should be limited to the situations where no alternative exists, and *in vitro* susceptibility pattern of the isolate should be considered for the choice of the drugs. A strict correlation between intestinal colonization and endogenous infection by XDR gram-negative bacteria has been observed in immunocompromized patients. In particular, a high rate of severe infections (about 30%) has been reported in allo-HCT patients with a documented CRE colonization. In this specific setting, the administration of a tailored, empiric therapy including the above mentioned unconventional antibiotics and guided by the susceptibility pattern of the colonizing microorganism may be considered at the onset of febrile neutropenia. In the present era of growing resistance, while new antibiotic associations will be increasingly used in the HCT setting, antibacterial strategies should be managed in the context of an antimicrobial stewardship, aiming to minimize unnecessary broad spectrum antibiotic use and further resistance selection.

SUMMARY

- Infections are frequent and life threatening complications in HCT recipients, particularly those submitted to allo-HCT.

- Fluroquinolones still represent the drugs of choice in the antibacterial prophylaxis during the engraftment period, but the phenomenon of fluoroquinolone resistance and the proficiency of the practice of antibacterial prophylaxis should be periodically re-evaluated.

- Vaccination against *Streptococcus pneumoniae*, *Haemophilus influenzae*, and meningococci are needed at 3–6 months after allo-HCT. Penicillin prophylaxis should be administered, in addition to vaccination, in patients with cGvHD until receiving immunosuppressive therapy.

- Prevention strategies of IFDs are based on environmental precautions and antimicrobial prophylaxis and should be guided by an accurate risk stratification.

- Prophylactic strategies with antiviral agents have been defined only for herpesviruses and HBV while vaccine schedules against several viral infections have been established (see Table 39.6).

- Targeted treatment of infections is frequently preceded or replaced by early empiric or preemptive antimicrobial approaches.

- In view of the emergence of infections by MDR gram negative bacteria the use of non-conventional antibacterial associations may be required in the context of an antimicrobial stewardship.

Table 39.6 Summary of prophylactic/preventive strategies against certain infections after HCT: approach at the Department of Hematology of the Policlinico Umberto I of Rome, Italy.

Prophylaxis	Auto-HCT	Allo-HCT
Bacterial	Ciprofloxacin 500 mg b.i.d. until engraftment to prevent bacterial infections during neutropenia	Engraftment period • Ciprofloxacin 500 mg b.i.d. to prevent bacterial infections during neutropenia After engraftment • After 3 months from transplant vaccination against *S. pneumoniae, H. influenzae*, and meningococcus. In addition to vaccination and until the completion of the vaccination course, benzylpenicillin 1,200,000 U i.m. every 4 weeks.
Fungal	No prophylaxis in patients without mucositis. In patients with mucositis Fluconazole 400 mg QD till engraftment to prevent superficial and deep Candida infections. Secondary prophylaxis according to pre-transplant fungal infection.	Engraftment period. • In patients at low risk of mold infections: Fluconazole 400 mg QD till day 70 from transplant or longer if immunosuppressive therapy to prevent superficial and deep Candida infections. • In patients at high risk of early mold infections: liposomal AmB 1 mg/kg QD, or micafungin 50 mg QD, or voriconazole 200 mg b.i.d. until engraftment followed by fluconazole 400 mg QD until day 70 from transplant or longer if immunosuppressive therapy to prevent mold and yeast infections. • Secondary prophylaxis according to pre-transplant fungal infection. After engraftment • In patients with acute or chronic GvHD and at high risk of mold infections: Posaconazole oral suspension, 200 mg t.i.d. or Posaconazole tablets 300 mg b.i.d. × 2 doses then 300 mg QD till immunosuppression discontinuation, to prevent mold and yeast infections.
Viral	Acyclovir 250 mg i.v. t.i.d. for prevention of HSV and VZV.	Engraftment period • Acyclovir 5–10 mg/kg i.v. t.i.d. After engraftment: • Valacyclovir 1–2 g orally b.i.d. in transplants from unrelated or mismatched-related donor; acyclovir 200–800 mg t.i.d. in transplant from matched related donor. For prevention of HSV and VZV. CMV potentially covered with higher doses
PCP	After engraftment: Trimethoprim-sulfametoxazole DS one tablet b.i.d. 2 consecutive days/week until immunosuppressive therapy	After engraftment: Trimethoprim-sulfametoxazole DS one tablet b.i.d. 2 consecutive days/week until immunosuppressive therapy

Selected reading

1. Averbuch D, Cordonnier C, Livermore DM et al. European guidelines for empirical antibacterial therapy for febrile neutropenic patients in the era of growing resistance: summary of the 2011 4th European Conference on Infections in Leukemia. *Haematologica.* 2013;**98**:1826–1835.
2. Engelhard D, Akova M, Boeckh MJ et al. Bacterial infection prevention after hematopoietic cell transplantation. *Bone Marrow Transplant.* 2009;**44**:467–470.
3. Freifeld AG, Bow EJ, Sepkowitz KA et al. Clinical practice guideline for the use of antimicrobial agents in neutropenic patients with cancer: 2010 update by the Infectious Diseases Society of Americainfectious diseases society of America. *Clin Infect Dis.* 2011;**52**:e56–93.
4. Girmenia C, Viscoli C, Piciocchi A, et al. Management of carbapenem resistant resistant Klebsiella pneumoniae infections in stem cell transplant recipients: an italian multidisciplinary consensus statement. *Haematologica.* 2015;**100**: e373–376.
5. Girmenia C, Barosi G, Piciocchi A, et al. Primary prophylaxis of invasive fungal diseases in allogeneic stem cell transplantation: revised recommendations from a consensus process by Gruppo Italiano Trapianto Midollo Osseo (GITMO). *Biol Blood Marrow Transplant.* 2014;**20**:1080–1088.
6. Ljungman P, Hakki M, Boeckh M. Cytomegalovirus in hematopoietic stem cell transplant recipients. *Hematol Oncol Clin North Am.* 2011;**25**:151–169.
7. Mikulska M, Nicolini L, Signori A et al. Hepatitis B reactivation in HBsAg-negative/HBcAb-positive allogeneic haematopoietic stem cell transplant recipients: risk factors and outcome. *Clin Microbiol Infect.* 2014;**20**:694–701.
8. Tomblyn M, Chiller T, Einsele H et al. Guidelines for preventing infectious complications among hematopoietic cell transplantation recipients: a global perspective. *Biol Blood Marrow Transplant.* 2009;**15**:1143–1238.

CHAPTER 40

Early non-infectious complications after hematopoietic cell transplantation

Piyanuch Kongtim and Stefan O. Ciurea

Department of Stem Cell Transplant and Cellular Therapy, The University of Texas MD Anderson Cancer Center, Houston, TX, USA

Introduction

Allogeneic hematopoietic cell transplantation (allo-HCT) is an effective therapy for patients with advanced hematologic malignancies and hemoglobinopathies. However, a major limitation of this form of treatment has been treatment-related mortality (TRM). Although, TRM has improved in time with modifications of the conditioning regimen, primarily after the introduction of reduced-intensity conditioning (RIC) protocols as well as advances in supportive care, it still represents a major limitation in extending this potentially curative form of treatment to more patients in need. Organ toxicity caused by conditioning chemotherapy given pre-transplant and inflammatory processes occurring early post-transplant is still major obstacle for successful transplantation especially in patients with advanced age. The main aim of this chapter is to present an overview of early transplant complications related to preparative regimens, and to provide recommendations regarding their prevention and early treatment, while other transplant-related complications, such as acute and chronic graft-versus-host-disease (GvHD) are mentioned elsewhere. A summary of these potential chemotherapy regimen-related complications occurring early post-transplant is provided in Table 40.1.

How can we grade regimen-related toxicities?

Morbidity and even mortality following high-dose chemo-radiotherapy, although less frequent than in the past, is still common today, usually occurs early post-transplant (mostly within the first 28 days) and may set up the stage for other complications that can occur later in the course of allo-HCT. The Bearman Toxicity Score is a validated scoring system that was initially developed and widely used to assess toxicity during allo-HCT. In this system, grade I toxicity is reversible without treatment, grade II is not life-threatening but required treatment, grade III requires life-support intervention and grade IV is fatal toxicity. However, because more organ-specific criteria are needed, the Bearman Toxicity Score was subsequently replaced by the Common Terminology Criteria for Adverse Events (CTCAE, also called "common toxicity criteria"), which has been developed by The National Cancer Institute (NCI) of the National Institutes of Health (NIH) (Table 40.2). The CTCAE is graded as mild (Grade I), moderate (Grade II), severe (Grade III), or life-threatening (Grade IV), with specific parameters according to the organ system involved. Death (Grade V) is used for some of the criteria to denote a fatality. While a detailed description of all toxicities cannot be provided in the chapter, it can be found on the web at https://evs.nci.nih.gov/ftp1/CTCAE/CTCAE_4.03_2010-06-14_Quick Reference_8.5x11.pdf. Of note, an adverse event is defined as any abnormal clinical finding temporally associated with the use of chemotherapy.

Oral mucositis

Oral mucositis is one of the most common early complications of HCT (both allogeneic and autologous) that negatively affect the quality of life (QoL). Mucositis and esophagitis are a direct consequence of conditioning chemotherapy resulting in tissue damage manifested by erythema, edema, and ulceration along the gastrointestinal mucosa and disruption of the protective barrier. Mucositis occurs early post-chemotherapy and tends to resolve after the neutrophil count recovery.

Clinical Manual of Blood and Bone Marrow Transplantation, First Edition. Edited by Syed A. Abutalib and Parameswaran Hari.
© 2017 John Wiley & Sons Ltd. Published 2017 by John Wiley & Sons Ltd.

Table 40.1 Summary of early post-transplant complications related to the high-dose chemotherapy prior to hematopoietic cell transplant.

Common Complications	Management and Prevention
Oral complications	
• Oral mucositis	• Pre-, peri-, and post-transplant oral care • Palifermin IV for mucositis prevention in patients received TBI-based myeloablative conditioning regimen • Adequate hydration • Pain control • Preventive intubation in patients with severe mucositis
• Xerostomia and hyposalivation	• Maintain oral moisture • Use sialagogues
Gastrointestinal complications	
• Gastritis and esophagitis	• Elevation of head of bed • Treatment with antacids: calcium carbonate, aluminum-magnesium hydroxide, PPIs
• Nausea and vomiting	• Medical treatment and prevention with serotonin antagonists, dopamine antagonists, anticholinergics, antihistamine, benzodiazepine, or cannabinoids
• Diarrhea	• Rehydration • Antidiarrheal drugs for non-infectious diarrhea, e.g. loparamide, diphenoxylate/atropine
Hepatic complications	
• Drug induced hepatitis	• Avoiding hepatotoxic agents in high-risk patients
• SOS	• Maintaining fluid and electrolyte balance • Aggressive diuresis • Prevention with ursodiol in high-risk patients • Treatment with defibrotide in patients with moderate to severe SOS
Pulmonary complications	
• Diffused alveolar hemorrhage	• Correct thrombocytopenia and coagulopathy • Adequate respiratory support • High-dose corticosteroid
• Idiopathic pneumonia syndrome	• Adequate respiratory support • High-dose corticosteroid • Empirical antimicrobial treatment
Kidney and bladder complications	
• Acute kidney injury	• Hyperhydration, allopurinol, rasburicase for TLS prevention • Use standard dose DMSO for cryopreservation (see Chapter 7) • Renal toxic drug dose adjustment and monitoring
• Hemorrhagic cystitis	• Hyperhydration • Prophylaxis with Mesna in patients received ifosfamide or high-dose cyclophosphamide • Antiviral treatment in patients with viral-associated HC

Comprehensive HCT oral supportive care not only reduces patient suffering, but also can substantially reduce health-care resource utilization and may improve long-term outcomes after transplantation.

Pathophysiology

Mucositis may be a direct consequence of a more intense conditioning chemotherapy regimen, which can damage the epithelial surfaces and subsequent disrupt the integrity of the epithelial layer. Multiple proinflammatory cytokines such as TNF-α, IL-1, IL-6 are released from destructive mucosal cells, cause further tissue damage and delayed healing process. Also, disruption of mucosal barrier is a greater risk for colonization and invasion of microorganisms. Besides mucositis, pre-transplant chemotherapy also causes salivary hypofunction and xerostomia that promote bacterial overgrowth and the development of serious infections.

Table 40.2 NCI-CTCAE Grading Scale. Source: Common Terminology Criteria for Adverse Events (CTCAE) 2009, U.S.DEPARTMENT OF HEALTH AND HUMAN SERVICES NIoH.

Grade I	Asymptomatic or mild symptoms; clinical or diagnostic observations only; intervention not indicated.
Grade II	Moderate; minimal, local, or noninvasive intervention indicated; limiting age-appropriate instrumental ADL*.
Grade III	Severe or medically significant but not immediately life-threatening; hospitalization or prolongation of hospitalization indicated; disabling; limiting self-care ADL**.
Grade IV	Threatening consequences; urgent intervention indicated.
Grade V	Death related to adverse events.

Note: *Instrumental ADL refer to preparing meals, shopping for groceries, or clothes, using the telephone, managing money, etc. **Self-care ADL refer to bathing, dressing, and undressing, feeding self, using the toilet, taking medications, and not bedridden.

Risk factors
- Higher intensity conditioning regimens
- Poor oral/dental hygiene
- Emesis
- Immunosuppressive drugs
- Medications that cause xerostomia such as opiates, diuretics
- Prolonged antibiotic usage
- Poor nutritional status
- Underlying conditions such as diabetes, obesity
- Total body irradiation (TBI)

Prophylaxis
Pre-transplant dental evaluation and cleaning:
- All sources of infection should be corrected before the beginning of conditioning. Decayed teeth and dental caries may require extraction.
- Patients receiving IV bisphosphonates should avoid dental procedures that can disrupt oral mucosa and gum to reduce risk of osteonecrosis of jaw related to bisphosphonate treatment.
- Dental procedures should be done 2 weeks before conditioning to allow wound healing before transplant.
- Avoid the use of dental appliances if possible. Orthodontic bands should be removed.

Peri-transplant oral care:
- Brushing with soft toothbrush and fluoride toothpaste twice daily.
- Oral cryotherapy: patients receiving high-dose melphalan ($\geq$140mg/m^2), as a single agent, should suck on ice chips for 15–30 minutes prior to, during, and for at least 4–6 hours after completion of the melphalan infusion.

- Palifermin (Kepivance™) is recommended for use in patients with hematologic malignancies undergoing allo-HCT to reduce the incidence and duration of severe oral mucositis. The recommended dose of palifermin is 60 µg/kg/day by IV bolus injection for 3 consecutive days before starting myeloablative conditioning chemotherapy and for 3 consecutive days after graft infusion. Palifermin should not be administered less than 24 hours before or less than 24 hours following myelotoxic therapy. It is currently used primarily with TBI-based myeloablative regimens in the allo-HCT setting.
- Maintain adequate hydration.
- Avoid using ill-fitting dentures.

Post-transplant oral care:
- Use saline rinse for at least 6 months post-transplant.
- Begin flossing once platelet count is more than 50,000/mm^3.
- Return to routine professional dental care after 6 months post-transplant, although serious dental procedures should be delayed for at least 12 months post-transplant.

Management
The management of mucositis is based on severity of symptoms:
- Mild (Grade II): normal saline rinse every 2 hours, ice chips, sponge swab.
- Moderate (Grade III): topical analgesia such as viscous lidocaine 5–10 ml. Swish and spit every 2 hours or phenol throat spray, one spray every 4 hours or combination oral rinse (Maalox + Benadryl + Viscous Lidocaine) 5–10 ml. Swish and spit every 2 hours. Continuous IV narcotic therapy might be needed.
- Severe (Grade IV): preventive intubation and pain control with continuous IV narcotics or patient controlled analgesia.

Management of xerostomia and hyposalivation:
- Maintain oral moisture by using normal saline, sodium bicarbonate solution, sponge swab, or half-strength hydrogen peroxide, swish and rinse.
- Use of sialagogues such as artificial saliva, pilocarpine, cavimeline, bethanecol, or biotene mouthwash.
- Xerostomia decay prevention by plaque removal, remineralization with tropical high-concentration fluoride, diet modification to reduce exposure to refined carbohydrate and sugar.

Gastrointestinal and hepatic complications

Gastrointestinal (GI) and hepatic complications are common in HCT (GI complications after auto-HCT as well). Conditioning chemotherapy as well as immunosuppressive agents (in allo-HCT setting) can directly damage GI mucosa and hepatic parenchymal leading to organ dysfunction and increase risk of serious opportunistic infections.

Nausea, vomiting, and anorexia

Myeloablative chemotherapy conditioning regimens are highly emetogenic and cause nausea and anorexia in most patients early post-transplant. This usually leads to delayed gastric emptying time and poor oral intake with a nadir at day 10–12 post-transplant, but often extending to day 20. Emetogenic potential of common chemotherapy agents is summarized in Table 40.3.

Treatment
- Serotonin (5HT3) antagonists: prevention of acute nausea and vomiting from highly emetogenic chemotherapy or TBI.
- Corticosteroids: use in combination with 5HT3 antagonist for prevention of nausea and vomiting; are most effective for delayed nausea and vomiting.

Table 40.3 Emetogenicity of variety of agents used during hematopoietic cell transplantation.

Emetogenicity	Chemotherapy Agent
Very high (>90%)	Cisplatin Carmustine Cyclophosphamide > 1000 mg/m^2 or > 24.7 mg/kg Cytarabine (Ara-C) > 1000 mg/m^2 or > 24.7 mg/kg Nitrogen Mustard
High (60–90%)	Carboplatin > 1000 mg/m^2 or > 24.7 mg/kg Cyclophosphamide 500 to 1000 mg/m^2 or 12.4 to 24.7 mg/kg Cytarabine (Ara-C) > 250 to 1000 mg/m^2 or 6.2 to 24.7 mg/kg Doxorubicin > 75 mg/m^2 or > 1.9 mg/kg Doxorubicin (in combination) > 40 mg/m^2 or > 1 mg/kg Etoposide > 200 mg/m^2 or > 4.9 mg/kg
Moderate (30–60%)	Azacitidine Busulfan > 3.2 mg/kg/day Carboplatin < 1000 mg/m^2 or < 24.7 mg/kg Clofarabine Cyclophosphamide < 500 mg/m^2 or 12.4 mg/kg Daunorubicin Doxorubicin < 75 mg/m^2 or < 1.9 mg/kg Idarubicin Ifosfamide IL-2 Melphalan (high dose) Methotrexate 250 to 1000 mg/m^2 or 6.2 to 24.7 mg/kg Thiotepa (high dose)
Low (10–30%)	Busulfan < 3.2 mg/kg/day Decitabine Etoposide < 200 mg/m^2 or < 4.9 mg/kg Fludarabine Gemcitabine Mitoxantrone < 15 mg/m^2 or < 0.4 mg/kg Pentostatin
Minimal (<10%)	Bleomycin Bortezomib Cytarabine (Ara-C) < 250 mg/m^2 or < 6.2 mg/kg Hydroxyurea L-asparaginase or Pegaspargase Methotrexate < 50 mg/m^2 or < 1.2 mg/kg Nelarabine Paclitaxel Vincristine

- Dopamine antagonists: prevention of acute nausea and vomiting from low emetogenic chemotherapy.
- Anticholinergics and antihistamines: adjuvant therapy for delayed nausea and vomiting in patients with vestibular symptoms. Management or prevention of extrapyramidal symptoms (EPS) caused by dopamine antagonists.
- Benzodiazepines/cannabinoids: prevention of anticipatory nausea and vomiting and treatment of delayed nausea and vomiting.

Esophagitis and gastritis

Most chemotherapy and immunosuppressive agents used in allo-HCT can cause esophagitis and gastritis, which occur during the first week post-transplant and may last longer if patients develop GvHD or infections. The diagnosis of these conditions is usually based on symptoms such as heartburn, epigastric pain, nausea, and vomiting. Poor oral intake and preexisting peptic ulcer may promote the severity of symptoms.

Treatment of esophagitis and gastritis is usually symptomatic and supportive.

First-line treatments

- Elevation of head of bed
- Antacids
  - Calcium carbonate (Tums): 1–2 tabs PO Q4 hours PRN
  - Aluminum-magnesium hydroxide (Maalox): 30 ml. PO Q4 hours PRN

Proton-pump inhibitors (PPIs)

- *Contraindications and cautions*
  - Symptoms have an infectious cause (such as fungal or viral esophagitis).
  - PPIs in the transplant setting may be harmful.
    - Eliminate the acid barrier to microbial colonization of the upper gut.
    - May lead to bacterial and fungal colonization and increased nosocomial infections of the upper airway and intestine.
    - Length of administration should be limited to 7–10 days.
    - Use of PPIs should be restricted to patients who most need potent antisecretory effects, that is, those with persistent peptic esophagitis or peptic ulcer.
  - There are reports of increased rates of *C. difficile* colitis and nosocomial pneumonia in patients on PPI therapy.
- **Inappropriate indications**
  - Prophylaxis against stress ulcers
  - Oro-pharyngeal mucositis
  - Episodic heartburn
  - Nausea and vomiting
  - Diarrhea

- Nonspecific abdominal pain
- Gastrointestinal bleeding of uncertain etiology
- **Appropriate indications**
  - Use of corticosteroids
  - Persistent acid-peptic symptoms despite maximal antacid therapy
  - Unable to tolerate oral antacid therapy
- **Dosing**
  - Pantoprazole 40 mg PO or IV daily for 7–10 days
  - Lansoprazole 30 mg PO daily for 7–10 days
  - Twice daily dosing of PPIs is generally not more effective. PPIs take up to 7 days to reach maximal acid suppression, so increasing to twice daily after a day or so of once daily therapy is ineffective and is not advised
  - Antacid PRN therapy should be continued (allowing PPI to reach steady state)

H2 antagonists (ranitidine, famotidine, nizatidine, cimetidine)

These should be avoided in the early post-transplant period as they may cause blood cell count suppression.

Sucralfate

Sucralfate is ineffective in the treatment of esophagitis in the transplant setting, and is not recommended.

Diarrhea

Diarrhea can occur anytime during the process of HCT (both auto and allo-HCT). The common etiologies of diarrhea include direct effect of chemotherapy and immunosuppressive agents, mucositis, infection, or early development of GvHD. Infections must be ruled out before treatment by stool culture. Rectosigmoidoscopy and tissue biopsy might be needed in refractory cases.

Treatments

- Identify and treat the underlying cause.
- Rehydration and treatment of electrolyte imbalances.
- For non-infectious diarrhea, *loperamide* (Imodium) 4 mg. PO, then 2 mg. after each loose stool (not to exceed 16 mg. per day) or *diphenoxylate/atropine* (Lomotil) 1–2 tablets PO TID-QID (not to exceed 8 tablets per day) might be effective to relieve symptom.
- Antidiarrheal agents should be avoided in patients with infectious diarrhea.
- Patient on MMF can also develop diarrhea; caution is advised before attributing diarrhea to GvHD.

Sinusoidal obstruction syndrome (SOS)

SOS is a clinical syndrome characterized by hepatomegaly, right upper quadrant pain, elevated serum bilirubin, fluid retention, and weight gain that occurs during the first 3 weeks following conditioning, usually prior to engraftment. This syndrome results from direct injury to sinusoidal endothelial cells and hepatocytes of toxins in certain conditioning chemotherapy (primarily alkylating agents especially busulfan or cyclophosphamide) or irradiation. Endothelial injury leads to occlusion of the terminal hepatic venules and hepatic sinusoids.

Risk factors

- Preexisting hepatic diseases: liver iron overload, viral hepatitis, cirrhosis
- Heavily chemotherapy pre-treated patients
- Use of certain monoclonal antibodies prior to transplant conditioning (inotuzumab ozogamicin)
- Certain diseases (more common in acute lymphoblastic leukemia)
- Myeloablative conditioning
- Chemotherapy agents (busulfan, high-dose cyclophosphamide) or TBI part of conditioning even in auto-HCT setting, although rare
- Abdominal irradiation
- Allo-HCT
- Second transplant
- Older age or younger age in children

Diagnosis

The diagnosis of SOS is primarily based on achievement of established clinical criteria including both the Modified Seattle and the Baltimore criteria (Table 40.4). Other causes of liver dysfunction and weight gain such as sepsis-related cholestasis, other cholestatic liver diseases, and GvHD must be excluded before the diagnosis of SOS is made. Abdominal ultrasound with liver Doppler may be helpful in the exclusion of other disorders. It usually shows hepatomegaly, ascites, and in advanced stages reversal of portal blood flow. A liver biopsy is not necessary for diagnosis of SOS. However, a transvenous liver biopsy with measurement of hepatic venous pressure gradient is the most accurate

diagnostic test that might be useful in case where the cause of liver dysfunction is unclear. Hepatic venous pressure gradient above 10 mmHg is highly specific for SOS. The risks of severe bleeding (in the setting of thrombocytopenia early post-transplant and live dysfunction) must be weighed against the need to make a diagnosis.

The severity of SOS is defined by using clinical criteria. It has been classified as mild (SOS that is clinically obvious, requires no treatment, and resolves completely), moderate (SOS that causes signs and symptoms requiring treatment such as diuretics or pain medications, but that resolves completely), or severe (SOS that requires treatment but that does not resolve before death or day 100 post-transplant).

Prevention and treatment

Identification of patients who are at risk and avoiding exposure to known risk factors are the most important strategy to prevent this complication. Supportive care is the standard treatment including maintaining fluid and electrolyte balance, providing aggressive diuresis, and avoiding hepatotoxic agents. To date there are no satisfactory therapies for severe SOS. Results from numerous small studies have shown that ursodeoxycholic acid (Ursodiol®) 300 mg PO TID from start of conditioning until approximately 1 week after engraftment effectively reduces the incidence of SOS in patients undergoing allo-HCT. The potential mechanism of ursodeoxycholic acid in SOS prevention is replacing hepatotoxic bile acids. However, this drug does not show efficacy in treatment for existing SOS. Defibrotide is a potent anti-thrombotic, anti-inflammatory agent that has been used successfully in the prevention and treatment of SOS. In a historically-controlled phase III study, a survival advantage has been noted for patients with severe SOS who received this drug early in the course of their disease. Defibrotide 6.25 mg/kg IV four times daily is currently recommended for treatment of patients who develop moderately to severe SOS.

Table 40.4 Clinical criteria of SOS.

Modified Seattle Criteria	Baltimore Criteria
Two of the following criteria must be present within 20 days of transplant: • Bilirubin > 34.2 μmol/1 (2 mg/dL) • Hepatomegaly or right upper quadrant pain • Weight gain (>2% from pre-transplant weight)	Bilirubin must be > 34.2 μmol/1 (2 mg/dL) within 21 days of transplant and two of the following criteria must be present: • Hepatomegaly • Ascites • Weight gain (>5% from pre-transplant weight)

Pulmonary Complications

Despite advances in post-transplant supportive cares, diffuse lung injury remains a significant problem following allo-HCT both in the immediate post-transplant period and in the months that follow. This chapter is focusing on non-infectious lung injuries that develop early post-transplant.

Diffused alveolar hemorrhage

Diffused alveolar hemorrhage (DAH) usually develops in the first 3 weeks post-transplant and is often a catastrophic clinical syndrome causing respiratory failure. Risk factors of DAH are advanced age, preexisting pulmonary diseases, severe acute GvHD, myeloablative conditioning regimen, TBI containing regimens, thrombocytopenia, and coagulopathy.

The pathogenesis of DAH in allo-HCT recipients has not yet to be clearly established, but it has been suggested that alveolar tissue injury caused by conditioning chemotherapy or radiation with or without associated infection, and the associated cytokine release play important roles.

Diagnosis

Clinical findings of DAH are nonspecific and sometimes are mistaken as infectious causes such as hemoptysis, fever, chest pain, cough, and dyspnea. Also, hemoptysis may be absent initially in approximately one third of the patients. Chest X-ray and CT-scan often show bilateral alveolar opacities, which can be seen in many other conditions. Bronchoscopy with bronchoalveolar lavage (BAL) shows progressive bloody return is the diagnostic confirmation. Cytology with Prussian blue staining usually shows more than 20% of hemosiderin-laden machophages. However, the utility of this test is limited if DAH occurred less than 48 hours as machophages may not take up enough red blood cells. Histologic result from lung biopsy shows diffused alveolar damage and alveolar hemorrhage.

Treatment

Patients with DAH should be managed in the medical intensive care unit given that respiratory failure can develop rapidly.

- Mechanical ventilation with low tidal volume is needed in patients who have respiratory failure or acute respiratory distress syndrome (ARDS).
- Correction of underlying coagulopathy by the maintaining a platelet count above 50,000–80,000/mm^3 and normalization of PT and aPTT.
- High-dose corticosteroids is the mainstay of treatment for patients with DAH, although, its effectiveness remains uncertain. Doses of up to 1 g of methylprednisolone divided into 2–4 doses administered daily for 3–5 days, followed by a slow taper over 1–3 months is recommended.
- Antibiotic therapy is usually applied if an associated infectious cause is suspected.
- Role of activated factor VII is not well established but few reassuring anecdotal data is present.

Idiopathic pneumonia syndrome

Idiopathic pneumonia syndrome (IPS) is an umbrella under which many non-infectious and non-transfusion related lung injuries are categorized. The injuries include widespread alveolar damage following HCT that develops in the first 2 months post-transplant with the absence of an active lower respiratory tract infection or cardiogenic causes. However, delayed onset IPS has been reported. Multiple inflammatory cytokines such as TNF-α, IL-8, monocyte chemoattractant protein-1 (MCP-1) and IFN-ϒ as well as donor-derived T-cells play a major role in pathogenesis of IPS.

Diagnosis

The diagnosis of IPS is based on clinical signs and symptoms of pneumonia, non-lobar radiographic infiltrates, abnormal pulmonary function. In 1993 National Heart Lung and Blood Institute workshop proposed the following criteria for the diagnosis of IPS: symptoms and signs of pneumonia, evidence of abnormal pulmonary physiology such as increased alveolar to arterial oxygen gradient or increased restrictive pulmonary test physiology, evidence of widespread alveolar injury suggested by multilobar infiltrates on chest radiography or computed tomography, and absence of active lower respiratory tract infection. According to the most recent diagnostic criteria of IPS updated by the American Thoracic Society, newly described pathogens determined by lung biopsy or BAL or other pathogen-specific tests such as polymerase chain reaction are considered. Moreover, IPS has been further classified into specific entities based on the primary anatomical sites of inflammation and dysfunction (pulmonary parenchyma, vascular endothelium, and airway epithelium) as shown in Table 40.5. The intent is to better characterize the clinical spectrum of disease and to more carefully match subtypes of IPS with specific preclinical models that have been developed to mimic and ultimately understand them.

Treatment

There is no specific treatment for IPS. Current standard treatment regimens for IPS include supportive care in conjunction with broad-spectrum antimicrobial agents and intravenous corticosteroids. Nevertheless, efficacy of corticosteroid in this setting has not been proved.

Table 40.5 Categorization of idiopathic pneumonia syndrome (IPS) by presumed site of primary tissue injury.

Pulmonary Parenchyma	Vascular Endothelium	Airway Epithelium
• Acute interstitial pneumonitis (AIP) • Acute respiratory distress syndrome (ARDS)* • Delayed pulmonary toxicity syndrome (DPTS)	• Peri-engraftment respiratory distress syndrome (PERDS) • Noncardiogenic capillary leak syndrome (CLS) • Diffuse alveolar hemorrhage (DAH)	• Cryptogenic organizing pneumonia (COP)/Bronchiolitis obliterans organizing pneumonia (BOOP) • Bronchiolitis obliterans syndrome (BOS)

Table 40.6 Clinical criteria for diagnosis of engraftment syndrome.

Spitzer Criteria	Maiolino Criteria
3 major, or 2 major, and 1 minor, within 96 hours of engraftment. *Major*: non-infectious fever, skin rash, pulmonary edema and hypoxemia. *Minor*: weight gain, hepatic or renal dysfunction and transient encephalopathy	Non-infectious fever plus: • skin rash, or • pulmonary infiltrates, or • diarrhea, commencing 24h before or at any time after the first appearance of neutrophils

Etanercep, a TNF-alpha inhibitor with or without corticosteroid has been used to reduce severity of IPS. However, the benefit of this agent is not clear.

Engraftment syndrome

Engraftment syndrome or peri-engraftment respiratory distress syndrome (PERDS) is characterized by fever, erythrodermatous rashes, noncardiogenic pulmonary edema, and hypoxemia that occur within 5–7 days of neutrophil engraftment, also falls within the definition of IPS. The pathogenesis of the syndrome is dependent upon the intensity of the preparative regimen, donor source of the stem cells and type of HCT. ES has usually been described following autologous HCT. It is postulated that the release of proinflammatory cytokines and the influx of neutrophils into the lungs during engraftment play a primary role. The use of G-CSF and rapid neutrophil engraftment are risk factors for development of ES. Two clinical diagnostic criteria of ES have been described (Table 40.6).

Treatment
Therapeutic guidelines for ES have not been well established. Mild ES following autologous HCT may not require therapy as resolution of these clinical signs following full hematologic recovery and discontinuation of growth factor is common. For patients with progressive

or severe ES, corticosteroids are often dramatically effective. Supportive care of patients with ES should include appropriate anti-infective prophylaxis.

Kidney and bladder complications

The time course of renal and urologic complications varies from early after conditioning to months or years after engraftment. Herein, we will discuss only the early onset or acute injuries of kidney and bladder.

Acute kidney injury
Acute kidney injury (AKI) is defined as an increase in serum creatinine or decrease in urine output that usually develop within the first 100 days after HCT. However, there is still no consensus definition for AKI. Most criteria use a 1.5-fold increase in serum creatinine from baseline or oliguria. The incidence of AKI varies from 20% in autologous, 30% in non-myeloablative allo-HCT, and up to 70% in myeloablative allo-HCT.

Common etiologies and managements
Multiple transplant-related factors as well as patient's underlying conditions can contribute to this complication. AKI that develops in the induction period may result from chemotherapy, tumor lysis syndrome, stem cell infusion toxicity, intra-vascular volume depletion, SOS, thrombotic microangiopathy (TMA), or renal toxic agents commonly used after transplant (like foscarnet, cidofovir, or Bactrim).

• Tumor lysis syndrome is caused by lysis of tumor cells results in hyperkalemia, hyperuricemia, hyperphosphatemia, hypocalcemia, and AKI. The mechanism of AKI caused by uric acid and calcium phosphate crystal precipitation in renal tubules results in renal epithelial and endothelial cell injury. This renal complication can be prevented by aggressive intravenous hydration. Allopurinol has been used to decrease uric acid formation in patients who are at risk of developing tumor lysis syndrome. Recombinant urate oxidase (Rasburicase™) helps increasing the conversion of uric acid to water-soluble allantoin. It is recommended for treatment and prevention of tumor lysis syndrome when allopurinol is contraindicated or in patients with severe hyperuricemia. Rasburicase™ is contraindicated in patients with G6PD deficiency.

- Graft infusion toxicity may cause AKI from DMSO in the product. There is a recent trend in reducing DMSO concentration or replacing it by other non-toxic cryo-protectant to prevent this complication although it is not a routine practice.
- Renal toxic agents used in HCT processes including chemotherapy, antibiotics, antifungals, and calcineurin inhibitors are the major cause of AKI in HCT setting. Renal function monitoring is crucial when these agents are prescribed. Dose adjustment and drug level monitoring are required in patients who are at risk or with preexisting renal dysfunction.
- HCT-related TMA may be the result of the conditioning chemotherapy, tacrolimus and or sirolimus, or infection, and results in acute tubular necrosis from hemoglobinuria. Treatment of this condition is mainly supportive. Plasmapheresis may not be as effective in HCT-related TMA. Eculizumab has been investigated in this setting with few reassuring anecdotal data. Some patients may develop chronic kidney disease.

Hemorrhagic cystitis

Hemorrhagic cystitis (HC) is defined as an inflammatory condition of the bladder resulting in bleeding from the bladder mucosa. Clinical symptoms are ranging from mild dysuria and non-visible microscopic hematuria, to bladder pain, severe hematuria, potential clot retention, and renal failure.

HC can be classified as early- or late-onset based on the time of appearance. Early-onset HC is usually induced by toxic effect of chemotherapy agents used in conditioning regimens. Cyclophosphamide is the most common cause of hemorrhagic cystitis in patients undergoing HCT. A urotoxic metabolite of cyclophosphamide, acrolein is responsible of causing this complication. Hydration and the use of mesna during administration may decrease toxic effects on the bladder. Other drugs used in HCT processes that can also cause HC such as ifosfamide, busulfan, and thiotepa. Radiation-induced HC is also common and can occur in early or late after the exposure. Another important cause of HC in the early post-transplant period is due to viruses, like BK virus (BKV) or adenovirus (predominantly in children). Symptoms of BKV cystitis occur usually after day 30; however, an earlier and later onset is possible.

Diagnosis of HC is based on symptoms, basic laboratory tests such as urine analysis and exclusion of other conditions primarily infection. A bladder scan, retroperitoneal ultrasound to detect hydronephrosis or a CT scan of the abdomen/pelvis may be useful for evaluating this condition and effects on the upper urinary tract.

Prevention

- Hyperhydration is an effective strategy in preventing HC associated chemotherapy such as cyclophosphamide or ifosfamide. It helps decrease the occurrence and severity of HC.
- Mesna is a synthetic sulfhydryl compound designated as sodium-2-mercaptoethane sulfonate, which can bind acrolein. It is indicated as a prophylaxtic agent in reducing the incidence of ifosfamide- or high-dose cyclophosphamide-induced HC.

Treatment

Treatment of HC often involves supportive care, hyperhydration with 5% dextrose normal saline and diuresis. Continuous bladder irrigation (CBI) with normal saline has been used to treat hematuria with clots. The use of appropriate analgesia to treat dysuria is also important. Maintaining a higher platelet count threshold and prevention of upper urinary tract involvement are also important while treatment with antiviral agents may be useful in viral-associated cystitis.

Fluid overload

Fluid overload is common during hospitalization for HCT and is associated with weight gain, edema, and other symptoms such as shortness of breath. Significant fluid overload is strongly associated with mortality and worse survival. Fluid overload is likely related to the rate of intravenous fluid administration and other factors such as oncotic pressure, capillary leak, and major organ dysfunction post-transplant. Prevention of excessive fluid accumulation is important for the management of HCT patients, since the chemotherapy or radiation used for pre-transplant conditioning may lead to small vessel injury and subsequent extravascular fluid extravasation, including pulmonary edema. However, HCT patients are at increased risk for fluid overload, as they often require frequent blood product infusions, total parenteral nutrition, high-volume infusions for multiple antibiotics, and white cell-stimulating factors. Treatment with diuretic might be necessary in patients who develop clinical significant fluid overload such as shortness of breath or edema.

Selected reading

1. Gooley TA, Chien JW, Pergam SA, Hingorani S, Sorror ML, Boeckh M, et al. Reduced mortality after allogeneic hematopoietic-cell transplantation. *N Engl J Med.* 2010;**363**(22): 2091–2101.
2. Bearman SI, Appelbaum FR, Buckner CD, Petersen FB, Fisher LD, Clift RA, et al. Regimen-related toxicity in patients undergoing bone marrow transplantation. *J Clin Oncol.* 1988;**6**(10):1562–158.
3. U.S.DEPARTMENT OF HEALTH AND HUMAN SERVICES NIoH, National Cancer Institute. Common Terminology

Criteria for Adverse Events (CTCAE) 2009 [updated June 14, 2010; cited 2015 May 19]. 4.3: Available from: http://evs.nci.nih.gov/ftp1/CTCAE/CTCAE_4.03_2010–06–14_QuickReference_8.5x11.pdf (accessed December 21, 2016).

4. Mehta J, Powles RL, Treleaven J, Shields M, Agrawal S, Rege K, et al. Cimetidine-induced myelosuppression after bone marrow transplantation. *Leuk Lymphoma*. 1994;**13**(1–2): 179–181.

5. Agura ED, Vila E, Petersen FB, Shields AF, Thomas ED. The use of ranitidine in bone marrow transplantation. A review of 223 cases. *Transplantation*. 1988;**46**(1):53–56.

6. McDonald GB, Hinds MS, Fisher LD, Schoch HG, Wolford JL, Banaji M, et al. Veno-occlusive disease of the liver and multiorgan failure after bone marrow transplantation: a cohort study of 355 patients. *Ann Intern Med*. 1993;**118**(4): 255–267.

7. Shulman HM, Hinterberger W. Hepatic veno-occlusive disease--liver toxicity syndrome after bone marrow transplantation. *Bone Marrow Transplant*. 1992;**10**(3):197–214.

8. Jones RJ, Lee KS, Beschorner WE, Vogel VG, Grochow LB, Braine HG, et al. Venoocclusive disease of the liver following bone marrow transplantation. *Transplantation*. 1987;**44**(6): 778–783.

9. Clark JG, Hansen JA, Hertz MI, Parkman R, Jensen L, Peavy HH. Idiopathic pneumonia syndrome after bone marrow transplantation. *American Review of Respiratory Disease*. 1993;**147**(6_pt_1):1601–1606.

10. Panoskaltsis-Mortari A, Griese M, Madtes DK, Belperio JA, Haddad IY, Folz RJ, et al. An Official American Thoracic Society Research Statement: Noninfectious Lung injury after hematopoietic stem cell transplantation: idiopathic pneumonia syndrome. *American Journal of Respiratory and Critical Care Medicine*. 2011;**183**(9):1262–1279.

11. Spitzer TR. Engraftment syndrome following hematopoietic stem cell transplantation. *Bone Marrow Transplant*. 2001;**27**(9):893–898.

12. Maiolino A, Biasoli I, Lima J, Portugal AC, Pulcheri W, Nucci M. Engraftment syndrome following autologous hematopoietic stem cell transplantation: definition of diagnostic criteria. *Bone Marrow Transplant*. 2003;**31**(5): 393–397.

13. Rondon G, Saliba RM, Chen J, Ledesma C, Alousi AM, Oran B, et al. Fluid Overload as new toxicity category has a strong impact on non relapse mortality and survival in allogeneic hematopoietic stem cell transplantation. *Blood*. 2015;**126**(23):4321.

14. Michael M, Kuehnle I, Goldstein SL. Fluid overload and acute renal failure in pediatric stem cell transplant patients. *Pediatr Nephrol*. 2004;**19**(1):91–95.

CHAPTER 41

Post-transplant lymphoproliferative disorders

Michael D. Keller, Conrad R. Cruz, and Catherine M. Bollard

Children's National Medical Center and The George Washington University, Washington, DC, USA

Introduction

Post-transplant lymphoproliferative diseases (PTLD) following hematopoietic cell transplantation (HCT) are an aggressive and potentially fatal group of disorders. Most PTLDs after HCT arise from lymphoproliferation of Epstein–Barr virus (EBV)-infected B-cells, which occurs as a result of (1) unchecked B-cell proliferation driven by viral proto-oncogenes, (2) absent T-cell response following HCT (i.e., from immunosuppressive therapy; IST), and sometimes (3) secondary genetic mutations in somatic oncogenes. Though the incidence of PTLD after HCT is lower than following solid organ transplantation, it is associated with a higher mortality rate. The clinical presentation can range from an infectious mononucleosis-like disorder to aggressive lymphoma.

As EBV is highly prevalent in the population and establishes lifelong latency, PTLD is a potential risk in many recipients of HCT. Key risk factors include: T-cell depleted graft, *in vivo* T-cell depletion (TCD), HLA-mismatched HCT (longer IST), and/or development of graft-versus-host disease (longer IST). Successful therapies have included targeted destruction of the B-cell viral reservoir and prompt reconstitution of antiviral T-cell immunity.

EBV biology

EBV (HHV4) is a highly ubiquitous member of the human herpesvirus family, and was the first described human oncovirus. EBV is an enveloped, double strand DNA virus, with a 172 kb genome which encodes over 90 proteins and 25 microRNAs. It is a member of the gamma-herpesvirus family (genus *Lymphocryptovirus*). EBV has tropism for B-lymphocytes and nasopharyngeal epithelial cells, and enters cells via interactions between viral gp350 and CD21 (also known as CR2), with viral gp42 serving as a coreceptor, which binds to MHC class II ligands.

Though average age of exposure varies by region and ethnicity, 90–95% of adults are EBV seropositive by the third decade of life. EBV maintains lifelong latency in B-lymphocytes, and in the absence of the opposing T-cell antiviral response, can cause disease ranging from a lymphoproliferative disease to EBV-associated lymphoma.

Following infection, EBV establishes latency in B-lymphocytes, during which its genome is maintained as a nuclear episome. Though no viral particles are produced in latent cells, a variety of viral proteins are expressed, including latent membrane proteins (LMP1 and LMP2), six EBV nuclear antigens (EBNAs), two small noncoding RNAs (EBER), and several clusters of miRNAs. Latently infected B-cells are immortalized, and can proliferate indefinitely *in vitro* due to the combined effects of proliferation-inducing viral latency products (Table 41.1). Three stages of latency have been recognized due to the unique patterns of expressed viral products. Depending on which combination of viral proteins are expressed (from the gene products encoding two latent membrane proteins 1 and 2 (LMP1 and 2), six EBNAs, and two small, nuclear, noncoding RNAs), the infected B-cell displays three latency expression patterns. Different types of EBV latency are influenced by the individual's immune status. The complete expression of all latent proteins is called type III latency which is highly immunogenic, and typically is seen when the patient is immune suppressed (e.g., PTLD). Given the immunogenicity of these type III latently infected cells, they are highly susceptible to EBV-specific T-cell mediated killing. To become increasingly invisible to the EBV response, the virus undergoes several phases

Clinical Manual of Blood and Bone Marrow Transplantation, First Edition. Edited by Syed A. Abutalib and Parameswaran Hari.
© 2017 John Wiley & Sons Ltd. Published 2017 by John Wiley & Sons Ltd.

Table 41.1 EBV Antigens: Different viral latency phases are associated with unique types of malignancies.

| EBV Gene Products | Viral Phase | | | | Function | Immunogenicity |
| | Latency | | | Lytic | | |
	III	II	I			
EBNA1	+	+	+	+	Viral genome maintenance	Poor
EBNA2	+	-	-	-	Activator of viral and B-cell genes	High
EBNA3a/b/c	+	-	-	-	Inhibit tumor suppressors (p16, RBP-Jk)	High
EBNALP	+	+	-	-	Coactivator of transcription with EBNA2	High
LMP1	+	+	-	-	Mimics CD40L signaling	Moderate
LMP2	+	+	+	-	Activator of BCR pathways; activates NF-kb, STAT1	Moderate
BZLF1	-	-	-	+	Transcriptional activator	High
BARF1	+	-	+/-	+	Encodes CSF1 receptor	High
EBERs	+	+	+	-	Influence B-cell autocrine and antiapoptotic pathways	Unknown
miRNAs	+	+	+	+	Influence viral and host transcription	Unknown
Associated Malignancies:	LPD, PCNSL	HL, NPC	BL, GC			

of downregulating latent protein expression, expressing fewer (type II then type I) until no proteins are left (type 0).

Virus production and shedding occurs during lytic cycle, at which time viral transcriptional activators including *BZLF1* and *BRLF1* induce production of viral DNA polymerase, thymidine kinase, and structural proteins including viral capsid antigens (VCAs) that permit virion formation.

Pathogenesis

The majority of PTLDs after allogeneic HCT are of B-cell origin, and are EBV-positive. Following primary EBV infection, a robust primary T-cell response reduces but does not eliminate the initial pool of infected B-cells. In hosts lacking normal T-cell response due to congenital immunodeficiency or immunosuppression, outgrowth of latently infected cells can cause malignant lymphoproliferation. Different latency phases are associated with unique types of malignancies (Table 41.1). Following HCT, PTLD is associated with type III latency, and is most often of donor origin, which is in contrast to PTLD following solid organ transplant. Since latently infected B-cells do not express viral replication proteins, viral cell cycle inhibitors (acyclovir, gancliclovir) are generally ineffective.

The WHO classifications recognize four subtypes of PTLD based on histologic and immunologic phenotype: (1) early lesions, (2) polymorphic PTLD, (3) monomorphic PTLD, and (4) classic Hodgkin-lymphoma. Early lesions may occur soon following HCT, and show reactive plasmacytic hyperplasia in the interfollicular regions as well as paracortical expansion of immunoblasts mixed with T-cells and plasma cells, with otherwise intact lymph node architecture. Polymorphic PTLD involve effacement of lymph node architecture, with variable sized immunoblasts, lymphocytes, and plasma cells. Cellular atypia is often seen, as are Reed Sternberg-like cells. Monomorphic PTLD has histologically uniform neoplastic cells, which is subdivided into diffuse large B-cell lymphoma, Burkitt's lymphoma, plasma cell myeloma, plasmacytoma-like lesions, and others. Hodgkin-lymphoma type PTLD is more frequently seen post solid organ transplantation and can be indistinguishable from HL occurring in immunocompetent patients.

These stages are considered a spectrum of disease, with early lesions typically being polyclonal without cytogenetic abnormalities, whereas higher stage PTLD has an increasing degree of monoclonality with cytogenetic changes including trisomy 9, trisomy 11, 17p deletions, and rearrangements of 8q24(c-Myc).

PTLD originating from T-cells or Natural Killer (NK) cells is extremely rare after HCT, and are less commonly associated with EBV. T/NK-derived PTLD is usually monomorphic in appearance, and T-cell derived PTLD often have clonal rearrangements of the T-cell receptor. EBV-negative lesions are associated with poor response to therapy.

The antiviral immune response to PTLD involves both innate and adaptive responses, with a substantial T-cell response as well as NK-cell and suspected NK-T-cell involvement. The T-cell response is multifaceted with both CD4$^+$ and CD8$^+$ effector and memory responses. T-cells targeting is largely skewed toward the latency associated viral proteins, with EBNA3 being a predominant epitope.

Presentation and diagnosis

PTLD tends to occur in the first 6–12 months following allogeneic HCT, and occurs in 0.5–1% of all HCT recipients. Risk is increased in patients who receive therapies targeting T-cells, including ATG, alemtuzumab, calcineurin inhibitors, recipients of T-cell depleted allografts, and patients receiving partially HLA-matched allografts.

PTLD can initially resemble infectious mononucleosis with fever, lymphadenopathy, myalgias, and abdominal pain. Mass lesions are often detectable in lymph nodes, while extranodal disease can affect the liver, spleen, intestines, bone marrow, and CNS. The GI tract is the most common site of extranodal disease. More profoundly immunosuppressed patients can potentially present with a sepsis-like clinical picture with multi-organ infiltration. Studies have demonstrated detectable PTLD in more than half of all deaths following allogeneic HCT.

Diagnosis is ideally determined by histopathology. Depending on the setting, the positive predictive value of blood EBV viral count for detection of PTLD is modest, which likely reflects the finding that viral replication does not seem to be a significant contributor to pathology. Nonetheless, monitoring of EBV viral counts following HCT has proven to be helpful in early diagnosis of EBV-associated pathology.

Management of disease

The list of risk factors for developing PTLD suggest a central role for the immune response; consequently the most important therapies for this disorder all relate to augmenting immunity against the malignant B-cells. As a result of the extensive heterogeneity of PTLD, there is no single prescribed therapy for the disorder.

As previously discussed, the disease is believed to be the result of imbalances between EBV-associated malignant B-cells and effector T-cells. Therapy is therefore geared toward eliminating infected B-cells or expanding EBV-specific T-cell immunity. Thus, removal of immune suppression, the use of the anti-CD20 monoclonal antibody rituximab, and the use of EBV-specific T-cells as cellular immunotherapy comprise treatment strategies that have shown some measure of clinical success. Other therapies include treatment with cytokines, radiation therapy, and chemotherapy.

Removal/reduction of immune suppression

Patients undergoing transplant are typically given immune suppressive drugs to either prevent rejection of the donor organ in solid organ transplants, or to prevent graft-versus-host disease in allogeneic hematopoietic cell transplants. The most straightforward method of treatment is the reduction of therapeutic immunosuppression, and its efficacy has made it the frontline treatment option especially for solid organ transplant recipients who develop PTLD.

Predictably, an exact regimen for reducing immune suppression remains to be identified. There is no optimal degree of the extent of reduction necessary, no clear choice of which drugs to discontinue or taper, and no clear indication as to which patient populations can benefit from this therapy alone. Additionally, reduction of immunosuppression may not be feasible due to risk of potential fatal solid organ rejection (e.g., recipients of orthotopic heart or lung transplants). Patient age at diagnosis, disease stage, presence of bulky disease, and clinical presentation of anorexia as initial symptom are all univariate predictors of response to use of reduction of immunotherapy alone.

In a study of 67 adult patients with PTLD, treatment by reducing immune suppression alone resulted in complete response rates of 37% and partial response rates of 8%. Some of the risk factors that are associated with poor response to reduction of immune suppression include elevated LDH, late-onset PTLD, patient age greater than 50 years old, presence of B symptoms, and systemic involvement of disease. Therefore, in some cases like low risk disease, reduction of immunotherapy alone can lead to successful clinical outcomes.

Monoclonal antibody against CD 20 receptor on B-cells

The anti-CD20 monoclonal antibody rituximab has changed the landscape of PTLD: since its introduction, disease outcomes have dramatically improved for the disorder. The antibody has been successfully used in PTLD and a variety of B-cell malignancies, either alone or in combination with other therapies – mediating complete and durable responses.

Rituximab is believed to act via several pathways; it is currently unclear which predominate in PTLD, and whether similar pathways are involved across different diseases. Signaling effects of CD20 antibody have been proposed and explored because the drug appears to be active in the absence of intact immune effectors. Binding of the antibody to CD20 receptor leads to inhibition of several pathways, including p38, NFkB, ERK1/2, and AKT – all of which are involved in survival of the malignant cells. Still, effector responses to the antibody likely contribute significantly to its activity. The antibody can lead to activation of the complement cascade, allowing for targeting of its bound B-cell. The Fc portion of the antibody can also be recognized by NK-cells, granulocytes, and macrophages expressing Fc receptors. These phagocytes not only directly lyse targeted B-cells, but also secrete cytokines that recruit additional immune effectors to the disease site.

PTLD following both solid organ transplants and hematopoietic cell transplants derive benefit from rituximab therapy. In a large multicenter retrospective study of four Chicago institutions (80 cases of PTLD), early treatment with rituximab-based regimens improved progression free survival and overall survival. Similarly, in a large retrospective study of 19 European Group for Blood and Marrow Transplantation centers (144 cases of PTLD), therapy with regimens based on rituximab resulted in the survival of two thirds of patients with PTLD after HCT.

Concerns were initially raised about the use of rituximab for PTLD since this agent is unable to discriminate between infected and healthy B-cells. Though plasma cells do not express CD19, hypogammaglobulinemia and lasting B-cell aplasia has been described in a small minority of patients. Further, infectious complications may arise in patients with PTLD, which may complicate their recovery. Fortunately, experience has shown that serious infectious complications only occur rarely in over half a million patients who have been treated with rituximab.

EBV-specific T-cell therapy

EBV-infected B-cells are presumably kept in check by antigen-specific T-cells, and early trials in PTLD after allogeneic HCT have demonstrated that immunity against EBV can be provided by donor lymphocytes (with responses up to 90%). Because most donors are EBV seropositive, they presumably possess EBV-specific T-cells among their lymphocyte populations. Nevertheless, there are few long term responses following DLI, and acute graft-versus-host disease is a persistent concern.

Providing EBV-specific immunity without GvHD has thus been explored using *ex vivo* manipulated EBV-specific T-cells. The expansion of EBV-specific T-cells *ex vivo* relies on a potent source of antigen;

fortunately, in the case of PTLD, this is provided by B95–8 virus-infected lymphoblastoid cell lines (LCL) – which are EBV-transformed cells manufactured in the laboratory and which express type III latency antigens that are frequently seen in the malignant cells of PTLD (see Table 41.1). Thus, using irradiated EBV LCL as antigen presenting cells (APC), investigators were able to readily activate and expand donor-derived EBV-specific T-cells to large numbers for the treatment of high-risk patients preemptively or therapeutically. Other methods to *ex vivo* expand EBV-specific T-cells include the use of APC pulsed with EBV peptide mixes, multimer selection, and IFNγ capture.

As numerous studies have shown, EBV-specific T-cell therapy is a potent treatment for PTLD, especially in the HCT setting.

The use of donor-derived EBV-specific T-cells to prevent or treat PTLD in high-risk patients after allogeneic stem cell transplant has been reported by multiple groups. For example, the group at Baylor College of Medicine showed that EBV-specific T-cells can mediate both protection against PTLD (none of the patients treated prophylactically (n = 101) developed PTLD) and as a treatment for active disease (11 of 13 patients achieved sustained complete remissions following T-cell therapy). More importantly, infusion of EBV-specific T-cells was predominantly safe and not associated with GvHD, with a single exception in a patient with multiple comorbidities who received expanded/non genetically modified T-cell immunotherapy.

A major limitation to the use of EBV-specific T-cells is the requirement for highly specialized centers to manufacture clinical grade cell products. To broaden use of T-cells, banks of virus-specific T-cells (including against EBV) have been established (containing the most common HLA types), and a clinical trial evaluating the efficacy of the most closely HLA-matched allogeneic T-cells specific for multiple viruses showed very promising results. In this trial, eight patients with refractory EBV PTLD received EBV-specific T-cells from the bank, and of these, two had complete responses, and four had partial responses.

In contrast, in the solid organ transplant setting, autologous EBV-CTLs were expanded and subsequently infused in patients post solid organ transplant at high risk for PTLD. In patients who had high EBV DNA post-transplant, T-cell infusions prevented the development of PTLD (in those at high risk for the disease) or resulted in decreases in PTLD size.

Current research efforts are aimed at developing faster and more efficient methods of manufacturing EBV-specific T-cells, as well as development of "off the shelf" third party CTL products.

Other therapies

Chemotherapy, with CHOP or MACE-CytaBOM has been used for PTLD, especially in the setting of poor responses to reduction of immune suppression. However, there are significant toxicities with chemotherapy, and it is therefore not recommended as a first line treatment for PTLD. However, to evaluate low-dose chemotherapy in combination with rituximab the Children's Oncology group conducted a phase II study in pediatric patients with EBV$^+$ CD20$^+$ PTLD. A complete remission rate of 69% and overall survival of 83% was obtained with a regimen consisting of rituximab, low-dose cyclophosphamide, and prednisone. Localized therapy, including surgery and radiotherapy may have roles in alleviating symptoms due to mass effects from PTLD lesions impinging on important systems.

Owing to disease heterogeneity in patients, as well as treatment resistance to rituximab, reduction of immune suppression, or EBV-specific T-cells, other therapies are currently being explored as adjuvants to the therapies discussed above or as novel approaches. For example, the use of cytokines (both antiviral cytokines that target virus-infected cells or antibodies targeting cytokines required by infected cells for their continued growth) have been studied, and have shown promising results. In addition, other immune targets (targeted either by monoclonal antibodies similar to rituximab, or antigen-specific T-cells similar to EBV-specific T-cell therapy) have been identified, including CD30 – present in up to 80% of PTLD. Some of the other therapies directed against PTLD are listed in Table 41.2.

Various clinical trials seeking to improve treatment for PTLD are currently open: some of these are highlighted in Table 41.3.

PRACTICE POINTS

Following allogeneic HCT, patients should be monitored for clinical signs of PTLD as well as EBV reactivation.

- Early screening by imaging and histopathologic analysis is essential in patients with clinical signs of PTLD and/or EBV reactivation.
- Reduction of immunosuppression and rituximab are first line therapies for early stage PTLD (Table 41.2).
- Higher grade PTLD often requires chemotherapy targeting B-cell proliferation.
- EBV-specific cytotoxic T-lymphocyte therapy is highly effective in both prevention and treatment of PTLD (Tables 41.2 and 41.3).

Table 41.2 Types of therapy for PTLD.

Therapy	Mechanism of Action	Notes
Reduction of immune suppression	Improve endogenous immune response to EBV	First line therapy effective but with slow onset of activity; durable responses uncommon
Monoclonal antibody against CD20 (rituximab)	Shift B-cell T-cell balance in favor of less B-cells; CD20 antibody targets B-cells by signaling induced cell death, complement dependent cellular cytotoxicity, or antibody dependent cellular cytotoxicity	Outcomes for PTLD have improved since the introduction of rituximab; limited to CD20+ PTLD; pre-emptive therapy improves outcomes
EBV-specific cytotoxic T-cells	Shift B-cell T-cell balance in favor of more T-cells; better than simple donor T-cell infusion because of decreased risk for GvHD from the antigen-specific T-cell product	Use of third party T-cells circumvents limitations of manufacturing expertise being available only in some centers
Cytokine therapy	Acts by decreasing viral infection with antiviral cytokines (e.g., IFNa) or by attacking B-cell reliance on cytokines (e.g., anti-IL6)	Limited experience/efficacy
Chemotherapy	Cytotoxic drugs to malignant cells	Often used for patients who are unresponsive/ineligible to treatment by reduction of immune suppression
Radiation therapy	For localized disease; indicated when PTLD produces local effects (e.g., mass effects)	May be used for patients requiring palliative therapy; often done in conjunction with reduction of immune suppression or rituximab

Table 41.3 Recent clinical trials for therapy of PTLD (from ClinicalTrials.Gov).

NCT Number	Drug/Intervention	Phase	Institution
NCT02042391	rituximab and immunochemotherapy	Phase II	Diako Ev. Diakonie-Krankenhaus gemeinnützige
NCT01760226	DA-EPOCH-R		Baylor College of Medicine/National Cancer Institute (NCI)/Texas Children's Hospital
NCT00895206	Individually Adapted Immunosuppression in de Novo Renal Transplantation Based on Immune Function Monitoring: a Prospective Randomized Study	Phase IV	University Hospital, Ghent/Roche Pharma AG
NCT02153580	CD19 CAR T-cell following cyclophosphamide	Phase I	City of Hope Medical Center/National Cancer Institute (NCI)
NCT01839916	donor T-cells	Phase II	University of Chicago/National Cancer Institute (NCI)
NCT01805037	brentuximab vedotin + rituximab	Phase I/II	Northwestern University/Seattle Genetics, Inc.
NCT01703949	brentuximab vedotin in treating patients with relapsed or refractory CD30+ lymphoma		University of Washington/National Cancer Institute (NCI)
NCT01434472	high-Dose Y-90-ibritumomab tiuxetan added to reduced-intensity allogeneic stem cell transplant	Phase II	Fred Hutchinson Cancer Research Center/National Cancer Institute (NCI)
NCT01261247	panobinostat	Phase II	Mayo Clinic/National Cancer Institute (NCI)
NCT01027702	donor lymphocyte infusion	Phase I/II	Andrew Gilman/Carolinas Healthcare System
NCT00621036	Idiotype-KLH conjugate vaccine and GM CSF	Phase II	Simmons Cancer Center/National Cancer Institute (NCI)

Selected reading

1. Bollard CM, Rooney CM, Heslop HE. 2012. T-cell therapy in the treatment of post-transplant lymphoproliferative disease. *Nature Reviews. Clinical Oncology* **9**:510–519.
2. Gottschalk S, Rooney CM, Heslop HE. 2005. Post-transplant lymphoproliferative disorders. *Annual Review of Medicine* **56**:29–44.
3. Al-Mansour Z, Nelson BP, Evens AM. 2013. Post-transplant lymphoproliferative disease (PTLD): risk factors, diagnosis, and current treatment strategies. *Current Hematologic Malignancy Reports* **8**:173–183.
4. Reshef R, Vardhanabhuti S, Luskin MR, Heitjan DF, Hadjiliadis D, et al. 2011. Reduction of immunosuppression as initial therapy for posttransplantation lymphoproliferative disorder(bigstar). *American Journal of Transplantation: Official Journal of the American Society of Transplantation and the American Society of Transplant Surgeons* **11**:336–347.
5. Weiner GJ. 2010. Rituximab: mechanism of action. *Seminars in Hematology* **47**:115–123.
6. Hutchinson L. 2010. Hematology: Rituximab improves survival for solid organ transplant recipients with PTLD. *Nature Reviews. Clinical Oncology* **7**:240.
7. Styczynski J, Gil L, Tridello G, Ljungman P, Donnelly JP, et al. 2013. Response to rituximab-based therapy and risk factor analysis in Epstein Barr Virus-related lymphoproliferative disorder after hematopoietic stem cell transplant in children and adults: a study from the Infectious Diseases Working Party of the European Group for Blood and Marrow Transplantation. *Clinical Infectious Diseases: An Official Publication of the Infectious Diseases Society of America* **57**:794–802.
8. Evens AM, David KA, Helenowski I, Nelson B, Kaufman D, et al. 2010. Multicenter analysis of 80 solid organ transplantation recipients with post-transplantation lymphoproliferative disease: outcomes and prognostic factors in the modern era. *Journal of Clinical Oncology: Official Journal of the American Society of Clinical Oncology* **28**:1038–1046.
9. Rouce RH, Louis CU, Heslop HE. 2014. Epstein-Barr virus lymphoproliferative disease after hematopoietic stem cell transplant. *Current Opinion in Hematology* **21**:476–481.
10. Leen AM, Bollard CM, Mendizabal AM, Shpall EJ, Szabolcs P, et al. 2013. Multicenter study of banked third-party virus-specific T-cells to treat severe viral infections after hematopoietic stem cell transplantation. *Blood* **121**:5113–5123.
11. Gross TG, Orjuela MA, Perkins SL, Park JR, Lynch JC, et al. 2012. Low-dose chemotherapy and rituximab for post-transplant lymphoproliferative disease (PTLD): a Children's Oncology Group Report. *American Journal of Transplantation: Official Journal of the American Society of Transplantation and the American Society of Transplant Surgeons* **12**:3069–3075.

CHAPTER 42

Survivorship issues after transplantation

Vanessa E. Kennedy[1,2], Madan Jagasia[1,3], and Bipin N. Savani[1,3]

[1] *Vanderbilt University School of Medicine, Nashville, TN, USA*

[2] *Department of Medicine, Vanderbilt University Medical Center, Nashville, TN, USA*

[3] *Hematology and Stem Cell Transplantation Section, Division of Hematology/Oncology, Department of Medicine, Vanderbilt University Medical Center and Veterans Affairs Medical Center, Nashville, TN, USA*

Introduction

Since the first successful allogeneic HCT in 1968, the number of HCTs performed annually has increased steadily. In the USA, the number of allogeneic transplants recently surpassed 8,000 per year, with a cumulative total of 340,000 transplants (Figure 42.1 a).

At the same time, post-transplant survival is also increasing due to a combination of better supportive care, less toxic conditioning regimens, and early recognition and management of transplant-related complications. Currently, more than 30,000 transplant recipients are surviving beyond 5 years. Should transplant survival rates remain unchanged, by 2030 there may be over half a million long-term survivors in the USA, and up to one million world-wide (Figure 42.1 b).

As patients survive long-term after HCT, they are at risk for developing multiple late complications. These complications cause significant patient and healthcare burden, impair quality of life (QoL), and lead to late morbidity and mortality. The majority of deaths in HCT recipients occur within the first 2 years post-transplant, after which the 10-year survival is approximately 80–90%. However, several studies indicate that survival rates among HCT recipients remain lower than the general population for at least 10–30 years.

What are the late complications after HCT?

As HCT survivorship increases, the focus of care has shifted to the identification and treatment of complications affecting long-term survival and QoL. Two important aspects of care in long-term survivors are surveillance and preventive care for secondary malignancies and late infections. Several organizations (e.g., National Comprehensive Cancer Network [NCCN], United States Preventive Services Task Force) have developed standardized cancer screening methods and vaccination guidelines that are currently implemented as part of routine health evaluation and disease prevention in the general population. However, we continue to lack literature and guidelines on how these preventive measures apply to long-term HCT survivors. This chapter focuses on long-term screening, surveillance, and preventive care in HCT survivors.

Secondary malignancies

Due to prior conditioning chemotherapy, total body irradiation (TBI), and an altered immune environment, HCT recipients are at a high risk for secondary malignancies, including post-transplant lymphoproliferative diseases (PTLD), secondary myeloid malignancies, and secondary solid cancers.

PTLD

PTLD occurs almost exclusively in allo-HCT recipients and is associated with the Epstein–Barr virus and intensive immunosuppression. In allo-HCT recipients, incidence of PTLD is approximately 1–2% (proportional to the recipient's immunosuppressive state), an increase of 30–182-fold over the general population. The majority of cases occur in the first 6 months post-transplant, and incidence declines steeply in patients more than one year post-HCT (see Chapter 41).

Secondary AML/MDS

Secondary AML and MDS are associated with auto-HCT recipients, treatment with high-dose chemotherapy, and treatment with alkylating agents. Cumulative incidence of secondary AML/MDS is between 1.4 and 8.9%

Clinical Manual of Blood and Bone Marrow Transplantation, First Edition. Edited by Syed A. Abutalib and Parameswaran Hari.

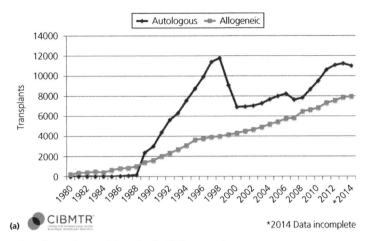

*2014 Data incomplete

Figure 42.1 (a) Annual number of transplant recipients in the US by transplant type.

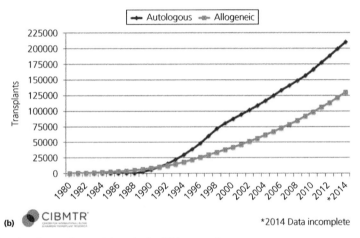

*2014 Data incomplete

Figure 42.1 (b) Cumulative plot of transplant recipients in the US by transplant type.

and 300-fold above the general population. Secondary myeloid malignancies tend to occur later than PTLD, with a median presentation ranging between 12 and 40 months.

Secondary solid malignancies

The incidence of secondary solid tumors increases throughout the survival time of HCT recipients and never reaches a plateau. In a cohort of over 28,000 allo-HCT recipients, cumulative risk of developing new solid malignancies was 1% at 10 years, 2.2% at 15 years, and 3.3% at 20 years post-HCT (Figure 42.2). HCT recipients develop new solid cancers at twice the rate of the general population in the first five years post-transplant and at three times the rate of the general population >15 years post-transplant. Overall, secondary solid malignancies represent the fourth most common cause

of non-relapse mortality (NRM) in patients surviving more than two years post-transplant. However, in HCT recipients more than 20 years post-transplant, secondary solid malignancies represent the number one cause of excess death over the general population.

Which type of secondary solid malignancies occur after HCT?

Nearly all cancer types have been described after HCT. When compared to the general population, HCT recipients are at highest risk for cancers of the skin, thyroid, oropharynx, esophagus, liver, nervous system, and connective tissues. Notably, the most common secondary malignancies, including skin, cervical, and oropharyneal cancer, have established links to human papillomavirus (HPV). More than one-third of female long-term survivors after allo-HCT develop cervical dysplasia, most of

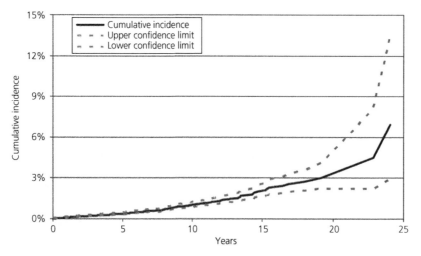

Figure 42.2 Cumulative incidence of secondary solid malignancies after allo-HCT.

which is associated with high-risk HPV subtypes. Currently, the Center of Disease Control and Prevention recommends HPV vaccination in patients who are immunocompromised. Given the prevalence of HPV-associated secondary malignancies, many transplant centers recommend three doses of HPV vaccination starting at one year post-allo-HCT in male and female patients aged 9–26, and potentially older patients as well (Table 42.1). Additional studies are needed linking common secondary malignancies in allo-HCT recipients to HPV and in evaluating the effectiveness of HPV vaccination in the population.

What are the risk factors for secondary solid malignancies?

Pre-transplant risk factors

Pre-transplant risk factors include patient age, gender, previous exposures and underlying diagnosis. The absolute risk of secondary solid malignancy increases with age at transplant; however, when compared to age-matched controls, relative risk of secondary solid malignancy is highest for patients under age 40. Pediatric transplant recipients have a particularly high risk for thyroid carcinoma and breast cancer. Previous exposures, including exposure to high-risk subtypes of HPV, are also associated with increased risk of secondary malignancies.

Transplant-associated risk factors

The most potent transplant-associated risk factor is radiation exposure, which doubles the risk of secondary solid malignancies. TBI increases the risk of non-squamous secondary malignancies, particularly sarcoma, breast

adenocarcinoma, and thyroid cancers. This risk is particularly pronounced for younger patients. In patients receiving TBI, the relative risk of non-squamous secondary malignancies was 9 times that of non-radiated patients in patients irradiated at <30 years old, compared to only 1.1 times in patients irradiated at >30 years old. In patients receiving non-radiation conditioning regimens, risk of secondary malignancy remains higher than the general population, although the link is not as pronounced as in patients receiving TBI.

Post-transplant risk factors

Chronic GvHD is thought to increase the risk of secondary neoplasms through chronic persistent inflammation and genetic changes in epithelial cells. At the same time, immunosuppression leads to decreased surveillance of dysplastic epithelial cells, allowing for development of neoplasia. Development of chronic GvHD and long-term (>24 months) immunosuppressive therapy are related to the development of squamous cell, basal cell, oropharyngeal, esophageal, and cervical carcinomas. This risk is further increased with severe chronic GvHD and in patients with preceding acute GvHD.

Screening for secondary malignancies: What are the recommendations?

Recently, a working group established through the CIBMTR published consensus-based recommendations applicable for screening and prevention of secondary solid cancers, summarized in Table 42.2. Given the lack of randomized trials testing diagnostic guidelines and treatment approaches, this consensus approaches offers

Table 42.1 Our practice for vaccination post-HCT.

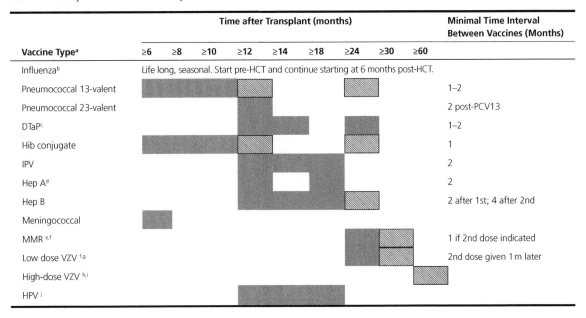

Vaccine Type[a]	Time after Transplant (months)									Minimal Time Interval Between Vaccines (Months)
	≥6	≥8	≥10	≥12	≥14	≥18	≥24	≥30	≥60	
Influenza[b]	Life long, seasonal. Start pre-HCT and continue starting at 6 months post-HCT.									
Pneumococcal 13-valent										1–2
Pneumococcal 23-valent										2 post-PCV13
DTaP[c]										1–2
Hib conjugate										1
IPV										2
Hep A[d]										2
Hep B										2 after 1st; 4 after 2nd
Meningococcal										
MMR [e,f]										1 if 2nd dose indicated
Low dose VZV [f,g]										2nd dose given 1 m later
High-dose VZV [h,i]										
HPV [j]										

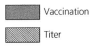   Vaccination

Titer

[a] Live vaccines should be administered > 5 months after last dose of IVIG. Inactive vaccines can be administered at > 2 months after last dose of IVIG.

[b] If < 9 years old, give 2 doses at least 1 month apart. Live attenuated vaccine is contraindicated.

[c] If only Tdap is available (e.g., because DTaP is not licensed for adults), administer Tdap. Acellular pertussis is preferred, but whole-cell pertussis can be used if it is the only pertussis vaccine available.

[d] Patients who do not respond to the primary vaccine series should receive a second three-dose series.

[e] Check serology before immunization and immunize if seronegative. Patients who do not respond to the primary vaccine should be re-vaccinated.

[f] "2-1-5 rule": do not give until > 2 years post-HCT, > 1 year off all immunosuppressive therapy, and > 5 months since last dose of IVIG/VZIG.

[g] Check varicella serology before immunization and immunize only if seronegative. Repeat titers after second dose of low dose VZV vaccine and re-vaccinated if negative.

[h] Check varicella serology before immunization and immunize only if seronegative. Only give if > 60 years of age.

[i] "5-1-5 rule": do not give until > 5 years post-HCT, 1 year off all immunosuppressive therapy, and > 5 months since last dose of IVIG/VZIG.

[j] Data for post-transplant HPV vaccination is limited and recommendations are center-specific.

practical advice on preventative care. However, due to the diversity of risk factors, future studies are needed to individualize screening for specific pre-transplant, transplant, and post-transplant factors. For example, heightened awareness is warranted for pediatric long-term survivors, TBI recipients, and patients with chronic GvHD.

Late infectious complications

Infections are the leading cause of NRM among long-term HCT survivors, and are second only to secondary malignancies in cause of excess death over the general population. The risk of infectious complications is highest in the first 1–2 years after transplant. However, due to delayed immune reconstitution and impaired cellular and humoral immunity, increased susceptibility to infection often persists long-term. This is especially true in patients with chronic GvHD, which is characterized by mucosal damage, organ dysfunction, and impaired immunity. Strategies to prevent late infections include repeat vaccinations and administration of prophylactic antimicrobials against common pathogens. Patients and family members should be educated about long-term infection risks and encouraged to seek prompt medical treatment for signs of contagion.

Table 42.2 Screening recommendations for secondary malignancies.

Screening Recommendations for Secondary Malignancies CIBMTR published consensus-based recommendations	
Site	Recommendation
Breast	-Annual mammogram and clinical breast exam starting at age 40 -If prior radiation >20 Gy, begin at age 25 or 8 years after radiation, whichever comes first
Cervix	-Annual Pap test and HPV DNA test -HPV vaccination
Colorectal	-Fecal occult blood annually starting at age 50 -Flexible sigmoidoscopy or barium enema every 5 years or colonoscopy every 10 years starting at age 50
Esophageal	-Upper GI endoscopy in patients with persistent GERD or dysphasia, particularly in patients with prolonged immunosuppression or chronic GvHD
Lung	-Yearly pulmonary exam -Counseling on smoking cessation
Oropharyneal	-Yearly exam, particularly in patients with chronic GvHD or history of local radiation
Skin	-Yearly skin exam, particularly in patients with TBI or chronic GvHD -Counseling on photoprotection and regular self-examination
Thyroid	-Yearly thyroid exam, particularly in patients transplanted <20 years of age or who received TBI

Adapted from Inamoto Y et al. *BMT* **50**, 1013–1023 2015.

Bacterial infections

Multiple factors lead to impaired humoral immunity and increased susceptibility to bacterial infections. Although hypogammaglobinemia is common, even normal or near-normal levels of IgG may in actuality be obscuring low IgG2 and IgG4 levels. In addition, HCT recipients have persistently low IgA levels, leading to increased susceptibility to conjunctivitis, sinusitis and bronchitis.

The presence of chronic GvHD often leads to functional asplenia and impaired opsonization. This creates an increased susceptibility to encapsulated bacteria, such as *Streptococcus pneumonia, Hemophilus influenza,* and *Neisseria meningitidis*. Patients with chronic GvHD should be treated with prophylaxis against encapsulated organisms for as long as they are receiving immunosuppression. In adult patients, prophylaxis with penicillin VK 250 mg twice daily is commonly used, although trimethoprim-sulfamethoxazole and levofloxacin may be considered based on local resistance patterns. While necessary, this prophylaxis is becoming increasingly problematic as bacteria develop antimicrobial resistance.

Fungal infections

Invasive fungal infections in HCT recipients are associated with significant morbidity and a low one-year survival. Although invasive candidiasis is most common in the early post-transplant period, late infections may be seen in patients with severe mucositis and neutropenia. Invasive aspergillus is seen in patients with profound T-cell deficiency due to chronic GvHD and high-dose steroids. Clinical trials have shown that posaconazole 200 mg three times daily is well tolerated and highly effective against invasive fungal infections. *Pneumocystis jiroveci* is also seen in long-term survivors, and without specific prophylaxis, develops in up to 30% of patients with chronic GvHD. Prophylaxis with trimethoprim-sulfamethoxazole is recommended until the discontinuation of immunosuppression.

Viral infections

Varicella zoster virus (VZV)

VZV is a serious pathogen in HCT recipients, and develops in approximately one third of HCT recipients without specific prophylaxis. Notably, visceral disease can occur with or without cutaneous manifestations and may be difficult to diagnose. Although the risk for VZV infection is greatest in the first 6 months post-HCT, antiviral prophylaxis with acyclovir 800 mg twice daily is recommended for the first 12 months post-transplant, and may exceed 12 months in patients with chronic GvHD.

Herpes simplex virus (HSV)

HSV can cause local and disseminated infections after HCT, and often manifests with atypical pain of the mucous membranes rather than classic vesicular lesions. Antiviral prophylaxis is indicated in all HSV seropositive HCT recipients with 800 mg of acyclovir twice daily, patients with a history of HSV reactivation prior to HCT, and patients with chronic GvHD.

Cytomegalovirus (CMV)

Late CMV reactivation is strongly associated with NRM. Risk factors include early CMV reactivation and chronic GvHD. Close monitoring, early CMV detection, and preemptive (positive CMV by PCR without organ involvement) therapy with ganciclovir or valganciclovir has become an effective strategy for prevention of symptomatic CMV. Prophylactic therapy with 2 g of valacyclovir four times daily has also been shown to reduce the risk of CMV infection and the need for preemptive therapy by 50% and may be considered in certain high-risk HCT recipients.

More recently, focus has shifted to CMV-specific antiviral drugs, many of which are now incorporated into phase III clinical trials. These novel agents have the potential to shift our current therapeutic strategy from molecular surveillance to a prophylactic approach, similar to that used in HSV or VZV.

Hepatitis B Virus (HBV)

Hepatitis B virus can reactivate in previously hepatitis B-infected patients, especially during prolonged immunosuppression for chronic GvHD, and can result in a severe acute hepatitis. If HBV reactivation occurs, HCT recipients should receive antiviral therapy. Ideally, patients should receive HBV immunization prior to transplant and chemotherapy. Patients who do not respond to pre-transplant vaccination should be re-immunized 6–12 months post-transplant.

Community-acquired viral respiratory infections

Due to their prevalence in the community, high transmission rates, and virulence in this susceptible population, community-acquired respiratory viruses are of particular concern. The most commonly acquired respiratory viral infections in HCT recipients are rhinovirus, parainflenza virus, respiratory-syncytial viruses (RSV), human metapneumovirus (hMPV), and influenza A or B. RSV, hMPV, parainfluenza, and influenza frequently cause pneumonia in HCT recipients. Even with appropriate treatment and supportive care, the case-fatality rate for these viral pneumonias is 25–45%. Education of the HCT recipient and their close contacts is key for preventing the spread of these pathogens. HCT recipients should practice frequent hand hygiene, avoid contact with individuals with infectious symptoms, and consider wearing a surgical mask, especially if the HCT recipient has chronic GvHD.

Influenza

Starting prior to transplant, and continuing indefinitely, the trivalent inactivated influenza vaccine should be administered annually to all HCT recipients and their close contacts. To further decrease risk of influenza, chemoprophylaxis with neuramidase inhibitors (zanmivir or oseltamir) is indicated for all HCT recipients exposed to influenza who are either within 2 years of their transplant or have chronic GvHD. Prophylaxis should begin as soon as possible after influenza contact and continue for 7–10 days after the exposure. Close contacts should also receive prophylaxis after exposure to influenza. There is no evidence supporting the use of antiviral prophylaxis or preemptive treatment for parainfluenza or RSV.

What are the vaccination recommendations for HCT recipients?

Re-immunization is critical for all HCT recipients because they lose immunity to infections to which they were previously vaccinated or exposed. After transplant, newly generated B-cells have limited capability to undergo somatic mutation and isotype switching, and naïve T-cells capable of responding to new antigens only start to be generated at 6–12 months post-transplant. The rate and degree of T-cell recovery depend on diagnosis, patient age, T-cell depletion of the graft, administration of rituximab during transplantation, and chronic GvHD.

The Center for Disease Control-Advisory Committee on Immunization Practice (CDC/ACIP) has provided guidelines for vaccination schedules post-transplant. Recently, the ACIP updated these recommendations to reflect the prevalence of pneumococcal disease observed in transplant recipients. The CDC vaccination and titer guidelines, ACIP updates, and center-specific HPV guidelines (see the section on Secondary Solid Malignancies) are summarized in Table 42.2.

What are the vaccination recommendations for close contacts?

Close contacts should be vaccinated per the usual immunization schedule, although special precautions are necessary regarding live vaccines. After transplant, HCT recipients are susceptible not only to wild-type infections, but also to infections by live attenuated viruses shed by immunized contacts. Oral polio vaccines, live attenuated influenza, cholera, and oral typhoid vaccines are not recommended for HCT recipients or their close contacts. There is no significant data indicating that the viruses in the live Measles, Mumps, and Rubella (MMR) vaccine are transmissible, although HCT recipients should avoid contact with individuals who develop fever, myalgias, or rash after receiving the MMR vaccine. Similarly, although there are no reported cases of virus transmission after live attenuated Rotavirus vaccines, HCT recipients should minimize contact with infants vaccinated with Rotavirus for 2–4 weeks after vaccination. Live varicella vaccines are available to prevent both chickenpox and shingles. Close contacts are encouraged to receive the chickenpox vaccine as indicated; however, the quantity of virus is greater in the shingles vaccine. Thus, some experts recommend delaying administration of the shingles vaccine to close contacts for 2 years post-transplant.

New considerations: Pre-transplant vaccines

Due to the delay in T-cell recovery in HCT recipients, new studies have examined whether pre-transplant vaccination of recipients and/or donors might offer additional immunoprotection. In the first 6–12 months post-transplant, most of the circulating T-cells are derived from the donor graft and capable of reacting to antigens exposed to the donor prior to transplant. Future directions include thorough evaluation of donor immunization status and development of more immunogenic vaccines so that patients can develop a more robust pre-transplant response.

Models for providing long-term care

As the number of long-term survivors after HCT increases, new, innovative care models must be developed to provide for their long-term care. These care models should focus on screening, prevention, and early treatment of late effects that impair quality of life and lead to late morbidity and mortality (Table 42.3).

Many institutions have created HCT-specific long-term survivor clinics, which provide regular multidisciplinary follow-up. These HCT-specific clinics are particularly important for HCT recipients with chronic GvHD, which has specific complications and may require multiple support services for management. Another potential solution for long-term follow-up is an umbrella model for all cancer survivors, similar to that proposed by the Children's Oncology Group. Many long-term survivors, however, have difficult or no access to survivorship clinics and will return to their local general hematologist or primary care physician for follow up care. As the number of HCT survivors increase, care models focusing on collaboration with non-transplant physicians will become increasingly important.

Table 42.3 High yield points about survivorship issues in allo-HCT recipients.

- The number of long-term HCT survivors is dramatically increasing and will continue to do so.
- Survival rates for HCT recipients remain lower than the general population for at least 10–30 years post-transplant.
- The two most common causes of excess death in HCT recipients are secondary malignancies and late infections.
- The incidence of secondary solid malignancies increases with time after HCT, never reaching a plateau.
- cGvHD is associated with secondary carcinomas; TBI-based conditioning is associated with non-squamous secondary malignancies. Many secondary malignancies are associated with HPV.
- Post-HCT, prophylactic antimicrobials against common pathogens are required. This is especially true in patients with cGvHD.
- Post-HCT, re-immunization is required.
- Precautions are indicated for vaccination of close contacts with live vaccines.

Selected reading

1. X. PMaZ. Current uses and outcomes of hematopoietic stem cell transplantation: 2015 CIBMTR Summary Slides. Available at: www.cibmtr.org (accessed December 2016).
2. Savani BN. *Blood and Marrow Transplantation Long-Term Management: Prevention and Complications*. Wiley-Blackwell, 2014, 414 p.
3. Majhail NS, Tao L, Bredeson C, Davies S, Dehn J, Gajewski JL, et al. Prevalence of hematopoietic cell transplant survivors in the United States. *Biology of Blood and Marrow Transplantation: Journal of the American Society for Blood and Marrow Transplantation* 2013,**19**:1498–1501.
4. Savani BN, Griffith ML, Jagasia S, Lee SJ. How I treat late effects in adults after allogeneic stem cell transplantation. *Blood* 2011,**117**:3002–3009.
5. Socie G, Stone JV, Wingard JR, Weisdorf D, Henslee-Downey PJ, Bredeson C, et al. Long-term survival and late deaths after allogeneic bone marrow transplantation. Late Effects Working Committee of the International Bone Marrow Transplant Registry. *The New England Journal of Medicine* 1999,**341**:14–21.
6. Bhatia S, Robison LL, Francisco L, Carter A, Liu Y, Grant M, et al. Late mortality in survivors of autologous hematopoietic-cell transplantation: report from the Bone Marrow Transplant Survivor Study. *Blood* 2005,**105**:4215–4222.
7. Pond GR, Lipton JH, Messner HA. Long-term survival after blood and marrow transplantation: comparison with an age and gender-matched normative population. *Biology of Blood and Marrow Transplantation: Journal of the American Society for Blood and Marrow Transplantation* 2006,**12**:422–429.
8. Majhail NS, Brazauskas R, Rizzo JD, Sobecks RM, Wang Z, Horowitz MM, et al. Secondary solid cancers after allogeneic hematopoietic cell transplantation using busulfancyclophosphamide conditioning. *Blood* 2011,**117**:316–322.

9. Tomblyn M, Chiller T, Einsele H, Gress R, Sepkowitz K, Storek J, *et al.* Guidelines for preventing infectious complications among hematopoietic cell transplant recipients: a global perspective. Preface. *Bone Marrow Transplantation* 2009,**44**:453–455.

10. Small TN, Cowan MJ. Immunization of hematopoietic stem cell transplant recipients against vaccine-preventable diseases. *Expert Review of Clinical Immunology* 2011,**7**:193–203.

11. Ljungman P, Cordonnier C, Einsele H, Englund J, Machado CM, Storek J, *et al.* Vaccination of hematopoietic cell transplant recipients. *Bone Marrow Transplantation* 2009,**44**: 521–526.

12. Wingard JR, Majhail NS, Brazauskas R, Wang Z, Sobocinski KA, Jacobsohn D, *et al.* Long-term survival and late deaths after allogeneic hematopoietic cell transplantation. *Journal of Clinical Oncology: Official Journal of the American Society of Clinical Oncology* 2011,**29**:2230–2239.

13. Majhail NS, Rizzo JD, Lee SJ, Aljurf M, Atsuta Y, Bonfim C, *et al.* Recommended screening and preventive practices for long-term survivors after hematopoietic cell transplantation. *Bone Marrow Transplantation* 2012,**47**:337–341.

14. Rizzo JD, Curtis RE, Socie G, Sobocinski KA, Gilbert E, Landgren O, *et al.* Solid cancers after allogeneic hematopoietic cell transplantation. *Blood* 2009,**113**:1175–1183.

15. Savani BN, Griffith ML, Jagasia S, Lee SJ. How I treat late effects in adults after allogeneic stem cell transplantation. *Blood* 2011,**117**:3002–3009.

Index
